Essentials of
Nuclear Medicine Imaging

Essentials of Nuclear Medicine Imaging

FIFTH EDITION

FRED A. METTLER, JR., MD, MPH
Clinical Professor, Radiology and Nuclear Medicine
Radiology and Nuclear Medicine Service
New Mexico Federal Regional Medical Center
University of New Mexico School of Medicine
Albuquerque, New Mexico

MILTON J. GUIBERTEAU, MD
Professor of Clinical Radiology and Nuclear Medicine
University of Texas Medical School at Houston
Chairman, Department of Nuclear Medicine
St. Joseph Hospital
Houston, Texas

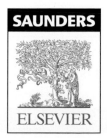

SAUNDERS

ELSEVIER

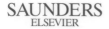

1600 John F. Kennedy Boulevard
Suite 1800
Philadelphia, Pennsylvania 19103-2899

Essentials of Nuclear Medicine Imaging

ISBN13: 978-0-7216-0201-1
ISBN10: 0-7216-0201-0

Fifth Edition

NOTICE

Knowledge and best practice in this field are constantly changing. As new research and experience broaden our knowledge, changes in practice, treatment, and drug therapy may become necessary or appropriate. Readers are advised to check the most current information provided (i) on procedures featured or (ii) by the manufacturer of each product to be administered, to verify the recommended dose or formula, the method and duration of administration, and contraindications. It is the responsibility of the practitioner, relying on his or her own experience and knowledge of the patient, to make diagnoses, to determine dosages and the best treatment for each individual patient, and to take all appropriate safety precautions. To the fullest extent of the law, neither the Publisher nor the Authors assume any liability for any injury and/or damage to persons or property arising out or related to any use of the material contained in this book.

The Publisher

Previous editions copyrighted 1998, 1991, 1985, 1983.

Library of Congress Cataloging-in-Publication Data
Mettler, Fred A., 1945–
   Essentials of nuclear medicine imaging / Fred A. Mettler, Jr., Milton J. Guiberteau.—5th ed.
     p. ; cm.
   Includes bibliographical references and index.
   ISBN 0-7216-0201-0
   1. Radioisotope scanning.   2. Diagnostic imaging.   I. Guiberteau, Milton J.   II. Title.
   [DNLM: 1. Nuclear Medicine.   2. Radionuclide Imaging. WN 445 M595e 2006]
   RC78.7.R4M47 2006
   616.07′575—dc22

                             2005050028

Acquisitions Editor: Allan Ross
Senior Project Manager: Cecelia Bayruns
Marketing Manager: Emily Christie

Printed in China.

Last digit is the print number: 9 8 7 6 5 4 3 2 1

This book is dedicated to our parents,

our families, and those who spend their time

teaching residents.

Contents

Preface

Seven years have elapsed since publication of our fourth edition, and it has been 22 years since our first edition. In this fifth edition, we have made substantial revisions while trying to keep to essentials and to keep the book affordable. We have updated the chapters to include newer aspects of instrumentation and radiopharmaceuticals and have removed outdated material. Tables on dosimetry have been moved from the chapters and placed in the appendix on examination protocols and techniques.

We have added a dedicated PET chapter. Although the rest of the book is predominantly organized by organ system, we felt that many experienced readers would be interested in PET only and that appropriate cross-referencing in other chapters would suffice. The advent of PET/CT and other forms of fusion imaging has also required the addition of color images.

At the end of the text, we have included sets of unknown cases that span the gamut of nuclear medicine. Review of the sets will allow the readers to assess their knowledge in a common testing format. This has added almost 70 pages to the text but we hope our readers find it worthwhile.

Fred A. Mettler, Jr.
Milton J. Guiberteau

Acknowledgments

We would particularly like to acknowledge the help and expertise of Dr. Michael Hartshorne who is a true pioneer of the fusion imaging techniques used in this edition. We are also indebted to Drs. William Spies and Tom Milller, who provided some cases. We also would like to recognize the many residents, technologists, and others who provided suggestions. Finally, images are crucial, and we would like to acknowledge Ruth Anne Bump, who provided many hours of help and expertise with the illustrations.

Radioactivity, Radionuclides, and Radiopharmaceuticals

1

BASIC ISOTOPE NOTATION

The atom may be thought of as a collection of protons, neutrons, and electrons. The protons and neutrons are found in the nucleus, and shells of electrons orbit the nucleus with discrete energy levels. The number of neutrons is usually designated by N. The number of protons is represented by Z (also called the atomic number). The atomic mass number, or the total number of nuclear particles, is represented by A and is simply the sum of N and Z. The symbolism used to designate atoms of a certain element having the chemical symbol X is given by $^A_Z X_N$. For example, the notation $^{131}_{53}I_{78}$ refers to a certain isotope of iodine. In this instance, 131 refers to the total number of protons and neutrons in the nucleus. By definition, all isotopes of a given element have the same number of protons and differ only in the number of neutrons. For example, all isotopes of iodine have 53 protons.

NUCLEAR STABILITY AND DECAY

A given element may have many isotopes, and some of these isotopes have unstable nuclear configurations of protons and neutrons. These isotopes often seek greater stability by decay or disintegration of the nucleus to a more stable form. Of the known stable nuclides, most have even numbers of neutrons and protons. Nuclides with odd numbers of neutrons and protons are usually unstable. Nuclear instability may result from either neutron or proton excess. Nuclear decay may involve a simple release of energy from the nucleus or may actually cause a change in the number of protons or neutrons within the nucleus. When decay involves a change in the number of protons, there is a change of element. This is termed a *transmutation*. Isotopes attempting to reach stability by emitting radiation are *radionuclides*.

Several mechanisms of decay achieve stability. One of these is *alpha-particle emission*. In this case, an

1

alpha (α) particle, consisting of two protons and two neutrons, is released from the nucleus, with a resulting decrease in the atomic mass number (A) by four and reduction of both Z and N by two. The mass of the released alpha particles is so great that they travel only a few centimeters in air and are unable to penetrate even thin paper. These properties cause alpha-particle emitters to be essentially useless for imaging purposes.

Beta-particle emission is another process for achieving stability and is found primarily in nuclides with a neutron excess. In this case, a beta (β⁻) particle (electron) is emitted from the nucleus accompanied by an antineutrino; as a result, one of the neutrons may be thought of as being transformed into a proton, which remains in the nucleus. Thus, beta-particle emission decreases the number of neutrons (N) by one and increases the number of protons (Z) by one, so that A remains unchanged (Fig. 1–1). When Z is increased, the arrow in the decay scheme shown in Figure 1–1 points toward the right, and the downward direction indicates a more stable state. The energy spectrum of beta-particle emission ranges from a certain maximum down to zero; the mean energy of the spectrum is about one third of the maximum. A 2-MeV beta particle has a range of about 1 cm in soft tissue and is therefore not useful for imaging purposes.

In cases in which there are too many protons in the nucleus (a neutron-deficient nuclide), decay may proceed in such a manner that a proton may be thought of as being converted into a neutron. This results in *positron* (β⁺) *emission*, which is always accompanied by a neutrino. This obviously increases N by one and decreases Z by one, again leaving A unchanged (see Fig. 1–1). The downward arrow in the decay scheme again indicates a more stable state, and its leftward direction indicates that Z is decreased. Positron emission cannot occur unless at least 1.02 MeV of energy is available to

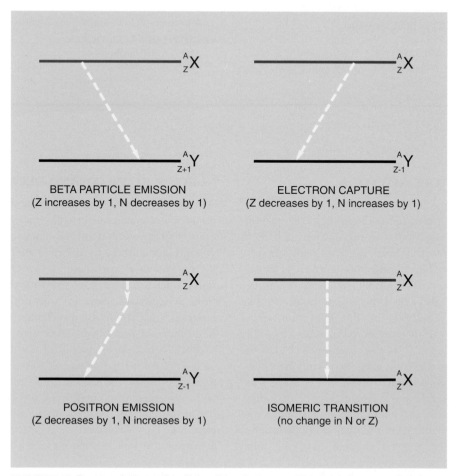

FIGURE 1–1. Decay schemes of radionuclides from unstable states (*top line* of each diagram) to more stable states (*bottom line*).

the nucleus. When positron emission occurs, the positron usually travels only a short distance and combines with an electron in an annihilation reaction. When this happens, two photons of 511 keV are emitted in opposite directions (annihilation radiation). This radiation can be imaged and results from the conversion of the masses of the positron and electron to energy.

Electron capture occurs in a neutron-deficient nuclide when one of the inner orbital electrons is captured by a proton in the nucleus, forming a neutron and a neutrino. This can occur when not enough energy is available for positron emission, and electron capture is therefore an alternative to positron decay. Because a nuclear proton is essentially changed to a neutron, N increases by one, and Z decreases by one; therefore, A remains unchanged (see Fig. 1–1). Electron capture may be accompanied by gamma emission and is always accompanied by characteristic radiation, either of which may be used in imaging.

If, in any of these attempts at stabilization, the nucleus still has excess energy, it may be emitted as nonparticulate radiation, with Z and N remaining the same. Any process in which energy is given off as gamma rays and in which the numbers of protons and neutrons are not changed is called *isomeric transition* (see Fig. 1–1). An alternative to isomeric transition is *internal conversion*. In internal conversion, the excess energy of the nucleus is transmitted to one of the orbital electrons; this electron may be ejected from the atom, which is followed by characteristic radiation when the electron is replaced. This process usually competes with gamma-ray emission and can occur only if the amount of energy given to the orbital electron exceeds the binding energy of that electron in its orbit.

The ratio of internal conversion electrons to gamma-ray emissions for a particular radioisotope is designated by the symbol α. (This should not be confused with the symbol for an alpha particle.) For an isotope such as Technetium-99m (^{99m}Tc), α is low, indicating that most emissions occur as gamma rays with little internal conversion. A low conversion ratio is preferable for in-vivo usage because it implies a greater number of gamma emissions for imaging and a reduced number of conversion electrons, which are absorbed by the body and thus add to the patient's radiation dose.

In many instances, a gamma-ray photon is emitted almost instantaneously after particulate decay. If there is a measurable delay in the emission of the gamma-ray photon and the resulting decay process is an isomeric transition, this intermediate excited state of the isotope is referred to as *metastable*. The most well-known metastable isotope is ^{99m}Tc (the m refers to metastable). This isotope decays by isomeric transition to a more stable state, as indicated in Figure 1–2. In the decay scheme, the arrows point straight down, showing that there is no change in Z. Also, ^{99m}Tc may decay by one of several routes of gamma-ray emission.

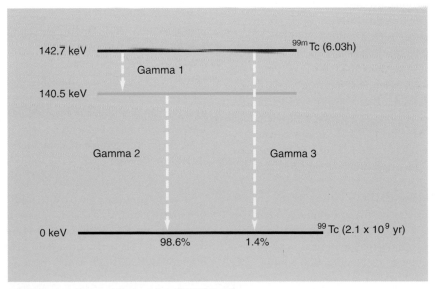

FIGURE 1–2. Decay scheme of technetium-99m.

RADIONUCLIDE PRODUCTION

Most radioactive material that does not occur naturally can be produced by particulate bombardment or fission. Both methods alter the neutron-to-proton ratio in the nucleus to produce an unstable isotope. Bombardment essentially consists of the irradiation of the nuclei of selected target elements with neutrons in a nuclear reactor or with charged particles (alpha particles, protons, or deuterons) from a cyclotron. Bombardment reactions may be summarized by equations in which the target element and bombarding particle are listed on the left side of the equation and the product and any accompanying particulate or gamma emissions are indicated on the right. For example,

$$_Z^A X + n(\text{neutron}) \rightarrow _Z^{A+1} X + \gamma \text{ or, more specifically,}$$

$$_{42}^{98}\text{Mo} + n(\text{neutron}) \rightarrow _{42}^{99}\text{Mo} + \gamma$$

These equations may be further abbreviated using parenthetical notation. The molybdenum reaction presented previously is thus represented as $^{98}\text{Mo} (n, \gamma)\ ^{99}\text{Mo}$. The target and product are noted on the outside of the parentheses, which contain the bombarding particle on the left and any subsequent emissions on the right.

Once bombardment is completed, the daughter isotope must be physically separated from any remaining and unchanged target nuclei, as well as from any target contaminants. Thus, it is obvious that the completeness of this final separation process and the initial elemental purity of the target are vital factors in obtaining a product of high specific activity. Because cyclotron isotope production almost always involves a transmutation (change of Z) from one element to another, this process aids greatly in the separation of the radionuclides to obtain *carrier-free* isotopes (i.e., isotopes that have none of the stable element accompanying them). Radionuclides made by neutron bombardment, which does not result in a change of elemental species (e.g., $^{98}\text{Mo} [n, \gamma]\ ^{99}\text{Mo}$), are not carrier free because the chemical properties of the products are identical, and thus radionuclides are not as easily separated.

Fission isotopes are simply the daughter products of nuclear fission of uranium-235 (^{235}U) or plutonium-239 (^{239}Pu) in a reactor and represent a multitude of radioactive materials, with atomic numbers in the range of roughly half that of ^{235}U. These include iodine-131 (^{131}I), xenon-133 (^{133}Xe), strontium-90 (^{90}Sr), molybdenum-99 (^{99}Mo), and

cesium-137 (^{137}Cs), among others. Because many of these isotopes are present together in the fission products, the desired isotope must be carefully isolated to exclude as many contaminants as possible. Although this is sometimes difficult, many carrier-free isotopes are produced in this manner.

Neutron bombardment and nuclear fission almost always produce isotopes with neutron excess, which decay by beta emission. Some isotopes, such as ^{99}Mo, may be produced by either method. Cyclotron-produced isotopes are usually neutron deficient and decay by electron capture or positron emission. Some common examples of cyclotron-produced isotopes include iodine-123 (^{123}I), fluorine-18 (^{18}F), gallium-67 (^{67}Ga), indium-111 (^{111}In), and thallium-201 (^{201}Tl). In general, cyclotron-generated radionuclides are more expensive than are those produced by neutron bombardment or fission.

RADIOACTIVE DECAY

The amount of radioactivity present (the number of disintegrations per second) is referred to as *activity*. In the past, the unit of radioactivity has been the curie (Ci), which is 3.7×10^{10} disintegrations per second. Because the curie is an inconvenient unit, it is being replaced by an international unit called a becquerel (Bq), which is one disintegration per second. Conversion tables are found in Appendices B-1 and B-2. *Specific activity* refers to the activity per unit mass of material (mCi/g or Bq/g). For a carrier-free isotope, the longer the half-life of the isotope, the lower is its specific activity.

Radionuclides decay in an exponential fashion, and the term *half-life* is often used casually to characterize decay. Half-life usually refers to the *physical half-life*, which is the amount of time necessary for a radionuclide to be reduced to half of its existing activity. The physical half-life (T_p) is equal to $0.693/\lambda$, where λ is the decay constant. Thus, λ and the physical half-life have characteristic values for each radioactive nuclide.

A formula that the nuclear medicine physician should be familiar with is the following:

$$A = A_0 e^{-0.693/T_p(t)}$$

This formula can be used to find the activity (A) of a particular radioisotope present at a given time (t) and given a certain activity (A_0) at time 0. For instance, if you had 5 mCi (185 MBq) of ^{99m}Tc at 9 AM today, how much would remain at 9 AM tomorrow? In this case, T_p of ^{99m}Tc is 6 hours, t is 24 hours, and e is a mathematical constant. Thus,

$$A = A_0 e^{\frac{-0.693}{T_p}(t)}$$

$$A = A_0 e^{\frac{-0.693}{6\,\text{h}}(24\,\text{h})}$$

$$A = 5\ \text{mCi}\ e^{\frac{-0.693}{6\,\text{h}}(24\,\text{h})}$$

$$A = 5\ \text{mCi}\ e^{-0.1155(24\,\text{h})}$$

$$A = 5\ \text{mCi}\ e^{-2.772}$$

$$A = 5\ \text{mCi}\ e^{\frac{1}{2.772}}$$

$$A = 5\ \text{mCi}\ \left(\frac{1}{15.99}\right)$$

$$A = 0.31\ \text{mCi}\ (11\ \text{MBq})$$

Thus, after 24 hours, the amount of ^{99m}Tc remaining is 0.31 mCi (11 MBq).

In addition to the physical half-life or physical decay of a radionuclide, two other half-life terms are commonly used. *Biologic half-life* refers to the time it takes an organism to eliminate half of an administered compound or chemical on a strictly biologic basis. Thus, if a stable chemical compound were given to a person, and half of it were eliminated by the body (perhaps in the urine) within 3 hours, the biologic half-life would be 3 hours. The *effective half-life* incorporates both the physical and biologic half-lives. Therefore, when speaking of the effective half-life of a particular radiopharmaceutical in humans, one needs to know the physical half-life of the radioisotope used as a tag or label as well as the biologic half-life of the tagged compound. If these are known, the following formula can be used to calculate the effective half-life.

$$T_e = (T_p \times T_b)/(T_p + T_b)$$

where

T_e = effective half-life

T_p = physical half-life

T_b = biologic half-life

If the biologic half-life is 3 hours and the physical half-life is 6 hours, then the effective half-life is 2 hours. Note that the effective half-life is *always* shorter than either the physical or biologic half-life.

RADIONUCLIDE GENERATOR SYSTEMS

A number of radionuclides of interest in nuclear medicine are short-lived isotopes that emit only gamma rays and decay by isomeric transition. Because it is often impractical for an imaging lab-

oratory to be located near a reactor or a cyclotron, generator systems that permit on-site availability of these isotopes have achieved wide use. Some isotopes available from generators include technetium-99m, indium-113m (^{113m}In), krypton-81m (^{81m}Kr), rubidium-82 (^{82}Rb), strontium-87m (^{87m}Sr), and gallium-68 (^{68}Ga).

Inside the most common generator (^{99}Mo-^{99m}Tc), a radionuclide "parent" with a relatively long half-life is firmly affixed to an ion exchange column. A ^{99}Mo-^{99m}Tc generator consists of an alumina column on which ^{99}Mo is bound. The parent isotope (67-hour half-life) decays to its radioactive daughter, ^{99m}Tc, which is a different element with a shorter half-life (6 hours). Because the daughter is only loosely bound on the column, it may be removed, or washed off, with an elution liquid such as normal (0.9%) saline. Wet and dry ^{99}Mo-^{99m}Tc generator systems are available and differ only slightly. A *wet system* has a saline reservoir and a vacuum vial that draws saline across the column. With a *dry system*, a specific amount of saline in a vial is placed on the generator entry port and drawn across by a vacuum vial (Fig. 1–3).

After the daughter is separated from the column, the build-up process is begun again by the residual parent isotope. Uncommonly, some of the parent

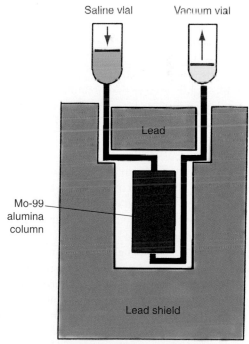

FIGURE 1–3. Schematic of dry molybdenum-99/technetium-99m generator system.

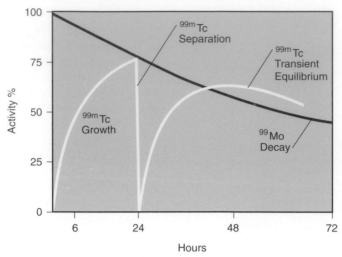

FIGURE 1–4. Molybdenum-99 decay and technetium-99m buildup in a generator eluted at 0 hours and again at 24 hours.

isotope (^{99}Mo) or alumina is removed from the column during elution and appears in the eluate containing the daughter isotope. This is termed *breakthrough*, and its significance and consequences are addressed in Chapter 3.

To make efficient use of a generator, elution times should be spaced appropriately to allow for reaccumulation of the daughter isotope on the column. The short-lived daughter reaches maximum activity when the rate of decay of the daughter equals its rate of production. At this equilibrium point, for instance, the amount of daughter ^{99m}Tc is slightly greater than the activity of the parent ^{99}Mo (Fig. 1–4). When the parent isotope has a half-life slightly greater than that of the daughter, the equilibrium attained is said to be a *transient equilibrium*. This is the case in a ^{99}Mo-^{99m}Tc generator.

Most generators used in hospitals have ^{99}Mo activity levels of about 1 to 6 Ci (3.7 to 22.0 GBq). The amount of ^{99m}Tc in the generator reaches about half the theoretical maximum in one half-life (6 hours). It reaches about three fourths of the theoretical maximum in about two half-lives, and so on (see Appendix C-1). This indicates that if one elutes all of the ^{99m}Tc daughter from an ^{99}Mo generator, 24 hours later (four half-lives), the amount of ^{99m}Tc present in the generator will have returned to about 95% of the theoretical maximum.

Other, much less common photon-emitting radionuclide generator systems include rubidium-81 (^{81}Rb) (4.5 hours)/^{81m}Kr (13 seconds), tin-13

(^{113}Sn) (115 days)/^{113m}In (1.7 hours), and yttrium-87 (^{87}Y) (3.3 days)/^{87m}Sr (2.8 hours). Although generator systems are most often used to produce photon-emitting radionuclides, certain generators can produce positron emitters. These include strontium-82 (^{82}Sr) (25 days)/^{82}Rb (1.3 minutes). ^{82}Rb is a potassium analog and can be used for myocardial perfusion imaging employing position emission tomography. Gallium-68 (6.5 hours) is another positron emitter that can be produced from a germanium-69 (^{69}Ge) (271 days) generator.

RADIONUCLIDES FOR IMAGING

In evaluating the choice of a radionuclide to be used in the nuclear medicine laboratory, the following characteristics are desirable:

Minimum of particulate emission
Primary photon energy between 50 and 500 keV
Physical half-life greater than the time required to prepare material for injection
Effective half-life longer than the examination time
Suitable chemical form and reactivity
Low toxicity
Stability or near-stability of the product

The basic characteristics of radionuclides most commonly used for imaging are given in subsequent sections and in Table 1–1. Many of these are radiopharmaceuticals in their own right and can be administered without alteration to obtain useful

TABLE 1–1.	Characteristics of Commonly Used Radionuclides			
	SYMBOL	**PHYSICAL HALF-LIFE**	**APPROXIMATE ENERGY**	
Photon-Emitting Radionuclides for Imaging			**Gamma (keV)**	
Technetium-99m	$^{99m}_{43}Tc$	6 hr	140	
Molybdenum-99	$^{99}_{42}Mo$	67 hr	181, 740, 780	
Iodine-123	$^{123}_{53}I$	13.2 hr	159	
Iodine-131	$^{131}_{53}I$	8.0 day	364	
Xenon-133	$^{133}_{54}Xe$	5.3 day	81	
Gallium-67	$^{67}_{31}Ga$	78.3 hr	90, 190, 290, 390	
Indium-111	$^{111}_{49}In$	67 hr	173, 247	
Indium-113m	$^{113m}_{49}In$	1.7 hr	392	
Thallium-201	$^{201}_{81}Tl$	73.1 hr	69, 81 (x rays from mercury daughter)	
Krypton-81m	$^{81m}_{36}Kr$	13 sec	191	
Positron-Emitting Radionuclides for Imaging			**Positron (MeV)**	
Carbon-11	$^{11}_{6}C$	20 min	0.960	
Nitrogen-13	$^{13}_{7}N$	10 min	1.190	
Oxygen-15	$^{15}_{8}O$	2 min	1.730	
Fluorine-18	$^{18}_{9}F$	110 min	0.635	
Rubidium-82	$^{82}_{32}Rb$	1.3 min	3.150	
Unsealed Radionuclides Used for Therapy			**Emissions**	
Phosphorus-32	$^{32}_{15}P$	14.3 day	1.71 MeV max; 0.7 McV mean beta	
Strontium-89	$^{89}_{38}Sr$	50.5 day	1.46 MeV max; 0.58 MeV mean beta; 910 keV gamma (0.01%)	
Yttrium-90	$^{90}_{39}Y$	64 hr	2.2 MeV max; 0.93 MeV mean beta	
Iodine-131	$^{131}_{53}I$	8.0 day	0.19 MeV mean beta; 364 keV gamma (82%)	
Samarium-153	$^{153}_{62}Sm$	46 hr	0.81 MeV max; 0.23 McV mean beta; 103 keV gamma (28%)	
Rhenium-186	$^{186}_{75}Re$	90 hr	0.34 MeV mean beta; 186 keV gamma (9%)	
Gold-198	$^{198}_{79}Au$	2.7 day	0.96 McV max; 0.31 MeV mean beta; 412 keV gamma (96%)	

Note: The approximate range (cm) of beta particle in tissue is the energy (MeV) divided by two.

images. The biologic behavior of most of these radionuclides can be markedly altered by combination with additional substances to form other radiopharmaceuticals.

Technetium-99m

Technetium-99m fulfills many of the criteria of an ideal radionuclide and is used in more than 70% of nuclear imaging procedures in the United States. It has no particulate emission, a 6-hour half-life, and a predominant (98%) 140-keV photon with only a small amount (10%) of internal conversion.

Technetium-99m is obtained by separating it from the parent ^{99}Mo (67-hour half-life) in a generator system. Molybdenum 99 for generators is generally produced by neutron irradiation of ^{98}Mo or by chemical separation of ^{235}U fission products. In the latter case, ^{99}Mo is nearly carrier free and has a high specific activity.

In the alumina generator system, the molybdenum activity is absorbed on an alumina column. By passing physiologic saline over the column, ^{99m}Tc is eluted or washed off as *sodium pertechnetate* (Na ^{99m}TcO$_4^-$).

Technetium can exist in a variety of valence states, ranging from −1 to +7. When eluted from an alumina column generator, ^{99m}Tc is present primarily as heptavalent (+7) pertechnetate (TcO$_4^-$). In the preparation of radiopharmaceuticals, ^{99m}Tc pertechnetate can be reduced from +7 to a lower valence state, usually +4, to permit the labeling of various chelates. This is generally accomplished with stannous (tin) ions.

As pertechnetate, the technetium ion is a singly charged anion and is similar in size to the iodide ion. After intravenous injection, ^{99m}Tc pertechnetate is loosely bound to protein and rapidly leaves the plasma compartment. More than half leaves the plasma within several minutes and is distributed in the extracellular fluid. It rapidly concentrates in the salivary glands, choroid plexus, thyroid gland, gastric mucosa, and functioning breast tissue; during pregnancy, it crosses the placenta.

Excretion is by the gastrointestinal and renal routes. Although ^{99m}Tc pertechnetate is excreted by glomerular filtration, it is partially reabsorbed by the renal tubules; as a result, only 30% is eliminated in the urine during the first day. The ion is also secreted directly into the stomach and colon, with a much smaller amount coming from the small bowel. The colon is the critical organ and receives 1 to 2 rad/10 mCi (0.02 mGy/MBq) of ^{99m}Tc pertechnetate administered. The biodistribution of ^{99m}Tc pertechnetate is shown in Figure 1–5. The principal emission (140-keV photon) of ^{99m}Tc has a half-value layer (HVL) of 0.028 cm in lead and

4.5 cm in water. Because tissue is close to water in terms of attenuation characteristics, it is clear that about 2 inches of tissue between the radionuclide and the detector removes about half of the photons of interest, and 4 inches removes about three fourths.

Iodine-123 and -131

Two isotopes of iodine (^{123}I and ^{131}I) are clinically useful for imaging and may be administered as iodide. Iodine-123 has a 13.3-hour half-life and decays by electron capture to tellurium-123 (^{123}Te). The photons emitted are 28-keV (92%) and 159-keV (84%) gamma rays. Iodine-123 is usually produced in a cyclotron by bombardment of antimony-121 (^{121}Sb) or tellurium-122 or -124 (^{122}Te or ^{124}Te). Another method is to bombard iodine-127 (^{127}I) to produce ^{123}Xe and let this decay to ^{123}I. The cyclotron production and short half-life make ^{123}I expensive and its distribution on a nationwide basis difficult. Iodine-123 has a whole-body dose of 0.04 rad/mCi (0.01 mGy/MBq) and a thyroid dose of 16 rad/mCi (4.3 mGy/MBq). Contamination with ^{124}I may increase the radiation dose; because ^{124}I is long lived, its proportion in an ^{123}I preparation increases with time.

Iodine-131 is a much less satisfactory isotope from an imaging viewpoint because of the high radiation dose to the thyroid and its relatively high photon energy. However, it is widely available, is relatively inexpensive, and has a relatively long shelf life. Iodine-131 has a half-life of 8.06 days and decays by beta-particle emission to stable ^{131}Xe. The principal mean beta energy (90%) is 192 keV. Several gamma rays are also emitted, and the predominant photon is 364 keV (82% abundance) (HVL in water of 6.4 cm). Iodine-131 gives a whole-body dose of 0.5 to 3.5 rad/mCi (0.14 to 0.95 mGy/MBq) and a thyroid dose of 1000 to 2000 rad/mCi (270 to 540 mGy/MBq).

When iodine is orally administered as the iodide ion, it is readily absorbed from the gastrointestinal tract and distributed in the extracellular fluid. It is concentrated in a manner similar to that for ^{99m}Tc pertechnetate in the salivary glands, thyroid, and gastric mucosa. As with pertechnetate, there is renal filtration with significant tubular reabsorption. Urinary excretion is the predominant route (35% to 75% in 24 hours), although there is some fecal excretion as well. Iodide trapped and organified by the normal thyroid has an effective half-life of about 7 days. Iodine is a useful radionuclide because it is chemically reactive and is used to

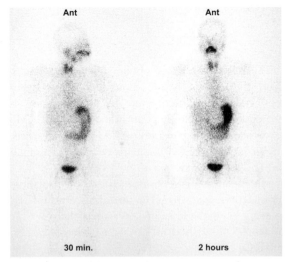

FIGURE 1–5. Whole-body distribution of technetium-99m sodium pertechnetate. Activity is seen in the salivary glands, thyroid gland, saliva, stomach, and bladder.

produce a variety of radiopharmaceuticals, which are discussed in later clinical chapters.

Xenon-133

Xenon is a relatively insoluble inert gas and is most commonly used for pulmonary ventilation studies. Xenon is commercially available in unit-dose vials or in 1-Ci (40-GBq) glass ampules. Xenon is highly soluble in oil and fat, and there is some adsorption of xenon onto plastic syringes.

Xenon-133 has a physical half-life of 5.3 days. The principal gamma photon has an energy of 81 keV and emits a 374-keV beta particle. With normal pulmonary function, its biologic half-life is about 30 seconds. Some disadvantages of ^{133}Xe include its relatively low photon energy, beta-particle emission, and some solubility in both blood and fat.

Gallium-67

Gallium is a metal with only one stable valence state (+3) in aqueous solution. Similar to iron, gallium binds to the plasma protein transferrin. Gallium-67 has a half-life of 78 hours. It can be produced by a variety of reactions in a cyclotron. The principal gamma photons from ^{67}Ga are 93 keV (40%), 184 keV (24%), 296 keV (22%), and 388 keV (7%). An easy way to remember these energies is to round off the figures (i.e., 90, 190, 290, and 390 keV).

Gallium is usually administered as a citrate and has a 12-hour half-life in the blood pool, where it is largely bound to plasma proteins, especially transferrin, lactoferrin, and ferritin. It ultimately leaves the blood pool to localize primarily in the liver, spleen, bone marrow, and skeleton. Tumor localization is not well understood, but lysosome binding appears to be involved, as does possible tumor concentration of the previously mentioned gallium–protein complexes. The biologic half-life of gallium is about 2 to 3 weeks, and about 40% of the dose is excreted in the first 5 days. Renal excretion (10% to 30%) is most common in the first 24 hours. Fecal excretion (about 10%) occurs primarily through the bowel wall.

Indium-111

Indium is a metal that can be used as an iron analog; it is similar to gallium. Isotopes of interest are ^{111}In and ^{113m}In. Indium-111 has a physical half-life of 67 hours and is produced by a cyclotron. The principal photons are 173 keV (89%) and 247 keV (94%). Indium-113m can be conveniently pro-duced by using a ^{113}Sn generator system. It has a physical half-life of 1.7 hours and a photon of about 392 keV. Indium-111 can be prepared as a chelate with diethylenetriaminepenta-acetic acid (DTPA). Because of its long half-life, the ^{111}In chelate can be used for intracranial cisternography. Indium-111 is also used to label platelets, white cells, monoclonal antibodies, and peptides.

Thallium-201

When a thallium metal target is bombarded with protons in a cyclotron, lead 201 (^{201}Pb) is produced, which can be separated from the thallium target and allowed to decay to ^{201}Tl. Thallium-201 has a physical half-life of 73.1 hours and decays by elec-tron capture to mercury 201 (^{201}Hg). Mercury-201 emits characteristic x-rays with energies from 68 to 80 keV (94.5%) and much smaller amounts of gamma rays with higher energies. The relatively low energy of the major emissions can cause sig-nificant attenuation by tissue between the radionu-clide and the gamma camera. The HVL in water is about 4 cm. For these reasons, attenuation correction methodologies have been developed (see Chapter 2). Because ^{201}Tl is produced by a cyclotron, it is expensive. Thallium-201 is normally administered as a chloride and rapidly clears from the blood with a half-life between 30 seconds and 3 minutes. Because it is roughly a potassium analog, it is rapidly distributed throughout the body, par-ticularly in skeletal and cardiac muscle. Thallium-202 (95% photon at 439 keV) contamination should be less than 0.5% and, if present in greater quantities, can significantly degrade images.

Positron-Emitting Radionuclides

These are discussed later in Chapter 13.

UNSEALED RADIONUCLIDES USED FOR THERAPY

Radionuclides can be administered to patients for therapeutic purposes in sealed or unsealed forms. Unsealed radionuclides may be given orally, admin-istered intravenously, or placed directly into a body cavity (such as a knee joint or peritoneum). Most unsealed radionuclides are predominantly beta emitters. As such, they usually present little hazard to the public or family members. A few radionu-clides also emit gamma photons, which can be helpful in imaging the localization of the material; however, a large amount of gamma emissions will present a radiation hazard and give a significant radiation dose to nontarget tissues. Physical properties of these are shown in Table 1–1. Issues related to release of patients in accordance with U.S. Nuclear Regulatory Commission regulation are included in Appendix G. Sealed radionuclides are administered to patients in an encapsulated form for regional radiotherapy. As they are generally used in the practice of radiation oncology, sealed radionuclides will not be discussed in this text.

Phosphorus-32, Yttrium-90 and Gold-198

All three of these radionuclides have been used for radioisotopic therapy. Currently, they are rarely used in colloidal form for intracavitary administration for abdominopelvic serosal metastases or knee joint synovectomy. Intravenous phosphorus-32, as an ionic phosphate, has been used in the past to treat polycythemia vera, but has largely been replaced by non-radiosotopic drugs. Yttrium-90 (^{90}Y) can be coupled with a localization agent to deliver antineoplastic therapy. Yttrium-90 labeled microspheres, injected through a transfemoral catheter into the hepatic artery, lodge in the small blood vessels of liver neoplasms to deliver a therapeutic dose. A ^{90}Y-labeled monoclonal antibody can be injected intravenously to treat some non-Hodgkin's lymphomas.

Iodine-131

Iodine-131 is discussed earlier in the section on imaging radionuclides; however, large administered activities of sodium ^{131}I are commonly used for treatment of hyperthyroidism and thyroid cancer. Although ^{131}I is a beta emitter, there is a predominant energetic gamma emission (364 keV), which can be used to image the biodistribution. This gamma photon also can result in measurable absorbed radiation doses to persons near the patient. Because excretion is via the urinary tract, and to a lesser extent via saliva and sweat, special radiation protection precautions need to be taken for days after these patients are treated. These are discussed further in Chapter 5 in the section on thyroid therapy and in Appendix G.

Strontium-89, Samarium-153 and Rhenium-186

All three of these radionuclides are administered intravenously and used to treat painful osseous metastases from prostate and breast cancer. Strontium-89 (^{89}Sr) is essentially a pure beta emitter and poses virtually no hazard to medical staff or patient

families, except for urinary precautions for a few days. Both samarium-153 (^{153}Sm) and rhenium-186 (^{186}Re) also emit small amounts of relatively low energy gamma photons, which can be used to image distribution. These are discussed in more detail at the end of Chapter 9.

RADIOPHARMACEUTICALS

A radionuclide that has desirable imaging properties can usually be used to make a variety of radiopharmaceuticals. This is done by coupling the radionuclide with various stable compounds that are localized by organs or disease states. Mechanisms of localization for some of these radiopharmaceuticals are listed in Table 1–2. The various radiopharmaceuticals used in imaging procedures are discussed in the appropriate chapters. Although the localizing properties of radiopharmaceuticals are generally sufficient to obtain adequate diagnostic images, the localizing mechanisms may be altered by various conditions in an individual patient, including the administration of other medications. A list of these agents and their effects on the distribution of particular radiopharmaceuticals is given in the Appendix E–2.

Monoclonal Antibodies

During the past several years, much interest has been generated in the development of labeled antibodies for the immunodetection and immunotherapy of a variety of diseases, particularly those of an oncologic nature. However, it was not until the development of methods of producing and labeling monoclonal antibodies that the clinical potential of such agents could be seriously explored. In addition to oncologic agents, radiopharmaceuticals for the evaluation of non-neoplastic diseases, such as myocardial infarction (anticardiac myosin monoclonal antibodies) and inflammation (antigranulocyte antibodies), are currently of interest.

Monoclonal antibodies are so named because when developed against a given antigen, they are absolutely identical to one another. The technique for producing monoclonal antibodies first involves the immunization of an animal, generally a mouse, with a specific antigen (Fig. 1–6). This antigen can be virtually anything capable of inducing the B lymphocytes to begin producing antibodies against the injected substance. Once this is done, the B lymphocytes are harvested from the mouse and placed in a tube containing mouse myeloma cells. Fusion of these myeloma cells with the B lympho-

TABLE 1–2.	Mechanisms of Localization and Examples
Capillary blockade	Macroaggregated albumin in lung
Diffusion	Filtration of DTPA by kidney
Sequestration	Leukocytes for abscess scanning
	Labeled platelets (damaged endothelium)
	Heat-damaged red blood cells for splenic scanning
Phagocytosis	Colloid scanning for liver and spleen, bone marrow, and lymph nodes
Receptor binding	Neuroreceptor imaging
Active transport	Iodocholesterol in adrenal scanning
	Iodine or pertechnetate (accumulation by choroid plexus, Meckel's diverticulum, salivary gland, stomach, and thyroid)
	Technetium-99m IDA analogs in liver/biliary tract
	Orthoiodohippurate in renal tubules
	Thallous ions in myocardium
Metabolism	Fluorodeoxyglucose imaging of brain, tumor, and myocardium
Compartmental containment	Labeled red blood cells for gated blood pool studies
Compartmental leakage	Labeled red blood cells for detection of gastrointestinal bleeding
Physicochemical adsorption	Phosphate bone-scanning agents
Antibody–antigen reactions	Tumor imaging, monoclonal antibodies

DTPA, diethylenetriaminepenta-actetic acid; IDA, iminodiacetic acid.

cytes then takes place, forming what is known as *hybridoma*. This hybridoma has the ability to continue producing antigen-specific antibodies based on the B-lymphocyte parent and, at the same time, to perpetuate itself based on the characteristic of continual mitosis conferred on it by the myeloma cells.

Hybridomas can then be grown in clones and separated out until a clone is developed that produces an antibody of particular interest. When such clones are developed, they are grown in the peritoneal cavities of mice, and the antibody produced is secreted into the ascitic fluid. This ascitic fluid is harvested and processed to provide a puri-

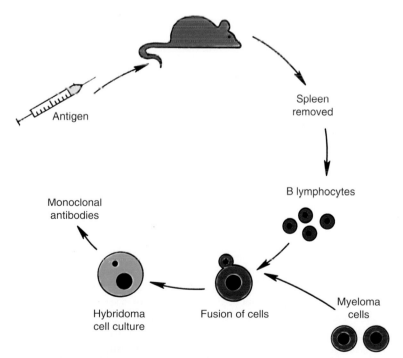

FIGURE 1–6. Schematic for production of monoclonal antibodies.

fied form of the antibody. Large quantities of monoclonal antibodies can be obtained in this way. Bulk production of monoclonal antibodies is also possible by using a synthetic approach in vitro.

Once produced, monoclonal antibodies, or fragments thereof, may be labeled with radionuclides and used to map the distribution of specific antigens in vivo. Although the concept initially appears simple, substantial problems exist that limit the clinical application of monoclonal antibodies for tumor imaging. Not the least of these problems is the selection of an appropriate specific antigen, the successful labeling of the antibody, significant cross-reactivity with other antigens, and poor target-to-nontarget ratios in vivo. Immune responses to the foreign antibody protein in humans have provided a further barrier to successful widespread use. When the antibodies are produced in a murine system, human antimouse antibody (HAMA) develops in up to 40% of patients receiving a single dose of whole antibody. HAMA limits the success of future administrations by complexing with the antibody radiopharmaceutical, thereby reducing the amount of antibody available for imaging. Monoclonal antibody fragments or antibodies of human or chimeric origin (human–mouse) appear to reduce HAMA production. As solutions to these drawbacks are devised, monoclonal antibodies are gradually becoming part of the radiopharmaceutical armamentarium of diagnostic and therapeutic nuclear medicine. Radiolabels currently include radioiodines, ^{111}In, ^{99m}Tc, and ^{90}Y.

Adverse Reactions

As drugs, radiopharmaceuticals are extremely safe: mild reactions are uncommon, and severe reactions are very rare. There are less than 200 serious reactions reported in the worldwide literature even though tens of millions of doses are administered annually. An *adverse reaction* may be defined as an unanticipated patient response to the nonradioactive component of a radiopharmaceutical; this reaction is not caused by the radiation itself. Overdoses of radioactivity represent reportable events and are not adverse reactions. The only adverse effect of a radiopharmaceutical that is required to be reported is one associated with an investigational drug.

The incidence of reactions to radiopharmaceuticals in the United States is about 2.3 per 100,000 administrations. Most reported adverse reactions are allergic in nature, although some vasovagal reactions have occurred. The clinical manifesta-

tions of most reactions are rash, itching, dizziness, nausea, chills, flushing, hives, and vomiting. These reactions may occur within 5 minutes or up to 48 hours after injection. Late-onset rash or itching, dizziness, and/or headache have most commonly been reported with ^{99m}Tc bone agents. Severe reactions involving anaphylactic shock or cardiac arrest are reported in less than 3% of adverse reactions. In addition to allergic or vasomotor reactions, adverse effects with albumin particulates have been reported owing to pulmonary capillary vascular blockage in patients with diminished pulmonary vascular capacity. Positron emission tomography (PET) radiopharmaceuticals are also extremely safe, with no reported adverse reactions in more than 80,000 administered doses.

Reactions related to pyrogens or additives have become exceedingly rare because of the extensive quality control used in the manufacture and preparation of radiopharmaceuticals. Pyrogen reactions may be suspected if more than one patient receiving a dose from a single vial of a radiopharmaceutical has experienced an adverse effect.

Common nonradioactive pharmaceuticals used in nuclear medicine are dipyridamole and glucagon. Severe reactions to these occur in about 6 per 100,000 administrations and include prolonged chest pain, syncope (dipyridamole), and anaphylaxis (glucagon).

Investigational Radiopharmaceuticals

Any new radiopharmaceutical must be treated as an investigational new drug (IND) and must go through the process outlined in the *Guidelines for the Clinical Evaluation of Radiopharmaceutical Drugs* of the Food and Drug Administration (FDA). Either manufacturers or health practitioners can file an IND application. Initially, the application must include complete composition of the drug, source, manufacturing data, and preclinical investigations, including animal studies.

Clinical investigation of INDs occurs in three phases. Phase one is early testing in humans to determine toxicity, pharmacokinetics, and effectiveness. These studies usually involve a small number of people and are conducted under carefully controlled circumstances. Phase two trials are controlled trials to test both for effectiveness in treatment of a specific disease and for evaluation of risk. Phase three, clinical investigation, involves extensive clinical trials, provided that information obtained in phases one and two demonstrates reasonable assurance of safety and effectiveness.

Phase-three studies acquire necessary information for complete drug labeling, including the most desirable dose and the safety and effectiveness of the drug. Most reimbursement organizations and third-party payers will not pay for a drug unless it is fully approved by the FDA.

SUGGESTED READINGS

Bushberg JT, Seibert JA, Leidholdt EM, Boone JM: The Essential Physics of Medical Imaging, 2nd ed. Baltimore, Williams & Wilkins, 2002, chapters 18–20.

Hendee WR, Ritenour ER, Medical Imaging Physics, 4th ed. New York, Wiley-Liss, 2002, chapters 2–4.

Silberstein EB: Positron-emitting radiopharmaceuticals: How safe are they? Cancer Biother Radiopharm 16:13–15, 2001.

Silberstein EB, Ryan J: Pharmacopeia Committee of the Society of Nuclear Medicine: Prevalence of adverse reactions in nuclear medicine. J Nucl Med 37:185–192, 1996.

Simpkin DJ: The AAPM/RSNA Physics Tutorial for Residents: Radiation Interactions and Internal Dosimetry in Nuclear Medicine. RadioGraphics 19:155–167, 1999.

Instrumentation

The most widely used imaging devices in nuclear medicine are the simple gamma scintillation (Anger) camera, single-photon emission (SPECT)–capable gamma cameras, and positron emission (PET) scanners. Several other instruments are commonly used in the nuclear medicine laboratory, including the dose calibrator, well counter, and thyroid probe. PET instrumentation is discussed separately in Chapter 13.

GAMMA SCINTILLATION CAMERA

A gamma camera converts photons emitted by the radionuclide in the patient into a light pulse and subsequently into a voltage signal. This signal is used to form an image of the distribution of the radionuclide. The basic components of a gamma camera system (Fig. 2–1) are the collimator, the scintillation crystal, an array of photomultiplier tubes (PMTs), preamplifiers, a pulse-height analyzer (PHA), digital correction circuitry, a cathode ray tube (CRT), and the control console. A computer and picture archiving systems (PACs) are also integral parts of the system. Gamma cameras may be classified as either analog or digital. An analog signal is used throughout the analog camera; this signal has an infinite range of values and is inherently noisy. A digital signal, on the other hand, only has a discrete number of values. The main advantages of digital cameras are that they are much faster, can interact directly with the computer, and generally require less maintenance. Most of the newer cameras incorporate digital features. Even the most advanced digital cameras, however, start with the analog signal in the scintillation crystal and return to an analog signal for CRT or PACs display of the image.

Collimator

The collimator is made of perforated or folded lead and is interposed between the patient and the scintillation crystal. It allows the gamma camera to localize accurately the radionuclide in the patient's body. Collimators perform this function by absorbing and stopping most radiation except that arriving almost perpendicular to the detector face. Most radiation striking the collimator at oblique angles is not included in the final image. Of all the photons emitted by an administered radiopharmaceutical, more than 99% are "wasted" and not recorded by the gamma camera; less than 1% are used to generate the desired image. Thus, the collimator is the "rate limiting" step in the imaging chain of gamma camera technology.

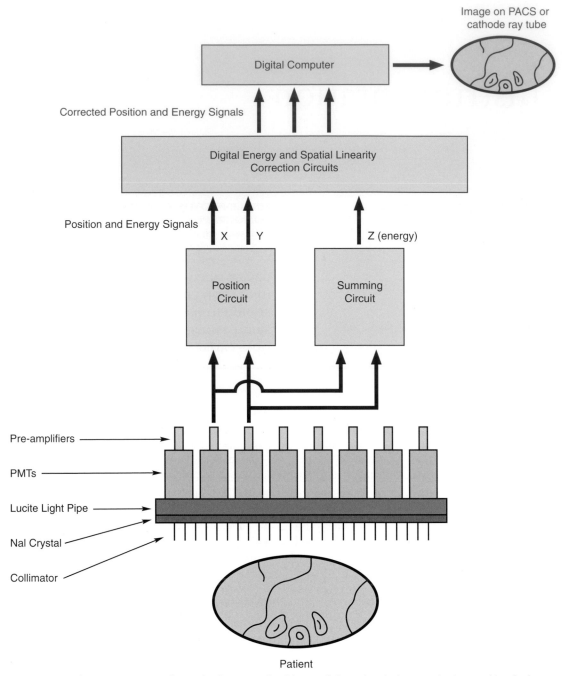

FIGURE 2–1. Gamma camera schematic. A cross-sectional image of the patient is shown at the *bottom*, with a final image seen on the cathode ray tube at the *top*.

The two basic types of collimators are *pinhole* and *multihole*. A *pinhole collimator* operates in a manner similar to that of a box camera (Fig. 2–2). Radiation must pass through the pinhole aperture to be imaged, and the image is always inverted on the scintillation crystal. Because little of the radia-tion coming from the object of interest is allowed to pass through the pinhole over a given time period, the pinhole collimator has very poor sensi-tivity. Collimator sensitivity refers to the percentage of incident photons that pass through the collima-tor. The poor sensitivity of a pinhole collimator

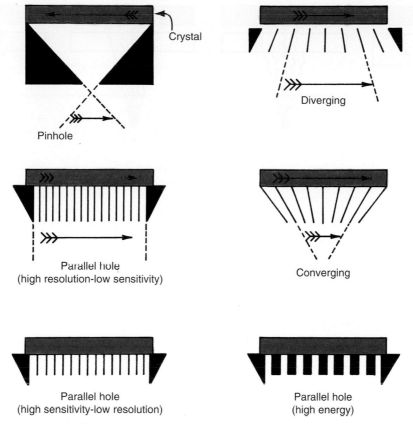

FIGURE 2–2. Types of gamma camera collimators.

makes placement near the organ of interest critical, and bringing the object of interest close to the pinhole magnifies the image. Because magnification is a function of distance, if the object of interest is not relatively flat or thin, the image may be distorted. Pinhole collimators are routinely used for very high resolution images of small organs, such as the thyroid, and for certain skeletal regions, such as hips or wrists.

The holes in a *multihole collimator* may be aligned in a diverging, parallel, or converging manner (see Fig. 2–2). The *parallel-hole collimator* is the most widely used multihole collimator in nuclear medicine laboratories. It consists of parallel holes with a long axis perpendicular to the plane of the scintillation crystal. The lead walls between the holes are referred to as *septa*. The septa absorb most gamma rays that do not emanate from the direction of interest; therefore, a collimator for high-energy gamma rays has much thicker septa than does a collimator for low-energy rays. The septa are generally designed so that septal penetration by

unwanted gamma rays does not exceed 10% to 25%.

A parallel-hole collimator should be chosen to correspond to the energy of the isotope being imaged. Low-energy collimators generally refer to a maximum energy of 150 keV, whereas medium-energy collimators have a maximum suggested energy of about 400 keV. Collimators are available with different lengths and different widths of septa. In general, the longer the septa, the better the resolution but the lower the count rate (sensitivity) for a given amount of radionuclide. The count rate is inversely proportional to the square of the collimator hole length. If the length of the septa is decreased, the detected count rate increases and resolution decreases (Fig. 2–3).

The difference between typical low-energy, general-purpose collimators and low-energy, high-sensitivity collimators is that high-sensitivity collimators may allow about twice as many counts to be imaged, although the spatial resolution is usually degraded by about 50%. A high-resolution, low-

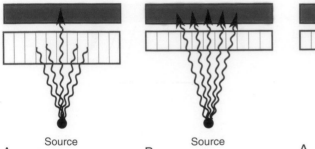

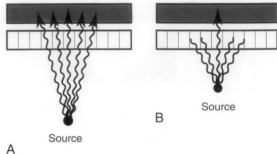

FIGURE 2–3. Effect of septal length on collimator sensitivity and resolution. *A,* Longer septa in the collimator attenuate most photons, except those exactly perpendicular to the crystal face. This increase in selectivity increases the resolution and decreases the count rate detected. *B,* Shortening the length of the septa allows more photons to reach the crystal; thus, the count rate is higher. The spatial resolution, however, is decreased because the photons coming through a hole in the collimator are from a larger area.

FIGURE 2–4. Effect of different source-to-camera distances. *A,* With the source a long distance from the camera head, a large number of photons can reach the crystal in an almost perpendicular fashion. The large area of impact on the crystal increases uncertainty about the exact location of the source. *B,* As the source is brought closer to the camera head, the correspondence of the scintillation event in the crystal with the actual location is much better, and resolution is improved.

energy collimator has about three times the resolving ability of a high-sensitivity, low-energy collimator. Most collimators are designed with hexagonal rather than round holes. Because hexagonal hole collimators have overall thinner septa, they have greater sensitivity but more septal penetration than do collimators with square or round holes.

With a parallel-hole collimator, neither the size of the image nor the count rate changes significantly with the distance of the object of interest from the collimator. This is because as the object is moved small distances away from the crystal, the inverse square law reduces the number of counts. However, this is compensated for by the increased

viewing area of the collimator. On the other hand, resolution is best when the object of interest is as close to the collimator face as possible (Figs. 2–4 and 2–5), and scans with multihole collimators are usually obtained with the collimator in contact with or as close as possible to the patient. Remember that with a parallel-hole collimator, scattered photons emitted from the patient perpendicular to the crystal face may be imaged (Fig. 2–6). These photons and those that penetrate the septa degrade spatial resolution.

A *diverging collimator* has holes and septa that begin to diverge from the crystal face. Generally, use of a diverging collimator increases the imaged area by about 30% over that obtained with a

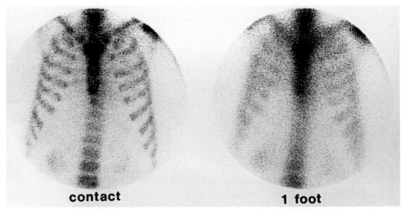

FIGURE 2–5. Effect of increasing the patient-to-detector face distance on clinical images. When the camera is in contact with this patient, who is having a bone scan, the osseous structures are well defined. Increasing the distance to 1 foot has a major adverse effect on resolution.

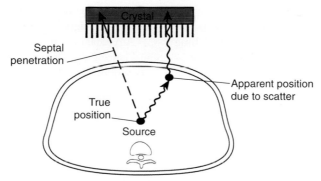

FIGURE 2–6. Scintillation events that degrade images. Both septal penetration and photon scattering within the patient's body cause events to be recorded in locations other than their true positions.

parallel-hole collimator. The image itself, however, is slightly minified. With a diverging collimator, both the sensitivity and resolution worsen as the object of interest moves away from the collimator. The sensitivity worsens because the area being imaged gets larger but the object imaged does not get larger, and the inverse square law predominates. Diverging collimators are used particularly on cameras with small crystal faces to image large organs, such as the lungs.

A *converging collimator* has holes that converge toward a point (usually 50 cm) in front of the collimator. This convergence forms a magnified image in the crystal. Sensitivity increases as the object of interest moves away from the collimator face until it reaches the focal point, beyond which the sensitivity begins to decrease. Resolution, however, decreases with distance. A converging collimator may be used for examination of small areas. A *fan-beam collimator* is sometimes used for SPECT.

Crystal

Radiation emerging from the patient and passing through the collimator may interact with a thallium-activated sodium iodide crystal. Interaction of the gamma ray with the crystal may result in ejection of an orbital electron (photoelectric absorption), producing a pulse of fluorescent light (scintillation event) proportional in intensity to the energy of the gamma ray. PMTs situated along the posterior crystal face detect this light and amplify it. About 30% of the light from each event reaches the PMTs. The crystal is fragile and must have an aluminum housing that protects it from moisture, extraneous light, and minor physical damage.

The crystal may be circular and up to about 22 inches in diameter, or it may be square or rectangular. Crystals are usually $\frac{1}{4}$ to $\frac{5}{8}$ inch thick. For most cameras, a $\frac{3}{8}$-inch-thick crystal is used. A larger-diameter crystal has a larger field of view and is more expensive but has the same inherent resolution as does a smaller-diameter crystal. The thicker the crystal becomes, the worse the spatial resolution but the more efficient the detection of gamma rays. In general, with a $\frac{1}{2}$-inch-thick crystal, the efficiency for detection of gamma rays from xenon-133 (^{133}Xe) (81 keV) and technetium-99m (^{99m}Tc) (140 keV) is almost 100%; that is, few of the photons pass through the crystal without causing a light pulse. As the gamma energy of the isotope is increased, the efficiency of the crystal is markedly reduced. For example, with iodine-131 (^{131}I) (364 keV), efficiency is reduced to about 20% to 30%. With a thinner crystal, the overall sensitivity (count rate) decreases by about 10% because more photons pass through, but there is about a 30% increase in spatial resolution because the PMTs are closer to the event and thus can localize it more accurately, and because there is an increase in light collection.

Photomultiplier Tubes

A PMT converts a light pulse into an electrical signal of measurable magnitude. An array of these tubes is situated behind the sodium iodide crystal and may be placed directly on the crystal, connected to the crystal by light pipes, or optically coupled to the crystal with a silicone-like material. A scintillation event occurring in the crystal is recorded by one or more PMTs. Localization of the event in the final image depends on the amount of light sensed by each PMT and thus on the pattern of PMT voltage output. The summation signal for each scintillation event is then formed by weighing the output of each tube. This signal has three components: spatial coordinates on x- and y-axes as well as a signal (*z*) related to intensity (energy). The x- and y-coordinates may go directly to instrumentation for display on the CRT or may be recorded in the computer. The signal intensity is processed by the PHA.

The light interaction caused by a gamma ray generally occurs near the collimator face of the crystal. Thus, although a thicker crystal is theoretically more efficient, the PMT is farther away from the scintillation point with a thick crystal and is unable to determine the coordinates as accurately. Therefore, spatial resolution is degraded. The number of PMTs is also important for the accurate localization of scintillation events; thus, for spatial resolution, the greater the number of PMTs, the greater the resolution. Most gamma cameras use about 40 to 100 hexagonal, square, or round PMTs.

Pulse-Height Analyzer

The basic principle of the PHA is to discard signals from background and scattered radiation or radiation from interfering isotopes, so that only photons known to come from the photopeak of the isotope being imaged are recorded. The PHA discriminates between events occurring in the crystal that will be displayed or stored in the computer and events that will be rejected. The PHA can make this discrimination because the energy deposited by a scintilla-

tion event in the crystal bears a linear relation to the voltage signal emerging from the PMTs.

A typical energy spectrum from a PHA is shown in Figure 2–7. The photopeak is the result of total absorption of the major gamma ray from the radionuclide. If the characteristic K-shell x-ray of iodine (28 keV) escapes from the crystal after the gamma ray has undergone photoelectric absorption, the measured gamma-ray energy for ^{99m}Tc would be only 112 keV (140 minus 28 keV). This will cause an *iodine escape peak.*

A *backscatter peak* may result when primary gamma rays undergo 180-degree scatter and then enter the detector and are totally absorbed. This can occur when gamma rays strike material behind the source and scatter back into the detector. It may also occur when gamma rays pass through the crystal without interaction and Compton scatter from the shield or PMTs back into the crystal.

The *lead x-ray peak* is caused by primary gamma rays undergoing photoelectric absorption in the lead of shielding or the collimator; as a result, characteristic x-rays (75 to 90 keV) are detected. The effect of Compton scattering in the detector gives a peak from 0 to 50 keV. The sharp edge at 50 keV is called the Compton edge. If the source of radiation is within a patient, Compton scattering occurs within the patient's tissue, and some of these scattered gamma rays travel toward the detector with an energy from 90 to 140 keV. These scattered photons from within the patient cause imaging difficulties because the Compton scatter overlaps with the photopeak distribution.

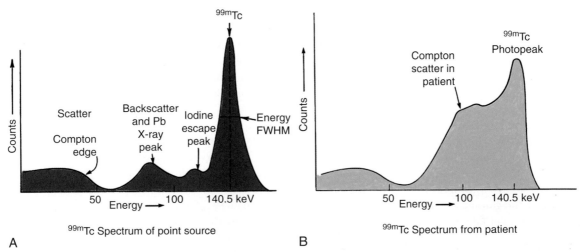

FIGURE 2–7. Energy spectra for technetium-99m when viewed by the gamma camera as a point source (*A*) and in a patient (*B*). Note the marked amount of Compton scatter near the photopeak that occurs as a result of scatter within the patient's body. FWHM, full width at half-maximum.

Signal intensity information is matched in the PHA against an appropriate *window*, which is really a voltage discriminator. To allow energy related to the desired isotope photopeak to be recorded, the window has upper and lower voltage limits that define the window width. Thus, a 20% symmetric window for 140-keV photopeak means that the electronics will accept 140 ± 14 keV (i.e., 140 keV $\pm 10\%$) gamma rays (Fig. 2–8*A*). Any signals higher or lower than this, particularly those from scattered radiation, are rejected. Some cameras have multiple PHAs, which allow several photopeaks to be used at once. This is particularly useful for radionuclides such as gallium 67 (^{67}Ga). On newer cameras, the signal processing circuitry, such as preamplifiers and PHAs, is located on the base of each PMT, so that there is little signal distortion between the camera head and the console.

Console Controls

Most gamma cameras allow for a fine adjustment known as *automatic peaking* of the isotope. This essentially divides the photopeak window into halves and calculates the number of counts in each half. If the machine is correctly peaked, each half of the window has the same number of counts from the upper and lower portions of the photopeak. Occasionally, an *asymmetric window* is used to improve resolution by eliminating some of the Compton scatter (see Fig. 2–8*B*).

Image exposure time is selected by console control and is usually a preset count, a preset time, or preset *information density* for the image accumulation. Information density refers to the number of counts per square centimeter of the gamma camera crystal face. Other console controls are present for orientation and allow the image to be reversed on the x- and y-axes.

In addition, the CRT image may be manipulated by an intensity control, which simply affects the brightness of the image, or by a persistence control, which regulates the length of time the light dots composing the image remain on the screen. Most gamma camera systems have two CRTs—one for operator viewing and another for photographic purposes. The photographic CRT is not persistent (i.e., the bright spots on the tube display disappear almost immediately). Hard-copy images on film may be obtained directly from the computer, although many institutions now display digital images on monitors and store the images in a picture archiving system.

Resolution

Resolution is one of the common performance parameters for gamma cameras. Typical performance characteristics of state-of-the-art cameras are shown in Table 2–1. Resolution usually refers to either spatial or energy resolution. *Energy resolution* is the ability to discriminate between light pulses caused by gamma rays of differing energies. *Spatial resolution* refers to the ability to display discrete but contiguous sources of radioactivity. The spatial resolution of various gamma camera systems is usually given in terms of either inherent or overall resolution. *Inherent spatial resolution* is the ability of the

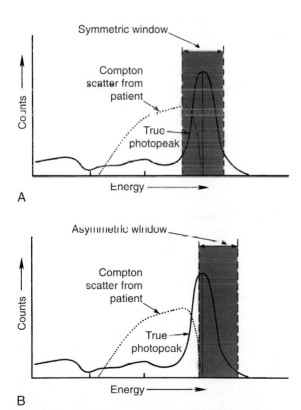

FIGURE 2–8. Use of a symmetric window (*A*) allows some of the Compton scatter to be counted and displayed. Theoretically, use of an asymmetric window (*B*) obviates this problem.

TABLE 2–1.	Typical Intrinsic Gamma Camera Performance Characteristics
Spatial resolution (full width at half-maximum)	3–5 mm
Energy resolution	10%–14%
Temporal resolution	100–350 k counts/sec
Field uniformity	2%–5%

crystal PMT detector and accompanying electronics to record the exact location of the light pulse on the sodium iodide crystal. Gamma cameras have an inherent resolution of about 3 mm.

Statistical variability is particularly important in resolution. An event occurring exactly between two PMTs does not always give the same number of photons to each tube; thus, for any single event, the distribution of photons is statistically variable. Statistical variation is relatively greater when fewer light photons are available. In other words, the inherent resolution of a system or its ability to localize an event is directly related to the energy of the isotope being imaged. When radioisotopes with low-energy gamma rays are used, the camera has less inherent spatial resolution.

Compton scatter also affects inherent resolution to a minor extent. When the gamma ray interacts with the crystal, there is usually photoelectric absorption, which results in a light pulse at the point of interaction. With higher-energy gamma rays, however, the initial event may be a Compton interaction or scatter within the crystal (i.e., a collision between a gamma ray and a loosely bound orbital electron). This results in scattered photons with light coming from several points, even though only a single gamma ray interacted with the crystal initially.

Overall spatial resolution is the resolution capacity of the entire camera system, including such factors as the collimator resolution, septal penetration, and scattered radiation. The simplest method of examining overall spatial resolution is to determine the full width at half-maximum (FWHM) of the line spread function. This refers to the profile response of the gamma camera to a single point source of radioactivity and reflects the number of counts seen by the crystal at different lateral distances from the source (Fig. 2–9*A*). The source is often placed 10 cm from the crystal for these measurements. The FWHM is expressed as the width in centimeters at 50% of the height of the line spread peak. The narrower the peak, the better the resolution. When state-of-the-art cameras and ^{99m}Tc are used, the position of scintillation events can be determined to within 3 to 5 mm. A typical high-resolution collimator has three times better resolution than does a representative high-sensitivity collimator but allows only one-tenth as many counts per minute for a given activity.

Although spatial FWHM is useful for comparing collimators, it often does not give other desirable information and does not necessarily relate to

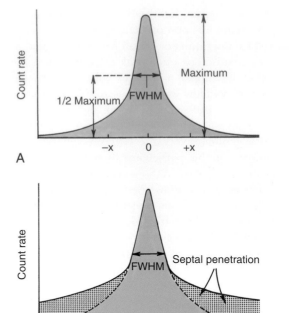

FIGURE 2–9. *A,* **The full width at half-maximum (FWHM) is the response in count rate to a single point source of radioactivity at different lateral distances from the point source.** *B,* With septal penetration, the image may be significantly degraded even though FWHM is unchanged.

the overall clinical performance of the collimator. More difficult but perhaps more encompassing measurements of collimator performance are modulation transfer functions, which take other factors for optimizing collimator design, such as the presence of scattering material and septal penetration, into account. The value of this can be seen in Figure 2–9*B*, which illustrates that the septal penetration occurring in the collimator may be completely undetected by the measurement of FWHM alone.

When the overall spatial resolution of the system with high-energy isotopes is considered, the limiting resolution is that of the collimator. When low-energy isotopes are imaged, the inherent resolution becomes more important than the collimator resolution. As the energy of the incident gamma ray decreases, the inherent resolution of the crystal decreases markedly because the lower-energy gamma rays provide less light for the PMTs to record; thus, there is more statistical uncertainty regarding the origin of the gamma ray. Although the inherent resolution of cameras is often championed by salespeople, the overall resolution determines the quality of the image because it is a combination of the resolutions of each of the components in the imaging chain, including the collimator, the inherent resolution, septal penetration, and scatter. The overall system resolution (R_s) is

$$R_S = \sqrt{R^2_i + R^2_c}$$

where R^2_i is inherent resolution and R^2_c is collimator resolution.

Another category of resolution is *energy resolution,* or the ability of the imaging system to separate and distinguish between the photopeaks of different radionuclides. If the energy resolution is good, the photopeaks are tall and narrow; if energy resolution is poor, the photopeaks appear as broad bumps in the energy spectrum. The FWHM concept is also used to examine energy resolution and is usually quoted for the relatively high energy (662-keV) photon of cesium-137 (^{137}Ce). With lower-energy photons, the energy resolution is worse. Most gamma cameras have energy resolution of 10% to 15%, allowing use of 15% to 20% energy windows to encompass all the photons of interest.

Count Rate and Dead Time

As with any detection system, it is important that scintillation events do not occur so fast that the electronic system is unable to count each as a separate event. If two equal light pulses occur too close together in time, the system may perceive this as one event with twice the energy actually present. Such an occurrence of primary photons would be eliminated by the energy window of the PHA, and none of the information from the two events would be imaged; thus, the sensitivity of the system would be diminished. A more significant problem is loss of spatial resolution when several scattered (low-energy) photons strike the crystal at the same time, so that their light production is summed and appears as a photon of interest. The time after an event during which the system is unable to respond to another event is referred to as *dead time.* Dead time can be important in high–count-rate dynamic studies (in the range of 50,000 counts/second), particularly with single-crystal cameras. An example is a first-pass cardiac study.

Field Uniformity

Despite the efforts of manufacturers to produce high-quality collimators, crystals, PMTs, and electronics, nonuniformity inevitably occurs. Accept-able field nonuniformity is on the order of 2% to 5%. Much of this can be corrected by the computer system. Analysis of field uniformity is discussed in Chapter 3.

Image Acquisition: Memory and Matrix Size

Data may be acquired either by *frame mode* or by *list mode.* In the frame mode, incoming data are placed in a spatial matrix in the memory that is used to generate an image. In the list mode, all data are put in the memory as a time sequence list of events. At regular intervals, a special code word is inserted into the list. This list is flexible and can be sorted or divided into images at a later time. The list mode has the disadvantage of a low acquisition rate and a large memory requirement. Frame mode uses much less memory than does the list mode and is more commonly used, except for gated cardiac studies. All data for images that are collected in the frame mode are acquired in a matrix. The usual image matrix sizes are 64×64 and 128×128, although 32×32 and 256×256 matrix sizes are occasionally used. The main disadvantage of frame mode is that the identity of individual events within a time frame is lost.

Matrix size refers to the number of picture elements along each side of the matrix. These elements may be either bytes or words. In an 8-bit computer, both a byte and a word are composed of 8 bits. In a 16-bit computer, a byte is 8 bits and a word is 16 bits. The maximum number of counts that can be represented by an 8-bit picture element (pixel) is 2^8, or 0 through 255 (256 different values). Ordinarily, 16-bit collections are used; the maximum size is 2^{16}, or 0 through 65,535 (65,536 different values) per pixel.

The matrix size determines the image resolution. Although the matrix size and the number of counts desired have a significant impact on memory required, the ultimate memory requirements depend on what the computer system is being used for and how many cameras it is interfaced with simultaneously. The matrix size has nothing to do with the final size of the displayed image. A 32×32 matrix has relatively few pixels; therefore, the final image is coarse. An image obtained in a 256×256 acquisition matrix is much more detailed. Remember that an image resolution of 256×256 may refer to either the memory acquisition matrix or the CRT display matrix. Some manufacturers take a 64×64 matrix image from the memory and display it on the CRT in a $256 \times$

256 or 1024 × 1024 matrix, using interpolation methods.

The 32 × 32 matrix occupies less memory and therefore less disk space. In addition, it can be acquired faster than can a finer matrix. Thus, there is a trade-off between spatial and temporal resolution. In a 32 × 32 matrix, the spatial resolution is poor, but because it can be acquired rapidly, the temporal resolution is excellent. For a given computer system, the matrix size desired for acquisition and the read–write speed of the hard disk dictate the maximum framing rate that is possible.

As mentioned previously, if all 16 bits in a 16-bit computer are used, 65,535 (2^{16}) counts per pixel are possible. This allows for statistical identification of small differences in function. To increase the matrix size, it is possible to address the memory at the byte level (8 bits/pixel). If this is done, twice as many pixels can be accommodated, and the image matrix will be finer but the number of counts possible in each pixel is reduced to 255 (2^8).

The amount of memory determines the number of frames that can be collected in the electro-cardiographic R-R interval on electrocardiogram-gated cardiac studies. For optimum measurement of ejection fraction, at least 25 frames/second are needed. If peak ejection or peak filling rate is to be measured, 50 frames/second are needed.

Image Display and Processing

Image display and processing is necessary in all nuclear medicine computer systems. The computer plays an extremely important role in lesion detectability, and it can perform this function in a number of ways, including reduction of noise, background subtraction, construction of cine loops, and production of tomographic images. Data are normally collected in 64 × 64 byte images. Although a 32 × 32 byte mode can be used, the decrease in spatial resolution is usually intolerable. Even in 64 × 64 pixel images, there is a noticeable saw-toothed appearance to the image edges. Because the pixel matrix achieved on a display video is 1024 × 1024 with 256 levels of gray, the data are usually processed to use all the pixels. The simplest method to fill in the extra pixels is linear interpolation.

To reduce the effects of statistical variation, particularly in low-count images, the image can be smoothed. Smoothing is accomplished through the use of filters, which may be either spatial or temporal. Temporal filters are used for dynamic acquisition, and spatial filters are used on static images.

Spatial filters attempt to remove statistical fluctuations of the image by modifying values of data points within various pixels.

Spatial Filters

The processing performed by spatial filters is done according to the spatial frequencies of the information. By attenuating or augmenting parts of the spatial frequency spectrum, an image should be obtained that is easier to interpret or that has more diagnostic value. The simplest smoothing method is nine-point smoothing. This takes 9 pixels of information and, by taking weighted averages of the 8 pixels on the edge of a central pixel, changes the value of that central pixel.

Other kinds of filters that are commonly used are low-pass, high-pass, and band-pass filters. A low-pass filter selectively attenuates high frequencies and smoothes the image by removing high-frequency noise. This filtering improves the statistical quality of an image but degrades the sharpness and spatial resolution. Figure 2–10A shows an example of low-pass filtering applied to data from a SPECT liver scan. High-pass filtering enhances edges to some extent but also augments the noise (see Fig. 2–10B). This type of filtering is important in cardiac nuclear medicine when locating the edge of the ventricle is needed. A band-pass filter is a combination of low-pass and high-pass filters that effectively suppresses high-frequency and low-frequency signals and transmits only signals that are in a given spatial frequency window.

A simple way of performing low-pass filtering is by addition of dynamic images. Remember that dynamic images have a low number of counts in each pixel and are therefore usually in the byte mode. Thus, the highest number of counts that can be stored in a pixel is 255. When adding images, it is necessary to change from the byte mode to the word mode so that the maximum number of counts that can be accommodated in each pixel is expanded. If the computer is in the byte mode and the number of counts per pixel exceeds 255, the computer begins counting at 0 again for that pixel. This results in a negative defect (rollover artifact) in areas that would normally have a high count rate. An example of this is seen in Figure 2–10.

Temporal Filters

Temporal filters are used on dynamic images and involve a weighted averaging technique between each pixel on one image and the same pixel from the frames before and after. Temporal filtering

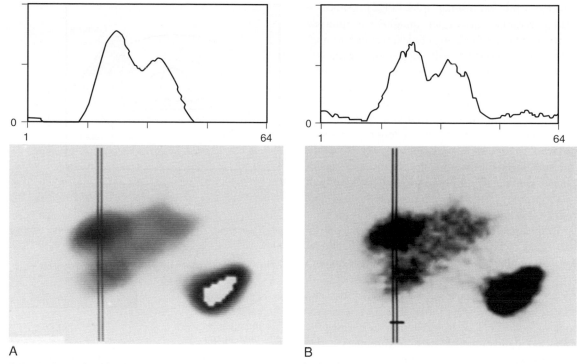

FIGURE 2–10. Application of spatial filtering to a coronal single-photon emission computed tomography (SPECT) image of the liver and spleen. Histograms of the activity defined in a linear region of interest are shown in the upper portions of *A* and *B*. The reconstructed tomographic images are shown in the lower portions (*left*, liver; *right*, spleen). (*A*) A low-pass filter removes high frequencies and smooths the image. Rollover artifact is seen as the white area in the central portion of the spleen. (*B*) With a high-pass filter, the image appears more noisy, but edges are enhanced. (Case courtesy of Michael Hartshorne, M.D.)

causes a loss of spatial resolution but allows a cine loop to be viewed without flicker. Remember that temporal filtering of dynamic studies does not preclude spatial filtering of the same study, and in fact, the two processes are frequently performed together.

Frame Manipulation

Another common computer image-processing application is frame subtraction. This method may be used for background subtraction and for subtraction of studies performed simultaneously with two different radionuclides. Although less commonly used, additional computer capabilities include frame multiplication and division. Combinations of the maneuvers may be used to produce the so-called functional parametric images obtained from radionuclide ventriculography.

Operator Interaction

The operator interacts with the computer in one of two ways, either by selecting from a menu or by using a command structure. The menu system requires sequential choices from a list or menu pre-sented on the video terminal. Although the menu system is somewhat slower than is the command system, the operator does not need to be familiar with all of the possible commands (usually about 100 commands that are chosen through use of a two- or three-letter mnemonic).

Interaction of the operator with the computer also occurs when a region of interest is selected. This can be done by moving a cursor, light pen, trackball, mouse, or joystick. Once a region of interest is defined, the operator can perform various functions: the most common of which is determining the total number of counts within the region of interest. A region of interest can be maintained over multiple frames to produce a dynamic time-activity curve.

SINGLE-PHOTON EMISSION COMPUTED TOMOGRAPHY (SPECT)

The successful application of computer algorithms to x-ray imaging in computed tomography (CT) has led to their application to radionuclide techniques and to the advent of single-photon emission computed tomography (SPECT) and positron emission tomography (PET). Although planar radionuclide organ imaging in multiple views is sufficient for many clinical settings, tomography offers several readily apparent advantages over two-dimensional planar images. The most obvious advantage of tomography is improved image contrast because it focuses on a thin slice of an organ, thus minimizing overlying and underlying activity that may obscure a lesion or area of interest. In addition, SPECT and PET permit absolute three-dimensional localization of radiopharmaceutical distribution, with the possibility of quantification and three-dimensional cinematic representation of the organ imaged.

Emission CT can be accomplished by one of two main techniques: (1) transverse or rotational tomography or (2) fixed-ring detector. Although both approaches have been clinically applied with success, rotational techniques have enjoyed widespread application. The purpose of this section is to describe SPECT instrumentation and principles. Clinical applications of each technique are discussed later in the organ system chapters. PET is covered in Chapter 13.

Instrumentation

In its simplest form, rotational SPECT is accomplished by using a conventional gamma (Anger) camera detector head and a parallel hole or hybrid collimator fitted to a rotating gantry. The detector is capable of orbiting around a stationary patient on a special imaging table, with the camera face continually directed toward the patient. The camera head rotates around a central axis called the *axis of rotation* (AOR). The distance of the camera face from this central axis is referred to as the *radius of rotation* (ROR). The orbit may be circular, with a 360-degree capacity, although elliptical (Fig. 2–11) or body contour motions are also used. Rotational arcs of less than 360 degrees may be used, particularly for cardiac studies. The detector electronics are coupled with a computer capable of performing acquisition and processing of the image data according to preselected parameters. The gamma camera is capable of acquiring data from a large volume of the patient during a single orbit, and multiple slices (sections) are produced from just one data acquisition sequence. More complex systems using multiple camera heads are becoming common. The various camera head configurations are shown in Figure 2–12.

Minor artifacts and inconsistencies can be tolerated in planar imaging, but they cause major prob-

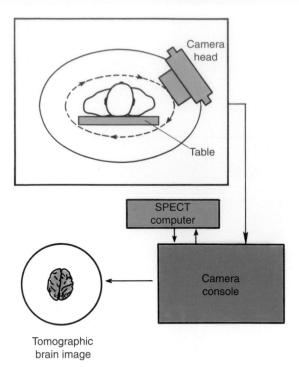

FIGURE 2–11. Schematic representation of a single-photon emission computed tomography (SPECT) system using a single camera head. The camera detector usually rotates around the patient in a noncircular orbit while acquiring data to be fed to the computer. The tomographic computer-reconstructed images are subsequently displayed.

lems with SPECT. As the principal component of the SPECT imaging system, the gamma camera must be state of the art, with an intrinsic resolution of at least 3 to 4 mm, an absolute linearity deviation of less than 1 mm, and a basic uncorrected uniformity deviation of 3% to 5% or less across the useful field of view of the detector. A system with excellent energy resolution is needed to permit adequate rejection of scattered radiation, a major degrader of contrast in SPECT images. This is enhanced by an autotune feature, which continually tunes and balances the PMTs of the detector during the operation. Although count rate capacity of the camera is not critical in SPECT, the system should be able to handle significantly high count rates to avoid any field uniformity distortion caused by high–count-rate effects.

The rotation of the detector on the gantry subjects the camera head to thermal, magnetic, and gravitational forces not experienced by planar instruments, and the system construction must take these factors into consideration. This includes shielding of the PMTs with a mu metal to protect against changing magnetic fields during rotation.

is detected by the PMT, which feeds into a scalar. The scalar readout directly reflects the amount of radioactivity in the sample and is usually recorded in counts for the time period during which the sample is measured.

Reflected light and scattering inside the well surface and the thickness of the crystal limit the energy resolution of the standard well counter. Because the sample is essentially surrounded by the crystal, the geometric efficiency for detection of gamma rays is high. *Geometric efficiency* is defined as the fraction of emitted radioactivity that is incident on the detection portion of the counter, in this case, the crystal. Because the crystal is relatively thick, most low-energy photons undergo interaction, and few pass through undetected. As a result, in the energy ranges below 200 keV, the overall crystal detection efficiency is usually better than 95%.

Because the top of the well in the crystal is open, it is important to keep the sample volume in the test tube small. If varying sample volumes are placed in the well counter, different amounts of radiation escape near the top of the crystal, resulting in unequal geometric efficiencies. Absorption of gamma rays within the wall of the test tube is a factor when lower-energy sources, such as iodine-125 (^{125}I), are counted; therefore, the sample tubes should also be identical.

Because sodium iodide well counters have such a high detection efficiency, there is a serious problem with electronic dead time. If high levels of activity are used, much of the radiation is not detected. In general, well counters can typically count only fractions of a microcurie (μCi) or rates of about 5000 counts/second. Attempts to measure amounts of activity greater than this in a well counter can lead to serious errors.

SINGLE-PROBE COUNTING SYSTEM

Single-probe counting systems using only one crystalline detector are useful for measuring not only thyroid uptake of radioactive iodine but also cardiac output. The probe used for thyroid counting is actually similar to the standard well counter in concept (Fig. 2–16), although it does not have the central hole in the sodium iodide crystal. The typical crystal is 5 cm in diameter and 5 cm in thickness, with a cone-shaped (flat-field) collimator. As with the well counter, a PMT is situated at the crystal base. When these probes are used, it is important for quantitative consistency to maintain a fixed distance from the object being measured to the face of the crystal and to eliminate all extraneous sources of background radiation.

DOSE CALIBRATOR

Because it is extremely important to calibrate a dose of isotope before injection, the dose calibrator is an essential piece of equipment in any nuclear medicine laboratory. A standard well counter is not useful because the upper limit of sample activity that can be measured accurately is in the microcurie range. A dose calibrator is essentially a well-type ionization chamber capable of measuring quantities in the millicurie range. It does not contain a sodium iodide crystal. The chamber is cylindrical and holds a defined volume of inert gas (usually argon). Within the chamber is a collecting electrode (Fig. 2–17). As radiation emanates from the radiopharmaceutical in the syringe, it enters the chamber and interacts with the gas, causing ionization. An electrical differential applied between the chamber and the collecting electrode causes the ions to be captured and measured.

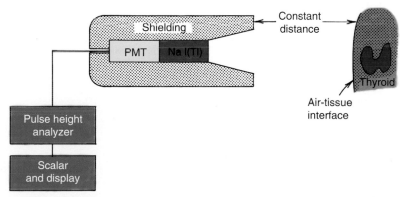

FIGURE 2–16. Schematic diagram of a single-crystal thyroid probe. PMT, photomultiplier tube.

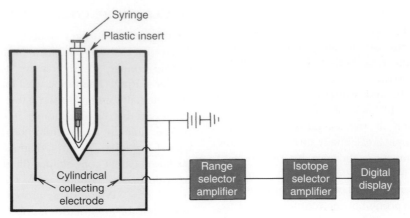

FIGURE 2–17. Schematic diagram of a dose calibrator.

PEARLS & PITFALLS

A well counter is a cylindrical sodium iodide crystal with a hole drilled in it and a PMT on the end (see Fig. 2–15).

A thyroid probe has a single sodium iodide crystal, a PMT on the end, and a single-hole collimator (see Fig. 2–16).

The dose calibrator is a gas-filled ionization chamber (see Fig. 2–17).

A gamma camera has a single large, flat sodium iodide crystal and multiple PMTs (see Fig. 2–1).

A GM counter has a gas-filled probe and is used to perform low-level surveys to detect small amounts of contamination. For high activities or dose-rate surveys, an air-filled ionization survey meter is used.

SPECT myocardial perfusion acquisition is usually done over 180 degrees; for most other studies, 360-degree acquisition is used.

SPECT reconstruction uses the same basic Fourier transformation back-projection method as does CT.

Most dose calibrators have a digital readout that indicates the amount of activity in microcuries or millicuries when the specific radionuclide being measured has been specified. Because not all radionuclides generate the same number of photons per radioactive decay, the dose calibrator must be recalibrated for each radionuclide that is to be measured.

The dose calibrator response must be linear over the activity range of interest; thus, a stable voltage supply is critical. In addition, for patient safety, a dose calibrator must have careful quality control (see Chapter 3).

SUGGESTED READINGS

Bushberg JT, Seibert JA, Leidholdt EM, Boone JM: The Essential Physics of Medical Imaging, 2nd ed. Baltimore, Williams & Wilkins, 2002.

Hendee WR, Ritenour ER, Medical Imaging Physics, 4th ed. New York, Wiley-Liss, 2002, chapter 12.

Ranger NT: The AAPM/RSNA Physics Tutorial for Residents: Radiation Detectors in Nuclear Medicine. RadioGraphics 19:481–502, 1999.

Royal HD, Parker JA, Holman BL: Basic principles of computers. In Sandler MP, Coleman RE, Patton JA, et al. (eds): Diagnostic Nuclear Medicine, 3rd ed. Baltimore, Williams & Wilkins, 1996, chapter 8.

Quality Control

3

A quality control program is especially important in two main areas: instrumentation and radiopharmaceutical preparation. The importance of such a program has been stressed by professional groups, governmental agencies, and hospital accreditation groups.

INSTRUMENTATION

Before any equipment is installed, it is important to ensure that there is a suitable environment to house it; otherwise, attempts at quality control will be ineffective. Most nuclear medicine equipment and computers generate a tremendous amount of heat, and all aspects of ventilation and temperature control need to be examined. Consoles should never be placed close to a wall, and dust and smoke also cause serious problems, especially for computers. In addition, shutting down newer imaging and computer systems at night prolongs the useful life of many components.

Instrument quality control takes place on several temporal levels. Well counters, dose calibrators, thyroid probes, and gamma cameras should be calibrated on receipt of a new machine and annually thereafter. For most instruments, this can often be done by plotting the energy spectrum of an isotope, such as cesium-137 (^{137}Cs). If a narrow window width is used and the number of counts at each 10-keV increment are recorded and plotted, an energy spectrum is demonstrated. The full width at half-maximum of the photopeak (see Chapter 2) is then measured and should be less than 10% of the peak height. Daily calibration also may be done by using a similar source at a specified window and adjusting the voltage so that the maximum count rate is obtained. If this information is recorded daily, subtle changes in the electronics may be identified.

Dose Calibrator

The dose calibrator is a particularly important instrument for patient protection. It assures the user that the appropriate amount of radiopharmaceutical is about to be administered to the patient. It is the physician's responsibility to determine that the correct dosage is being given to the patient. If the radiopharmaceutical has been prepared at an outside licensed radiopharmacy as an individual patient unit dosage, this may be done either by assay of the dosage or by decay correction. The U.S. Nuclear Regulatory Commission (NRC) requires that all other radiopharmaceuticals be assayed for activity before administration, and the accuracy must be within ± 10% of the intended dosage.

The dose calibrator should be tested daily. Consistency of the circuits may be evaluated with 100 to 200 μCi (3.7 to 7.4 MBq) of ^{137}Cs (662 keV; similar in energy to molybdenum-99 [^{99}Mo]) and with 2 to 5 mCi (74 to 185 MBq) of cobalt 57 (^{57}Co) (122 keV; similar to technetium-99m [^{99m}Tc]). After decay corrections are made, the observed activity should agree with the actual calibration source activity by ± 5%. Daily background count rates should also be measured and recorded. The dose calibrator must function over a range of 30 μCi (1.1 MBq) to 2 Ci (74 GBq) and must be linear over a wide range of activity. Linearity may be tested by using a high-activity ^{99m}Tc source measured periodically over 24 hours of decay. The dose calibrator readings should closely agree with activity levels calculated from decay tables for ^{99m}Tc. An alternative procedure is to use several lead shields, which attenuate a high-activity ^{99m}Tc source by a known amount. This latter method reduces the time to perform the linearity test from 1 day to a few minutes. It also ensures that the sample size remains the same and that there is no possibility of dilution errors. Such linearity measurements should be made quarterly.

The volume of a sample and the type of syringe or vial used can alter the sensitivity of a dose calibrator or scintillation well counter. With low-energy gamma-ray emitters, such as thallium- 201 (^{201}Tl), xenon-133 (^{133}Xe), and iodine-125 (^{125}I), the use of plastic or glass syringes may change readings by as much as 100%. When these instruments arrive at the laboratory, measurements are made with the various volumes and syringes used in clinical practice to derive geometric correction factors. Measurement of the threshold response of the calibrator (lower sensitivity limit) is also important, particularly for ^{99}Mo.

Gamma Cameras

Scintillation camera systems are subject to a variety of detector and associated electronic problems that can cause aberrations of the image and may not be detected by the casual observer. Thus, quality control procedures are especially important to ensure high-quality, accurate diagnostic images. The three parameters usually tested are (1) spatial resolution, or the ability to visualize an alternating, closely spaced pattern of activity; (2) image linearity and distortion, or the ability to reproduce a straight line; and (3) field uniformity, or the ability of the imaging system to produce a uniform image from the entire crystal surface. In general, these determinations can be made with or without the collimator.

For gamma camera quality control, the source of radioactivity used is either a solid disk (sheet source) large enough to cover the detector surface with radionuclide dispersed homogeneously throughout (uniform to 1%), or a thin Lucite or Plexiglas chamber with a central area filled with radioactive liquid (flood source). The radionuclides used for evaluation of most gamma camera systems are ^{99m}Tc and ^{57}Co. Technetium-99m has the advantage of being inexpensive, and it tests the electronic circuitry for the photopeak of ^{99m}Tc, which is used in most of the clinical imaging procedures. Because of its short (6-hour) half-life, ^{99m}Tc has the disadvantage that the flood phantom must be prepared daily. Other disadvantages include nonuniformity if the ^{99m}Tc liquid is not mixed thoroughly and the possibility of contamination if any of the liquid leaks out. Cobalt-57 (122 keV) has a half-life of 270 days and thus does not have to be prepared daily. The cobalt sheet source is also light-weight and solid (spill-free), and can be used for checking sensitivity of the instruments. Disadvantages of ^{57}Co are that it is more expensive and does not accurately test the photopeak electronics for ^{99m}Tc. Another disadvantage is that the cobalt source initially may have too much activity for electronic handling by the camera system. This may necessitate calibration with the collimator in place to reduce the activity seen by the crystal. Most single-crystal gamma cameras are subject to activity limitations, and a source in excess of about 1.2 million counts/minute should not be used.

Spatial Resolution and Linearity Testing

To test for spatial resolution, several phantoms have been developed. In general, they are either Lucite sheets embedded with lead bars or a sheet of lead with holes in it. The phantom is placed between the camera or collimator face and a radioactive flood or sheet source, and a transmission image is then obtained. Two types of available phantoms (the Hine-Duley and the parallel-line, equal-space phantom) have lead bars that extend completely across the detector face. This allows some measurement of detector spatial resolution, distortion, uniformity, and linearity. A more common four-quadrant bar phantom has four sets of bars of different widths and spacing in each quadrant, which are arranged at 90-degree angles to each other. The four quadrants test a spectrum of resolution ranging from relatively coarse to fine. Spatial resolution measurements require that the phantom be rotated 90 degrees and reimaged to check the spatial resolution in all areas of the crystal (Fig. 3–1). Linearity and distortion problems are manifested when the otherwise straight bars are depicted as wavy lines (Fig. 3–2). All of these phantoms come

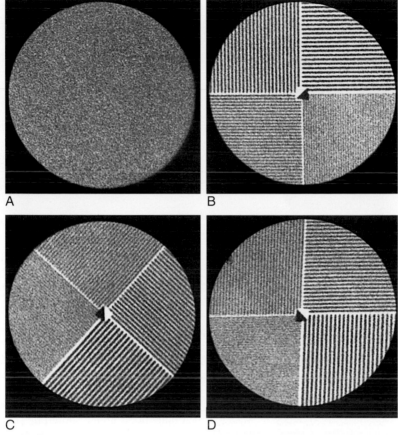

FIGURE 3–1. Normal flood-field (*A*) and bar phantom (*B*) images. The bar phantom should be rotated (*C, D*) to check all portions of the detector.

in different sizes to best define the resolution capabilities of a particular system.

Field Uniformity Assessment

Field uniformity is tested extrinsically (with the collimator) or intrinsically (without the collimator). Extrinsic field uniformity is evaluated by using a flood-field image obtained by presenting the collimator–crystal combination with a uniform planar source of activity. The planar source is usually a ^{57}Co solid plastic sheet source or a plastic tank filled with ^{99m}Tc in liquid. Covering the detector head with a plastic cover is an excellent way to avoid collimator and crystal contamination if a liquid source is used. If the flood field is obtained by mixing ^{99m}Tc and water in a plastic flood tank, there must be adequate mixing (Fig. 3–3). After mixing, all air bubbles must be removed to prevent inhomogeneity.

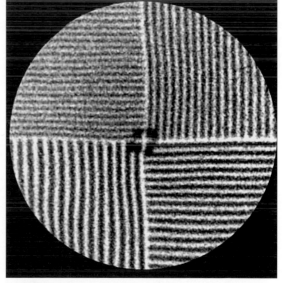

FIGURE 3–2. Linearity and distortion problems. The four-quadrant bar phantom demonstrates wavy lines seen particularly in the left lower quadrant.

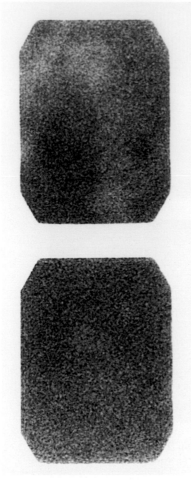

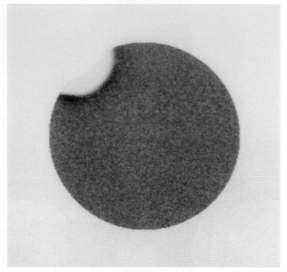

FIGURE 3–4. Photomultiplier defect. The flood field image shows a peripheral cresentic defect due to a non-functioning photomultiplier tube (PMT).

FIGURE 3–3. Inadequate mixing of technetium in the flood-field phantom. *Top,* This panel demonstrates an inhomogeneous appearance because the technetium was not adequately mixed with the water in the phantom. *Bottom,* This panel demonstrates a much better homogeneity and was obtained after the phantom was shaken several times.

For intrinsic uniformity evaluation, either a planar or a point source can be used after the collimator has been removed. The point-source method uses a small volume of ^{99m}Tc in a tuberculin syringe at a sufficient distance (1 to 2 m) from the detector.

When obtaining the images for evaluation of uniformity, 2 million counts should be accumulated on a standard-field-of-view camera and up to 6 million on a large-field-of-view camera. The flood-field image is visually evaluated for uniformity. If the collimator has been removed, an area of increased activity is often seen around the edge of the image; this is referred to as *edge-packing*. This artifact results in part from more efficient collection of scintillation events near the edge of the crystal because there is some reflection from the side of the crystal back toward the phototubes. Edge-packing is not normally visible on the cathode ray display. A daily flood image should be placed in a logbook to assess any changes in uniformity and for accreditation inspections. A variety of abnormalities can be identified on flood-field images, including cracks in the crystal (Fig. 3–5), collimator defects (Fig. 3–6), and electronic or photomultiplier abnormalities (Fig. 3–4).

Most cameras have microprocessor and computer circuits to correct for image nonuniformity. An initial flood-field image is obtained and stored in the computer memory. Field uniformity is then obtained by adjusting subsequent clinical images based on the initial image in its memory (Fig. 3–6). A flood field should also be obtained without the use of the computer correction so that the operator can see the status of the detectors and whether there is degradation over time or need for adjustment. If this is not done, data losses of up to 50% may result in prolonged imaging times. Other computer correction systems are also available.

A number of other steps are required in the daily evaluation of the gamma scintillation camera. These include assurance that the correct energy window for the imaged radionuclide is being selected and that the photopeak is included in the energy window. Centering the energy window too high or too low results in nonuniform images (Fig.

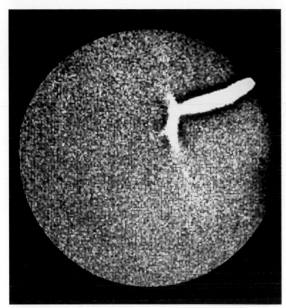

FIGURE 3–5. Large crack in the sodium iodide crystal. The branching white pattern is caused by a crack and because no scintillations are occurring in this region. The dark edges are due to the edge-packing phenomenon.

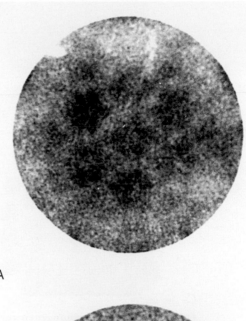

A

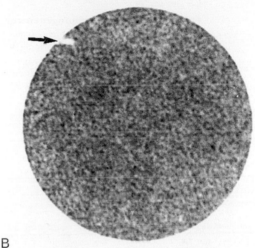

B

FIGURE 3–6. Effect of computer correction. *A,* The flood-field image was obtained without computer correction. The lower image (*B*) was done with computer correction and demonstrates a much more homogeneous flood field. A defect (*arrow*), however, remained. This was because of a deformity of the lead septa of the collimator.

3–7). Whether the phototubes appear hot or cold when the energy window is off-peak depends on the specific manufacturer. Images obtained off-peak or with malfunctioning computer correction circuits can be seriously misinterpreted (Figs. 3–8 and 3–9). Because scattered radiation may result in improper peaking, peaking should never be done using a patient or a dose syringe in contact with the collimator as the radioactive source.

A summary of quality control procedures and frequency is given in Table 3–1.

Single-Photon Emission Computed Tomography Quality Control

To ensure high performance standards of single-photon emission computed tomography (SPECT) cameras, routine detector quality control procedures should be performed weekly, as with any gamma camera, including tests of intrinsic uniformity, extrinsic uniformity (collimator in place), resolution, and linearity. Regular meticulous quality control of SPECT imaging systems is absolutely essential for the production of clinically useful, artifact-free images. Although even significant deviations from optimum performance can be tolerated in routine planar imaging, more minor departures from performance standards in SPECT

imaging may produce unacceptable or even misleading images.

Field Uniformity Assessment and Correction

Because rotational SPECT images are produced from planar views and because that process amplifies any suboptimal characteristics introduced by the instrumentation, quality control of SPECT imaging begins with assurances that the imaging system is operating at the highest intrinsic performance standards. This is especially true of

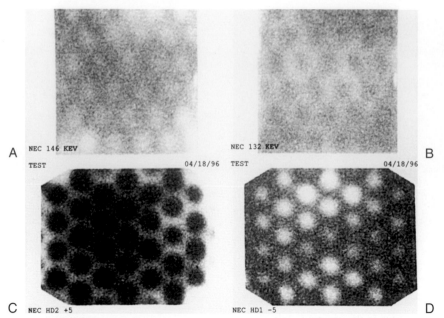

A NEC 146 KEV

B NEC 132 KEV

TEST   04/18/96   TEST   04/18/96

C NEC HD2 +5

D NEC HD1 -5

FIGURE 3–7. Effect of improper energy peaking. The field uniformity images on the upper (*A and B*) and lower (*C, D*) rows were obtained on different cameras. In each row, the images were obtained with the cameras off-peak on the left too high (*A, C*), and on the right too low (*B, D*). Note that in both cameras, off-peak imaging causes the photomultiplier tubes (PMTs) to be imaged too hot or too cold. It is obvious that the PMT response varies among cameras.

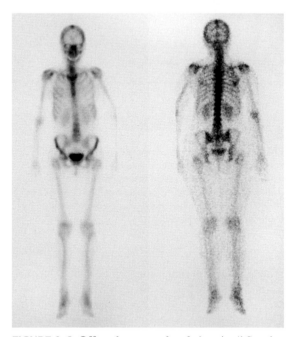

FIGURE 3–8. Off-peak camera head. Anterior (*left*) and posterior (*right*) images from a bone scan were obtained with a moving dual-headed gamma camera and a fixed table. The camera head anterior to the patient was properly peaked for the radionuclide energy, whereas the posterior camera was improperly peaked, resulting in poor spatial resolution. The individual photomultiplier tubes are not seen because of the moving detector head.

system uniformity, which is governed by multiple factors in the imaging chain: principally, detector uniformity of response (intrinsic uniformity), collimator integrity (extrinsic uniformity), and the quality of the analog/digital signal conversions at the camera–computer interface. Significant camera field nonuniformities can result in image artifacts, the most common of which is the *ring artifact*.

In ordinary planar imaging, system uniformity variation of 3% to 5% may be acceptable. Nonuniformities that are not apparent in planar images, however, can give rise to significant errors in the reconstructed tomographic views, which may appear as full or partial ring artifacts. A 5% detector or collimator nonuniformity on the axis of rotation (AOR) can produce a 35% cold or hot spot on the reconstructed image. The farther the nonuniformity is from the AOR, the less intense is the artifact. In addition, use of noncircular orbits minimizes nonuniformity artifacts. Because the back-projection process used in SPECT amplifies nonuniformities inherent in the imaging system, a uniformity deviation in SPECT imaging must be 1% or less to produce artifact-free images. This is significantly less than that achievable because of inherent system inhomogeneity, so system nonuniformity must be corrected.

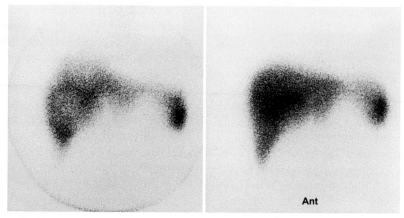

FIGURE 3–9. Off-peak camera. An anterior view from a liver and spleen scan (*left*) demonstrates a mottled appearance of the liver, suggesting metastatic tumor. The patient was transferred to another camera in the department, and a subsequent image (*right*) demonstrates a much more homogeneous appearance.

TABLE 3–1.   Quality Control Parameters for Gamma Cameras

PERFORMANCE PARAMETERS	QUALITY CONTROL PROTOCOL	FREQUENCY*
Spatial resolution	Resolution phantom (quadrant bar phantom, rotate 90 degrees between acquisitions)	Weekly
Uniformity	Intrinsic or extrinsic flood evaluated qualitatively	Daily (before first patient)
Image linearity	Subjective evaluation from bar phantom resolution test	Weekly
Energy resolution	Full width at half-maximum of technetium-99m photopeak expressed as percentage	Annually
Count rate response	20% data loss, resolving time, maximum count rate for 20% window	Annually
Sensitivity	Count rate per microcurie through all collimators with 20% window; calculate absolute sensitivity for available collimators	Annually
Collimator integrity	10 million count floods through each collimator for evaluation of collimator defects	Annually or when suspicious of damage
Formatter performance	Flood images at all locations and for all image sizes	Annually
Whole-body accessory	Scan bar phantom along diagonal, and compare with stationary image; calibrate speed	Annually
Window setting	Confirm energy window for specific radionuclide used	For each patient
ADDITIONAL QUALITY ASSURANCE NECESSARY FOR SPECT GAMMA CAMERAS		
Center of rotation	Point or line source	1–2 wk
High count uniformity	30–120 million count floods	1–2 wk
Head tilt angle	Bubble level	Quarterly
System performance	SPECT phantom	Quarterly
	Cylindrical phantom	Monthly
Spatial resolution	Point source reconstructed	Quarterly

*The frequency may be shorter if problems have been encountered recently.
SPECT, single-photon emission computed tomography.

To correct system nonuniformity, a superior uniformity correction is needed. This is attained by the weekly acquisition and computer storage of a high-count reference flood-field image performed with the collimator in place for uniformity correction of each planar view acquired before reconstruction. Typically, 30 million counts for a 64×64 matrix and 120 million counts for a 128×128 matrix are required. The flood field must be performed under conditions and acquisition parameters (e.g., collimators, matrix size, radioisotope) specific for the examination to which it will be applied. Thus, separate flood fields must be acquired for each set of parameters. Cobalt-57 plastic sheet sources, with their high intrinsic uniformity and ease of use, are best used for this activity. Technetium-99m flood tanks can also be used but must be thoroughly mixed. Although high flood-field uniformity correction rectifies inhomogeneity caused by most sources in the imaging chain, it should not be viewed as a substitute for correction of faulty detector electronics or collimators, or for adequate camera service and maintenance.

Center of Rotation Determination and Correction

The center of rotation (COR) of the imaging system is superficially determined by the mechanical construction of the camera and gantry, as well as by the electronics of the system. Thus, the apparent COR may be affected by mechanical aberrations in the detector or gantry alignment, electronic instabilities in the detector system, or nonlinearities between the camera–computer coupling analog-to-digital converter (ADC). In fact, the apparent COR as perceived by the computer may differ from the actual mechanical COR because of conditions affecting the system electronics. Thus, it is necessary to align the electronic center (center of computer matrix) with the mechanical COR (camera COR) properly to prevent COR misalignment artifacts. Any significant misalignment (>0.5 pixel for a 64×64 matrix) results in increasing losses of contrast and resolution in the reconstructed images, and often gross image distortion (Fig. 3–10). The maximum acceptable uncorrected error in the COR is 0.5 pixel.

Evaluation of the COR of the system is a relatively simple procedure, typically consisting of placing a ^{99m}Tc or ^{57}Co point or line source near the COR of the camera and performing a SPECT scan of the source. With a small COR misalignment, the point source appears blurred; but with a large misalignment, it has a doughnut appearance. Most commercial SPECT systems have software programs capable of calculating the apparent COR and any offset from the computer matrix center and storing these data for later COR correction as needed in clinical acquisitions. If a misalignment is found, a correction can be made by the computer software to realign the rotation and matrix centers by shifting the rotational axis of the camera to the center of the computer matrix.

COR calibration must be performed for each collimator, zoom factor, and usually matrix size used for clinical imaging. Furthermore, COR calibration factors based on ^{99m}Tc may be valid only for other radionuclides if energy registration circuits have been properly calibrated. With a newly installed camera, COR calibration should probably

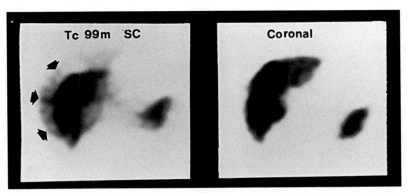

FIGURE 3–10. Center of rotation artifact demonstrated on a coronal sulfur colloid liver-spleen scan. *Left,* Image obtained with a 1-pixel center-of-rotation misalignment, resulting in blurring and halo artifact. *Right,* With correction, the image is markedly improved.

be performed frequently (perhaps daily) until system stability is established and then every 1 to 2 weeks. Frequent fluctuations in COR values suggest a problem requiring professional servicing of the instrument.

X- and Y-Gain (Pixel Size) Calibration

The gains in the x and y directions must be matched so that each pixel has the same size in both dimensions. Dimensional discrepancies may produce inaccurate reconstructions in standard and oblique planes, erroneous attenuation correction, and even shifts in the perceived COR. Usually, calibration software is provided by the system vendor. However, x and y pixel dimensions may be calculated by imaging two- or three-point or line sources of ^{99m}Tc separated by a known distance. X- and y-gain calibration should be performed every 6 months or after repair involving components that could change pixel size.

Detector Head Alignment with the Axis of Rotation

To produce accurate back-projected images without loss of resolution or contrast, the planar images must be acquired in planes perpendicular to the AOR of the camera. This requires the camera face to be level and untilted from the AOR. A 1% tilt at a distance of 14 cm produces a shift of about 1 pixel in a 64 × 64 matrix. Head tilt may be assessed by using the camera and computer to collect a set of 36-point source images over 360 degrees and adding selected frames together. If no tilt is present, the images describe a straight line parallel with the x-axis.

Alternatively, a simple check independent of system electronics may be performed by using a carpenter's (bubble) level to evaluate camera face position at the 12-o'clock and 6-o'clock positions on the gantry. The latter test presumes that the crystal face, detector housing, and AOR are all parallel with the earth's surface in the above positions. Camera head tilt should be assessed quarterly and corrections made as necessary.

Collimator Evaluation

For optimum image production, the collimator should be as close to the manufacturer's specifications as possible and free of obvious defects. Damaged collimator septa may introduce significant field nonuniformity, which can degrade image quality. Various methods have been described to evaluate collimator integrity and may be used when a serious problem is suspected. Routinely, collimator inspection should be performed through the actual visual examination of the collimator and inspection of high-count extrinsic flood images. Defective collimators should be replaced.

System Performance

Overall system performance under different acquisition parameters can be assessed by using a variety of commercially available ^{99m}Tc-filled phantoms, including the Jaszczak or Carlson phantoms. These are best used according to the manufacturer's protocols but usually are performed monthly. Parameters evaluated may include object contrast and image noise, field uniformity, and accuracy of attenuation correction. Each view should contain at least 200,000 counts in a 64 × 64 or 128 × 128 matrix. The angular sampling (number of views) should match the matrix size. System evaluation using phantoms can be repeated and compared with previous acquisitions to check system performance over time and after hardware or software upgrades or major repairs. The same radius of rotation, filter, and cutoff frequency should be used each time.

RADIOPHARMACY QUALITY CONTROL

Quality control in radiopharmaceutical preparation is important to protect the patient and to ensure that the radiopharmaceutical localizes in the intended area. As with any parenteral substance, radiopharmaceuticals must be sterile and free of pyrogens and chemical, radiochemical, or radionuclide impurities.

Regulations or recommendations for radiopharmaceutical quality control have been published by at least two groups: the NRC and the U.S. Pharmacopeia (USP). The USP regulations are important only if a true dedicated pharmacy is being operated, not if a nuclear medicine physician is labeling cold kits for injection in the laboratory. The NRC regulations, on the other hand, must be strictly adhered to because they are a provision of licensing.

The quality control of radiopharmaceuticals throughout the preparation process is primarily performed on ^{99m}Tc radiopharmaceuticals. The other radionuclides used (and, increasingly, many ^{99m}Tc radiopharmaceuticals) are commonly obtained directly from the manufacturer or from a centralized radiopharmacy, and typically, the only quality controls performed in the department are dose calibration and photopeak analysis at the time of imaging.

Generator and Radionuclide Purity

The first step in quality control is to ensure that the radionuclide is pure. This is expressed as the percentage of activity present that is due to the radionuclide of interest. Because ^{99m}Tc normally is obtained by "milking" a molybdenum generator, there must be assurance that only ^{99m}Tc is eluted. Most ^{99}Mo-^{99m}Tc generators are fission produced, and radionuclide impurities such as ^{99}Mo, iodine-131 (^{131}I), and ruthenium-103 (^{103}Ru) may be present. The amount of ^{99}Mo contamination, or breakthrough, during elution is normally determined by placing the eluate from the generator in a lead shield and measuring the penetration of any ^{99}Mo (740- and 780-keV) photons. The presence of other radionuclides may be determined by multichannel analysis or by counting of the eluate at different times to allow for decay. The latter method indicates whether the half-life of the contaminant is or is not consistent with that of ^{99}Mo.

The NRC and USP regulations allow no more than 0.15 µCi (0.005 MBq) of ^{99}Mo per 1 mCi (37 MBq) of ^{99m}Tc at the time of administration. Because ^{99m}Tc decays much faster than ^{99}Mo, the relative amount of any molybdenum contaminant rises with time. Thus, if the ^{99}Mo in an eluate from a generator was barely acceptable at 8 AM, it will likely become unacceptable later the same day.

The elution column inside the generator is made of alumina (Al_2O_3). If, during elution, sufficient alumina breaks through, the eluate may become cloudy. The presence of aluminum ion (Al^{3+}) should be ascertained at the time of eluting ^{99m}Tc from the generator. Small amounts of aluminum ion may be detected with an indicator paper similar to the pH paper used in chemistry. If aluminum ion is present, a red color develops. The maximum permissible amount of aluminum ion is 10 µg/mL of ^{99m}Tc eluate with a fission generator. If too much aluminum is present, technetium–aluminum particles form, which are manifested clinically by hepatic uptake. Excessive aluminum ion may also cause aggregation of sulfur colloid preparations, resulting in lung uptake (Fig. 3–11). The purpose of ethylenediaminetetra-acetic acid (EDTA) in sulfur colloid kits is to bind excess Al^{3+} and thus to prevent such problems. Agglutination of red blood cells may also occur when inordinate amounts of alu-

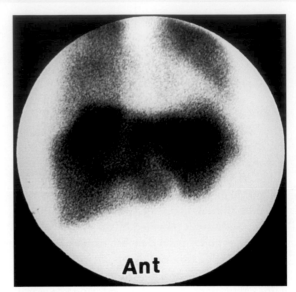

FIGURE 3–11. Excessive aluminum levels in preparation. A liver and spleen scan demonstrates activity above the liver and both lungs owing to aggregation of the sulfur colloid, causing larger particles.

minum ion are contained in ^{99m}Tc pertechnetate solutions.

Radiochemical Labeling

Once radionuclide purity is ensured, a prepackaged kit containing an unlabeled pharmaceutical may be used to produce a radiochemical compound. The biodistribution of that radiochemical in a patient can then easily be visualized with a gamma camera system. Assessment of chemical purity of ^{99m}Tc radiopharmaceuticals is performed by determining the degree of successful tagging of the agent contained in the kit and the amount of residual (unbound ^{99m}Tc) in the preparation. The degree of purity may reflect the proficiency of those who prepare the kits or simply any lot-to-lot or manufacturer-to-manufacturer variability in the kits.

Instant thin-layer chromatography is usually performed to assess radiochemical purity, using silica gel impregnated in glass fiber sheets or strips. By using various solvents, impurities can be identified by their different migrations in the particular solvent used.

A drop of the radiochemical compound to be analyzed is placed on the strip, and the solvent is applied. As the solvent approaches the end of the sheet, an assessment is made of the radioactivity present at the point of origin and at the advancing solvent front. Although this may be performed by various scanning methods, the simplest way is to cut the fiber strip into segments and count them individually in a well counter. If this is done, the technician must be extremely careful to put only a very small amount of activity at the spot of origin because well counters are efficient and it is easy to exceed their count rate capability.

The most common ^{99m}Tc radiopharmaceuticals are prepared by adding ^{99m}Tc freshly eluted from a generator to a cold kit as prescribed by the kit manufacturer. The eluate of the generator should be ^{99m}TcO$_4^-$(+7) (i.e., pertechnetate). Because pertechnetate in this valence state is relatively stable, it cannot tag a cold kit preparation and must be reduced to a lower valence state (+3, +4, +5). This is done by using a reducing agent such as stannous chloride, which is generally present in the reaction vial.

Most radiochemical impurities obtained in kit preparation are the result of interaction of either oxygen or water with the contents of the kit or vial. If air reaches the vial contents, stannous chloride may be oxidized to stannic chloride even before introduction of ^{99m}Tc into the vial. If this happens, production of reactive technetium is no longer possible, and free pertechnetate becomes an impurity. If moisture reaches the vial contents, stannous chloride becomes hydrolyzed, and the formation of stannous hydroxide, a colloid, results.

Reactive reduced technetium may also become hydrolyzed, forming technetium dioxide. This hydrolyzed reduced form of technetium is insoluble and is another impurity that must be tested. Technetium that has been tagged to a compound can reoxidize and revert to pertechnetate.

To minimize oxidation problems, most cold kits are purged with nitrogen, and additional antioxidants, such as ascorbic acid, may also have been added. It is still extremely important not to inject air into the reaction vial when preparing a radiopharmaceutical. An often overlooked source of problems is the sterile saline used in preparation of the kits. This saline should be free of preservatives because bacteriostatic agents often interfere with the tagging process.

To check for the presence of free pertechnetate, the radiopharmaceutical is placed on the chromatographic strip, and acetone is used as the solvent. Most tagged radiopharmaceuticals remain at the origin, whereas the free pertechnetate advances with the solvent front (Fig. 3–12). To assess the presence of hydrolyzed technetium or technetium dioxide, saline is used as the solvent. In

this case, technetium dioxide remains at the origin, whereas those radiopharmaceuticals that are soluble in saline, such as diethylenetriaminepentaacetic acid (DTPA) and pertechnetate, advance with the solvent front. For some compounds that are insoluble in saline, such as macroaggregated albumin, it is not possible to assess the presence of technetium dioxide by using instant thin-layer chromatography.

USP regulations define the lower limits of acceptability for radiochemical purity as 95% for pertechnetate, 92% for ^{99m}Tc sulfur colloid, and 90% for all other ^{99m}Tc radiopharmaceuticals. Once the chromatographic procedures are established, they take little time to perform and ideally should be done before patient injection.

One reason for performing thin-layer chromatography before patient injection is that simple errors can cause the radiolabeling to be completely ineffective. For example, in production of sulfur colloid, one kit normally calls first for injection of syringe A and then for injection of syringe B into the reaction vial. If these two injections are reversed, no sulfur colloid is produced, and there is a large amount of free ^{99m}Tc pertechnetate. Thus, a liver scan is not possible with the agent. Free ^{99m}Tc pertechnetate is seen as unexpected activity in both the thyroid and stomach (Fig. 3–13).

The ^{99m}Tc radiopharmaceuticals that are produced with stannous chloride reduction or stannous chelates include macroaggregated albumin, phosphate compounds, and glucoheptonate. The only one in common use that is produced without reduction or chelation by tin is sulfur colloid. The compounds in which the presence of hydrolyzed technetium (Tc dioxide) may need to be checked are DTPA, phosphate compounds, glucoheptonate, and iminodiacetic acid (IDA) derivatives.

Excessive stannous agents can cause quality control problems during radiopharmaceutical preparation that become evident in the actual clinical images. Excess stannous ions (tin) may cause liver uptake on bone scans by formation of a tin colloid (Fig. 3–14). Residual stannous ions in the blood may also cause red blood cell labeling. Stannous ions may remain in the blood after a bone scan, so that a ^{99m}Tc pertechnetate thyroid or Meckel's diverticulum scan attempted within 1 week may result in red blood cell labeling.

Particle size of certain compounds may be checked by a hemocytometer as part of the quality control procedure. The USP maximum diameter recommendation for macroaggregated albumin

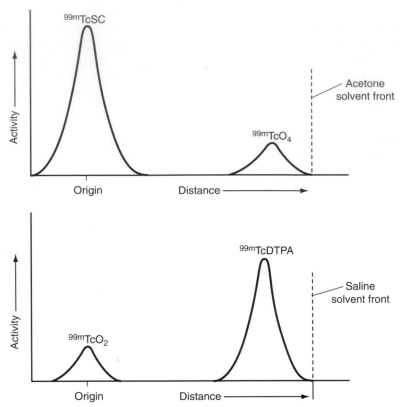

FIGURE 3–12. *Top,* **Acetone chromatography is used to check for the presence of free pertechnetate, which migrates with the acetone solvent front.** *Bottom,* To check for technetium dioxide, saline is used; those radiopharmaceuticals that are soluble in saline advance with the solvent.

is 150 μm, with 90% of particles between 10 and 90 μm. Most physicians prefer particles less than 100 μm in size for pulmonary perfusion imaging. Slightly large particle size in preparations of ^{99m}Tc sulfur colloid results in relatively more uptake in the spleen and may give a false impression of hepatocellular dysfunction.

Sterility

Most compounds provided in kits are sterile and pyrogen-free. USP regulations call for microbiologic testing, including growth on a culture media for 14 days. This is clearly a problem for ^{99m}Tc compounds with a 6-hour half-life and is generally not performed. Pyrogen testing according to USP recommendations includes intravenous injection of three rabbits, after which any rise in body temperature during the next 3 hours is noted. This is clearly impractical for most nuclear medicine laboratories, and thus pyrogen testing is usually limited to the evaluation of Gram-negative endotoxins in

compounds that are being injected in the central nervous system or cerebral spinal fluid. Gram-negative endotoxins may be conveniently and quickly evaluated by the limulus amebocyte lysate test. This material is derived from the horseshoe crab; in the presence of an extremely small amount of a Gram-negative endotoxin, an opaque gel is formed.

ARTIFACTS

Areas of Decreased Activity

There are really no problems in radiopharmaceutical preparation or administration that lead to a focal area of decreased activity. If there is something between the radiopharmaceutical and the gamma camera that causes attenuation of the photons, however, this appears as an area of focal photopenia. The key to recognition of these artifacts is that they do not persist in the same location with respect to the organ on differing or orthogo-

PEARLS & PITFALLS—cont'd

Poor spatial resolution can result from an insufficient amount of injected activity (inadequate counts), use of a high-energy or a particularly low-energy radionuclide, poor background clearance of the radiopharmaceutical, a patient too distant from the detector face, or an off-peak energy window.

For SPECT cameras, uniformity and COR checks are done weekly, and gantry and table alignment is checked quarterly.

Ring artifacts on SPECT images are usually produced by flood-field inhomogeneity.

COR artifacts usually cause cold defects and blurring. When extreme, ring artifacts may be caused.

Negative defects caused by COR artifacts on SPECT images may have a tail of activity extending peripherally.

Molybdenum breakthrough in a generator eluate is detected by the penetration of 740- and 780-keV photons through a lead shield that attenuates the 140-keV photons of technetium.

Aluminum ion breakthrough in the eluate from a ^{99}Mo-^{99m}Tc generator is detected by using a special test paper that changes color. Excessive aluminum indicates lack of stability of the generator column.

Radionuclide purity of a sample is performed by examining the energy of the photons emitted and comparing it to those expected for a given radionuclide.

Radiochemical purity related to radiopharmaceutical labeling is tested by using thin-layer chromatography with either acetone or saline as the solvent. Usually, 95% tagging is required.

Free ^{99m}Tc pertechnetate is usually seen as unexpected activity in the stomach, thyroid, and salivary glands.

only common instrumentation or computer problem that causes apparent increased activity in an organ or in the body as a whole is an improper high-intensity setting of the cathode ray tube.

SUGGESTED READINGS

Freeman LM, Blaufox MD: Pitfalls and artifacts in radionuclide imaging. Semin Nucl Med 26:75–76, 1996.

Saha GP: Fundamentals of Nuclear Pharmacy, 3rd ed. New York, Springer-Verlag, 1992.

Cerebrovascular System

4

RADIONUCLIDE BRAIN IMAGING
  Planar Brain Imaging
  SPECT Brain Perfusion Imaging

CEREBROSPINAL FLUID IMAGING
  Radiopharmaceuticals and Technique
  Normal Examination
  Clinical Applications

RADIONUCLIDE BRAIN IMAGING

Nuclear medicine imaging of the central nervous system has been largely eclipsed by the widespread availability of computed tomography (CT) and magnetic resonance imaging (MRI). In certain clinical settings, however, radionuclide planar, single-photon emission computed tomography (SPECT) or positron emission tomography (PET) brain imaging can provide valuable functional and perfusion information about suspected cerebral abnormalities or cerebrospinal fluid (CSF) dynamics that is not obtained through anatomic imaging. For this reason, an understanding of the techniques and principles involved in radionuclide brain imaging remains important.

In the normal cerebrum, passage of most substances from the cerebral capillaries into the extravascular space is severely restricted, constituting what has been referred to as the *blood-brain barrier*. The degree of permeability of this barrier varies with the nature of the material attempting to pass and with the numerous complex carrier mechanisms used to facilitate or hinder passage through the cell membranes involved.

The most common nuclear medicine imaging procedures of the brain can be divided into three different approaches relative to this principle:

Planar brain imaging, which uses radiopharmaceuticals that are perfusion agents. Planar imaging is usually only performed for brain death studies.
SPECT brain perfusion imaging, which uses lipophilic radiopharmaceuticals that routinely cross the blood-brain barrier to localize in normal brain tissue and pathologic processes in proportion to cerebral blood flow. This is the most commonly used radionuclide brain imaging technique.
PET metabolic brain imaging, which uses functional positron-emitting radiopharmaceuticals, such as radiolabeled fluorodeoxyglucose (a glucose analog) and neuroreceptor agents. PET glucose techniques are available in clinical practice. They are discussed in Chapter 13.

Planar Brain Imaging

Technique

Planar radionuclide cerebral imaging generally consists of two phases: (1) a dynamic or angiographic study composed of rapid sequential images of the arrival of the radioactive bolus in the cerebral hemispheres, which essentially constitutes a qualitative measure of regional brain perfusion; and (2) delayed static images, which provide a record of the distribution of the radiopharmaceutical in the sagittal sinus and cerebral regions, including any abnormal concentrations or absences.

The radionuclide angiogram is routinely performed in the anterior position. After a rapid bolus intravenous injection of 15 to 20 mCi (555 to 740 MBq) of a ^{99m}Tc-labeled brain imaging agent, sequential 2- to 3-second images are obtained for 30 to 60 seconds. Imaging is usually begun when the radiopharmaceutical first appears in the proximal carotid arteries. Static images routinely consist of 500,000-count views obtained after a delay of 15–60 minutes, depending on the radiopharmaceutical used, in the anterior, posterior, and right and left lateral positions as needed to determine any intracerebral activity and its distribution.

The most common application of planar technique is in the setting of suspected brain death. A sample protocol giving details of the technique and associated radiation doses are given in Appendix E–1.

Normal Planar Brain Scan

Most brain scans are performed with either a transient perfusion agent (technetium-99m [^{99m}Tc]–diethylenetriaminepenta acetic acid [DTPA], ^{99m}Tc-pertechnetate) or a perfusion agent that is extracted by the brain on the first pass (^{99m}Tc–hexamethylpropyleneamine oxime [HMPAO], ^{99m}Tc–ethylene L-cysteinate dimer [ECD]). Normally, on the angiographic images performed with either type of agent, there is

prompt symmetric perfusion that in the anterior projection looks similar to a trident. The middle cerebral arteries are seen to the right and left, and the anterior cerebral arteries are seen as a single midline vertical line of activity. Perfusion should extend to the calvarial convexities bilaterally (Fig. 4–1). Although symmetry is the hallmark of the arterial-capillary phase of a normal perfusion scan, asymmetry in the venous phase is common because of variations in venous anatomy. Care should be taken not to overinterpret lack of symmetry in the venous phase in the absence of an arterial abnormality.

On the static images of a ^{99m}Tc-DTPA or ^{99m}Tc-pertechnetate scan, radioactivity does not normally lie within the brain itself because of the integrity of the blood-brain barrier, but rather is located in the overlying scalp soft tissues, calvarium, and sub-arachnoid spaces that outline the cerebral hemi-

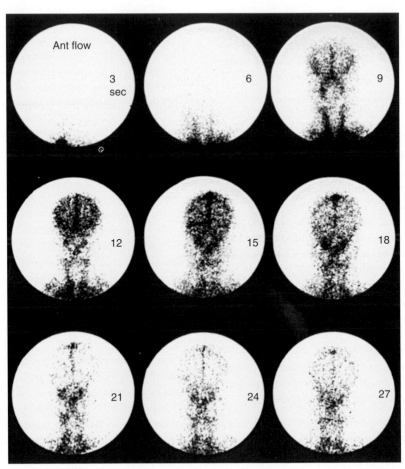

FIGURE 4–1. Normal anterior radionuclide angiogram (^{99m}Tc DTPA). The anterior and middle cerebral arteries are clearly visualized on the 9-second frame. The sagittal sinus is easily seen by 15 seconds.

spheres. Activity is also seen in the larger blood pool accumulations, such as the sagittal and transverse sinuses. Thus, the normal static brain images include a number of consistent landmarks (Fig. 4–2). On the posterior view, the transverse sinuses are generally symmetric, although it is not uncommon for the right sinus to be dominant. On the lateral views, activity in the suprasellar and sylvian regions is noted, although it is less constant and less well defined than activity in the venous sinuses. Occasionally, activity in the soft tissues of the ears may be identified, overlapping or just anterior to the sigmoid sinus region. When ^{99m}Tc-pertechnetate is used, the choroid plexus of the lateral ventricles will be normally visualized.

If the integrity of the blood-brain barrier is compromised for any reason (e.g., cerebrovascular accident, tumor, abscess, herpes encephalitis), the delayed static images usually show increased activity in the area of the abnormality. In contrast to ^{99m}Tc-DTPA or ^{99m}Tc-pertechnetate imaging, normal static planar images obtained with a first-pass extraction perfusion agent (^{99m}Tc-HMPAO, ^{99m}Tc-ECD) will demonstrate activity in the brain substance (primarily gray matter) (Fig. 4–3).

Brain Death

The radionuclide angiogram is a simple, noninvasive method of determining the presence or absence of intracerebral perfusion and thereby of confirming a clinical diagnosis of brain death. The radiopharmaceuticals most widely used for radionuclide cerebral angiography are the usual planar brain imaging agents, ^{99m}Tc-pertechnetate and ^{99m}Tc-DTPA. Sometimes, in difficult cases, the cerebral brain perfusion imaging agents ^{99m}Tc-HMPAO or ^{99m}Tc-ECD, which normally localize in

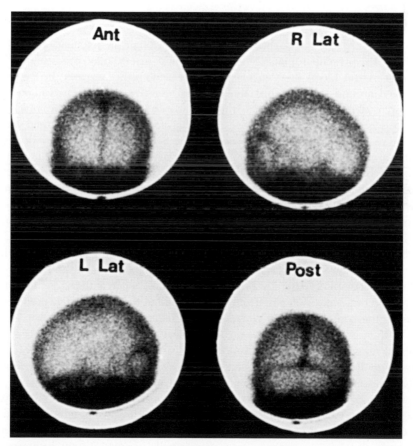

FIGURE 4–2. Normal planar static brain scan (^{99m}Tc-DTPA). A large amount of activity is normally seen in the face and base of the skull. The sagittal and transverse sinuses are normally prominent.

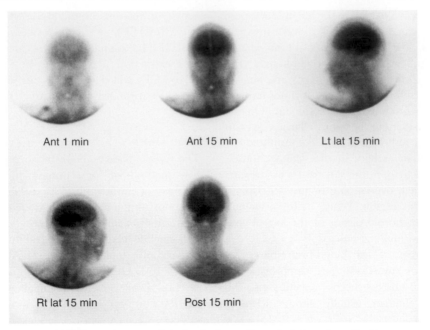

Ant 1 min   Ant 15 min   Lt lat 15 min

Rt lat 15 min   Post 15 min

FIGURE 4–3. Planar images of the brain done after administration of a first-pass extraction agent (^{99m}Tc HMPAO). The images show activity primarily in the gray matter.

perfused brain tissue, are used with planar or SPECT scanning. To prevent mistaking scalp perfusion for intracerebral blood flow, an elastic band can be placed around the head just above the orbits. This may diminish blood flow to the superficial scalp vessels.

In the presence of cerebral death, the injected activity typically proceeds through the carotid artery to the base of the skull, where the radioactive bolus stops, owing to increased intracranial pressure (Fig. 4–4). As with all radionuclide arteriograms, injection of a good bolus is important. If distinct activity in the common carotid artery is not identified, the injection should be repeated. The absence of intracerebral flow is strong corroborative evidence of cerebral demise. Generally, a single anterior or lateral cerebral view is obtained within 5 to 10 minutes of the completion of the angiographic portion of the study to determine the presence of any sagittal sinus activity. The significance of such activity without an obvious arterial phase is somewhat controversial, but it may represent a small amount of intracerebral flow. Most of these patients have a grave prognosis. The presence of slight dural sinus activity does not contradict the diagnosis of brain death.

When intracranial carotid blood flow ceases in the setting of brain death, increased or collateral flow through the maxillary branch of the external carotid artery may produce markedly increased perfusion projecting over the nasal area in the anterior view, as seen on the radionuclide angiogram and subsequently on static images. This so-called "hot-nose" sign cannot be used specifically to indicate brain death, but it may be used as a secondary sign when intracerebral perfusion is absent. This sign may also occur with a generalized decrease of cerebral perfusion from various causes, including severe cerebrovascular or carotid occlusive disease or increased intracranial pressure of any cause.

Radionuclide techniques are independent of interfering conditions and do not require withdrawal of medical therapy. They may be especially helpful in the settings of hypothermia; intoxication with fentanyl, barbiturates, or pancuronium; hypovolemic shock; when electroencephalogram recording is not possible because of significant head injury; or in instances in which clinical examination is inconclusive.

If clinical evaluation of the patient suggests brain death and no cerebral perfusion is demonstrated on the radionuclide study, brain death is virtually certain. Although an actual diagnosis of brain death should not be made by using nuclear imaging techniques alone, these techniques are

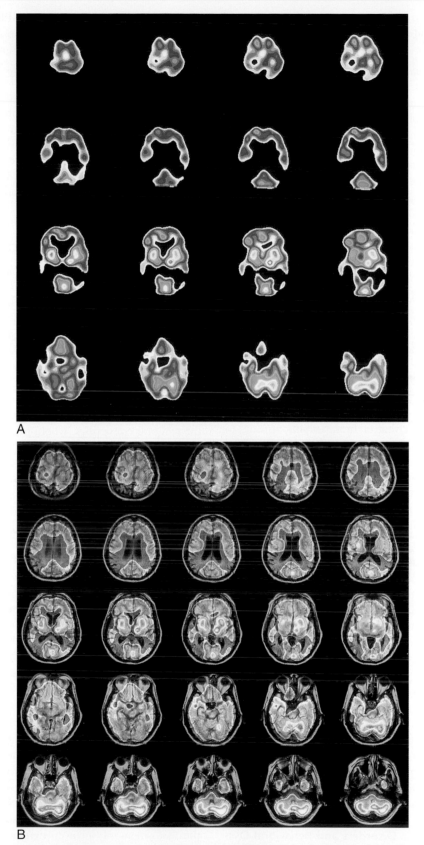

FIGURE 4–11. Alzheimer's disease. Multiple transaxial SPECT HMPAO images (*A*) demonstrate decreased perfusion in both temporal parietal regions. Fusion images of the SPECT and MRI scans (*B*) help with anatomic localization of the abnormalities.

schizophrenia, depression, progressive supranuclear palsy, and Pick's disease.

Acquired Immunodeficiency Syndrome Dementia Complex. Up to half of patients with acquired immunodeficiency syndrome (AIDS) demonstrate neurologic involvement. The study may be useful in distinguishing subtle AIDS dementia complex from depression, psychosis, or focal neurologic disease. Because these findings may occur even in the presence of normal CT and MRI scans, SPECT imaging may constitute the only objective evidence of AIDS dementia complex. The SPECT perfusion pattern is that of multifocal or patchy cortical and subcortical hypoperfusion deficits. Lesions are most frequent in the frontal, temporal, and parietal lobes and basal ganglia. These perfusion abnormalities may resolve with therapy, and SPECT may provide a role in monitoring improvement. Because the brain perfusion patterns seen in AIDS dementia complex may also be seen in chronic cocaine or multidrug users, interpretation in this setting should be made with caution.

Head Trauma. Although SPECT brain perfusion imaging in the setting of brain trauma appears to be more sensitive and able to detect abnormalities earlier than can CT, its clinical utility is less clear. The size and number of perfusion abnormalities may have prognostic value in predicting the amount of permanent damage and may suggest patients who will develop post-traumatic headache.

Substance Abuse. Both acute and chronic cocaine use result in alterations in cerebral blood flow. Chronic cocaine use frequently presents as multifocal alterations in rCBF without underlying structural damage on CT or MRI scans. On SPECT perfusion imaging, typical findings include multiple perfusion defects of small and moderate size in the cerebral cortex (especially the frontal lobes), diminished blood flow to the basal ganglia, and generalized reduction in cerebral blood flow. The findings may occur in asymptomatic patients and may be partially reversible with abstinence or opioid antagonist (buprenorphine) therapy. The SPECT imaging patterns are not specific and are often indistinguishable from those of early AIDS-related dementia.

Neuropsychiatric Disorders and Behavioral Dysfunction. Various neuropsychiatric disorders have been evaluated by using PET and SPECT imaging, but clearcut diagnostic or prognostic functional abnormalities have not been consistently described, and the clinical utility of such imaging techniques in this setting remains uncertain. There are a few studies of children with attention-deficit hyperactivity disorder (ADHD) that show increased perfusion in the motor, premotor, and anterior cingulate cortex when the children were withdrawn from their medication, methylphenidate, and effective treatment with methylphenidate was associated with increases in perfusion in the prefrontal cortex and caudate nucleus.

CEREBROSPINAL FLUID IMAGING

About 400 to 500 mL/day of CSF is formed in the normal adult, largely in the choroid plexus of the cerebral ventricular system. CSF is essentially an ultrafiltrate of plasma with an actively secreted component added by the choroid plexus. The total CSF volume ranges between 120 and 150 mL, of which about 40 mL are contained within the ventricular system. After exiting the ventricles by way of the fourth ventricular foramina, the CSF flows cephalad through the subarachnoid spaces to the cerebral convexities, where primary resorption occurs in the arachnoid villi. Absorption also occurs across the meninges of both the brain and the spinal cord as well as through the ependymal lining of the ventricular system. These latter pathways are probably of great importance in pathologic states in which there is blockage of normal absorption through the arachnoid villi.

The principle involved in imaging the CSF consists of intrathecal administration of a substance that is miscible with and diffusible in the CSF and that remains in the CSF compartment until it is absorbed through the normal pathways. Any such substance must be nontoxic and nonpyrogenic. Strict pyrogen testing of all intrathecally administered agents should be routinely performed.

Radiopharmaceuticals and Technique

The most widely used agent for studies of CSF dynamics is indium-111 (^{111}In)–labeled DTPA, with a physical half-life of 2.8 days. The short (6-hour) half-life of ^{99m}Tc-labeled agents, principally ^{99m}Tc-DTPA, renders them of limited use in studies of CSF dynamics, which may take several days to complete. They are commonly used, however, in the assessment of intraventricular shunt patency and cisternography in children, who normally demonstrate more rapid CSF flow dynamics than do adults.

The administration of 500 μCi (18.5 MBq) of ^{111}In DTPA is accomplished by lumbar puncture with a small-bore (22-gauge) needle into the subarachnoid space. To minimize leakage from the puncture site, it is wise to postpone such procedures for about 1 week after the most recent diagnostic lumbar puncture.

Initial posterior images over the thoracolumbar spine may be obtained at 2 to 4 hours to discern the success of injection. For evaluation of CSF dynamics, anterior, posterior, and lateral gamma camera images of the head are obtained at 6, 24, and 48 hours and at 72 hours or longer, if necessary. For CSF leaks, early imaging at 1–24 hours is preferred in projections that are most likely to demonstrate the site of the leak and/or position that provokes or encourages flow at the leakage site.

For CSF shunt patency studies, 1–3 mCi (37–111 MBq) of ^{99m}Tc-DTPA or 500 μCi (18.5 MBq)

of ^{111}In DTPA may be injected into the shunt reservoir or tubing.

A sample technical protocol is presented in Appendix E–1.

Normal Examination

After injection of approximately 500 μCi (18.5 MBq) of ^{111}In-DTPA into the lumbar subarachnoid space, the activity ascends in the spinal canal and reaches the basal cisterns at 2 to 4 hours in adults (Fig. 4–12). Subsequent images obtained during the next 24 hours demonstrate ascent of the radiopharmaceutical through the intracranial subarachnoid spaces, with identification of activity in the sylvian and interhemispheric cisterns. At 24 hours, there should be complete ascent of the radiopharmaceutical, which consists of distribution of the activity over the cerebral convexities and the parasagittal region, with relative clearance from the basilar cisterns.

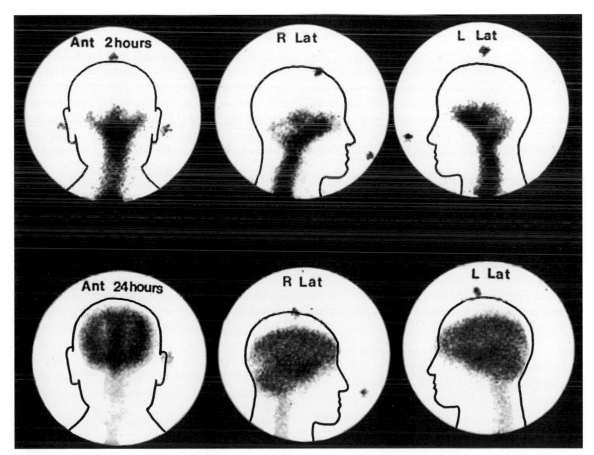

FIGURE 4–12. Normal cisternogram. The images obtained at 2 hours demonstrate activity in the basal cisterns as well as some activity in the sylvian and interhemispheric cisterns. The images obtained at 24 hours demonstrate that there has been normal ascent of activity over the convexities.

The presence of radioactivity in the lateral ventricles at any point in the examination should be viewed as abnormal. However, transient entry noted at 4 hours and disappearing by 24 hours is of questionable pathologic significance and is considered by some to be a normal variant flow pattern. Failure of the radionuclide to achieve complete ascent over the cerebral convexities or activity in the ventricles at 24 hours is an indication for further evaluation at 48 hours and/or 72 hours.

Clinical Applications

The major indications for radionuclide imaging of the CSF are the following:

- Investigation of suspected communicating hydrocephalus (normal-pressure hydrocephalus)
- Evaluation of suspected CSF leaks
- Verification of diversionary CSF shunt patency

Communicating Hydrocephalus

Normal-pressure hydrocephalus characteristically presents as a clinical triad of ataxia, dementia, and urinary incontinence. By definition, hydrocephalus without significant atrophy is noted on CT scans, with a normal CSF pressure determination. If the diagnosis of normal-pressure hydrocephalus can be established, CSF shunting from the ventricular system may provide prompt relief of symptoms in selected patients. CSF imaging may provide corroborative evidence of the diagnosis and aid in selecting patients most likely to benefit from shunt therapy.

Hydrocephalus with normal lumbar pressures often presents a problem of differentiation between cerebral atrophy and normal-pressure hydrocephalus. CT or MRI studies can generally provide the answer. In some patients with mild degrees of atrophy and dilated ventricles, radionuclide CSF imaging provides additional differential information. The classic pattern of scintigraphic findings in normal-pressure hydrocephalus (Fig. 4–13) consists of the following:

Early entry of the radiopharmaceutical into the lateral ventricles at 4 to 6 hours

Persistence of lateral ventricular activity at 24, 48, and even 72 hours

Considerable delay in the ascent to the parasagittal region, with or without delayed clearance of activity from the basilar cisterns

In general, patients who demonstrate these characteristic findings are among those most likely to benefit from diversionary shunting. Although varying degrees of ventricular entry and persistence, with or without delay in convexity ascent, may be noted, these so-called mixed patterns are of questionable value in establishing a firm diagnosis of normal-pressure hydrocephalus or in predicting therapeutic success.

Noncommunicating Hydrocephalus

Because the radiopharmaceuticals injected into the lumbar space normally do not enter the ventricular system, a radionuclide cisternogram cannot be used to distinguish communicating from noncommunicating hydrocephalus. By injecting the material directly into the lateral ventricles, however, communication between the ventricles and the subarachnoid space can be discerned. This method may rarely be of value in the investigation of enlarged lateral ventricles noted on CT when noncommunicating disease is suspected.

Cerebrospinal Fluid Leaks

Radionuclide cisternography is frequently used to substantiate the presence of a CSF leak from the nose or ear or to localize more precisely the site of a leak. The most common sites of CSF fistulas are in the region of the cribriform plate (Fig. 4–14) and ethmoid sinuses, from the sella turcica into the sphenoid sinus, and from the sphenoid ridge into the ear (Fig. 4–15). Because these leaks are frequently intermittent, the results of the radionuclide cisternogram greatly depend on whether the leak is active at the time of the examination.

The radionuclide evaluation of CSF leaks should consist of (1) imaging the site of the leak and (2) measuring differential activity in pledgets placed deep into each nostril or ear, as appropriate. It is important to image for a CSF leak at the time the radioactivity reaches the suspected site of origin of the leak. Because most of these leaks develop near the basilar cisterns, imaging between 1 and 3 hours is typical. Imaging at half-hour intervals after lumbar puncture may better allow determination of the optimal time to detect a leak. Likewise, if any position or activity is known by the patient to provoke or aggravate the leak of CSF, such should be accomplished immediately before or during imaging.

Pledgets placed before lumbar injection of the radiopharmaceutical are removed 4 to 24 hours after placement and counted in a well counter. Concurrent blood serum samples should be obtained and counted. Sample counts should be expressed in

PEARLS & PITFALLS—cont'd

Herpes encephalitis can be seen as increased activity in the temporal lobe.

Epileptic seizure foci show increased perfusion (^{99m}Tc-HMPAO or ^{99m}Tc-ECD) and metabolism (^{18}FDG) during seizure activity but decreased or normal activity interictally.

A normal radionuclide angiographic examination of the brain presents a trident appearance of intracranial flow in the anterior cerebral and right and left middle cerebral territories. In brain death, there is no obvious arterial phase (the trident is absent) and only scalp activity is seen, which is often accompanied by a hot-nose sign. These studies can also be performed by using ^{99m}Tc-HMPAO or ^{99m}Tc-ECD (SPECT or planar).

A Diamox challenge study evaluates cerebral vascular reserve. It is analogous to use of dipyridamole in myocardial perfusion studies. In areas of vascular disease, regional perfusion worsens after Diamox compared with perfusion without Diamox.

Cerebrospinal Fluid Imaging

Common indications for CSF imaging are for evaluation of a CSF leak or for differentiating normal-pressure hydrocephalus from other causes of hydrocephalus. These studies are done with intrathecal administration of ^{111}In-DTPA.

Most CSF leaks occur in the ear, paranasal sinuses, or nose. Substantial leaks can be imaged by noting asymmetric activity around the region of the ears on the frontal view or activity in the nose on the lateral view. Some leaks are detected only by removing and counting cotton pledgets that were placed in the area of concern.

Cisternography images are usually obtained anteriorly. Six hours after injection, these images normally show a trident appearance of activity produced by labeled CSF in the anterior interhemispheric and right and left sylvian cisterns. Any abnormal entry into the lateral ventricles is seen as heart-shaped activity. Early ventricular entry with stasis, accompanied by lack of activity over the superior surface of the brain after 24 to 48 hours, supports a diagnosis of normal-pressure hydrocephalus.

The classic clinical triad of normal-pressure hydrocephalus includes ataxia, incontinence, and dementia.

SUGGESTED READINGS

Bernard F, Romsa J, Hustinx R: Imaging gliomas with positron emission tomography and single photon emission computed tomography. Semin Nucl Med 33:148–162, 2003.

Bonte FJ, Devous Sr. MD: SPECT Brain imaging. In Sandler MP, Coleman RE, Patton JA, et al. (eds): Diagnostic Nuclear Medicine, 4th ed. New York, Lippincott, Williams and Wilkins, 2003, pp 757–782.

Camargo EE: Brain SPECT in neurology and psychiatry; continuing education. J Nucl Med 42:611–623, 2001.

Catafau A: Brain SPECT in clinical practice, part 1: perfusion, continuing education. J Nucl Med 42:259–271, 2001.

Conrad GR, Sinha P: Scintigraphy as a confirmatory test of brain death. Semin Nucl Med 33: 312–323, 2003.

Henry TR, Van Heertum RL: Positron emission tomography and single photon emission computed tomography in epilepsy care. Semin Nucl Med 33:88–104, 2003.

Lawrence SK, Delbeke D, Partain CL, Sandler MP: Cerebrospinal fluid imaging. In Sandler MP, Coleman RE, Patton JA, et al. (eds). Diagnostic Nuclear Medicine, 4th ed. New York, Lippincott, Williams and Wilkins, 2003, pp 835–850.

Minoshima S, Frey KA, Cross DJ, et al.: Neurochemical imaging of dementias. Semin Nucl Med 34:70–82, 2004.

Norfray JF, Provenzale JM: Alzheimer's disease: neuropathic findings and recent advances in imaging. AJR Am J Roentgenol 182:3–13, 2004.

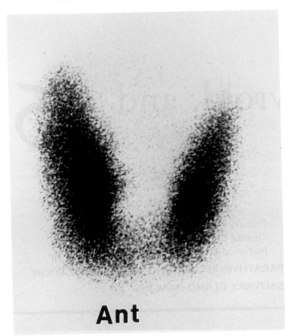

FIGURE 5–1. Normal iodine-123 scan of the thyroid.
The normal bilobed gland with an inferior isthmus is easily
appreciated. Note that no salivary gland activity is seen.

gamma emission of ^{123}I allows excellent imaging
($\approx 80\%$ efficiency for a ½-inch-thick crystal) with low
background activity. It provides considerably lower
doses of radiation to the thyroid with comparable
activity than does ^{131}I. The major disadvantages of
^{123}I are high cost, because it is produced by
cyclotron, and occasional problems with availability and delivery. Despite these restrictions, ^{123}I is the
iodine of choice for thyroid imaging (Fig. 5–1).

Technetium-99m

Technetium-99m pertechnetate is trapped by the
thyroid in the same manner as iodides but is not
organified; therefore, it is released over time as
unaltered pertechnetate (^{99m}TcO$_4^-$) ion. Its short
physical half-life of 6 hours and principal gamma
energy of 140 keV are ideal for gamma camera
imaging (>90% efficiency with a ½-inch-thick
crystal). These physical characteristics and its ready
availability are distinct advantages for thyroid scanning. In addition, the low absorbed dose to the
thyroid permits administration of higher doses and
therefore allows for more rapid imaging of the
gland with minimal motion artifact. Only 1% to
5% of administered ^{99m}Tc-pertechnetate is normally trapped by the thyroid, so image background
levels are higher than those with radioiodine. On a
^{99m}Tc-pertechnetate scan, the salivary glands are

usually well seen in addition to the thyroid. As a
result, unless a patient is hyperthyroid, a ^{99m}Tc scan
can usually be distinguished from an ^{123}I scan by
excellent visualization of the salivary glands (see
Fig. 5–6A). Technetium-99m pertechnetate is preferred over radioiodine when the patient has been
receiving thyroid-blocking agents (such as iodinated
contrast agents) or is unable to take medication
orally or when the study must be completed in less
than 2 hours.

Dosimetry

Radiation doses to the adult thyroid and whole
body for the radioiodines and ^{99m}Tc-pertechnetate
are presented in Appendix E with imaging protocols. With the usual administered activities for
scanning, the radiation to the thyroid gland is
comparable for ^{123}I and ^{99m}Tc, and the whole-
body dose is only slightly greater with ^{99m}Tc. Both
agents provide considerably less radiation dose to
the thyroid and to the total body than does
^{131}I. The dose to the thyroid from ^{131}I is about 100
times greater than that from ^{123}I for the same
administered activity ($\approx$ 1 rad/μCi versus 1 rad/
100 μCi). The absorbed thyroid dose from ^{99m}Tc-
pertechnetate is about 1 rad/5000 μCi.

Because both ^{99m}Tc and the various radioiodines
cross the placenta and because the fetal thyroid
begins accumulation of iodine at about the 12th
week of gestation, care must be taken when
administering these radiopharmaceuticals during
pregnancy. They are also secreted in breast milk
in lactating women and may be transferred to
nursing infants. Nursing can usually be resumed 12
to 24 hours after the administration of ^{99m}Tc-
pertechnetate and about 2 to 3 days after ^{123}I
administration. When ^{131}I is administered in any
form, nursing should be stopped and any pumped
breast milk discarded, because the Nuclear Regulatory Commission (NRC) recommends that
nursing should be discontinued entirely if administered activities of ^{131}I exceed about 1 μCi
(0.04 MBq).

On an administered activity basis, the dose to
the thyroid is significantly greater in infants and
children than in adults, and considerably smaller
scanning and uptake doses should be administered
to pediatric patients (see Appendixes D and E). In
addition, because the radiation dose to the pediatric
thyroid from ^{131}I nears the level shown to increase
the incidence of thyroid carcinoma, ^{131}I is not recommended for scanning children and is essentially
contraindicated for pregnant women.

Many physicians incorrectly assume that radiation dose to the thyroid from ^{131}I can be accurately determined by knowing the administered activity and the thyroid uptake. A complex of less easily determined factors (thyroid size, biologic half-life of iodine in the gland, size of the iodine pool, and spatial distribution of iodine in the gland) for a specific administered activity can change the absorbed dose by up to a factor of 10 in any given patient.

Iodine Uptake Test

The iodine uptake test is easily performed and gives a useful clinical index of thyroid function. The main purposes of an uptake examination before radioiodine therapy are to ensure that the thyroid will take up iodine and to determine how much. The diagnosis of hyperthyroidism or hypothyroidism, however, is not made by using radioactive iodine uptake but should be made by serum measurements of thyroid hormone and thyroid-stimulating hormone (TSH). However, the thyroid uptake can be used to differentiate Graves' disease from subacute thyroiditis or factitious hyperthyroidism.

Principle and Technique

Thyroid uptake is based on the principle that the administered radiopharmaceutical is concentrated by the thyroid gland in a manner that reflects the gland's handling of stable dietary iodine and therefore the functional status of the gland. The higher the uptake of the radiopharmaceutical, the more active the thyroid; conversely, the lower the uptake, the less functional the gland. Uptake is conventionally expressed as the percentage of the administered activity in the thyroid gland at a given time after administration (usually at 4 to 6 hours and 24 hours). Normal range is about 10% to 30% for 24-hour uptake determinations. The normal range for a 4- to 6-hour uptake is about 6% to 18%.

To aid absorption, it is advisable for patients to be NPO beginning at midnight the day before oral administration of the radionuclide. It is also helpful to determine the functional status of the gastrointestinal tract before administering the radiopharmaceutical because vomiting or diarrhea may hinder adequate absorption.

To begin the test, about 5 μCi (0.2 MBq) of ^{131}I-sodium or 10 to 20 μCi (0.4–0.7 MBq) of ^{123}I-sodium in either liquid or capsule form is administered. [123]I uptakes may also be performed in conjunction with an ^{123}I thyroid scan using the scanning dosage. An identical amount of activity,

called a *standard*, is placed in a neck phantom, and the activity is compared with that in the patient's thyroid, using a single-crystal counting probe with a flat-field collimator. Such standards obviate the use of decay constants or geometric corrections in calculating uptakes.

The distance from the face of the probe crystal to the anterior aspect of the neck (about 25 to 30 cm) and the method of counting the ^{131}I standard are the same for all patients. It is usually unnecessary to correct measurements for body blood pool activity in the neck at 24 hours, but this correction is employed, especially when uptakes before 24 hours are desired. Correction is approximated by measuring the activity in the patient's thigh in the same manner as the neck measurements are performed. The number of counts obtained may then be subtracted from the neck reading to estimate counts isolated in the thyroid gland.

All measurements are usually performed twice, for 1 to 2 minutes each, and are then averaged to calculate the percentage uptake, using the following formula:

$$\% \text{ Thyroid uptake} = \text{Neck counts} - \text{thigh counts}/\text{Counts in standard} \times 100\%$$

It is occasionally advantageous to perform a 4- or 6-hour radioiodine uptake in addition to the 24-hour determination, particularly for abnormalities in which the iodine turnover is rapid (Graves' disease) or in which organification of the trapped iodine is defective (congenital, antithyroid drugs, Hashimoto's thyroiditis). Occasionally, the uptake obtained at 6 hours may be significantly higher than that at 24 hours, owing to rapid uptake and secretion or enhanced washout from the gland.

A sample technical protocol for performing radioiodide uptakes can be found in Appendix E 1.

Factors Affecting Iodine Uptake

Increased circulating iodides compete with administered radioiodines for trapping and organification by the thyroid gland. An increase in the body iodide pool is most frequently caused by an increase in dietary intake of iodine, which may significantly reduce the uptake values obtained. Conversely, a decrease in ambient iodine produces an "iodide-starved gland," which traps and binds greater amounts of radioactive iodide, producing elevated uptake values. Some authors suggest a low-iodine diet for 3 to 10 days before the test, but this practice is not widespread. In addition, regional differ-

TABLE 5–1.	Compounds that may Decrease Thyroid Iodine Uptake	
MEDICATION		**TIME***
Adrenocorticosteroids		1 week
Amiodarone		
Bromides		
Butazolidine		
Mercurials		
Methimazole (Tapazole)		
Nitrates		
Perchlorate		
Propylthiouracil		
Salicylates (large doses)		
Sulfonamides		
Thiocyanate		
Iodine solution (Lugol's or SSKI)		2 weeks
Iodine-containing antiseptics		
Kelp		
Some cough medicines and vitamin preparations		
Tri-iodothyronine (Cytomel)		3 weeks
Thyroid extract (Synthroid, Proloid)		
Intravenous contrast agents		1–2 months
Oil-based iodinated contrast agents		3–6 months

*Time that patient should wait after medication is discontinued in order to obtain an accurate uptake. SSKI, saturated solution of potassium iodide.

TABLE 5–2.	Factors Affecting Iodine Uptake
Increased uptake	
Hyperthyroidism (diffuse or nodular goiter)	
Early Hashimoto's thyroiditis	
Recovery from subacute thyroiditis	
Rebound after abrupt withdrawal of antithyroid medication	
Enzyme defects	
Iodine deficiency or starvation	
Hypoalbuminemia	
Thyroid-stimulating hormone	
Tumor-secreted stimulators (gonadal and chorionic origin)	
Pregnancy	
Decreased uptake	
Hypothyroidism (primary or secondary)	
Iodine overload (especially radiographic contrast)	
Medications (see Table 5–1)	
Subacute or autoimmune thyroiditis	
Thyroid hormone therapy	
Ectopic secretion of thyroid hormone from tumors	
Renal failure	

ences in dietary iodide intake give rise to local variations in the normal range. These factors, along with differences in technical aspects of the procedure among laboratories, make it necessary for each facility to determine its own range of normal values.

Good renal function is essential to normal radioiodine uptake. In patients with chronic renal failure, iodides usually excreted by the kidneys are retained, producing an increase in the stable iodide pool. This dilutes the percentage of radioiodine taken up by the gland, resulting in low uptake determinations. Large meals shortly before or after oral administration of radioiodine can slow or decrease absorption and interfere with uptake measurements.

Numerous medications and iodinated contrast agents also affect radioiodine uptake (Tables 5–1 and 5–2). To perform a radioiodine uptake successfully, these medications must be withheld for appropriate periods before the uptake procedure is attempted. Also, careful interviewing of patients undergoing the uptake test is necessary to determine whether there is a history of antithyroid drugs, thyroid hormones, iodide preparations, or radiographic contrasts used in kidney and myelo-graphic studies, computed tomography scans and angiographic procedures. Notably, β-blockers, such as propranolol, which are commonly used to combat the clinical manifestations of hyperthyroidism, do not affect the function of the gland and therefore do not interfere with thyroid uptake of the radioactive iodine.

Clinical Considerations

Radioiodine uptake is used to estimate the function of the thyroid gland by measuring its avidity for administered radioiodine. In the absence of exogenous influences, glands demonstrating a poor avidity for iodide are generally considered to be hypofunctioning, and the converse is true for hyperfunctioning glands.

Elevated Radioiodine Uptake

Primary hyperthyroidism (Graves' disease or toxic nodular goiter) and secondary hyperthyroidism commonly produce elevated iodine uptakes. These uptakes are useful in determining the level of therapeutic ^{131}I doses for the treatment of Graves' disease. On the other hand, hyperthyroidism produced by toxic nodular goiters (Plummer's disease) may yield uptake values in the high, normal, or mildly elevated range. Therefore, a normal or borderline elevated radioiodine uptake alone cannot be used to exclude the diagnosis of hyperthyroidism when it is clinically suspected.

Elevated uptakes also may be produced by a variety of other conditions (see Table 5–2), including any state of the gland characterized by increased avidity of the organ for iodine. The so-called iodine rebound phenomenon may result from the release of TSH by the pituitary after sudden withdrawal from thyroid hormone suppression therapy. It may also result from hormone synthesis rebound after withdrawal of antithyroid drugs, such as propylthiouracil. High uptakes can also be the result of abnormally increased production of TSH by the pituitary or secretion of TSH-like hormones by gonadal or chorionic tumors (secondary hyperthyroidism), or may occur in the recovery phase of subacute thyroiditis.

Reduced Radioiodine Uptake

Primary or secondary hypothyroidism may produce decreased radioiodine uptake. Primary hypothyroidism is a failure of the gland to respond to TSH, whereas secondary hypothyroidism is caused by insufficient pituitary secretion of TSH. Because of the prevalence of iodine in the American diet, it has become increasingly difficult to use reduced radioiodine uptake as an indicator of hypothyroidism. Serum TSH and thyroid hormone assays are necessary to establish the diagnosis.

Of note in considering the causes of decreased radioiodine uptake are the numerous medications outlined in Table 5–1. Again, withdrawal of the medications for the times given in the table is necessary to obtain accurate measures of thyroid function. Rarely, well-differentiated thyroid cancers, teratomas, and struma ovarii can be sites of ectopic secretion of thyroid hormone and cause low thyroidal uptake.

Thyroid Gland Imaging

Although ^{131}I or ^{123}I may be used for obtaining thyroid uptakes, ^{99m}Tc-pertechnetate and ^{123}I-sodium remain the agents of choice for obtaining maximum morphologic detail of the thyroid gland with the gamma camera. Either radionuclide, however, provides images of excellent quality, although the higher energy photons of ^{131}I may be preferable for imaging deep ectopic tissue. Even though ^{123}I is more expensive than ^{99m}Tc, it has the advantage of being able to provide concurrent radioiodine uptake and images with relatively low radiation dose. In addition, ^{123}I images reflect both trapping and organification in the gland.

The indications for scintigraphic thyroid imaging include:

- To relate the general structure of the gland to function, particularly in differentiating Graves' disease from toxic nodular goiter. This distinction is important in determining therapeutic radioiodine dose.
- To determine function in a specific area, for example, to see if a palpable nodule is functional.
- To locate ectopic tissue, such as a lingual thyroid.
- To assist in evaluation of congenital hypothyroidism or organification defects.
- To determine that a cervical or mediastinal mass is thyroid tissue.
- To differentiate among the causes of thyrotoxicosis, that is, Graves' disease from subacute, silent, postpartum, or factitious hyperthyroidism. In the latter entities, there are symptoms of mild hyperthyroidism with elevated serum levels of thyroid hormone, but radioiodine studies reveal that the radioiodine uptake in the gland is low and visualization is poor.

Imaging with ^{99m}Tc-pertechnetate or radioiodine requires no prior preparation of the patient. As with uptake studies, a brief screening of patients for a possible history of recent medication or iodinated contrast administration is advisable. In addition, before imaging is begun, palpation of the thyroid gland, with the patient sitting upright, is recommended to assess any enlargement or nodules. The prior localization of palpable nodules within the gland makes it much easier to relocate these abnormalities with the patient in the supine scanning position, when marker localization may be required.

Even with a history of recent radioiodinated contrast or suppressive medication administration, it is frequently possible to obtain reasonably good anatomic assessment of the thyroid gland with ^{99m}Tc when it is not possible with radioiodine. This, in part, is related to the significantly greater allowable activity for pertechnetate scanning than for radioiodine. When feasible, however, the patient should return after an appropriate interval of withdrawal from the interfering drug for a more definitive examination.

Technique and Clinical Protocol

Technetium-99m

The thyroid is imaged 20 minutes after the intravenous administration of 5 to 10 mCi (185 to

370 MBq) of ^{99m}Tc-pertechnetate, using a scintillation camera with a pinhole collimator. Anterior and left and right anterior oblique images are then obtained for 100,000 to 300,000 counts (or 5 minutes) each, with the patient supine and neck extended. In addition, the position of palpable nodules under investigation should be documented and a view obtained with a radioactive marker placed on the lesion. This aids in an accurate correlation of the physical and scan findings. The oblique images are essential for the identification of laterally and posteriorly placed nodules that might be missed with simple anterior imaging.

In some laboratories, the static images are preceded by a blood-flow study of the thyroid. If this is to be done, at least 10 mCi (370 MBq) of ^{99m}Tc-pertechnetate should be injected as an intravenous bolus using a parallel-hole collimator. The field of view is from the level of the salivary glands to the upper sternum.

Iodine-123

Imaging with ^{123}I may be performed after the oral administration of 200 to 600 µCi (7.4 to 22.2 MBq) to a fasting patient. Imaging can be performed at 3 to 4 hours, but the images are better when done at 16 to 24 hours. Images of high quality are obtained employing 50,000- to 100,000-count or a 10-minute acquisition. Imaging 24 hours after administration may give a more accurate indication of the distribution of organified iodine within the gland than earlier images.

The complete technical protocols for performing thyroid scintigraphy using ^{99m}Tc-pertechnetate and ^{123}I can be found in Appendix E–1.

Normal Images

The normal thyroid gland is a bilobed organ with reasonably homogeneous distribution of activity in both lobes (see Fig. 5–1). The normal gland weighs 1.5 g at birth and about 6.5 g by 5 years of age. In adults, the entire gland weighs between 15 and 25 g, and each lobe measures about 2 × 5 cm. Slight asymmetry in the sizes of the lobes is common, with the right lobe generally dominating. The lobes are usually joined inferiorly and medially by the thyroid isthmus, which may demonstrate relatively decreased activity compared with the adjacent lobes. In some instances, complete absence of activity is noted in this region. In a small number of patients, a pyramidal lobe is identified that arises from the isthmus or medial aspect of one lobe and extends superiorly and medially. Although this is a common variation, it may be accentuated in partial thyroidectomy patients and in patients with diffuse thyroid abnormalities such as Hashimoto's thyroiditis or Graves' disease. Less common variants of thyroid configuration include congenital absence of one lobe, substernal extension of the gland, or a sublingual thyroid with functioning tissue at the base of the tongue.

The most common artifact of ^{99m}Tc-pertechnetate studies of the thyroid is produced by activity secreted by the salivary glands and swallowed by the patient. This usually presents as a linear area of esophageal activity in the midline of the image. If this complicates interpretation or causes confusion with an enlarged pyramidal lobe, repeat imaging should be performed using oblique images or after clearing the esophagus by drinking water.

Abnormal Images
Ectopic Thyroid Tissue

Ectopic thyroid tissue may occur in the neck, in the base of the tongue (lingual thyroid) (Fig. 5–2), in the pelvis (struma ovarii), or retrosternally in the region of the mediastinum (substernal goiter). When ectopic sites deep within the body are suspected, 24-hour imaging with ^{131}I-sodium is the method of choice (although ^{123}I also can be used). Because of interfering salivary gland activity in the neck, attenuation of 140-keV gamma rays by the sternum or soft tissues, and excessive blood pool activity, ^{99m}Tc-pertechnetate is generally not as useful.

Identification of an anterior mediastinal mass on chest radiograph is the most frequent benign indication for ^{123}I or ^{131}I imaging of the chest. Intrathoracic thyroid tissue most commonly presents as a substernal extension of a cervical thyroid goiter (Fig. 5–3). This occurs most commonly on the left, displacing the trachea to the right. Less commonly, it presents as a mediastinal mass anatomically unrelated to the thyroid gland. Thoracic thyroid tissue is most frequently found in middle-aged women but may occur in either sex at any age. Thyroid tissue in the chest may not demonstrate radioiodine uptake as intensely as that in the neck, and some mediastinal thyroid tissue may not function at all. Therefore, although uptake in a mediastinal or substernal mass indicates that the tissue is thyroid related, lack of concentration of radioiodine does not necessarily exclude that diagnosis.

Aberrant functioning thyroid tissue, struma ovarii, is rarely identified in some ovarian teratomas. Even more rarely, this tissue may hyper-

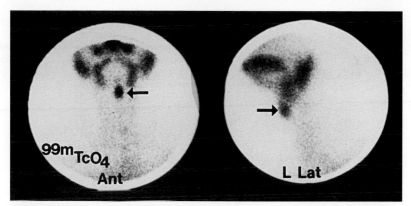

FIGURE 5–2. Lingual thyroid. Anterior and lateral views of the cervical region from a technetium-99m pertechnetate study demonstrate no activity in the region of the thyroid bed, but a focal area of increased activity is seen high in the midline of the neck near the base of the tongue (*arrows*), compatible with a lingual thyroid. The patient was clinically hypothyroid.

function, producing symptoms of hyperthyroidism with suppression of function in the normal thyroid.

Congenital Organification Defect
Congenital organification defects become apparent in the first months of life. The typical presentation is an infant with low serum thyroid hormone levels and a high TSH level. A 24-hour radioiodine scan usually shows no activity in the thyroid because without organification, the trapped iodine washes out of the gland and it is not possible to distinguish

this from an absent thyroid. A ^{99m}Tc-pertechnetate, or 2- to 4-hour ^{123}I scan, on the other hand, clearly shows the presence of the thyroid because the trapping mechanism of the gland is intact (Fig. 5–4).

Thyroid Nodules
Although fine-needle aspiration biopsy has largely supplanted radionuclide imaging as the initial investigative procedure for palpable thyroid nodules, imaging can be useful in selected patients. In patients with suppressed TSH levels or with

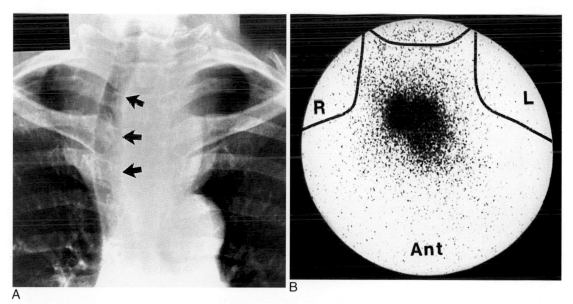

FIGURE 5–3. Substernal thyroid. *A*, Chest radiograph demonstrates a large soft-tissue mass at the thoracic inlet (*arrows*), deviating the trachea to the right. *B*, A radioiodine scan shows the left lobe of the thyroid extending inferiorly.

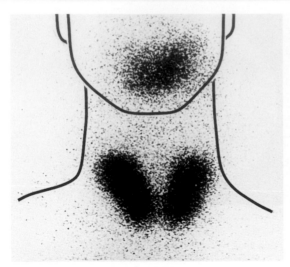

FIGURE 5–4. Congenital organification defect. This infant was clinically hypothyroid and had a thyroid-stimulating hormone concentration in excess of 400 mU/mL. This technetium-99m pertechnetate scan clearly shows the thyroid to be present and trapping. Normal activity in the mouth and salivary glands is seen superiorly. A 24-hour iodine-123 scan showed no thyroid activity.

TABLE 5–3.	Pathologies of Solitary Cold Thyroid Nodule	
PATHOLOGY		**INCIDENCE (%)**
Colloid cyst or adenoma		70–75
Carcinoma		15–25
Miscellaneous		<15%
Focal area of thyroiditis		
Abscess		
Hemorrhage		
Lymphoma, metastases		
Parathyroid adenoma		
Lymph nodes		

nodules with indeterminate cytology results, imaging provides information regarding the functional status of the nodule and may indicate the presence of additional nodules. Because hyperfunctional nodules are almost always benign, they can be managed medically with radioactive iodine therapy.

Conventionally, nodules are classified at imaging with respect to the relative amount of activity present. Cold nodules demonstrate an essential absence of activity, whereas hot nodules are iden-tified by focally increased activity compared with the normal thyroid parenchyma. Nodules that are neither hot nor cold but contain activity comparable to that of the surrounding gland are frequently termed *warm* nodules.

Cold Nodule. A nonfunctioning thyroid nodule is essentially a nonspecific finding and may be due to any of numerous pathologies (Table 5–3), the most common of which is a colloid cyst. Although most cold nodules are benign (Fig. 5–5), the small percentage that prove to be cancerous are sufficient to warrant further investigation or therapy, depending on the clinical circumstances. The reported percentage of solitary cold nodules harboring thyroid cancer varies depending on the clinical bias of the particular study but is generally thought to be about 20%. The likelihood of carcinoma significantly increases if the patient is young. Suspicion is further increased if associated lymphadenopathy is identi-

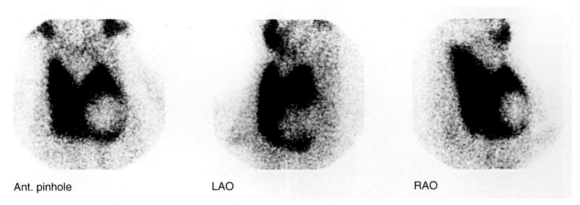

Ant. pinhole   LAO   RAO

FIGURE 5–5. Nonfunctioning thyroid adenoma. A technetium-99m pertechnetate scan shows a large "cold" area in the inferior left lobe. Left (LAO) and right (RAO) anterior oblique views show that the lesion projects within the gland on all images and is not an extrinsic abnormality. A thyroid carcinoma may present an identical appearance.

TABLE 5–4.	Clinical Factors Influencing Treatment of Cold Thyroid Nodule*

Factors tending toward benign
   Older patients
   Female sex
   Sudden onset
   Tender or soft lesion
   Multiple nodules
   Shrinkage on thyroid hormone
Factors tending toward malignant
   Young patients
   Male sex
   History of radiation to head or neck
   Hard lesion
   Other masses in neck
   No shrinkage on thyroid hormone
   Familial history of thyroid carcinoma

*None of these factors is absolute.

fied or if the nodule fails to decrease in size after a trial of thyroid hormone suppression. If a history of previous head and neck radiation therapy is elicited, a cold nodule has about a 40% chance of being malignant (Table 5–4).

Ultrasound may be of value in distinguishing between a benign cystic abnormality and a solid lesion, which may harbor a neoplasm. Ultrasound is not useful in differentiating malignant from benign solid nodules. An anterior radionuclide thyroid blood flow study performed with ^{99m}Tc-pertechnetate may also provide information regarding the perfusion status of the lesion. Definite evidence of perfusion in the region of a cold nodule is compatible with a solid lesion in need of further investigation or biopsy.

Hot Nodule. Most nodules that demonstrate increased radionuclide concentration are benign, although thyroid carcinoma has been described in a small percentage (<1%). Hot nodules almost always represent hyperfunctioning adenomas, of which up to half are autonomous. Autonomous nodules function independently of the thyroid pituitary axis feedback mechanism; thus, they are not suppressible with exogenous thyroid hormone. Autonomous hyperfunctioning nodules may produce enough thyroid hormone to inhibit pituitary secretion of TSH and secondarily to suppress function in the surrounding normal thyroid tissue (Fig. 5–6C).

Discordant Thyroid Nodule. By use of iodine imaging, a small number of cases of hot nodules on ^{99m}Tc-pertechnetate imaging have subsequently proved to be cold or "discordant," and a small number of those lesions have been shown to be thyroid carcinoma. Theoretically, the discordant images are produced either by the preservation of technetium trapping, but not of organification of iodine within the nodules, or by rapid turnover of organified iodine so that the nodule presents as a "cold" on a 24-hour radioiodine scan. Because the ^{99m}Tc-pertechnetate scan is performed at 20 minutes, the avid trapping of pertechnetate by the nodules renders a focal area of increased activity. With radioiodine imaging, however, which is normally performed at 24 hours, the trapped radiopharmaceutical has either not been organified or has been organified and rapidly secreted and has thus washed out of the nodule, giving rise to a cold area on the scan (Fig. 5–7). It has been recommended that patients demonstrating solitary hot nodules on pertechnetate scans be reimaged using an iodine agent to determine whether the lesion represents a discordant nodule or a true hyperfunctioning adenoma. If the lesion proves to be discordant, further investigation may be warranted, depending on the clinical status of the patient.

Warm Nodule. Although some warm nodules do function normally, many are actually cold nodules deep within the thyroid gland, with overlying normally functioning tissue. Oblique views often disclose the true nature of these abnormalities; however, frequently, the abnormality can be classified only as warm even after thorough imaging. Because of the risk of carcinoma in a cold nodule obscured by overlying tissue, it is probably prudent to classify these abnormalities as cold and in need of further investigation.

Multinodular Gland

Multinodular goiter typically presents as an enlarged gland with multiple cold, warm, and hot areas, which give the gland a coarsely patchy appearance (Fig. 5–8). These nodules generally constitute a spectrum of thyroid adenomas ranging from hyperfunctioning to cystic or degenerating lesions. This type of gland is most frequent in middle-aged women but may occur in younger patients, who are usually female. In adults, the cold lesions identified in a multinodular goiter are significantly less likely to represent carcinoma than are solitary cold nodules. Dominant or otherwise

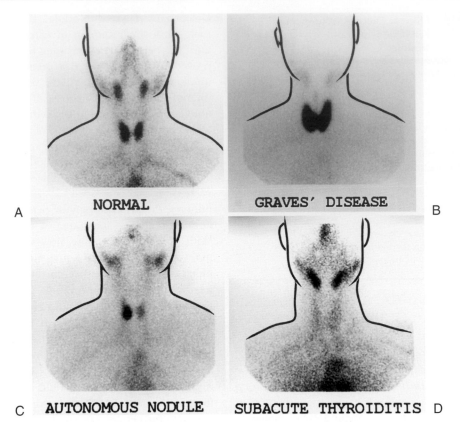

A   **NORMAL**

B   **GRAVES' DISEASE**

C   **AUTONOMOUS NODULE**

D   **SUBACUTE THYROIDITIS**

FIGURE 5–6. Appearance of the thyroid on technetium-99m pertechnetate scans. *A*, Normal. The thyroid is clearly visible, and the salivary glands are also seen but are somewhat less intense in activity. *B*, Graves' disease. The thyroid is enlarged and has accumulated much of the activity, so that the salivary glands are harder to see. *C*, Hyperfunctioning "hot" nodule. The nodule is seen as an area of intense activity, and its autonomous hormone production has suppressed the remainder of the thyroid gland, so that the normal thyroid is hard to see. *D*, Subacute thyroiditis. In this case, the inflammation has caused the thyroid to have difficulty trapping, and the amount of activity in the thyroid is lower than normally expected, whereas the salivary gland activity is normal.

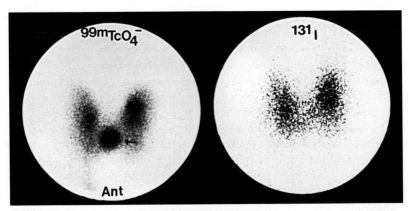

FIGURE 5–7. Discordant nodule. Two images obtained in a patient with a prominent nodule in the thyroid isthmus demonstrate increased technetium-99m pertechnetate activity in the region of the nodule (*arrow*) but no significant activity when imaged with radioiodine. At surgery, this lesion proved to be a mixed papillary follicular carcinoma.

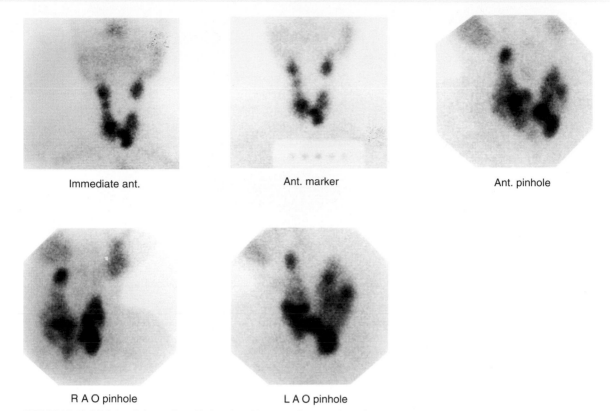

Immediate ant.   Ant. marker   Ant. pinhole

R A O pinhole   L A O pinhole

FIGURE 5–8. Multinodular goiter. Technetium-99m pertechnetate planar images of the neck (*top*) demonstrate patchy activity in both lobes of the enlarged thyroid. Anterior pinhole images (*bottom*) of just the thyroid gland show multiple "hot" and "cold" areas in the gland, compatible with the typical appearance of multinodular goiter.

suspicious cold nodules in a multinodular goiter warrant further characterization. Multinodular goiters with cold lesions are more likely to harbor malignant neoplasms in children than they are in adults, although the incidence is still low. In addition, any patient with a previous history of head and neck irradiation is also at higher risk for carcinoma.

Occasionally, multinodular goiter may be mimicked by thyroiditis with multifocal involvement of the gland (Fig. 5–9). However, differentiation on clinical and laboratory grounds is usually possible.

Diffuse Toxic Goiter (Graves' Disease)

Diffuse toxic goiter is thought to be of autoimmune origin. It usually presents with varying degrees of thyromegaly, with notably uniform distribution of increased activity throughout the thyroid gland, and often with a prominent pyramidal lobe (Fig. 5–10). On ^{99m}Tc-pertechnetate scan of a patient with Graves' disease, the thyroid has increased activity, and the salivary glands are difficult to

identify (see Fig. 5–6B). Because salivary glands are not normally seen on an ^{123}I scan, it is often difficult to differentiate Graves' disease from a normal scan without knowing the iodine uptake value. Twenty-four-hour iodine uptakes in patients with Graves' disease are usually in the range of 40% to 70%.

Although cold nodules are sometimes found in patients with diffuse toxic goiter, carcinoma under these circumstances is exceedingly uncommon. It is still prudent, however, to further evaluate any solitary cold nodules occurring in this setting.

Thyroiditis

Chronic thyroiditis (Hashimoto's thyroiditis) is the most common form of inflammatory disease of the thyroid. The disease is thought to be autoimmune in origin and is much more common in female patients. Thyromegaly is usually the presenting finding, although occasionally symptoms of mild hyperthyroidism or hypothyroidism may be present, depending on the stage and severity of the disease.

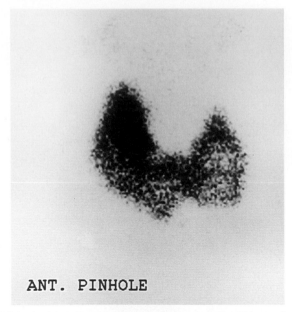

FIGURE 5–9. Chronic thyroiditis. A pinhole image of the thyroid from an iodine-123 scan shows patchy or inhomogeneous activity throughout the gland. This pattern is also seen with multinodular goiter.

The scan appearance of the thyroid varies from diffusely uniform increased activity in the gland early in the disease (which may resemble Graves' disease) to a coarsely patchy distribution of activity within the gland later in the disease (which may mimic multinodular goiter).

The more uncommon diseases of acute (bacterial) and subacute (viral or autoimmune) thyroiditis have such typical clinical features that they are usually diagnosed on physical and clinical grounds, and scanning generally plays little role in their evaluation. Subacute thyroiditis usually presents as a painful swollen gland with elevated circulating thyroid hormone levels but with markedly depressed radioiodine uptake. Attempts at imaging with radioiodine or ^{99m}Tc-pertechnetate (see Fig. 5–6D) usually show little or no localization of radiopharmaceutical in the gland.

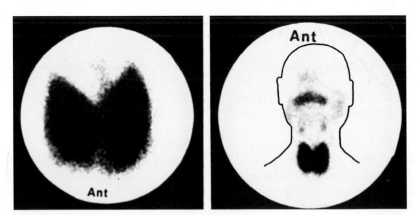

FIGURE 5–10. Diffuse goiter in a patient with Graves' disease. *Left,* The pinhole collimator image (technetium-99m [^{99m}Tc] pertechnetate) demonstrates a large gland with increased activity and a pyramidal lobe arising from the superior aspect of the left lobe. *Right,* An image obtained with the parallel-hole collimator demonstrates the relatively increased trapping of ^{99m}Tc-pertechnetate in the thyroid compared with the salivary gland activity.

Thyroid Carcinoma

Ninety percent of all thyroid cancers are well differentiated and have the ability to concentrate radioiodine; therefore, thyroid cancer is usually amenable to adjunctive radioiodine therapy. Between 80% and 90% of well-differentiated thyroid cancers are papillary. These occur twice as often in female as in male patients and over a wide age range, with a mean age of about 45 years. These tumors almost always are seen on a thyroid scan as a single cold nodule but often are histologically multifocal. Papillary carcinoma commonly metastasizes to cervical lymph nodes. Ten percent to 20% of well-differentiated cancers are follicular. These also occur over a wide age group, but with a mean age of 50 to 55 years. These tumors most commonly metastasize hematogenously to the lungs and bone and less commonly to liver and brain.

The overall prognosis of patients with well-differentiated types of thyroid cancer is good, with a 5-year survival rate of more than 95% in properly treated patients. The metastases of either lesion may histologically present the characteristics of the other; that is, primary follicular lesions may give predominantly papillary metastases, or vice versa.

The remaining thyroid malignancies include anaplastic or poorly differentiated carcinomas (5%) and occur primarily in older patients. The prognosis is generally poor. Medullary carcinoma of the thyroid parenchyma constitutes about 5% of malignant thyroid lesions. This cancer may be associated with other endocrine lesions, such as pheochromocytoma; may actively secrete hormones (most notably thyrocalcitonin); and may be familial. Hürthle cell carcinoma (5%) is an unusual variant of follicular cell carcinoma, which is generally more aggressive with early distant metastases. Most of these latter types of tumors do not concentrate iodine well and therefore are not usually amenable to metastasis localization or radioiodine therapy.

Clinically and scintigraphically, primary carcinomas of the thyroid may initially present as discrete thyroid nodules or as enlargement of one lobe with or without cervical nodal or distant metastases. When discrete, the lesions are almost invariably demonstrated as cold areas on the radionuclide images. By use of a gamma camera, ^{99m}Tc-pertechnetate with a pinhole collimator, 80% of lesions 8 mm in diameter are detected.

Because the metastatic lesions of well-differentiated thyroid carcinomas with follicular

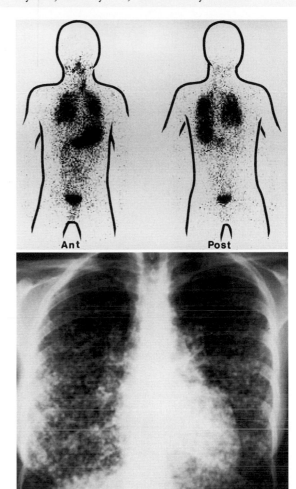

FIGURE 5–11. Metastatic disease from thyroid carcinoma. *Top,* Anterior and posterior images of a whole-body iodine-131 scan obtained 72 hours after injection. Normal physiologic activity is seen in the mouth and salivary glands, stomach, colon, and bladder. The activity in the lower neck represents functioning nodal metastases, and the activity in the lung is due to many tiny hematogenous pulmonary metastases, which are seen on the chest radiograph (*Bottom*).

elements frequently (65% to 85%) concentrate radioiodine, whole-body imaging with ^{123}I or ^{131}I is of value in monitoring post-thyroidectomy patients to detect functioning metastases or to assess the results of treatment of known metastatic lesions (Fig. 5–11). Non–radioiodine-avid thyroid carcinomas are not visualized with radioiodine imaging but can be successfully imaged using either ^{99m}Tc-sestamibi (Fig. 5–12) or fluorine-18 deoxyglucose (^{18}FDG) positron emission tomography (PET) (Fig 13–38).

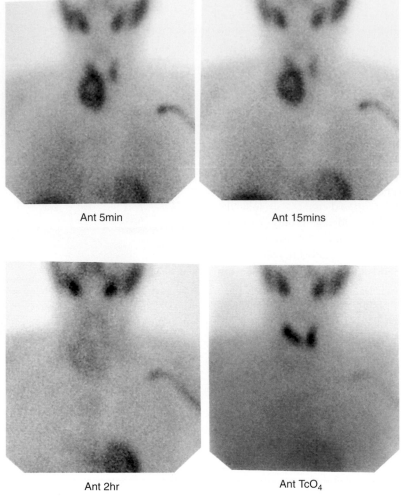

Ant 5min   Ant 15mins

Ant 2hr   Ant TcO₄

FIGURE 5–12. Thyroid carcinoma. A technetium-99m (^{99m}Tc) sestamibi scan (*top row*) shows a large area of increased uptake in the right lobe of the thyroid with a central cold area of necrosis. The activity decreases over 2 hours. A ^{99m}Tc pertechnetate scan shows the normal gland but no activity in this area because the cancer is unable to trap or organify.

Post-thyroidectomy Imaging. Whole-body evaluation for metastatic thyroid disease is first performed within 1 to 2 months after total or subtotal thyroidectomy. Thyroid hormone replacement is withheld during this period to allow for endogenous TSH stimulation of any remaining normal tissue in the thyroid bed and any functioning metastatic lesions. This stimulation allows even poorly functioning or small amounts of tissue to be maximally visualized. A serum TSH value of greater than 30 μU/mL is desirable, and a level greater than 50 μU/mL is optimal. After the oral administration of about 3 to 5 mCi (111 to 185 MBq) of ^{131}I-sodium iodide, sequential whole-body images are obtained for the next several days, generally at 48, 72, and, if necessary, 96 hours or longer. When ^{123}I whole-body scanning is used, 1.5 mCi (55.5 MBq) is administered orally and imaging is optimally performed at 24 hours, although earlier imaging at 6 hours is possible.

A whole-body imaging device or large-field-of-view gamma camera may be used (optimally with a high-energy collimator, although a medium-energy collimator may be used). If gamma camera spot images are the method of imaging, it is important to include adequate neck, chest, abdominal, and pelvic views in the anterior position as well as appropriate posterior images.

Knowledge of the normal distribution of radioiodine before and after thyroid ablation is

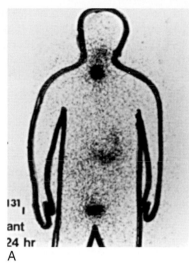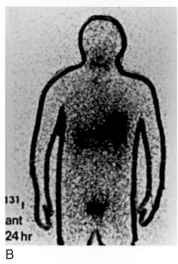

FIGURE 5–13. Whole-body distribution of iodine-123 displayed 24 hours after oral administration. A: Activity is present in the thyroid and salivary glands, stomach, and bladder in a patient who has residual thyroid tissue. **B:** After ablation or total thyroidectomy, activity is present in salivary glands, stomach, and bladder, and there is a moderate amount of background activity. Physiologic activity can also occur in the nose, mouth, liver, and colon.

essential (Fig. 5–13). Activity is commonly seen in the stomach, bowel, and bladder. Mild diffuse activity in the liver is also normal and is caused by clearance of bound iodine by the liver. Residual normal thyroid tissue in the neck may produce a star artifact when a medium-energy collimator is used. This is owing to septal penetration by the large number of high-energy gamma rays from the ^{131}I (Fig. 5–14).

When whole-body radioiodine imaging using a diagnostic administration of ^{131}I is performed after thyroidectomy for detection of residual thyroid tissue or functioning metastases, some concerns have been raised regarding the possibility of stunning these tissues. "Stunning" results in a decreased ability to uptake a subsequent therapeutic dose of ^{131}I, leading to less effective treatment. It has been postulated that this might result from a reduction in the number of functional cells, or more likely, a reduction in transport of radioiodine into the cells due to the beta radiation from the diagnostic dose. Because the severity of stunning is directly related to the amount of ^{131}I used, limiting the diagnostic dose to 3 to 5 mCi (111–185 MBq) for imaging before thyroid remnant ablation or treatment of functioning metastases has been recommended. If stunning is a major concern, imaging using 1.5 mCi (55.5 MBq) of orally administered ^{123}I can

be performed at 24 hours. The only drawback is that ^{123}I is more expensive than is ^{131}I.

Postradioiodine Therapy Imaging. If significant functioning thyroid tissue remains in the neck, as is frequently the case even after "total" thyroidectomy, ablation of the remaining tissue with high-dose ^{131}I therapy is indicated. Metastatic lesions are only infrequently visualized with ^{123}I or ^{131}I whole-body imaging when there is functioning thyroid in the neck. Ablation of residual tissue allows for sufficient TSH stimulation by the pituitary to permit functioning of distant metastatic sites, thus allowing their detection on follow-up ^{131}I imaging. Adequate endogenous TSH stimulation usually takes 4 to 6 weeks. Once all residual thyroid tissue in the neck has been ablated, follow-up whole-body imaging with ^{123}I or ^{131}I may be performed at 6-month to 1-year intervals. Although protocols vary by institution, such scanning is often done until the scans are negative for 2 years.

When follow-up ^{131}I imaging is performed, patients should undergo thyroid hormone withdrawal for 4 to 6 weeks to allow endogenous serum TSH levels to rise in excess of 30 µU/mL so that stimulation of any residual normal thyroid tissue or functioning metastases can enhance the likelihood of detection. However, because hormone with-

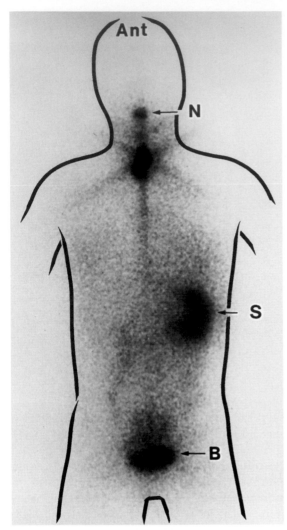

FIGURE 5–14. Star artifact. A residual thyroid remnant in this patient after thyroidectomy has accumulated a large amount of radioiodine. The high energy and activity of the radioiodine have caused a number of photons to penetrate the lead septa of the medium-energy collimator, causing a star pattern. Depending on the arrangement of the holes in the collimator, this pattern may be a six-pointed star or a cross pattern. Normal physiologic activity is seen in the nose (N), stomach (S), and bladder (B).

The dosage for Thyrogen in this setting is 0.9 mg given intramuscularly every 24 hours for 2 doses or every 72 hours for 3 doses, with diagnostic administration of ^{131}I given 24 hours after the last Thyrogen injection. Imaging is then performed 48 and/or 72 hours later. It should be recognized that the sensitivity of whole-body ^{131}I imaging after rhTSH is slightly less sensitive for both detection of residual thyroid tissue and tumor in the thyroid bed and for functioning metastases in 15% to 25% of patients compared with imaging after thyroid hormone withdrawal. Thus, in high-risk patients, hormone withdrawal may well be advised.

After all functioning tissue within the thyroid bed has been ablated, subsequent identification of functioning tissue in the neck should be considered as tumor recurrence and treated appropriately. It is important not to mistake the physiologic excretion of radioiodine in the salivary glands, saliva, nose, stomach, colon, liver, and bladder for metastases. Most physiologic activity in the liver is diffuse, whereas hepatic metastases usually are focal.

In addition to whole-body ^{131}I imaging, postablation thyroid cancer patients are also followed by monitoring serum thyroglobulin (Tg) levels. Serum Tg tests are the most accurate method of detecting recurrent thyroid cancer even if the patient is taking thyroid hormone. This glycoprotein is synthesized by follicular cells, and most well-differentiated thyroid cancers secrete Tg even if they do not concentrate radioiodine or if the patient is taking thyroid hormone. Measurement of Tg can vary from one laboratory to another, and it is best for the patient to have serial measurements performed by the same laboratory. Measurement of Tg before surgery and thyroid ablation is not useful. In addition, Tg levels can be high for the first 2 months after thyroidectomy, and tests should not be performed until after this period. A rising Tg level should raise serious concern about metastases or recurrence. A Tg level above 10 ng/mL is associated with metastases in more than 85% of patients. Whole-body radioiodine scans for follow-up are generally unnecessary in patients with negative serum Tg and no other signs of recurrent thyroid cancer.

In patients with suspected metastatic lesions to the skeleton, a radionuclide bone scan before the administration of a whole-body ^{123}I or ^{131}I scanning dose may be useful, although thyroid metastases to bone are not uncommonly photopenic and may go undetected on ^{99m}Tc-diphosphonate bone scans (Fig. 5–15).

drawal can be unpleasant and medically ill-advised in some patients, exogenous recombinant human thyrotropin (Thyrogen; rhTSH) may be used while continuing thyroid hormone replacement, thus avoiding the ill-effects of hypothyroidism. rhTSH may also be used to supplement endogenous TSH when the serum levels fail to respond sufficiently to the withdrawal of replacement thyroid hormone.

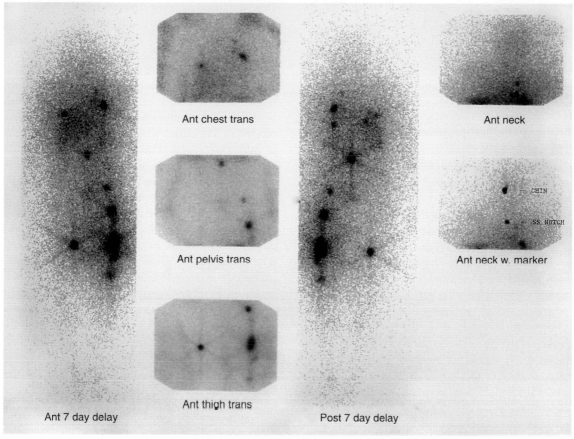

FIGURE 5–15. Metastatic thyroid cancer. This patient presented with a lytic pathologic fracture of the left femur. A technetium-99m methylene diphosphonate bone scan showed the fracture but no other abnormal areas. A whole-body iodine-131 scan demonstrates multiple areas of increased iodine uptake in the osseous metastatic lesions. (Also note the star artifacts).

IODINE-131 THERAPY IN THYROID DISEASE

Although this introduction to diagnostic radionuclide techniques is primarily restricted to imaging methods, a discussion of the use of ^{131}I in the treatment of thyroid disease is appropriate because ^{131}I plays an important role in the control and cure of certain thyroid diseases. Each institution should develop a protocol for patient care and personnel safety when patients are hospitalized for radioiodine therapy. This needs to comply with relevant local, state, and NRC requirements. A sample protocol is provided in Appendix H.

The primary therapeutic uses of ^{131}I are (1) the treatment of hyperthyroidism caused by either diffuse or nodular goiter, (2) the postsurgical ablation of the thyroid gland remnants, and (3) the treatment of functioning thyroid metastases.

Principle

Whether benign or neoplastic, any thyroid tissue capable of producing thyroid hormone will trap and organify stable iodine or its radioactive isotopes. Once a radioactive form of iodine has been taken up by the functioning tissue, therapeutic effects are made possible by the delivery of destructive ionizing radiation, primarily in the form of relatively high-energy beta emissions. Subsequent to irradiation, cell death occurs over a period of weeks to months. The beta-emitting properties of ^{131}I have made this radioisotope the most useful for the elimination of unwanted benign or malignant thyroid tissue.

Several factors influence the dose of radiation delivered to functioning thyroid tissue by ^{131}I and therefore govern its effectiveness as a therapeutic agent. These include (1) the degree of uptake of

[131]I, (2) the bulk of tissue to be destroyed, (3) the length of residence of ^{131}I within the tissue, (4) the distribution of ^{131}I within the tissue, and (5) the radiosensitivity of the particular cells. A serum pregnancy test should be performed on any woman of childbearing age for whom there may be a question of adequate birth control.

Primary Hyperthyroidism

The three basic approaches to the therapy of primary hyperthyroidism are (1) antithyroid drugs, such as the thioamides, propylthiouracil and methimizole; (2) surgery; and (3) [131]I therapy. Iodine-131 is regarded as the treatment of choice for hyperthyroidism in patients older than 30 years and in patients of any age in whom hyperthyroidism is accompanied by medical complications or in whom other treatments have failed. Although antithyroid drugs are frequently used as an initial approach to the control of diffuse toxic goiter (Graves' disease), such drugs are generally not used in the treatment of toxic nodules or multinodular goiter. In a significant number of patients with Graves' disease, antithyroid drug therapy produces intolerable side effects, does not adequately control the disease, or results in patient compliance problems. In these patients and in patients with toxic nodular disease, ^{131}I therapy is of considerable value. Iodine-131 therapy is also of value in patients with recurrent hyperthyroidism after previous thyroidectomy, when repeat surgery would cause enhanced risks; in children who have experienced toxicity to antithyroid drugs; and in patients who refuse other therapy.

Although most children with hyperthyroidism have Graves' disease, there is a certain amount of controversy regarding the treatment of children and adolescents with [131]I. The complication rate in children undergoing thyroid surgery is significantly higher than that in adults, and antithyroid therapy in children usually has poor compliance and carries a significantly higher risk of toxicity and relapse compared with that experienced in adults. As many as 80% of children and adolescents treated for Graves' disease with antithyroid drugs eventually require ^{131}I therapy. Even though there is little evidence to indicate significant radiation carcinogenesis from therapeutic doses of ^{131}I in these patients, a few physicians still choose not to use ^{131}I therapy routinely in children and in adults younger than 30 years.

Proposed methods of calculating doses for treating hyperthyroidism are numerous and varied.

Determination of dose follows one of two basic philosophies, commonly referred to as low-dose and high-dose therapy. Currently, low-dose therapy is rarely used. The difference in approaches is predicated on the likelihood of the induction of hypothyroidism. In low-dose therapy, there is an emphasis on reducing the resulting hypothyroidism in the first year after therapy and accepting any morbidity associated with the prolonged presence of hyperthyroidism. This method does not appear to alter the incidence of hypothyroidism after 1 year. The more commonly used high-dose therapy considers that hypothyroidism is an acceptable risk, indeed, almost an inevitable result, of ^{131}I therapy for Graves' disease. Rapid reduction in thyroid function is the most important objective of high-dose therapy. With this approach, the patient is normally rendered hypothyroid and put on replacement hormone as soon as possible. High-dose therapy is especially appropriate for patients with underlying medical conditions worsened by hyperthyroidism, such as cardiac congestive failure.

Formulas for the calculation of actual doses generally take into account one or more of the following: (1) the size of the gland, (2) the presence or absence of nodularity in the gland, and (3) the results of the ^{131}I uptake test. Palpation used to estimate the mass of the thyroid gland often introduces a substantial subjective error into the calculation of dose, although assessment of thyroid images and the occasional use of ultrasonography may aid in improving the estimate of gland size. With experience, a reasonable estimate can be made by palpation alone. Rather than calculate a specific dose for a given patient, some laboratories simply use a fixed dose for patients with diffuse toxic goiter, often in the range of 10 to 15 mCi (370–555 MBq). Studies have shown that there is little difference in the success of therapy between calculated and fixed dose treatment.

Most institutions use high-dose therapy, and doses in the range of 8 to 30 mCi (296 to 1110 MBq) or higher may be initially administered to allow for definitive therapy. Administered doses are also selected at the higher end of the dose range if the patients are severely hyperthyroid or have large glands, significant nodularity, or cardiac disease aggravated by their thyrotoxic state. With high-dose therapy, retreatment is usually unnecessary. In general, for treatment of diffuse goiter, therapy may be in the range of 15 mCi (555 MBq) of ^{131}I in patients with no evidence of thyroid nodularity. These doses may be repeated at 3- to

6-month intervals as necessary for the control of hyperthyroidism.

Hyperthyroidism related to toxic nodular goiter (Plummer's disease) is particularly resistant to radioactive iodine therapy and frequently requires doses two to three times larger than those applicable in diffuse toxic goiter. Thus, in addition to ^{131}I uptakes, thyroid imaging is usually used before ^{131}I therapy to distinguish toxic nodular goiter from Graves' disease. Large multinodular goiters may require doses in excess of 30 mCi (1.11 GBq), and multiple treatments may be needed. Solitary toxic nodules generally can be successfully treated with administered doses in the 15- to 25-mCi (555–925 MBq) range. Even with such large doses, it is not usual to induce hypothyroidism when there is significant suppression of function in the remainder of the thyroid gland by the autonomous nodules.

Regardless of the type of dose regimen used, it is often difficult to predict accurately the outcome of radioactive iodine therapy in a given patient. Results are frequently significantly affected by a number of variables:

- Nodular thyroids (including those of nodular Graves' disease) are usually more resistant and require larger doses.
- Bulkier thyroid glands demonstrate diminished response.
- Prior administration of antithyroid drugs increases resistance.
- Patients with severe hyperthyroidism may likewise be less responsive, possibly based on the rapid turnover of ^{131}I within the gland.

Although there is a clear correlation between the dose of radioiodine used and the onset of hypothyroidism in the first year after therapy, the incidence of hypothyroidism after that time shows less correlation with the dose used. At least half of patients exhibit hypothyroidism 10 years after therapy regardless of the ^{131}I dose regimen chosen. Therefore, careful follow-up is necessary in all patients who become initially euthyroid, to watch for the development of late hypothyroidism. In our experience, unless the gland is very large, a one-time orally administered activity of 15 mCi (555 MBq) is all that is needed to treat 90% to 95% of patients with Graves' disease successfully, and 25 mCi (925 MBq) cures about 80% to 90% of patients with a toxic nodular goiter. Aside from latent hypothyroidism, other complications of radioiodine therapy for hyperthyroidism are rare. There is no evidence of increased incidence of radiation-induced malignancies, including thyroid cancer and leukemia, after radioiodine therapy for hyperthyroidism. No change in fertility rates or genetic damage in offspring has been found. Thyroid storm occurs in less than 0.1% of patients, and clinically significant radiation thyroiditis is uncommon. In patients with Graves' disease and orbitopathy, the subsequent radiation-induced hypothyroidism confers an increased risk of exacerbation. This can be minimized by concurrent oral prednisone therapy or prompt T_4 replacement. Patients without orbitopathy are unlikely to develop it after radioiodine treatment.

Patient Preparation

Before the oral administration of a therapeutic dose of ^{131}I, the diagnosis of toxic goiter must have been firmly established on the basis of physical examination, history, and elevated circulating serum thyroid hormone levels and depressed TSH. An ^{131}I uptake should be routinely performed to exclude hyperthyroidism due to certain diseases, such as silent, painless thyroiditis, and to gauge the dose required. The patient should take nothing by mouth after midnight the evening before treatment. Female patients should be carefully screened for possible pregnancy, which is a contraindication for radioiodine therapy because of possible carcinogenic risk to the fetus and risk of injury to the fetal thyroid gland after the first trimester. In lactating mothers, therapy should be instituted only if the patient is willing to completely cease breastfeeding because the iodine is secreted in breast milk.

Severely hyperthyroid patients with marked symptoms may be pretreated with antithyroid drugs to avoid worsening the clinical status or causing thyroid storm, which results from the sudden release of hormone from the gland after radiation destruction of thyroid follicles. For most patients, however, this pretreatment is unnecessary.

If antithyroid drugs are already in use, they should be discontinued for 5 to 7 days before the ^{131}I treatment is administered, depending on the clinical status of the patient. If clinically necessary, these drugs may be readministered 7 to 10 days after therapy without adversely affecting the results of treatment. As an alternative, β-adrenergic blocking agents, such as propranolol, may be used throughout the therapy period because they do not affect thyroid function and therefore permit recirculation of ^{131}I in the gland for maximum radiation effect.

In the first week after a therapeutic dose of radioiodine, a patient may experience several symptoms, including sore throat, dysphagia, and an increase in hyperthyroid symptoms due to increased release of hormone from radiation-damaged follicles. Patients should drink as much fluid as possible and void often to reduce whole-body and bladder radiation doses.

Whichever dose regimen is used, there is generally no significant improvement in hyperthyroid symptoms for about 3 to 4 weeks after treatment. In adequately treated patients with diffuse toxic goiter, however, a significant shrinkage in the size of the gland is usually identified in the first month after therapy. If, after 3 to 4 months, the patient still has signs, symptoms, or laboratory evidence of hyperthyroidism, a repeat dose of ^{131}I may be administered.

Thyroid Carcinoma

Iodine-131 therapy remains a valuable adjunct in thyroid carcinoma therapy for ablation of postsurgical residual thyroid tissue in the neck and for eradication of functioning local and distant thyroid metastases. Although most thyroid cancers are well differentiated and have an excellent prognosis when treated appropriately, 75% of the deaths from thyroid cancer occur from these initially well-differentiated lesions. Because thyroid cancer may undergo transformation into more aggressive forms with time, it is very important to detect and eradicate the lesions in their early stage while they are capable of concentrating radioiodine and thus can be successfully treated with ^{131}I.

Postsurgical Ablation

Radioiodine "ablation" typically refers to the destruction of functioning remnants of normal thyroid tissue remaining after subtotal thyroidectomy. Whole-body thyroid imaging is usually performed 4 to 6 weeks after thyroidectomy to detect residual functioning tissue in the thyroid bed and any possible distant metastases. The scan assists in determining the size of the ablation dose needed, depending on the amount of residual thyroid tissue and any unsuspected metastatic foci.

Surgery is seldom able to effect removal of all of the functioning thyroid tissue, even in the best hands. Residual tissue may be confused with local nodal metastatic disease when postsurgical scan-

ning is performed. In addition, through suppression of endogenous TSH, residual thyroid tissue in the neck significantly reduces the likelihood that distant metastatic lesions will be visualized with follow-up whole-body ^{131}I scanning techniques. Therefore, ^{131}I ablation of remaining thyroid tissue in the neck is a convenient and relatively inexpensive method for obtaining the desired results of total thyroidectomy. Further, radioiodine ablation after surgical removal of the thyroid is associated with a deceased risk of recurrence and death in patients with well-differentiated thyroid cancer.

The amount of administered activity used after surgery to ablate residual normal thyroid is a matter of debate. In many hospitals, this depends on the particular characteristics of the tumor and the assumed risk level of recurrence. In lower-risk situations of residual postsurgical functioning tissue in which the primary tumor is less than 1.5 cm and has not invaded the thyroid capsule, ablation of a remnant can be done with 29.9 mCi (1.1 GBq) or less of ^{131}I.

In higher-risk patients, those with vessel, lymphatic or capsular invasion, a primary lesion of greater than 1.5 cm, poorly differentiated cell types, metastasis, or multifocal lesions, high-dose therapy (>30 mCi) in the range of 100 to 200 mCi (3.7 to 7.4 GBq), should be used. The rationales are that the residual normal thyroid remnant can be used as a source of radiation to nearby tissues and that the first chance at tumor cure will be the best chance. Because well-differentiated thyroid cancers tend to be more aggressive in older patients, high-dose therapy is also recommended for treatment of patients older than 45 years of age.

In the uncommon case in which a surgeon has actually removed all the normal thyroid tissue and in which the whole-body scan is negative, high-dose therapy can be used with some modifications. If the tumor was less than 1.5 cm, was well differentiated, and had no capsular invasion, the patient may be placed on thyroid hormone and monitored by serum Tg measurements. Whether a patient with no residual thyroid and no functioning metastases seen on imaging should be treated with ^{131}I remains a matter of controversy. In this setting, ^{131}I ablation may be desirable whether or not residual thyroid tissue or metastases are identified—the rationale being that such therapy may destroy undetectable, functioning micrometastases. On follow-up, patients with elevated Tg levels may show improvement with repeat high-dose ^{131}I therapy even in the presence of a negative ^{131}I scan. After ablation therapy, imaging may be performed 4 to 10 days after treatment by using the residual ^{131}I activity. Thyroid replacement may be instituted 3 to 5 days after the administration of therapy. Re-examination after ablation in 6 to 12 months is typical, and therapy is repeated if residual thyroid tissue is found.

Functioning Metastases

Doses for the eradication of well-differentiated thyroid metastases are high, usually 100 to 200 mCi (3.7 to 7.4 GBq). Iodine-131 may be administered up to 5 or 10 times, usually at about 6-month to yearly intervals. Typically, if metastases persist after three treatments, future therapy is not likely to be curative, although it may be palliative. In some institutions, increased radiation dose from ^{131}I to the functioning tissue is achieved by depleting the extracellular iodide pool using pretherapy low-iodine diets or drug-induced diuresis, although this is not a common practice. In any case, serum TSH levels should be in excess of 30 μU/mL after an appropriate period of thyroid hormone withdrawal to facilitate uptake of the therapy dose of ^{131}I by the functioning lesions. In preparing patients, rhTSH can be used at the physician's discretion to supplement endogenous serum TSH levels as needed.

When patients are treated for functioning pulmonary thyroid metastases, pulmonary fibrosis is a possible complication, especially as cumulative doses exceed 600 mCi (22 GBq). Further, repeat doses of ^{131}I may produce changes in salivary gland function, leading to the unpleasant and irreversible side effect of xerostomia (dry mouth). Thus, after each treatment patients should be instructed stimulate saliva flow over several days through the use of items such as hard candy (e.g., lemon drops) to reduce radiation to the salivary glands.

In patients with extensive metastatic lesions or in whom repeat therapeutic administrations are contemplated, monitoring of the hematologic status is desirable because bone marrow suppression may occur in patients with large absorbed radiation doses. Significant bone marrow depression is likely when cumulative administered activities exceed 800 mCi (29.6 GBq). Because of the high doses used in therapy, strict radiation protection procedures must be outlined and carefully followed. According to prior NRC regulations, any patient with ^{131}I activity in excess of 29.9 mCi (1.1 GBq) needed to be hospitalized. This is still true in some agreement states. Current NRC regulations permit release based on (1) administered activity (<33 mCi or 1.2 GBq) for ^{131}I, (2) measured dose rate at 1 m from the patient (<7 mrem/h for ^{131}I), or (3) patient-specific dose calculations that indicate that the maximum likely dose to another individual is no greater than 0.5 rem (5 mSv) in any 1 year (see Appendix H). Regulations regarding disposal of the radioactive urine vary from state to state. Patients are usually given thyroid hormone replacement several days later. Follow-up scanning is then performed at 6-month intervals, with ^{131}I therapy repeated as needed until the disease is eradicated. Patients may then be followed with serum Tg levels as described earlier.

An increase in secondary tumors as a result of ^{131}I therapy has been extensively examined. Most studies do not show an increase, although there have been suggested increases in leukemia after therapy for thyroid cancer, with a rate of about 5 per 1000 patients. Bladder and breast cancer incidence also may be slightly increased. Almost all of these cases have occurred in patients who received cumulative activities in excess of 800 mCi (29.6 GBq).

Radiation Safety Aspects

Regulations regarding release of patients after nuclear medicine therapy are presented in Appendix H; however, a few important points are presented here. After diagnostic nuclear medicine procedures, precautions for the public are rarely required, but after some therapeutic procedures doses to the public and family members and others may need to be limited. Because ^{131}I is a frequently used high-energy gamma emitter and has an 8-day physical half-life, it is the radionuclide that results in the majority of the dose to medical staff, the public, and family members after procedures involving therapeutic administration of unsealed radionuclides. The major aspect of radiation therapy that needs to be controlled when releasing a patient with radioiodine is external exposure of others. However, the typical doses that occur to other persons from patients treated with radioiodine only have a very low risk of cancer induction. Approximate dose rates at 1.0 m from a patient treated for hyperthyroidism are 0.185 mrem/mCi (0.05 μSv/MBq) immediately after administration, 0.11 mrem/mCi (0.03 μSv/MBq) at 2 to 4 days after administration, and 0.07 mrem/mCi

(0.02 μSv/MBq) at 5 to 7 days after administration. Patients treated for thyroid cancer metastases eliminate iodine more quickly and approximate values at the same times are 0.185 (0.05), 0.011(0.003), and 0.007 mrem/mCi (0.002 μSv/MBq), respectively.

Internal contamination of family members from bodily fluids is most likely 1 to 7 days after treatment. The risks from internal contamination of other adults are less significant than are those from external exposure. Incorporation of large activities of ^{131}I in an adult caregiver or family member that might cause hypothyroidism is extremely unlikely. However, thyroid cancer as a result of radiation exposure appears to be a significant risk for unborn children, infants, and persons under the age of 20, and particular care should be taken to avoid internal contamination of infants and children. Contamination of infants and young children with saliva from a treated patient during the first several days could result in significant doses to the child's thyroid and potentially raise the risk of subsequent radiation-induced thyroid cancer.

Very low activities of ^{131}I are observed in the environment as a result of medical uses. Even with direct release to sewer systems, the relatively short physical half-life results in doses to the public or sewer workers well below public dose limits and low compared with other sources. No environmental effects have been linked to the levels of radionuclides released as a result of medical uses of unsealed radionuclides.

The International Commission on Radiological Protection (ICRP) recommends the concept of a dose constraint of a few rem (a few mSv) per episode for caregivers and family, whereas the recommended international annual dose limit for the public is 100 mrem (1 mSv). Infants and young children as well as casual visitors should probably be excluded from the dose constraint and be limited to the public dose limit. Continuation of breastfeeding is absolutely contraindicated after radioiodine therapy. Because the patient may need to be retreated with radioiodine, pregnancy is contraindicated until at least 6 months after radioiodine therapy.

PARATHYROID IMAGING AND LOCALIZATION

Hyperparathyroidism occurs with a frequency of about 0.5 per 1000, with approximately half of the persons being asymptomatic and detected by serum calcium screening. Those with symptoms may have recurring nephrolithiasis, frank hypercalcemia with low serum phosphate, weakness, fatigue, and bone pain.

Because of the small size and location of the normal parathyroid glands, imaging with most modalities is difficult. Normally, there are two pairs of parathyroid glands usually located on the posterolateral surface of the upper and lower lobes of the thyroid. About 80% to 85% of parathyroid adenomas are found adjacent to the thyroid, but the remainder are ectopically placed and may be in the anterior or posterior superior mediastinum, within or next to the thymus, along the esophagus, along the carotid sheath, or even at the carotid bifurcation. This variation results in 5% of hyperfunctional parathyroid lesions being missed at the initial surgical procedure.

Hyperfunctioning glands, however, can be imaged by using nuclear medicine techniques. Eighty percent to 85% of cases of primary hyperparathyroidism are due to single or multiple hyperfunctioning adenomas. Hyperplasia accounts for 12% to 15% of cases and parathyroid carcinomas for about 1% to 3% of cases.

Technetium-99m sestamibi is the radiopharmaceutical of choice for imaging hyperplastic parathyroid glands and adenomas because of its good energy characteristics for imaging and its avid localization in the mitochondria of parathyroid tissue. Technetium-99m sestamibi has yielded sensitivity rates of about 90% in primary hyperparathyroidism but significantly lower rates in secondary hyperparathyroidism. No special patient preparation is necessary before these scans, but it is important to perform a physical examination specifically to palpate for nodular thyroid disease and other masses.

The basis of the examination is predicated on the selective uptake of ^{99m}Tc-sestamibi by both the thyroid and parathyroid glands. With this method, 20 mCi (740 MBq) is administered intravenously, and images are obtained at about 15 minutes and again at 1.0 to 3 hours. The complete technical/clinical protocol can be found in Appendix E–1.

Technetium-99m sestamibi initially concentrates in normal thyroid tissue, thyroid adenomas, parathyroid adenomas, and hyperplastic parathyroid glands. Activity in the normal thyroid tissue significantly decreases with time (Fig. 5–16). Thyroid adenomas and hyperplastic parathyroid glands initially have more intense activity than does

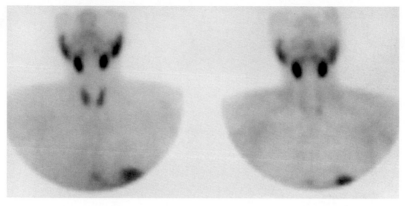

Ant immed   Ant 2hr

FIGURE 5–16. Normal parathyroid scan. An immediate technetium-99m sestamibi image of the chest and neck shows activity in the parotids, salivary glands, thyroid and left ventricle. On the 2-hour image the thyroid activity has faded almost completely, whereas the other areas remain mostly unchanged. The individual normal parathyroid glands are not seen.

the thyroid but also typically fade with time (Fig. 5–17). Most parathyroid adenomas are more intense than is the thyroid on the early images, but also retain much of their activity on the delayed images (Fig. 5–18) and become more visible. A majority of parathyroid adenomas greater than 500 mg can be detected with parathyroid scanning. Some thyroid adenomas may not fade as much as expected on delayed images, and some parathyroid adenomas may behave atypically by fading somewhat on delayed images. If delayed sestamibi images are inconclusive in either of these respects, it may be helpful to reinject the patient with ^{99m}Tc pertechnetate to see if the equivocal focus hyper-concentrates pertechnetate, as thus likely represents a thyroid adenoma, or presents as a relative defect, indicative of a parathyroid adenoma. It should be noted that ^{99m}Tc-sestamibi may also concentrate

and persist in thyroid cancers producing a false positive examination. Despite its established success in localizing hyperfunctioning parathyroid adenomas, ^{99m}Tc-sestamibi imaging is still unable to image hyperplastic or normal parathyroid glands consistently. Thus, some have advocated the use of single-photon emission computed tomography (SPECT) imaging to increase the sensitivity of ^{99m}Tc-sestamibi examinations for parathyroid lesions. Parathyroid imaging is especially useful in patients with negative neck explorations and recurrent or persistent hypercalcemia (Fig. 5–19). Because of the possibility of ectopic parathyroid adenomas, a routine large-field view of the chest and mediastinum should be performed.

Many surgeons will routinely use either ultrasound or radionuclide parathyroid imaging before surgery. However, radionuclide methods also are

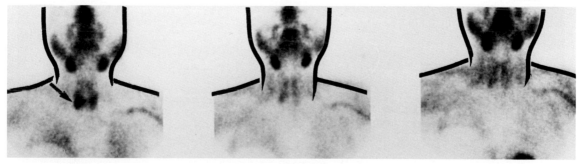

15 min   1 hour   3 hours

FIGURE 5–17. Thyroid adenoma on early and delayed technetium-99m sestamibi images. The thyroid adenoma (*arrow*) is initially seen as an area of increased activity relative to the thyroid. Both the normal thyroid and the adenoma fade significantly on the delayed images.

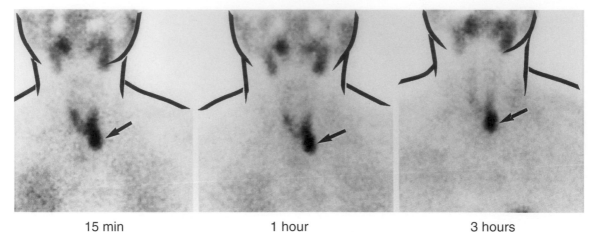

15 min   1 hour   3 hours

FIGURE 5–18. Parathyroid adenoma. The parathyroid adenoma (located at the inferior aspect of the left lobe of the thyroid) (*arrows*) is present as an area of increased activity relative to the thyroid on the early images. The parathyroid adenoma is persistent throughout the study as activity in the normal thyroid gland fades.

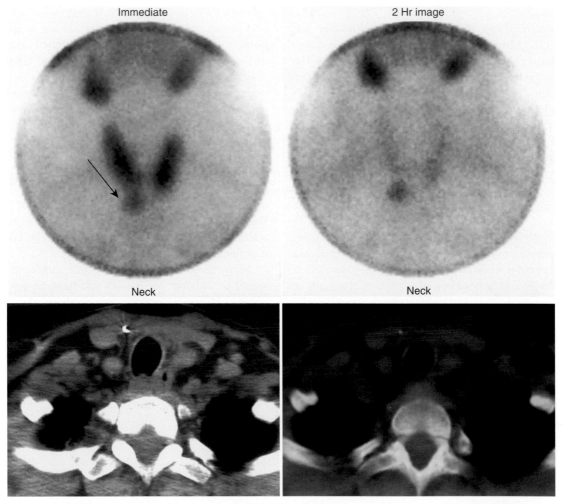

FIGURE 5–19. Ectopic parathyroid adenoma. In this patient who had unsuccessful surgery to find a parathyroid adenoma, technetium-99m sestamibi images show an area of increased activity below the thyroid (*arrow*). The activity persists on delayed 2-hour images. A single-photon emission computed tomography (SPECT)/computed tomography (CT) fusion study precisely localizes the lesion.

useful to locate the adenoma during surgery. The technique for intraoperative parathyroid localization involves injection of the patient with ^{99m}Tc-sestamibi about 2 to 4 hours before surgery and use of a small gamma probe during the operation to localize the parathyroid adenoma. This procedure is typically reserved for patients with a solitary parathyroid adenoma and a normal thyroid gland (to exclude confusion due to activity in a thyroid adenoma). After removal, the parathyroid adenoma should be counted and should be at least 20% and usually 50% higher than the thyroid background.

SALIVARY GLAND IMAGING

As noted in the discussion of thyroid imaging with ^{99m}Tc-pertechnetate, activity is seen in the parotid, submandibular, and sublingual glands. Although activity in these glands and in the saliva can be a source of confusion when imaging the thyroid, the concentration of pertechnetate in the salivary glands can help in the diagnosis and assessment of some salivary and parotid disorders.

Evaluation of suspected mass lesions of the salivary glands is best done by using computed tomog-raphy. Use of ^{99m}Tc-pertechnetate scans is generally reserved for functional evaluation, although most mass lesions, including primary tumors and metastases, are seen as areas of decreased activity. The exception to this is Warthin's tumor, which usually appears as a focal area of increased uptake. Warthin's tumors are benign parotid gland lesions, which predominate in elderly men and are frequently bilateral.

Functional assessment is performed by administering 5 to 15 mCi (185 to 550 MBq) of ^{99m}Tc-pertechnetate intravenously and obtaining 1-minute images of the salivary glands over about 20 minutes. Computer-generated regions of interest are placed over the glands of interest, and time-activity curves are generated for accumulation and clearance of activity. Trapping in the glands usually begins at 1 minute and reaches a peak in about 5 to 10 minutes. Stimulation of the glands with lemon juice usually results in rapid diminution of activity as saliva and ^{99m}Tc-pertechnetate are secreted. In patients with Sjögren's syndrome, there may be decreased accumulation of activity relative to the thyroid, as well as delayed clearance of activity from the glands. These findings may be asymmetric.

PEARLS & PITFALLS

A normal 24-hour iodine uptake in most laboratories ranges between 10% and 30% to 35%.

Common indications for radionuclide thyroid imaging are to differentiate between various types of hyperfunction (Graves' disease, toxic multinodular goiter, or autonomous adenoma) and to assess nodularity (cold or hot) and ectopic tissue.

Salivary glands are usually seen on ^{99m}Tc-pertechnetate scan unless the patient has Graves' disease. They are not seen on an ^{123}I scan.

A lingual thyroid is usually located in the midline at the base of the tongue, with no thyroid seen in the normal location. The ectopic gland is often hypofunctional.

A thyroid gland with an organification defect is usually seen as a normal gland on a ^{99m}Tc-pertechnetate scan but manifests no activity on an iodine scan in a child with a high TSH level.

A large gland with intense homogeneous activity is usually Graves' disease. A pyramidal lobe is commonly associated with Graves' disease.

A large gland with patchy activity is usually a multinodular goiter but could also be chronic thyroiditis or an infiltrative process.

Most hot nodules are benign hyperfunctioning adenomas. They can be single or multiple and can suppress the normal portions of the gland.

Chronic thyroiditis can mimic numerous thyroid conditions but on imaging is usually patchy and decreased in activity.

Subacute thyroiditis classically presents with a markedly depressed radioiodine uptake and nonvisualization of the gland in a patient with thyrotoxicosis and a tender, swollen thyroid.

Thyroid cancer is usually a single focal cold lesion and only rarely is seen to be diffuse or multifocal on thyroid scans.

Thyroid cancers may concentrate ^{99m}Tc-sestamibi and persist on delayed images. They are typically "cold" on ^{99m}Tc-pertechnetate scans.

PEARLS & PITFALLS—cont'd

If there is a rising serum Tg and a negative whole-body iodine scan, thyroid cancer can sometimes be visualized on a ^{99m}Tc-sestamibi or ^{18}FDG PET scan.

Activity in the bladder, stomach, and bowel and diffuse activity in the liver is usually normal on a whole-body iodine scan and is very unlikely to represent metastatic disease.

Whole-body thyroid scans may be performed with ^{123}I rather than ^{131}I. The ^{123}I scans have better resolution and may cause less stunning

Most patients with Graves' disease are treated with about 10 to 15 mCi (370–555 MBq) of ^{131}I, and most with toxic multinodular goiter are given about 15–29 mCi (555 MBq–1.1 GBq) of ^{131}I. Cancer treatment doses depend on the size and stage of disease, but most patients receive about 100 to 150 mCi (3.7–5.5 GBq) of ^{131}I.

After successful radioiodine ablation of residual thyroid tissue, serum Tg measurements are a sensitive method to detect recurrent thyroid cancer.

Iodine-131 treatment doses for thyroid cancer have been shown to be effective when using the following schedule:

Functioning tissue in the thyroid bed: 50 to 100 mCi (1.85–3.7 GBq) of ^{131}I

Cervical node metastases: 150 mCi (5.5 GBq) of ^{131}I

Lung or skeletal metastases: 200 mCi (7.4 GBq) of ^{131}I

The most common indication for parathyroid imaging is to localize the hyperfunctioning gland (adenoma) either in the thyroid bed or in an ectopic location (lower neck or mediastinum).

Parathyroid adenomas are usually single.

Parathyroid imaging is usually performed by using ^{99m}Tc-sestamibi with sequential mages over 2 hours. Normal thyroid tissue and thyroid adenomas usually fade over 2 hours, whereas parathyroid adenomas usually hyperconcentrate ^{99m}Tc-sestamibi and persist over time.

Decreased salivary uptake on a ^{99m}Tc-pertechnetate scan can be caused by the thyroid taking most of the activity (e.g., Graves' disease) or by a salivary problem (Sjögren's disease).

SUGGESTED READINGS

Intenzo CM, Capuzzi DM, Jabbour S, Kim SM, dePapp AE: Scintigraphic Features of Autoimmune Thyroiditis. Radio-Graphics 21:957–964, 2001.

Intenzo CM, dePapp AE, Jabbour S, Miller JM, Kim SM, Capuzzi DM: Scintigraphic Manifestations of Thyrotoxicosis. RadioGraphics 23:857–869, 2003.

McDonald DK, Parman L, Speights, Jr VO: Best Cases from the AFIP: Primary Hyperparaphyroidism Due to Parathyroid Adenoma. RadioGraphics 25:29–834, 2005.

Ma C, Xie, J, Kuang A: Is Empiric ^{131}I Therapy Justified for Patients with Positive Thyroglobulin and Negative ^{131}I Whole-Body Scanning Results? J Nucl Med 46:1164–1170, 2205.

Mariani G, Gulec SA, Rubello D, Boni G, Puccini M, et al: Preoperative Localization and Radioguided Parathyroid Surgery. J Nucl Med 44:1443–1458, 2003.

Martin WH, Sandler MP: Thyroid imaging. In Sandler MP, Coleman RE, Patton JA et al. (eds.), Diagnostic Nuclear Medicine, 4th ed. New York, Lippincott, Williams and Wilkins, 2003, pp 607–652.

Nguyen BD: Parathyroid Imaging with Tc-99m Sestamibi Planar and SPECT Scintigraphy. RadioGraphics 19:601–614, 1999.

O'Dougherty MJ: Radionuclide parathyroid imaging. J Nucl Med 38:840–841, 1997.

Robbins RJ, Schlumberger MJ: The Evolving Role of ^{131}I for the Treatment of Differentiated Thyroid Carcinoma. J Nucl Med 46:28S–37S, 2005.

Smith JR, Oates ME: Radionuclide Imaging of the Parathyroid Glands: Patterns, Pearls, and Pitfalls. RadioGraphics 24:1101–1115, 2004.

Tuttle RM, Becker DV, Hurley JR: Radioiodine treatment of thyroid diseases. In Sandler MP, Coleman RE, Patton JA et al. (eds.), Diagnostic Nuclear Medicine, 4th ed. New York, Lippincott, Williams and Wilkins, 2003, pp 653–670.

Cardiovascular System

6

INTRODUCTION

Clinical nuclear medicine studies play a pivotal role in the noninvasive evaluation of cardiac physiology and function. The widespread use of nuclear cardiovascular examinations permits the sensitive detection and diagnosis of numerous cardiac abnormalities as well as the determination of the functional consequences of disease.

Two general types of radionuclide imaging procedures constitute the primary thrust of cardiovascular nuclear imaging. These are designed to assess:

- Myocardial perfusion and viability
- Regional and global ventricular function

Extensive experience with these procedures in their appropriate clinical settings has proved them to be valuable noninvasive tools for the clinical assessment of cardiac disease with application to a broad spectrum of patients. Further, the addition of gated single-photon emission computed tomography (GSPECT) technique to myocardial perfusion imaging allows combined evaluation of coronary perfusion and left ventricular (LV) function in a single study.

ANATOMY AND PHYSIOLOGY

Because the heart functions predominantly as a pump, it is important to examine the physiology and anatomy related to this function. The volume of each chamber may be expressed as *end-diastolic volume* (EDV), which is the volume of the chamber after it is completely filled with blood at the end of diastole. Although the EDVs of the left and right ventricles are different, under normal circumstances, the *stroke volumes* (volume of blood ejected by each ventricle during systole) must be equal and normally range from 80 to 100 mL. *Cardiac output* is the volume of blood pumped by either ventricle over a period of 1 minute. It can be obtained by multiplying stroke volume by heart rate. The *ejection fraction* of a chamber is the measurement commonly used clinically, because it takes into account the EDV and the stroke volume. The ejection fraction is the percentage of EDV that is ejected by a ventricle during systole.

During systole, the LV normally shortens at least 20% along its long axis and 40% along the short axis as the various walls of the LV move inward. The apical portion of the LV moves inward the least, and the anterior wall moves the most and is the largest contributor to LV pump function. The septum thickens and moves slightly toward the center of the LV. Assessment of wall motion by nuclear medicine techniques depends largely on viewing ventricular wall segments in tangent. When identified, regional wall motion abnormalities are generally classified as hypokinetic (*diminished wall motion*), akinetic (*absent wall motion*), or dyskinetic. Dyskinesia indicates that a particular segment moves paradoxically outward rather than contracting inward during systole. It is associated with prior myocardial injury and usually indicates the presence of a cardiac aneurysm.

In the diastolic phase of the cardiac cycle, the myocardium first relaxes without a change in volume but with an exponential decline in LV pressure. This is referred to as *isovolumic relaxation*. As the ventricular pressure falls below that of the left atrium, the mitral valve opens, and the early, rapid-filling phase is initiated. This is followed by diastasis, the third and final phase of diastole, which begins with the decline of passive filling and ends with the onset of an atrial "kick" that concludes diastole (Fig. 6–1).

The heart muscle is supplied by the right and left coronary arteries. The major branches of the left coronary artery are the left anterior descending (LAD) and circumflex coronary arteries (Fig. 6–2). The LAD branch supplies the interventricular septum anteriorly, primarily through the first septal perforator branch, and the anterolateral wall of the

LV, primarily by multiple diagonal branches. The left circumflex branch supplies the left atrium and the posterolateral wall of the LV, primarily through its obtuse marginal branch. The right coronary artery has an acute marginal branch and often terminates as the posterior descending artery. It supplies the right atrium, the right ventricle, the inferior wall of the LV, and a variable portion of the interventricular septum. In 80% of people, the right coronary artery is dominant even though it is usually smaller. Dominance is determined by which main coronary artery, right or left, gives rise to the posterior descending coronary artery, which supplies the inferior wall of the heart.

The normal coronary blood flow is about 0.6 to 0.8 mL/min/g of myocardium. With exercise or pharmacologic stress, however, both the coronary flow and the cardiac output may increase four- to sixfold. Myocardial blood flow is greatest during diastole because at this time the blood flows fastest through vessels that are not being constricted by the surrounding cardiac muscle. These flow changes with the cardiac cycle are much more prominent in the left coronary artery than in the right, owing to the larger mass and higher pressure achieved by the LV muscle. When the narrowing of a coronary artery diameter is less than 50% of the diameter of the vessel, the effect on blood flow generally is clinically insignificant. As diameter narrowing approaches 70%, the lesions become much more hemodynamically significant, particularly during exercise. To be significant at rest, 90% or greater narrowing is usually required.

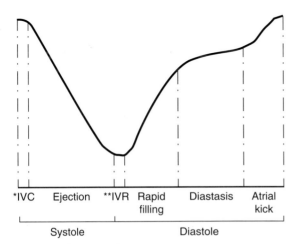

*IVC   Ejection   **IVR   Rapid   Diastasis   Atrial
                           filling   kick

        Systole   Diastole

* Isovolumic contraction

** Isovolumic relaxation

FIGURE 6–1. Time-activity curve obtained from a region of interest placed over the left ventricle. The curve reflects changes in left ventricular volume over one cardiac cycle.

SPECT MYOCARDIAL PERFUSION IMAGING

Imaging of myocardial perfusion with radiopharmaceuticals is the most commonly performed cardiac examination in clinical nuclear medicine practice. Its primary goal is to determine the adequacy of blood flow to the myocardium, especially in conjunction with exercise or pharmacologic stress for the detection and evaluation of coronary artery disease (CAD). Although the basic principles are similar, protocols for imaging vary among the radiopharmaceuticals used. Myocardial perfusion imaging may be performed by using one of several technetium-99m (⁹⁹ᵐTc)-labeled agents, thallium-201 (²⁰¹Tl) chloride, or positron-emitting radiopharmaceuticals. The state of the art for myocardial perfusion imaging is SPECT with electrocardiogram (ECG) gating (GSPECT). This

ANTERIOR

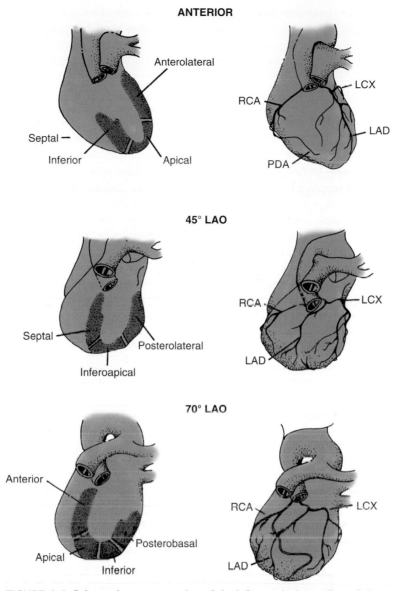

FIGURE 6–2. Schematic representation of the left ventricular walls and the associated blood supply. RCA, right coronary artery; PDA, posterior descending artery; LCX, left circumflex artery; LAD, left anterior descending artery; LAO, left anterior oblique view.

procedure is capable of producing excellent tomographic images of the myocardium reflective of regional perfusion in addition to LV functional parameters, which, taken together, provide enhanced physiologic assessment of the heart.

Principle

The diagnosis of occlusive coronary disease using radionuclide imaging is made by detection of relatively decreased myocardial perfusion distal to the site of vascular obstruction, compared with the more normally perfused surrounding myocardium.

The success of imaging depends on a number of factors, especially the degree of stenosis and its hemodynamic significance under conditions of increased myocardial metabolic demand, such as exercise. Because even severe stenosis may not produce detectable blood flow abnormalities at rest, some form of stress, either exercise or pharmacologic stress, is usually needed to render a flow differential that can be seen on myocardial perfusion imaging.

The myocardium is so efficient in extracting oxygen from the blood to meet metabolic demands that there is little room for improvement in extraction as metabolic demands increase during exercise. Thus, the heart satisfies increased oxygen requirements primarily by augmenting coronary blood flow, through the rapid dilatation of the vessels in response to oxygen deficit. This ability to increase blood flow from resting baseline to maximal levels is termed *coronary reserve*. In the presence of a fixed coronary stenosis, the ability of the vessel to dilate and thus the coronary reserve are diminished during conditions of stress. Under such circumstances, the myocardium supplied by the stenosed artery becomes apparent as a relative defect on myocardial perfusion images because perfusion to the involved area increases less than in the neighboring, relatively normally perfused tissue. Although stenoses of up to 90% of the arterial diameter may not produce a decrease in blood flow significant enough to be detected at rest (Fig. 6–3), stenoses of 50% or more are reliably detected with myocardial perfusion imaging under conditions of maximal myocardial stress. By comparing myocardial perfusion at rest (baseline perfusion) to perfusion under conditions of stress (maximal perfusion), areas of reduced coronary reserve indicative of stenoses and resultant stress-induced ischemia can be identified. These principles are the same regardless of the radiopharmaceutical or method of stress used.

Radiopharmaceuticals

Although ^{201}Tl was the first clinically successful myocardial perfusion imaging agent and is still used in many clinical settings, radiopharmaceuticals are now widely available with the imaging advantages of a ^{99m}Tc label. Because there are significant biokinetic differences among these radiopharmaceuticals, protocols for imaging vary, although the basic underlying physiologic principles and rationale for interpretation remain the same. A major determinant of protocol design is whether the administered radiopharmaceutical remains fixed in the myocardium, washes out, or redistributes in the myocardium over time. Because of these differences, the choice of radiopharmaceutical influences almost every aspect of the approach to imaging, including the timing and acquisition of image sequences. Thus, an understanding of the in vivo behavior of the radiopharmaceutical or combination of radiopharmaceuticals used to perform myocardial perfusion imaging is critical in determining the examination protocol and to the interpretation of the resulting images.

Thallium-201

Physical Characteristics. Thallium-201 is a cyclotron-produced radionuclide that decays by electron capture, with a half-life of about 73 hours. On decay, the major emissions are characteristic x-rays of the daughter product, mercury-201 (^{201}Hg), with an energy range of 69 to 81 keV. These are the primary photons used in myocardial imaging. Thallium-201 also emits smaller numbers of gamma rays at energies of 135 keV and 167 keV. The relatively long physical half-life of ^{201}Tl is advantageous, providing convenient shelf storage

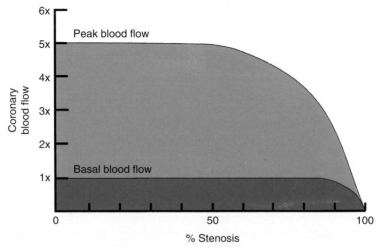

FIGURE 6–3. Relationship of coronary blood flow at exercise (peak blood flow) and rest (basal blood flow) relative to the percentage diameter of coronary artery stenosis (diameter narrowing).

and successful imaging over a period of hours. The long half-life, however, also increases absorbed dose to the patient and limits the amount that can be administered. The relatively low administered activity requires longer imaging acquisition times and results in lower-count densities with inferior contrast resolution compared to ^{99m}Tc-labeled radiopharmaceuticals. Further, soft-tissue absorption of the low-energy emissions of ^{201}Tl increases the likelihood of attenuation artifacts from overlying breasts and diaphragm, producing spurious defects that decrease the specificity of the study.

Biokinetics. Thallium is a group IIIA metallic element with biokinetic properties similar but not identical to potassium. Like potassium, thallium crosses the cell membrane by active transport mechanisms, especially the adenosine triphosphate (ATP)-dependent Na^+-K^+ pump. After intravenous administration, it ultimately has a mainly intracellular distribution. Thallium localizes in the myocardium in two phases: (1) initial distribution based on blood flow and cellular extraction by viable myocardium, and (2) delayed redistribution in the myocardium mediated by a dynamic equilibrium based on the continued extraction of thallium from the blood and ongoing washout of previously extracted thallium from the cells.

The extraction of thallium from the blood by viable myocardial cells is rapid, approaching 90% extraction efficiency. However, the total amount of thallium ultimately accumulating in the normal heart is limited by the concentration of thallium circulating through the coronary blood supply. Therefore, only about 3% to 5% of the total injected dose is localized in the heart.

Under resting and normal stress conditions, regional myocardial uptake of ^{201}Tl is linearly related to the regional coronary perfusion. Decreased perfusion to an area of myocardium results in a decrease in thallium accumulation in that region, compared with adjacent areas of relatively normal activity. Animal studies have shown that a flow differential between normally perfused and poststenotic ischemic myocardium of about 2 : 1 is required before a definite defect is noted on thallium imaging. At maximum exercise, a 50% stenosis is generally sufficient to consistently present as a defect.

After the rapid initial uptake of ^{201}Tl by the normal myocardium, there begins a slower process of washout of the thallous ion from the myocardial intracellular compartment back into the vascular compartment. At the same time, however, there is representation of additional bloodborne thallium to the myocardial cells for re-extraction provided by the large pool of the injected radioisotope that was initially held by other organs of the body. These simultaneous processes of thallium washout and re-extraction across the cell membrane provide a means for a dynamic equilibrium between intracellular and extracellular thallium, which defines the phenomenon known as *redistribution*. The washout component of redistribution depends strongly on coronary perfusion, with ischemic areas demonstrating much slower washout than normal regions.

Because of the more rapid washout of thallium from normally perfused tissue and the slower washout from myocardium that became ischemic at stress, the delayed redistribution images show an ultimate equalization of activity between the normal and ischemic tissue under most circumstances. Thus, on postexercise thallium images, a defect indicative of relatively decreased perfusion should disappear on later redistribution images if the initial defect was caused by transient reversible stress-induced ischemia. A nonreversible defect carries other implications and frequently indicates an area of scarring.

In addition to the myocardium, thallium is initially distributed in other tissues, especially those of the gastrointestinal tract, skeletal muscle, and kidneys, with only about 5% of the injected dose persisting in the blood 5 minutes after intravenous injection. This provides for myocardium-to-background ratios adequate for scintigraphic imaging. Exercise diminishes the activity within the gastrointestinal tract, particularly the liver, by reducing splanchnic blood flow. Thallium clearance from the body occurs mostly by urinary excretion, with only 4% to 8% cleared in 24 hours. About 3% of thallium localizes in the kidneys, which are the critical organs. The slow biologic clearance and long physical half-life result in an effective half-life in the body of 55 hours.

Technetium-99m Labeled Radiopharmaceuticals

The development of several classes of ^{99m}Tc-labeled radiopharmaceuticals that overcome the technical limitations of ^{201}Tl has led to their widespread use in myocardial perfusion imaging. These include principally isonitriles and diphosphines. Compared with ^{201}Tl, the technetium label confers the favorable characteristics of ready availability;

larger administered activity for better statistics, with reduced radiation dose to patients; and advantageous photon energy, producing higher-resolution SPECT images. The larger administered activity leading to higher myocardial count rates allows shorter acquisition times, with resultant decrease in patient motion and improved patient tolerance for the examination. The higher 140-keV photon of ^{99m}Tc also helps to minimize attenuation artifacts from the breast or diaphragm. In addition, good statistics and reasonably long retention in the myocardium of ^{99m}Tc-labeled radiopharmaceuticals optimizes GSPECT acquisition for evaluation of LV function and wall motion. Thus, myocardial perfusion and function can be assessed by using a single tracer.

In addition to the technetium label, a major distinction between the most commonly used ^{99m}Tc agents and ^{201}Tl is that, unlike thallium, the technetium agents do not undergo clinically significant redistribution and remain in a fixed myocardial distribution, reflecting regional perfusion at the time of injection. Thus, diagnostic evaluation comparing resting and poststress imaging requires two separate injections, one at rest and one at peak stress. In addition, whereas thallium localizes in the myocardium by active transport through the cell membrane, these lipophilic technetium agents enter the cells by passive diffusion. Nevertheless, like thallium, their deposition in the myocardium is proportional to regional blood flow, with regions of lower blood flow accumulating less of the radiopharmaceutical and thus presenting as areas of decreased activity (defects) compared with adjacent normal areas of relatively higher flow.

Whichever ^{99m}Tc agent is used, the overall sensitivity for the detection of CAD is comparable to that of thallium imaging, and the specificity may be improved, resulting in part from fewer attenuation artifacts.

Technetium-99m Sestamibi

Technetium-99m sestamibi (Cardiolite) is a lipophilic cationic isonitrile that is extracted by the myocardium with a first-pass efficiency of 60% and with lengthy myocardial retention (myocardial clearance half-time of >6 hours), primarily through binding to cytoplasmic mitochondria. Unlike thallium, there is minimal redistribution (<20%) over time in the myocardium. Advantages to this fixed distribution include the convenience of delaying imaging when necessary, without loss of sensitivity, and the ability to reimage in case of equipment malfunction, positioning error, or patient motion. However, lack of significant redistribution also means that imaging of myocardial perfusion under stress and rest conditions requires two separate injections of radiopharmaceutical. Because uptake of sestamibi in the myocardium requires viable cells with intact cell membranes, it has been advocated by some as a myocardial viability marker in addition to its primary use as a perfusion imaging agent. However, thallium is more commonly used in this setting.

After intravenous injection, initial concentration of sestamibi is highest in the heart and liver. Approximately 1% to 2% of the activity localizes in the heart at rest. Accumulation of sestamibi in the myocardium is directly proportional to blood flow at physiologic levels. However, at high flow rates (greater than about two to three times baseline flow), such as those achieved during pharmacologic stress, blood flow may be underestimated. Although there is minimal change in concentration in the heart, there is progressive clearance of liver activity through biliary excretion ($\approx 35\%$) into the bowel and ultimately into the colon, which receives the highest absorbed dose. There is also some ($\approx 25\%$) renal excretion (Fig. 6–4). Because adjacent or overlapping liver activity may interfere with cardiac imaging, enhanced clearance of activity from the liver and gallbladder may be accomplished by having the patient drink 8 ounces of milk or eat a fatty meal about 15 minutes after sestamibi injection. However, this may result in an increase in interfering bowel activity, especially when imaging is sufficiently delayed to allow passage of the radiopharmaceutical into the transverse colon and splenic flexure. When sestamibi is administered with the patient at rest, hepatobiliary clearance is slower but usually sufficient to permit imaging about 45 to 90 minutes after injection. Accumulation of sestamibi in the liver and gallbladder is relatively less with maximal exercise than at rest, so postexercise imaging may generally be obtained 30 to 45 minutes after injection. Postexercise hepatic activity is much higher if exercise is submaximal or pharmacologic stress is used.

Technetium-99m Tetrophosmin

Technetium-99m tetrofosmin (Myoview) is a cationic diphosphine with good myocardial uptake (1% to 2% of the injected dose with a first-pass extraction efficiency of $\approx 50\%$) and retention with little redistribution from the myocardium over time. Tetrophosmin underestimates myocardial blood

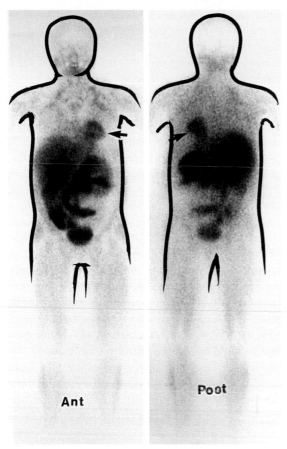

Ant

Post

FIGURE 6–4. Normal whole-body distribution of technetium-99m sestamibi. Postexercise anterior and posterior planar images demonstrate left ventricular (*arrow*) and skeletal muscle activity. There is also a large amount of activity in the liver, gallbladder, and bowel, as well as in the kidneys and bladder due to hepatobiliary and renal excretion routes.

TABLE 6–1.	Stress Myocardial Perfusion Scintigraphy

SOURCES OF FALSE-POSITIVE EXAMINATIONS
True Defects
Coronary anomaly
Coronary spasm (variant angina)
Noncoronary disease
   Mitral valve prosthesis
   Cardiomyopathies
   Aortic stenosis
   Myocardial bridge
   Idiopathic hypertrophic subaortic stenosis
   Conduction defects
   Left bundle-branch block (LBBB)
   Miscellaneous
   Long-distance runners
   Young females
   Ischemia of noncoronary origin
Apparent Defects
Artifacts
   Chest wall artifacts
   Breast tissue or pectoral muscles
   Breast prosthesis
   Electrocardiogram leads
   Braces
   Items in pockets, pendants, etc.
   Obesity
   High left hemidiaphragm
Excess patient motion (deep respiration)
Misinterpretation of normal variants
   Over- or underappreciation of apical defects
   Variant activity at cardiac base, proximal septal
     area, and posterolateral walls
   Papillary muscle attachments
   Small ventricular cavity

SOURCES OF FALSE-NEGATIVE EXAMINATIONS
Early or delayed redistribution
Submaximal exercise
Noncritical stenoses (<50%)
Small ischemic area
Isolated right coronary lesion
Coronary collaterals
Multivessel disease (balanced)
Overestimation of stenosis on angiogram
Interfering medication

flow at high flow rates (about two times baseline flow). There is rapid clearance of background activity from the blood pool. Similar to sestamibi, its cellular localization involves binding to cytoplasmic mitochondria. Its biokinetics are also in many ways similar to those of ^{99m}Tc-sestamibi. Less hepatic uptake and more rapid clearance from the liver after exercise, however, make imaging possible within 30 minutes of intravenous injection and minimizes the likelihood of artifacts associated with overlapping hepatic activity.

Imaging Protocols

SPECT is the standard for myocardial perfusion imaging with both ^{201}Tl- and ^{99m}Tc-labeled radiopharmaceuticals. As expected, SPECT imaging acquisition and processing protocols differ signifi-

cantly depending on the radiopharmaceutical used. However, regardless of the specifications, SPECT imaging is a technically demanding procedure. Strict compliance with SPECT quality-control measures and familiarity with study protocols established in each laboratory are essential for the standardization of the procedure and for achieving consistently accurate results. Some technical sources of error are listed in Table 6–1.

Exercise Thallium SPECT Imaging Protocol

Exercise is the most common form of stress for most patients undergoing myocardial perfusion imaging.

Because ^{201}Tl is the prototypical exercise myocardial perfusion radiopharmaceutical and because the protocol used elucidates the principles of stress myocardial perfusion imaging, a review of this technique is appropriate.

The SPECT thallium exercise test consists of an initial postexercise set of myocardial images and an identical set of delayed redistribution images. An outline of the procedure is presented in Figure 6–5.

Initial Postexercise Imaging. When using ^{201}Tl, 2 mCi (74 MBq) are administered intravenously at peak exercise. Because redistribution of thallium within the myocardium begins immediately at the termination of exercise and may be very rapid in some patients, imaging should commence as soon as possible, ideally within the first 10 to 15 minutes after exercise. This helps to ensure that the initial images reflect as nearly as possible the distribution of coronary perfusion at peak stress. In patients who exercise especially vigorously, a full delay of 15 minutes may be prudent to allow for respiration to calm so that artifacts from changes in the extent of diaphragmatic excursion are minimized.

For SPECT image acquisition, the patient is placed on the imaging table with the left arm over the head and with any interfering breast tissue uniformly compressed over the chest or elevated to minimize potential attenuation artifacts. Specific SPECT acquisition protocols vary among laboratories and depend largely on available instrumentation and the preferences of the imaging physician. When using a single-detector SPECT camera, a rotational arc of 180 degrees is commonly used, frequently beginning at the 45-degree

right anterior oblique (RAO) position and ending at the 45-degree left posterior oblique (LPO) position. When using a 64 × 64 computer matrix, 64 images are obtained over the 180-degree arc for a total study recording time of about 30 minutes. Although high-sensitivity or high-resolution collimators may be used, a low-energy, all-purpose collimator provides an adequate compromise between sensitivity and image resolution.

If available, multidetector cameras are preferable for SPECT acquisitions because they allow increased counts over the same imaging time or, alternatively, the same number of counts over a shorter acquisition than do single detector systems. Because the position of the patient during cardiac SPECT imaging is somewhat uncomfortable, and patient motion during image acquisition may severely compromise image quality, preference may be given to shortening acquisition times. Specific protocols vary with respect to the number of detectors used. After the completion of postexercise imaging and before the redistribution imaging, the patient is instructed to eat sparingly and to avoid strenuous exercise, even climbing stairs. In some laboratories, if the stress images are normal, the study is terminated; in others, a redistribution study is done routinely.

Redistribution SPECT Imaging. Redistribution images are obtained 3 to 4 hours after the initial set and reflect the staus of myocardial perfusion at rest. Ideally, these are performed on the same instrument that was used to perform postexercise imaging. Care is taken to reproduce the positioning of the patient so that it is as similar as possible to that used during postexercise imaging, especially with regard to breast and arm location. To ensure that adequate ambient thallium is available for redistribution, the administration of an additional

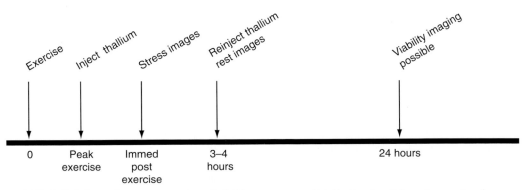

FIGURE 6–5. Schematic representation of thallium stress–redistribution (rest) imaging protocol.

dose of 1 mCi (37 MBq) of thallium before the second set of images (ranging from 1 hour before to immediately before reimaging) is helpful. In some laboratories, 24-hour repeat imaging may be performed in patients who exhibit nonreversible defects on the 4-hour redistribution images to determine with greater certainty any degree of reversibility of the postexercise defects.

Technetium-99m Radiopharmaceutical Exercise SPECT Imaging Protocol

The requirement of separate stress and rest injections of ^{99m}Tc sestamibi or ^{99m}Tc tetrophosmin to differentiate fixed from reversible defects has given rise to several different imaging protocols. These may be summarized as 1- and 2-day protocols (Fig. 6–6). The simplest approach is to perform the stress and rest examinations on two separate days. This allows the use of a full imaging dose of 15 to 30 mCi (555 MBq to 1.11 GBq) for each study, avoids interference in the subsequent study by residual myocardial activity from the first, and, if the stress study is performed first, permits omitting the rest study altogether if the stress images are entirely normal.

For reasons of patient convenience and timeliness of results, however, a 1-day protocol is the most frequently used. In this setting, either the stress or the rest study may be performed first, although the rest–stress sequence is the more widely used. Because of the long retention of sestamibi/tetrophosmin in the myocardium, it is necessary to adjust the administered doses so that activity from the first study does not interfere with the second. In the rest–stress, same-day protocol, 8 to 10 mCi (296 to 370 MBq) of ^{99m}Tc-sestamibi/tetrophosmin is administered at rest, with imaging performed about 30 to 60 minutes after injection, followed 1 to 4 hours later by stress imaging by using 25 to 30 mCi (925 MBq to 1.11 GBq), for a total administered dose of about 30 to 40 mCi (1.11 to 1.48 GBq). The patient should be encouraged to void frequently to decrease absorbed dose to the bladder and adjacent pelvic structures.

Image interpretation principles are virtually the same as for qualitative interpretation of thallium studies. Because hepatobiliary or other splanchnic activity may be a larger problem than with thallium imaging, any interfering activity should be taken

ONE DAY SESTAMIBI PROTOCOL

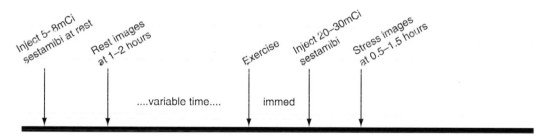

TWO DAY SESTAMIBI PROTOCOL

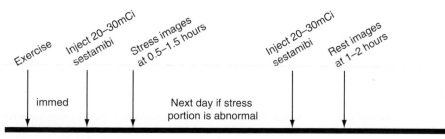

FIGURE 6–6. Schematic representation of 1- and 2-day technetium-99m (^{99m}Tc) sestamibi myocardial exercise protocols. The protocol using ^{99m}Tc-tetrophosmin is similar, except that rest images may be obtained as early as 30 minutes after injection of the radiopharmaceutical.

into account when evaluating the myocardial images, especially the inferior wall. In addition, since GSPECT is often performed with ^{99m}Tc sestamibi or tetrophosmin, the myocardial perfusion findings must be correlated with the LV wall motion and functional information obtained.

Dual Isotope Imaging: ^{201}Tl–^{99m}Tc Sestamibi/Tetrophosmin Protocol

Dual-isotope, 1-day, rest–stress imaging using separate ^{201}Tl and ^{99m}Tc sestamibi/tetrophosmin SPECT acquisitions is an efficient alternative to single isotope protocols. In this protocol (Fig. 6–7), a rest ^{201}Tl (2.5 to 4.0 mCi [92.5 to 148 MBq]) study is first obtained, followed shortly by a stress ^{99m}Tc sestamibi or tetrofosmin study (25 to 40 mCi [925 MBq to 1.48 GBq]), so that the entire examination can be completed within 90 minutes. The rest study is performed first with the lower-energy ^{201}Tl (68 to 80 keV) to prevent interference from the higher-energy ^{99m}Tc (140 keV). Because attenuation defects are generally more prominent on thallium imaging than with technetium agents, stress imaging is subsequently performed with ^{99m}Tc sestamibi or tetrofosmin to minimize false-positive examinations caused by such artifacts. Further, poststress GSPECT using ^{99m}Tc radiopharmaciticals may increase the specificity of any perfusion defects. Extra care should be taken in processing the two different sets of images because different parameters need to be used to optimize the image quality of each data set.

Myocardial SPECT Image Processing and Display

Image Processing

After acquisition, the poststress and rest (redistribution) images are reformatted in oblique planes. For structures with an oblique axis of symmetry in the body, such as the heart, the standard reconstructed cross-sectional views referencing the body are inadequate. Thus, image reconstruction of cardiac tomograms is performed in three planes that are perpendicular or parallel with the long-axis of the heart and oblique to the axis of the body; these include (1) short-axis (SA), (2) vertical long-axis (VLA), and (3) horizontal long-axis (HLA) images (Figs. 6–8 to 6–10). Generally, the primary operator input required for reconstruction is the identification of the long axis of the heart. This allows the computer to reconstruct tomographic images in three orthogonal planes relative to the orientation of the heart in the chest. Typically, the reconstructed slices are 1 to 2 pixels in thickness when a 64×64 matrix is used.

The quality of SPECT images is greatly enhanced by computer processing and display. The most frequent maneuvers applied to the raw data are background subtraction, contrast enhancement, and image filtering. These processes are meant to make the images more pleasing to the eye and to improve contrast by removing distracting, unwanted activity and statistical noise. A wide choice of image filters is available for image manipulation, commonly including Butterworth, Hamming, and Hanning filters. The specific filtering processes used vary greatly among laboratories and depend on the preferences of individual interpreters. Care must be taken not to overprocess images such that the data are distorted and artifacts are induced (Fig. 6–11).

SPECT Image Display

After processing is completed, the myocardial slices must be displayed in a fashion that facilitates com-

THALLIUM / SESTAMIBI PROTOCOL

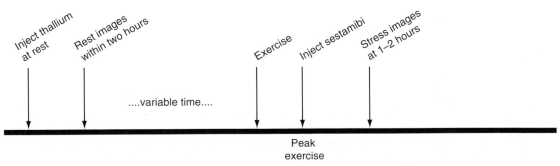

FIGURE 6–7. Schematic representation of 1-day thallium-201—technetium-99m (^{99m}Tc) sestamibi exercise imaging protocol. A similar protocol may be used using ^{99m}Tc tetrophosmin.

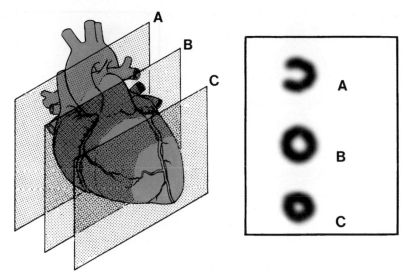

FIGURE 6–8. Short-axis sections through the left ventricle from the base of the heart to the apex are shown with corresponding single-photon emission computed tomograph (SPECT) slices of the myocardium. Note the considerable thinning of the proximal septal wall in plane A (the base of the heart) due to the membranous septum.

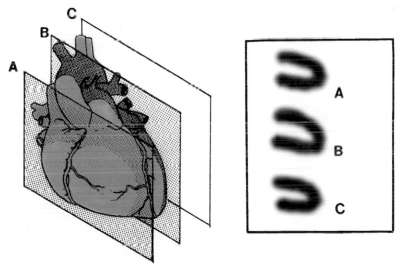

FIGURE 6–9. Vertical long-axis sections through the left ventricle from septum to free (lateral) wall are shown with corresponding single-photon emission computed tomograph (SPECT) slices of the myocardium.

parison of the stress and redistribution/rest image sets. It is attendant on the interpreter to ensure that corresponding slices between the two sets of images are displayed so that an accurate comparison is made. The orientation of the images obtained in each reconstruction plane is standardized to the generally accepted convention (Fig. 6–12). This is usually automatically performed by using the user software supplied by the equipment manufacturer. Generally, only tomographic sections that represent slices through both the myocardium and the cavity of the heart are used to avoid partial-volume artifacts. Subsequent interpretation is best performed by manipulation of the image intensity and contrast on the computer screen or the viewing station of a picture archiving system.

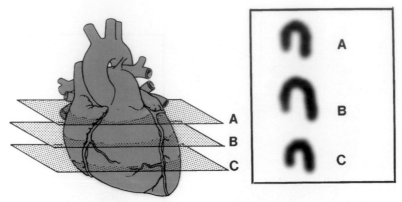

FIGURE 6–10. Horizontal long-axis sections through the left ventricle from the anterior to the inferior wall are shown with corresponding single-photon emission computed tomograph (SPECT) slices of the myocardium.

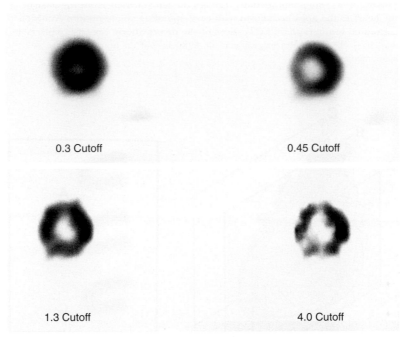

0.3 Cutoff

0.45 Cutoff

1.3 Cutoff

4.0 Cutoff

FIGURE 6–11. Effect of the cutoff value of a filter applied to a single short-axis image of the left ventricle. Sharpness of the image is improved with an increasing cutoff value, but artifactual defects may be created. The image becomes fuzzy with a low cut-off value, which may mask true defects. Obviously, the choice of filter may have great effect on the quality of the images and if not properly chosen, can produce false-positive or false-negative interpretation.

Bull's Eye (Polar Map) Display

In addition to the conventional display of tomographic slices, the entire three-dimensional perfusion distribution of a set of exercise or rest (redistribution) images may be condensed into one two-dimensional display by using a so-called polar or bull's eye map (Fig. 6–13). This display may be thought of as the heart viewed from its apex and opened up like an umbrella. Semiquantitative methods are applied to this bull's eye display of the SPECT perfusion data that compare the radiopharmaceutical distribution for each patient to a gender-matched normal database of distribution. Thus, regional activity less than that expected in a normal population identifies a perfusion deficit and

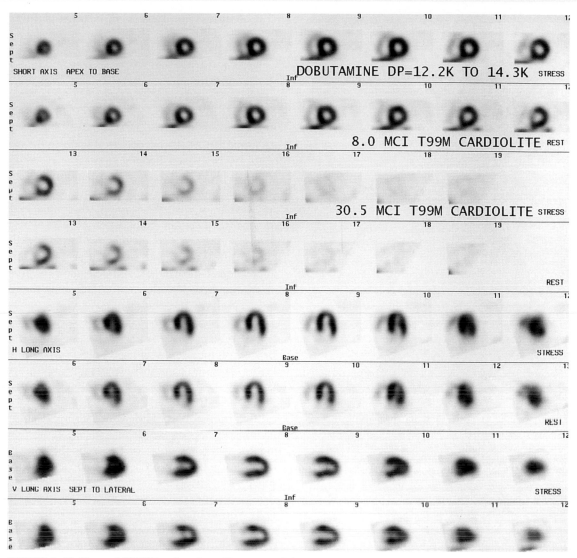

FIGURE 6–12. Normal SPECT technetium-99m sestamibi stress study. The upper four rows represent short-axis stress and short-axis rest images. These "slices" go from the apex on the left to the base of the heart on the right. The next two rows show horizontal long-axis stress and rest images, with the slices going from the inferior to the anterior left ventricular wall. The lower two rows are the vertical long-axis stress and rest images, going from the septum on the left to the lateral wall on the right.

is displayed as such on the polar map. The actual visual appearance of this deficit based on its severity is determined by the gray or color scale used. When using this display, however, the interpreter should be aware that perfusion defects at the base of the heart (outer circumference of the polar map) tend to be overemphasized, whereas centrally located defects, such as the LV apex, tend to be under-represented. The bull's eye representations of stress and rest (redistribution) myocardial perfusion can easily be visually compared in a third bull's eye display that shows the differences

in activity. This defines the reversibility or fixed nature of a perfusion defect. These bull's eye plots are a convenient tool to be used as an adjunct to standard visual image interpretation and to summarize a patient's perfusion pattern in a single image.

Interpretation

Approach to Interpretation

Consistent interpretation of SPECT myocardial perfusion images is best ensured by a systematic approach that includes the following elements:

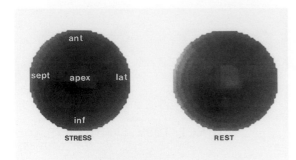

A

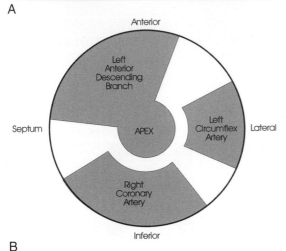

B

FIGURE 6–13. Normal polar (bull's eye) display of myocardial perfusion. *A,* Both the stress and rest images demonstrate relatively uniform activity without significant deviation from perfusion in age-matched controls. *B,* Approximate coronary artery distribution relative to the polar plot. The unshaded regions are areas of variable arterial supply. ant, anterior; lat, lateral; inf, inferior; sept, septum.

Proper alignment (co-registration) of the poststress and rest (redistribution) tomographic slices

Perusal of the images for obvious motion and attenuation artifacts, with review of sinogram or three-dimensional cine image as needed

Evaluation of the LV myocardium for the presence of perfusion defects and classification regarding size, severity, location, and degree reversibility, if any

Estimation of LV cavity size and any transient enlargement

Assessment of lung activity on thallium scans

Assessment of right ventricular activity

Assessment of interfering adjacent splanchnic (liver, spleen, or bowel) activity

Correlation with stress ECG findings and adequacy of stress

Correlation of findings with ancillary patient information, including history and clinical findings, prior coronary angiography or revascularization procedures, and previous myocardial perfusion studies

On GSPECT studies: evaluation of LV ejection fraction (LVEF) and LV wall motion with correlation with any perfusion abnormalities noted on the tomographic slices

Alignment of Images

An initial task of the interpreter is to assess the two series of processed images consisting of reconstructed stress and rest (redistribution) slices to ensure that they are properly aligned. Such co-registration of the slices in all three planes is essential for accurate comparison of perfusion in corresponding regions of the myocardium. Misalignment of the image sets may lead to a false impression of the fixed or reversible nature of areas of relative hypoperfusion and significantly reduce the accuracy of the examination.

Artifacts

Because tomographic images are composed of highly processed data, the interpreter should ascertain that the acquisition and resulting processed images are artifact free. If an artifact is suspected, careful examination of the raw data in a rotating cine display of the sequential planar projections aids in detecting gross patient motion, areas of significant soft-tissue attenuation and any superimposed liver or spleen activity. Other means for detecting patient motion, such as a sinogram (an abrupt break in the otherwise continuous sinogram stripe signifies patient motion), or a summed display of all the projections may be generated and viewed as needed. A thorough knowledge of SPECT imaging artifacts is critical in SPECT image interpretation (Table 6–2).

Attenuation Artifacts. Significant soft-tissue attenuation by large breasts or breast implants may produce spurious fixed anterior or lateral wall defects (Fig. 6–14) and considerable accumulation of adipose tissue in the lateral chest wall in obese patients may give rise to fixed lateral wall myocardial defects, if the patient is imaged identically in the postexercise and subsequent rest (redistribution) studies. Changes in positioning of the patient or of the patient's breasts in the rest (redistribution) images that make the attenuation defect less apparent than on the post-exercise images, however, may give rise to apparent reversible abnormalities.

Patients with left hemidiaphragmatic elevation may have spurious inferior wall defects due to focal

TABLE 6–2. **Single-Photon Emission Computed Tomography: Image Artifacts and Variants**

CAUSE	RESULT	RECOGNITION/CORRECTION
ACQUISITION		
Soft-Tissue Attenuation		
Breast or obesity	Anterior or lateral wall defect	Bind or elevate breast View rotating planar images View GSPECT 3D Cine (fixed defects) Use attenuation correction programs
Elevated left hemidiaphragm	Inferior wall defect	Prone imaging View rotating planar images View GSPECT 3D Cine (fixed defects) Use attenuation correction programs
Abdominal visceral activity (liver, gallbladder, spleen, bowel)	Relative increased inferior wall activity (overlap) Relative decreased inferior wall activity (reconstruction artifact)	Repeat study when activity passes
Patient motion	Myocardial defect (depends on type and direction of motion)	View rotating planar images or image sinogram Use computer motion correction algorithm
Postexercise respiratory motion ("Diaphragmatic Creep")	Reversible inferior wall defect	Delay immediate postexercise images 10–15 min
PROCESSING AND DISPLAY		
Oblique axis reconstruction; incorrect selection of LV long axis	Myocardial defects, frequently basal	Review long-axis selection
Scaling artifact	Apparent myocardial defect	Typical appearance; rescale images and compare appearance in different slice planes
INSTRUMENTATION		
COR Errors		
Rightward (+)	Posteroapical defect	Misaligned anteroposterior walls in horizontal-axis view
Leftward (−)	Anteroapical defect	Strict quality control and COR correction
Marked Flood-Field Nonuniformity	Ring artifacts	Strict quality control and field uniformity correction
NORMAL VARIANT		
Variable septal and apical thinning	Myocardial defects	Typical location
Papillary muscles	Focal myocardial hot spots	Typical location (2-o'clock and 7-o'clock positions in transverse images)
Cardiac Rotation		
Dextrorotation	Fixed relative lateral wall defect	History of congenital heart disease; hyperexpanded lungs; marked right or left selective chamber enlargement
Levorotation	Fixed relative septal defect	Inspect ECG and transaxial slices
NONCORONARY DISEASE		
LBBB	Reversible septal defect	Review ECG
Myocardial hypertrophy	Fixed relative lateral wall defect (lower lateral-to-septal count ratio)	Review ECG; history of hypertension or valvular heart disease

GSPECT, gated single-photon emission computer tomography; 3D, three-dimensional; LV, left ventricle; COR, center of rotation; ECG, electrocardiogram; LBBB, left bundle-branch block.

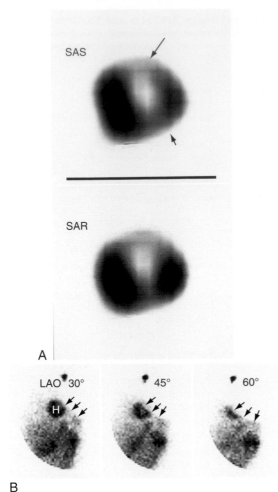

B

FIGURE 6–14. Single-photon emission computed tomography (SPECT) breast attenuation artifact. *A,* Both the short-axis stress (SAS) and short-axis rest (SAR) myocardial perfusion images demonstrate an anterior wall (*large arrow*) defect due to breast attenuation. The apparent defect is fixed because the breast position is similar on both the stress and rest images. There is a true defect in the inferior wall (*small arrow*). *B,* Soft-tissue attenuation of breast tissue can easily be appreciated on three-dimensional rotating views of the thorax. Here, selected planar image frames from the SPECT acquisition at different angles show the overlying breast tissue (*arrows*) having progressively more attenuation of the myocardial (H) activity as the SPECT camera rotates around the patient during acquisition. LAO, left anterior oblique view.

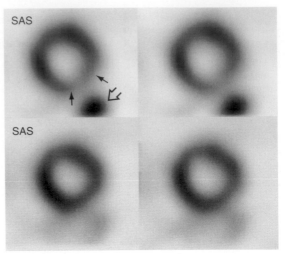

FIGURE 6–15. Reconstruction artifact. *Top,* Consecutive short-axis poststress images from a technetium-99m tetrophosmin myocardial perfusion study demonstrate a focal defect in the inferolateral wall of the left ventricle (*short arrows*) adjacent to a focus of intensely increased bowel activity (*open arrow*). *Bottom,* Repeat images after the bowel activity has passed from the area show the defect to have resolved. Such artifactual myocardial defects adjacent to areas of nearby extracardiac increased activity are a result of filtered back-projection, especially with the use of ramp filtration. SAS, short-axis stress.

attenuation. In addition to attenuation, intense liver, spleen, or bowel activity overlying the inferior wall of the LV may mask areas of decreased perfusion or may paradoxically produce an inferior wall defect (Fig. 6–15). This latter artifact is thought to be related to an inherent effect of filtered back projection on myocardial segments immediately adjacent to such areas of intense activity.

In addition to indirect approaches, such as review of the raw data as a rotating display of frames in a cine loop format, regional wall motion data available with GSPECT often allows differentiation of true fixed defects, substantiated as scars by locally diminished wall motion, from attenuation artifact with regionally preserved wall motion. Further, direct attenuation correction methods can greatly improve the specificity of SPECT imaging by eliminating or minimizing soft-tissue attenuation artifacts (Fig. 6–16). Although becoming more available, these technologies are not widely used. With the introduction of SPECT/CT hybrid scanners, however, this maneuver will likely become routine.

Motion Artifacts. Patient motion is a significant cause of artifactual myocardial defects, and the appearance of the scan artifact depends on the direction and degree of motion and whether it is abrupt or gradual. Motion-correction software may be used in many instances to salvage studies in which motion is not extreme. In patients who exercise vigorously, exaggerated diaphragmatic respiratory motion that persists after exercise and subsequently returns to normal may induce an

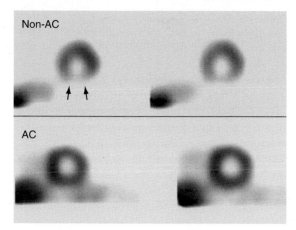

FIGURE 6–16. Attenuation correction. *Top*, Consecutive non–attenuation-corrected short-axis poststress myocardial perfusion images show an inferior wall defect (*short arrows*). Review of the rotating display of SPECT image frames suggested diaphragmatic attenuation. *Bottom*, Repeat imaging using an attenuation correction program corrects for the diaphragmatic attenuation and the defect is no longer seen. non-AC, non–attenuation-corrected; AC, attenuation-corrected.

artifact that mimics inferior wall ischemia, if the patient is imaged during this interval. This is produced as the diaphragm and thus, the heart subsequently "creep" upward during image acquisition. To avoid the upward *diaphragmatic creep artifact,* a delay in acquisition of immediate postexercise images for about 15 minutes to allow for hyperventilation to subside and the depth of respiration to return to normal is recommended.

Technical Artifacts. Artifacts during image reconstruction may occur if the long axis of the LV is incorrectly selected during processing. This generally results in overestimation or underestimation of activity at the apex. As expected, breaches in quality control of the imaging system, such as center of rotation malalignment and flood-field nonuniformity, may also produce significant image artifacts.

Normal Appearance and Variants

After myocardial perfusion images have been determined to be free of obvious artifacts or after any recognized artifacts have been accounted for and/or corrected, visual interpretation of SPECT images may proceed.

In the normal myocardial perfusion study, there is often slightly diminished activity at the LV apex, and in areas of anatomic thinning at the base of the intraventricular septum (membranous portion) and in the base of the inferior wall. Thinning at the base of the septum and inferior walls may be distinguished from true perfusion defects in that they are limited to the base of the heart and do not extend distally to the apex. These anatomic variants should not be mistaken for fixed perfusion defects. Defects that extend from the base to the apex should be considered abnormal. Furthermore, the lateral myocardium normally demonstrates more activity than do other myocardial territories, especially when compared with the septum in the short-axis slices. This likely results from the lateral wall being closest to the camera during much of the usable acquisition.

Areas of focally increased activity in and at the insertions of the papillary muscles frequently can be seen, especially on the short-axis images at about the 2-o'clock and 7-o'clock positions. These hot spots may give a false impression of a defect adjacent to or between them, owing to relative differential in activity, when in actuality the intervening activity is normal. The apparently diminished perfusion is often accentuated by the scaling of relative intensities in the displayed images based on the most intense pixel in the images (the markedly increased activity in the papillary muscles). This may artifactually suppress activity in the normal, but relatively less intense regions. These apparent differences in relative activity must be interpreted with caution. Generally, review of these areas in the long-axis slices, in which the papillary muscles are not as well seen, will demonstrate a homogeneous normal distribution in these regions, confirming a "scaling" artifact rather than a real perfusion deficit. However, significant perfusion defects which are also evident on the long-axis slices and are not attributable to artifact may be viewed as a positive finding.

Abnormal Scans

Visual Analysis

Myocardial Activity. Two distinct patterns of abnormal radiopharmaceutical distribution in the myocardium provide the basis for the detection and differential diagnosis of stress-induced ischemia and permanent myocardial damage. These patterns are referred to as (1) reversible (transient) defects and (2) nonreversible (fixed) defects. Defects may also be partially fixed with a reversible component. A third pattern, called *reverse redistribution (reverse perfusion defects)* is well documented, but its significance is less well defined.

True defects usually are visible on at least two of the three standard sets of reconstructed slices. In addition to the short-axis views, defects are often best seen on the long-axis image set in which the axis of the slices is perpendicular to the involved wall (i.e., the anterior or inferior wall on VLA images and the septum or posterolateral wall on HLA images).

Reversible (Transient) Defects. A reversible defect is virtually synonymous with stress-induced ischemia in patients with CAD. The abnormality is identified on the initial poststress images as an area of relatively decreased radiopharmaceutical activity that disappears or becomes significantly less apparent on the rest or redistribution views (Fig. 6–17).

Nonreversible (Fixed) Defects. Fixed defects demonstrate no significant change in activity between the poststress and rest or redistribution studies (Fig. 6–18). They most frequently indicate areas of scarring or fibrosis, usually after myocardial infarction, or areas of chronically ischemic, "hibernating" myocardium. Some fixed lesions identified on the initial poststress images may be partially reversible. Ischemia associated with a previous

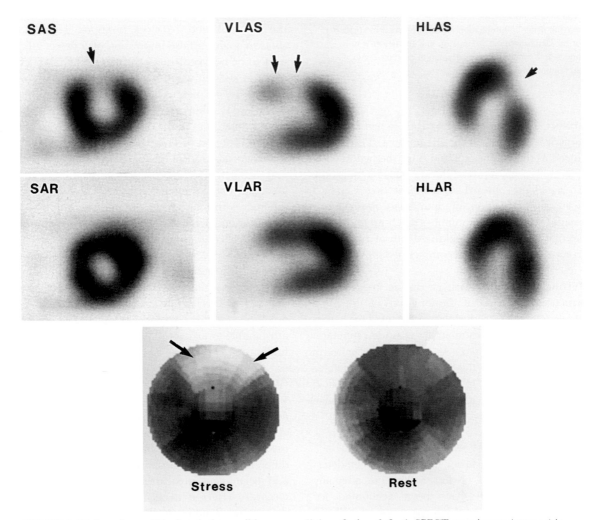

FIGURE 6–17. Anterior wall ischemia (reversible myocardial perfusion defect). SPECT stress images (*upper row*) in short-axis stress (SAS), vertical long-axis stress (VLAS), and horizontal long-axis (HLAS) stress images clearly demonstrate a perfusion defect (*arrows*). The rest images are seen on the *lower row*, and the perfusion defect has disappeared on the rest (redistribution) views. Bull's eye images confirm the perfusion defect at stress (*arrows*) but not at rest. SAR, short-axis rest; VLAR, vertical long-axis rest; HLAR, horizontal long-axis rest.

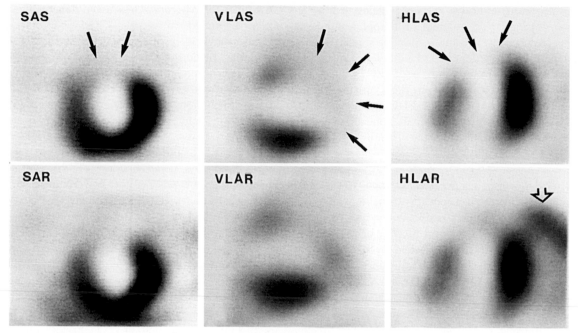

FIGURE 6–18. Left ventricular anterior/apical infarct (fixed perfusion defect). The *upper row* shows decreased perfusion (*arrows*) to the left ventricular anterior wall and apex on these short-axis stress (SAS), vertical long-axis stress (VLAS), and horizontal long-axis stress (HLAS) technetium-99m sestamibi SPECT images. The *lower row shows* that the anterior/apical defect persists on rest images in all three projections. Of note is activity (*open arrow*) on the horizontal long-axis rest (HLAR) image owing to sestamibi in the colon after hepatic excretion. SAR, short-axis rest; VLAR, vertical long-axis rest.

myocardial infarction with scarring (peri-infarct or "flanking" ischemia) commonly presents in this manner.

This straightforward approach to exercise–rest (redistribution) scan interpretation is complicated by the recognition that 30% to 60% of nonreversible, fixed defects on delayed thallium (3 to 4 hours) images or on rest images using technetium-labeled radiopharmaceuticals actually represent primarily viable myocardium rather than postinfarction scarring. In patients with severe coronary stenoses, these defects frequently represent chronically ischemic, but viable, "hibernating" myocardium that remains poorly perfused at rest with loss of functional wall motion. Fixed defects in viable myocardium may also be caused by "repetitive stunning," a chronic process of repeated, but transient episodes of ischemia in regions with or without normal resting perfusion that also leads to prolonged regional contractile dysfunction. There is some evidence that these conditions may be related and coexist in the same patient, and if recognized, both may be reversed by revascularization intervention with restoration of regional contractile function.

To differentiate hibernating myocardium from scar in patients with fixed myocardial perfusion defects, conditions that allow maximal accumulation of the radiopharmaceutical in the region must be provided. Thallium imaging offers a proven method to confirm myocardial viability in this setting, because thallium uptake in myocardial cells serves as an indicator preserved cell membrane function. Thallium uptake in a fixed perfusion defect with accompanying myocardial dysfunction predicts improvement of function after revascularization. If a stress–redistribution thallium imaging protocol was initially used, providing additional thallium, additional time for redistribution, or both is required. Reinjection of patients with additional thallium (1 mCi [37 MBq]) before 4-hour redistribution imaging and/or further delayed 18- to 24-hour imaging, are common approaches.

If the initial study was performed by using a technetium labeled agent, a thallium rest–redistribution protocol may be used on a separate day (to allow for radioactive decay). In this protocol, the patient is injected with thallium at rest and imaged immediately and again after a variable delay of 4 to 24 hours to image the chronically ischemic myocardium. Although delayed imaging at 3 to 4 hours using ^{99m}Tc-sestamibi or tetrophosmin has been advocated by some to provide similar information, it is less often used as a marker of myocardial viability. In addition to SPECT imaging, positron emission tomography (PET) imaging with fluorine-18 deoxyglucose (^{18}F-FDG) (as discussed in Chapter 13) may be used and appears to have improved accuracy for documenting regional myocardial viability.

Reverse Redistribution (Reverse Perfusion Defects). In

some instances, a scan appears normal or with only a slight defect on the poststress views and shows a new or worsened defect on the rest or redistribution images (Fig. 6–19). The exact mechanisms that produce this pattern and its significance are uncertain. However, reverse redistribution has been associated with prior myocardial infarction, especially after revascularization or thrombolytic therapy. This is likely to be due to some residual tissue viability, and some postulate that the regional hyperemic response to exercise may mask resting hypoperfusion in these areas. The finding does not indicate stress-induced ischemia.

Description of Myocardial Perfusion Abnormalities.

Once identified, myocardial perfusion defects should be described with reference to (1) the defect size (large, medium, or small), (2) severity of perfusion deficit (severe, moderate, or mild), (3) location (including the involved wall and expected coronary artery distribution, if possible), and (4) degree of reversibility, if any.

Lung Activity. The presence of excessive ^{201}Tl in the

lungs should be noted as part of the routine interpretation of postexercise and redistribution myocardial images. This activity may be visually assessed but is better quantified by calculating a ratio of lung-to-heart activity. This is performed by using counts from regions of interest created over the LV myocardium and the left mid-lung field just above the heart (Fig. 6–20). An anterior planar projection from a SPECT acquisition or a separately obtained anterior planar view of the thorax may be used. The accumulation of ^{201}Tl in the lung is variable, with a normal postexercise lung-to-heart activity ratio of about 30% to 50%. Abnormally increased lung activity (lung-to-heart ratio greater than 50%) on postexercise images has been consis-

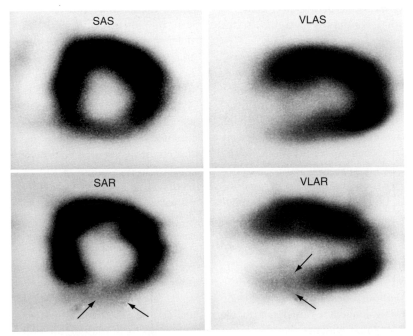

FIGURE 6–19. Reverse redistribution (reverse perfusion defect). The *upper row* shows SPECT myocardial perfusion stress images both in short-axis stress (SAS) and vertical long-axis stress (VLAS) projections that demonstrate slightly reduced perfusion of the inferior wall. However, rest (redistribution) images show that the defect is much more obvious (*arrows*). SAR, short-axis rest; VLAR, vertical long-axis rest.

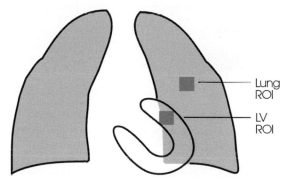

FIGURE 6–20. Schematic representation of regions of interest (ROI) for measuring lung-to-heart ratio of thallium 201. LV, left ventricle.

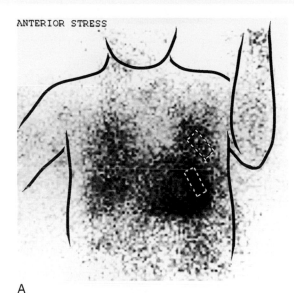

A

Normalized Counts	
Heart	: 22.600000
Lung	: 12.485437
Ratio	: 0.552453

B

FIGURE 6–21. Left ventricular dysfunction at exercise. *A.* An anterior view of the chest demonstrates abnormally increased thallium-201 activity in the lungs. *B.* Calculation of lung to-heart ratio using the regions of interest shown confirms an abnormally high lung-to-heart ratio of 55% during a ^{201}Tl exercise stress examination.

tently shown to be a marker of transient LV dysfunction at exercise (Fig. 6–21).

In the presence of CAD, the mechanism appears to be related to transient interstitial pulmonary edema caused by a rise in LV end-diastolic pressure secondary to stress-induced myocardial ischemia. Thallium leaking into the pulmonary interstitium appears as increased lung activity on the immediate postexercise images. As pulmonary pressure returns to normal and pulmonary edema subsides, the lung activity approaches normal on delayed images as thallium washes out of the lungs. Abnormally increased thallium uptake in the lungs correlates anatomically with multivessel CAD or high-risk disease involving either a high grade proximal LAD artery stenosis or a dominant left circumflex lesion. It correlates clinically with increased morbidity and mortality rates.

Because of differences in pharmacokinetics, increased lung activity is not generally seen under similar circumstances when ^{99m}Tc myocardial perfusion agents, such as sestamibi or tetrofosmin, are used, and calculation of a lung-to-heart ratios are not performed.

Transient Ischemic Dilatation (TID). Apparent transient LV cavity dilatation is present when the diameter of the LV cavity is visibly larger on poststress images (either with exercise or with pharmacologic stress) than on images obtained at rest. This should be distinguished from fixed cavity dilatation, which is present to equal degree on both sets of images and indicates pre-existing cavity enlargement. Underlying mechanisms for transient ischemic dilatation (TID) include transient stress-induced diffuse subendocardial hypoperfusion, producing

an apparent cavity dilatation (Fig. 6–22), ischemic systolic dysfunction and perhaps in some instances, physical cavity dilatation. In the presence of CAD, TID correlates with high risk disease (left main or multivessel involvement) and a worse prognosis.

Right Ventricular Activity. Right ventricular activity is a common normal finding on immediate poststress images, and is usually significantly less apparent on rest or redistribution views. Because of the greater administered activity and improved resolution on studies performed by using ^{99m}Tc radiopharmaceuticals, right ventricular activity may normally be more apparent compared with that on ^{201}Tl images. When the right ventricular myocardium is evident, any transient right ventricular defects should raise suspicion of right CAD. Significant right ventricular activity persisting on rest or redistribution imaging that approaches the intensity of the LV myocardium is abnormal and is often due to either right ventricular wall hyper-

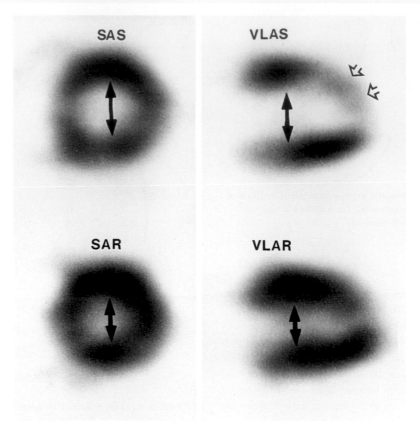

FIGURE 6–22. Left ventricular transient dilatation (TID) with exercise. The short-axis stress (SAS) and vertical long-axis stress (VLAS) images (*upper row*) show a much larger left ventricular cavity than seen at rest (*lower row*). This is a high-risk finding in this patient with coronary artery disease. Note the large reversible defect in the anterior wall consistent with stress-induced ischemia (*open arrows*). SAR, short-axis rest; VLAR, vertical long-axis rest.

trophy (Fig. 6–23) or increased workload ("strain") of the right ventricle in response to increased pulmonary vascular resistance.

Splanchnic Activity. Because splanchnic activity (liver and bowel) on postexercise studies generally decreases with increasing success of stress, the amount of such activity is a rough estimate of the adequacy of exercise. A large amount of activity suggests submaximal exercise, whereas minimal or absent activity suggests that significant exercise was achieved. Good myocardial activity-to-background activity ratios are also usually seen in patients with adequate exercise. With any myocardial perfusion radiopharmaceutical, a perusal of liver and bowel activity aids in identifying interfering activity that may affect image interpretation. Since the commonly used technetium-labeled radiopharmaceuticals are excreted into bowel by the liver through the biliary system, problematic intense activity may be seen in the liver, biliary tract, stomach (with bile reflux), transverse colon and splenic flexure, and occasionally the small bowel.

Quantitative Analysis. Visual interpretation of SPECT myocardial perfusion images is subject to considerable interobserver variability and depends markedly on the quality of the visual display. As an adjunct to visual assessment, computer quantitative analysis of myocardial perfusion images, primarily with the goal of exhibiting the relative distribution of the radiopharmaceutical in the myocardium as a function of space or time, may be used. These techniques permit a more objective and reproducible assessment of any change in activity within a given segment of myocardium between the poststress and rest (redistribution) images. This can be helpful in the documentation and quantitation of

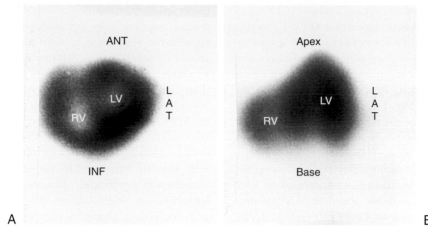

FIGURE 6–23. Right ventricular hypertrophy. On these SPECT myocardial perfusion rest images presented in both short-axis (*A*) and horizontal long-axis (*B*) views, the right ventricle (RV) myocardial activity is markedly increased so that it is equal to that of the left ventricle (LV). Ant, anterior; Inf, inferior; Lat, lateral.

areas of scarring or ischemia, especially for comparison with future studies obtained to assess the progression of disease or success of medical or revascularization therapy. Protocols for quantitative analysis of images, as well as the display of the derived information, vary from department to department and with different manufacturer processing software. In general, however, the principles underlying such programs are the same. Quantified data may include assessment of defect size, severity, and reversibility.

As previously discussed, bull's eye or polar maps are frequently used to display the processed data and to compare the perfusion data from a particular patient with a pooled database of gender-matched normal controls. A difference of more than 2.5 standard deviations below the mean is usually considered abnormal.

In addition to polar maps, numerical scoring to semiquantitate myocardial perfusion abnormalities can be used. One frequently used approach uses a 17- to 20-myocardial-segment scoring system based on dividing three short axis slices (distal, mid, and basal) selected to represent the entire LV into small regions, plus an additional apical segment. A five-point scoring per myocardial segment allows the calculation of summed scores, which can be used to represent global indices of myocardial perfusion. Each segment is scored visually as follows: 0, normal; 1, slight reduction of uptake (equivocal); 2, moderate reduction of uptake (usually implies a

significant abnormality); 3, severe reduction of uptake; and 4, absence of radioactive uptake. The summed stress score (SSS) is defined as the sum of the 17 to 20 stress perfusion scores (a measure of both fixed and reversible perfusion defects: infarcted and/or stress-induced ischemic myocardium), and the summed rest score (SRS) is the sum of the rest scores (a measure of fixed perfusion defects: infarcted and/or hibernating myocardium). The summed differences score (SDS) is defined as the difference between the SSS and the SRS and measures the degree of reversibility or ischemia, which reflects myocardium at risk. These scores provide a semiquantitative measure of the extent of total myocardial perfusion impairment as well as the amount of ischemic myocardium present, and allow risk stratification of patients depending on whether SSSs are mildly (SSS of 4 to 8), moderately (SSS of 9 to 13), or severely (SSS > 13) abnormal. Importantly, they also provide an objective expression of subjective visual interpretation as a means to compare serial studies with or without interval therapeutic interventions.

Gated SPECT (GSPECT) Imaging

GSPECT is the state of the art for myocardial perfusion imaging and is the most common mode of data acquisition and display in clinical practice. It combines all of the information contained in myocardial perfusion tomography discussed above in addition to relevant regional and global LV functional data. Nongated myocardial SPECT imaging is performed without respect to the cardiac cycle so that the images obtained represent data averaged during image acquisition by ventricular wall excursions of the beating heart. By synchronizing the collection of SPECT imaging data with the patient's ECG, the degrading effect of ventricular wall motion can be eliminated or reduced. In addition, cinematic display of the myocardial images is possible over the entire cardiac cycle, allowing the evaluation of wall motion and correlation with any evident perfusion abnormalities. LV parameters easily measured by GSPECT include LVEF and LV absolute volumes (end-systolic and end-diastolic). Because the RV myocardium is not adequately seen on the perfusion images, GSPECT is not used to evaluate RV function. Although GSPECT with ²⁰¹Tl is possible by using multidetector cameras, non-redistributing ⁹⁹ᵐTc-labeled myocardial perfusion agents are preferred because of higher count statistics, better imaging characteristics for the gamma camera, and more reliable and reproducible measurement of LV functional parameters.

Technique

The technique of gating to the cardiac ECG cycle is similar to that used during gated blood pool ventriculography (described in detail later in this chapter) but produces a dynamic image of the contracting myocardium rather than of the blood pool chamber. Definition of the LV walls uses automated computer software for detection of the epicardial and endocardial edges of the myocardium. Once the endocardial margins are detected, this defines the LV cavity throughout the cardiac cycle so that changes in LV volume can be measured and LVEF calculated. Depending on the time of acquisition, the GSPECT cine images reflect either resting or postexercise LV function. Because of the higher administered and thus higher myocardial activity, GSPECT is most frequently obtained during the postexercise acquisition, because the better imaging statistics permit more reliable definition of the LV wall. However, either or both the rest or poststress studies may be acquired in gated mode.

A typical poststress GSPECT acquisition requires 20 to 30 minutes. The study is usually acquired as 8 to 16 frames per cardiac cycle and is displayed in endless-loop cine format for visual analysis. Although 16-frame acquisition provides better temporal resolution, the increased number of frames requires a longer acquisition time. Thus eight-frame acquisition is more frequently used. It should be noted that an 8-frame acquisition results in about a 5% lower calculated ejection fraction than that obtained with a 16-frame acquisition. Software accomplishing automated reformatting of the SPECT slices into a three-dimensional cine representation is usually rapid, accurate, and reproducible. However, precise determination of the LV walls may be hampered by the presence of adjacent areas of significantly increased activity, usually splanchnic in origin, which are mistaken by the edge detection algorithm for myocardium (Fig. 6–24). Large severe perfusion defects, sizable LV aneurysms, or marked distortion of the LV for any reason may also create uncertainty for myocardial edge detection algorithms. These may lead to inaccurate results, especially when calculating LVEF and LV volumes. However, more focused operator input into the processing may overcome these problems in some instances.

Accuracy of the technique is also limited in patients with small hearts (often producing falsely high LVEF), such as some women and pediatric patients. Enlargement or zooming of the images may be helpful in these instances. In addition, poststress LVEF determinations (the most common GSPECT LVEF measurement) may be reduced from actual resting LVEF by the presence of stress-induced ischemia and accompanying wall motion abnormalities persisting into the poststress acquisition period and temporarily impairing LV function. This problem does not occur with ejection fractions obtained from a true resting gated acquisition. Thus, in reporting a GSPECT LVEF, it is important to specify whether it was obtained after stress or at rest.

As with all ECG-gated studies, severe arrhythmias (atrial fibrillation, heart block, frequent ectopic beats) may preclude successful gating so that nongated myocardial perfusion imaging is more appropriate. However, for less significant variations in cardiac rhythm, application of one of several software methods for rejection of aberrant beats allows valid data to be collected. This is usually accomplished by comparing the R-R interval of each beat during imaging to the average R-R interval of cardiac cycles (calculated prior to image acquisition) and excluding those cycles that vary by more than ±10% from the patient's mean. Although arrhythmia filtering increases imaging times, it is necessary, because the inclusion of "bad

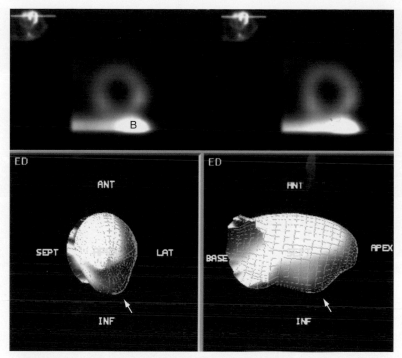

FIGURE 6–24. GSPECT edge detection uncertainty artifact. *Top,* Consecutive images from a ^{99m}Tc-sestamibi myocardial perfusion study show significantly intense bowel activity near the inferior wall of the left ventricle (LV). *Bottom,* The three-dimensional representation of the LV shows a bulge deformity (*arrow*) of the inferior contour of the LV with an accompanying wall motion abnormality. This bulge is a result of the myocardial edge detection algorithm confusing the adjacent bowel activity for myocardial activity, which was mistakenly incorporated into the contour of the LV. B, bowel activity.

beats" in the data set can invalidate results for both wall motion and calculated parameters such as LVEF.

Data Display and Interpretation

As expected, the routine display of coregistered sets of poststress and rest slices of the myocardium identical to that produced by nongated studies of myocardial perfusion are produced. In addition, a closed cine loop of cardiac wall motion can be displayed as both individual contracting slices as well as a three-dimensional representation of the entire LV viewed from multiple directions, such that all LV walls can be scrutinized (Fig 6–25). This allows correlation of segmental myocardial perfusion defects noted on the static slices with the presence or absence of wall motion abnormalities in the same region (Fig. 6–26). This permits more specific and accurate interpretation of suspected perfusion abnormalities.

Wall motion is visually assessed globally and regionally by the degree of endocardial excursion and by regional myocardial wall thickening during contraction. Wall motion abnormalities are categorized in the conventional manner as hypokinetic, akinetic, or dyskinetic. Because camera resolution and partial volume effect limit accurate measurement of actual wall thickness, wall thickening is inferred from local increases in count intensity or "brightening" during systole. Localized brightening has been shown to be proportional to regional wall thickening. To augment visual assessment, software programs supplying automated quantitative indices of regional wall motion and wall thickening are also available.

In addition to perfusion and wall motion, automated, user friendly computer programs supply values for LVEF and LV volumes, which add further significance to the results. As with all computer quantitation programs, the specific

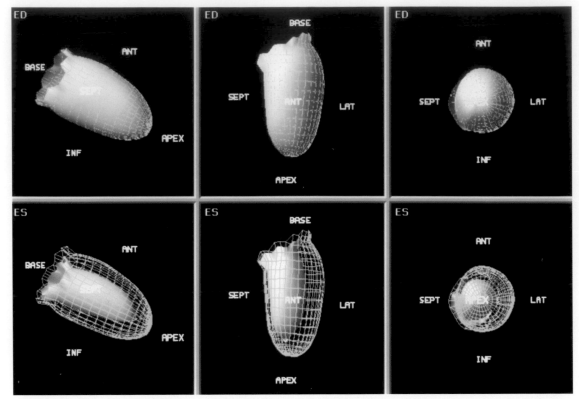

FIGURE 6–25. Normal GSPECT three-dimensional representation of the left ventricle. The upper row of images is a static display of the left ventricle in three of the projections of the LV normally reviewed in endless loop cine format to assess LV wall motion. These images are "frozen" at end diastole. The second row displays the same projections at end systole. The green mesh defines the endocardial surface at end-diastole as a reference to assess wall excursion during systole (between the two sets of images). In this case normal wall motion is implied and was also observed when these 3-D images were viewed in cine format.

definitions of normal limits and criteria for abnormalities of the program used are essential for the accurate interpretation of the processed data.

GSPECT Clinical Applications

The information provided by GSPECT regarding LV wall motion and LV function adds powerful adjunctive data to myocardial perfusion imaging in several well-defined settings. These are further discussed as relevant in the "Clinical Application" section of "Myocardial Perfusion Imaging." However, in summary, GSPECT is especially helpful in the following clinical situations:

■ Identification of suspected attenuation artifacts
■ Enhanced detection of multivessel CAD
■ Risk assessment of patients with known or suspected CAD
■ Assessment of myocardial viability
■ Follow-up of patients undergoing revascularization procedures

■ Distinguishing ischemic from nonischemic cardiomyopathy

Exercise Stress Protocol

In most patients, exercise is the most suitable method for stressing patients undergoing myocardial perfusion imaging. The basic exercise protocol used is the same regardless of the radiopharmaceutical used.

Patient Preparation

Patients should remain NPO for 4 to 6 hours before the exercise test. This allows for a decrease in splanchnic blood flow and, therefore, a reduction in uptake in the bowel and liver. Calcium-channel blockers and β-blockers such as propranolol should be discontinued, if possible, for a sufficient length of time before the examination to avoid any interference with obtaining an adequate stress examination by limiting heart rate response. Long-acting

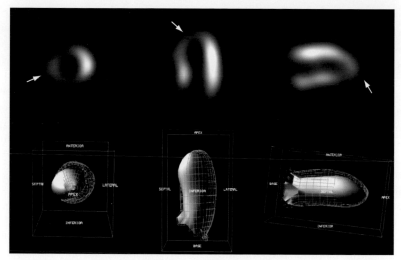

FIGURE 6–26. GSPECT correlation of perfusion and wall motion. *Top,* Short, horizontal long-axis and vertical long-axis poststress images from a GSPECT myocardial perfusion scan show a prominent perfusion defect (*arrows*) at the left ventricular apex extending into the inferior and septal walls. The defect persisted on rest images. The differential diagnosis includes a postinfarct scar and hibernating myocardium. *Bottom,* Three-dimensional representation (lower row) of the left ventricle at end-systole shows diminished wall motion at the apex and septum with a focal area of dyskinesia in the distal septum consistent with a scar with aneurysm formation.

nitrates should also be withheld on the day of testing. It is also advisable to avoid caffeinated beverages for 24 hours before the examination, so that if necessary, the exercise stress can be converted to pharmacologic stress using dipyridamole or adenosine without interference.

Exercise Protocol

The most common mode of stress used in myocardial perfusion imaging is a multistage treadmill exercise test based on a Bruce or modified Bruce protocol. Basically, this involves a consistent measured increase in the speed and grade (upward elevation) of the treadmill to provide gradually increasing levels of stress. Although bicycle ergometer exercise may be used, it often results in less optimal exertion levels that may compromise the sensitivity of the study.

Once exercise has begun, timing is critical. Regardless of the radiopharmaceutical used, it should be injected at peak stress, through a previously established intravenous line or heparin lock. Ideally, the patient continues to exercise for about 30 seconds to 1 minute after the injection to allow sufficient time for the radiopharmaceutical to localize in the myocardium under conditions of peak exercise. The determination of peak stress varies with the institution, but it is generally considered to be maximal when chest pain or significant ECG changes appear, when the patient's heart rate reaches 85% of predicted maximum heart rate (frequently defined as 220 beats/minute minus the patient's age in years), or when the heart rate-blood pressure product (maximum heart rate achieved multiplied by the maximum systolic blood pressure reached) exceeds a value of 25,000. If none of these conditions is met, the stress is generally deemed submaximal.

Maximal stress provides for optimal myocardial-to background ratios for imaging as well as for the most sensitive evaluation of myocardial perfusion. The most common cause of a false-negative examination and reduced test sensitivity is failure of the patient to achieve maximal stress. Still, a submaximal exercise myocardial perfusion study is more sensitive than is stress ECG alone for the detection of CAD. In patients who have recently sustained acute myocardial infarction, an intentionally submaximal exercise test may be performed for predischarge evaluation of residual stress-induced ischemia (myocardium still at risk).

Alternatives to Exercise: Pharmacologic Stress

In patients who cannot perform or tolerate adequate exercise, whose heart rate response may be limited by β-blockers or calcium-channel blockers, who have a pacemaker rhythm, or in whom the presence of left bundle-branch block (LBBB) may produce spurious, reversible exercise-induced septal perfusion defects, pharmacologic stress allows a successful myocardial perfusion study to be performed. Test sensitivity and specificity are comparable to that of maximal exercise studies, in the range of 85% to 90%, and image interpretation criteria are essentially the same.

Commonly used intravenous agents are (1) the non-nitrate vasodilators, dipyridamole (Persantine) and adenosine, and (2) the inotropic drug, dobutamine. Although pharmacologic stress may be safely performed in most patients, it is a good idea to use the technique only in patients who would otherwise be candidates for an exercise study. Pharmacologic stress should be used advisedly in patients with unstable angina, acute myocardial infarction (within 72 hours), hypotension, or refractive congestive heart failure, and is usually best avoided altogether. Because dipyridamole and adenosine may exacerbate or induce severe bronchospasm, they should not be used in patients with asthma or reactive airway disease. In addition, adenosine should not be used in patients with second- or third-degree heart block or sinus node disease.

Dipyridamole Stress Imaging

Dipyridamole is an adenosine deaminase inhibitor that allows the accumulation of endogenous adenosine, a potent vasodilator, in the myocardium by preventing adenosine degradation. This produces selective vasodilatation of normal coronary arteries, predominantly in the small, resistance vessels of the coronary bed. At the commonly used dosages, intravenous dipyridamole increases coronary blood flow by three to five times resting levels, compared with a one- to threefold increase with exercise.

Unlike normal coronary arteries, diseased stenosed vessels demonstrate no further dilatation because they are already maximally dilated secondary to autoregulatory mechanisms triggered by myocardial hypoperfusion. Therefore, although there is proportionally increased flow to the myocardium supplied by normal vessels, blood flow in the distribution of abnormal vessels is not increased as much, depending on the degree of stenosis. Thus, when dipyridamole is used in conjunction with myocardial perfusion imaging, there is radionuclide mapping of this discrepancy in perfusion, which results in a relative defect in the hypoperfused myocardium. For purposes of imaging, this accomplishes the effect of exercise on the coronary arteries with one important exception: there is minimal effect on cardiac work or myocardial oxygen demand, thus providing an additional margin of safety in patients with significant coronary stenosis.

Patient Preparation. Because they reverse the cardiovascular effects of dipyridamole, xanthine-containing medications, including theophylline (aminophylline), should be withheld for 48 hours, if tolerated by the patient, and caffeine-containing beverages should be withheld for 12 to 24 hours before the study. Stopping or altering any pre-existing oral dipyridamole therapy is generally not necessary.

Dipyridamole Protocol. Dipyridamole may be administered orally or intravenously, although the intravenous route is preferred because of its more predictable blood levels. Intravenous infusion through a large (antecubital) arm vein is performed over 4 minutes at a concentration of about 0.5 mg per kg in 20 to 40 mL of normal saline (an infusion rate of 0.14 mg/kg/min), with a total dose of 0.56 mg/kg. ECG, heart rate, and blood pressure should be monitored throughout the study. Patients may be supine, standing, or sitting, and low levels of exercise, including walking or isometric hand grip, may be used adjunctively if desired. The myocardial perfusion imaging agent is administered intravenously 3 to 4 minutes after the dipyridamole infusion is completed (7 to 8 minutes into the study, when maximal coronary dilatation occurs). Imaging is started at a time appropriate to the radiopharmaceutical used.

As with many interventional pharmaceuticals, significant undesirable side effects may occur in about 50% of patients. Dipyridamole may cause chest discomfort, headaches, dizziness, flushing, and nausea. These side effects may be rapidly reduced by the intravenous administration of aminophylline (100 to 200 mg). This antidote should be readily available during the procedure. Because the plasma half-life of dipyridamole (30 to 40 minutes) is longer than that of aminophylline, careful patient monitoring even after aminophylline administration is prudent.

Image Interpretation. Myocardial uptake of ^{201}Tl or ^{99m}Tc sestamibi is greater with dipyridamole than with exercise stress. When thallium is used for dipyridimole imaging, the pattern of liver, spleen, and splanchnic activity is the reverse of that noted with maximal-exercise thallium imaging; that is, increased activity in these regions is seen on initial images, but activity decreases on the delayed views.

The cardiac findings are interpreted identically to exercise examinations, with comparable sensitivity and specificity. As expected, however, important physiologic information such as ECG response, exercise capacity, and heart rate and blood pressure product obtained during conventional exercise stress is not available. Because normal thallium lung activity is slightly higher with dipyridamole or adenosine stress than with maximal exercise, the threshold for abnormal accumulation is somewhat higher. A lung-to-heart ratio of greater than 60% to 65% is generally considered abnormal and correlates with the presence of multivessel CAD.

Adenosine Stress Imaging

Because dipyridamole achieves coronary dilatation indirectly through the accumulation of adenosine in the coronary bed, an alternative method is the direct intravenous infusion of adenosine. The pharmacologic effect of adenosine is much more rapid than that of dipyridamole, but the degree of coronary dilatation is comparable, producing about three to five times baseline blood flow.

Patient Preparation. Contraindication to adenosine use and patient preparation are similar to those of dipyridamole. Caffeine should be avoided for 12 to 24 hours. Because dipyridamole potentiates the effects, and thus the side effects, of both endogenous and administered adenosine, its use should be withheld for 12 to 24 hours before adenosine infusion.

Adenosine Protocol. The usual dose is 0.14 mg/kg/min for 6 minutes, but doses may be titrated downward for unstable patients. The myocardial perfusion radiopharmaceutical is injected about halfway into the adenosine infusion (at 3 minutes), when maximal vasodilatation and myocardial hyperemia occur. No complementary exercise is usually used.

Side effects with adenosine are more common than those with dipyridamole and occur in 75% of patients. The three most common side effects are flushing, shortness of breath, and chest pain. These are usually transient and require no action or treatment. An uncommon, but more serious, side effect is atrioventricular block, which usually occurs in the first few minutes of infusion and is also transient. First-degree and second-degree block are more common. Because the biologic half-life of adenosine is extremely short (<10 seconds), its effects may be reversed by simply stopping infusion and beginning any specific treatments, if necessary.

Dobutamine Stress Imaging

The mechanism of action of dobutamine pharmacologic stress is different from the direct coronary vasodilatation produced by dipyridamole or adenosine. Dobutamine is a β_1-agonist that acts in a manner similar to exercise by increasing myocardial oxygen demand through increases in both heart rate and myocardial contractility and, at higher doses, through increases in systolic blood pressure. In response, normal coronary arteries dilate to increase blood flow and satisfy increased oxygen demand. Stenotic arteries cannot dilate as much as normal vessels can, so a relative perfusion defect is produced in the myocardium supplied by the stenotic vessel. The increased blood flow of three times the baseline levels is somewhat less than that produced by the vasodilators dipyridamole or adenosine. Further, the success of dobutamine stress is limited in patients on β-blocker medications. Dobutamine is best reserved for those patients in whom dipyridamole or adenosine stress is contraindicated, such as in patients with asthma or chronic obstructive pulmonary disease, in those who have had caffeine or methylxanthine medications within 12 hours of the study, and in those taking oral dipyridamole therapeutically before adenosine stress

Dobutamine Protocol. The administration protocol consists of a gradually increasing intravenous infusion, beginning with 5 to 10 μg/kg/min for 3 minutes, with the dose increasing every 3 minutes until a maximum dose of 40 μg/kg/min is reached. The maximum dose administered may be titrated downward if significant symptoms, heart rate or blood pressure effects, or ECG evidence of ischemia occurs. The myocardial perfusion radiopharmaceutical is injected 1 minute after beginning the highest tolerated dose of dobutamine, and the infusion is maintained for an additional 2 minutes while the radiopharmaceutical localizes in the myocardium. Imaging is started at a time appropriate to the radiopharmaceutical used.

About 75% of patients undergoing dobutamine infusion experience side effects. The most common are transient and similar to those of adenosine infusion, including palpitation, chest pain, flushing, headache, and dyspnea. More worrisome is the common occurrence of premature ventricular contractions and, less commonly, unsustained ventricular tachycardia and atrial fibrillation. Patients with baseline atrial tachycardia should be infused with caution. Because the biologic half-life of dobutamine (≈ 2 minutes) is longer than that of adenosine, the occasional use of a rapidly acting β-blocker may be needed to reverse its effects when a rare, persistent, adverse reaction occurs. Contraindications to dobutamine stress include significant ventricular arrhythmias, hypotension, marked hypertension, and LV outflow obstruction.

Clinical Applications

Coronary Artery Disease

Diagnosis of Coronary Artery Disease

SPECT Imaging Data. Stress and rest or redistribution myocardial perfusion is well recognized as an examination of high sensitivity and specificity for the detection of CAD. Its sensitivity for the detection of coronary artery stenosis increases directly with the severity of the stenoses and the extent of the disease (number of vessels involved). The overall sensitivity in the detection of stress-induced ischemia is about 80% to 90%, with a normalcy rate (percentage of normal patients with normal scans) of 85%. This represents a significant increase in sensitivity over exercise electrocardiography (60% to 70% sensitivity), with comparable or slightly increased specificity. This greater sensitivity is in large part due to the considerable number of patients with nondiagnostic exercise ECG tests because of baseline electrocardiographic abnormalities or inadequate stress. However, despite its superiority for the detection of CAD, radionuclide myocardial perfusion imaging should not replace routine stress ECG examinations for the general screening of patients for coronary disease.

Diagnostic stress myocardial perfusion imaging is most useful when it is applied to two broad groups of patients with suspected CAD: those in whom a routine exercise ECG test is nondiagnostic and those with an intermediate probability of disease. The latter group includes patients with high clinical suspicion of CAD based on symptoms and/or risk factors but with negative exercise ECGs, and those with a low pretest likelihood of CAD but with suggestive or positive ECGs at stress. Patients with underlying ECG abnormalities caused by left bundle-branch block, pacemakers, LV hypertrophy, baseline ST changes, or digoxin effect are also suitable candidates for myocardial perfusion imaging.

Although stress myocardial perfusion imaging is sensitive and specific for the diagnosis of CAD, it is less sensitive in determining the extent of disease. The presence of perfusion defects in more than one vessel distribution strongly indicates the presence of two- or three-vessel disease. However, a perfusion defect present in the distribution of only one vessel cannot be used to exclude the involvement of other vessels. False-negative studies may be caused by the phenomenon of balanced, symmetric, three-vessel CAD producing apparently normal, but uniformly reduced, flow through each artery. In this setting, transient LV dilatation or increased thallium lung activity may provide clues to the presence of underlying three-vessel CAD. Failure to reach adequate stress (>85% of maximum predicted heart rate during exercise stress) may also result in false-negative studies, especially in patients with moderate coronary stenoses.

GSPECT Functional Data. Assessing the severity of CAD can be enhanced by using the functional data derived from GSPECT. In most patients, any stress-induced ischemic segmental wall motion abnormalities quickly resolve after cessation of exercise. However, in approximately 30%, these areas of regional ischemic dysfunction persist as long as 1 hour after stress and are documented as focal wall motion abnormalities (stress-induced stunning) and/or LVEF reductions on GSPECT imaging. Such regional stress-induced hypokinesia in myocardial segments exhibiting reversible perfusion defects predicts high-grade stenosis and increased severity of disease.

Since a common cause of a false-positive SPECT myocardial perfusion scan is soft-tissue attenuation artifact, especially in women, the ability to differentiate between a true fixed perfusion defect (characterized by diminished or absent wall motion and/or thickening) and artifact (demonstrating normal wall motion and thickening) is important in improving the specificity of the study. GSPECT wall motion displays may demonstrate the presence of wall motion in an apparent fixed perfusion defect, thus establishing the spurious nature of the abnormality consistent with an attenuation artifact. Conversely, the presence of a wall motion abnormality is compatible with scar or viable but hibernating myocardium. It should be noted, however, that wall motion in the region of some true fixed defects, especially small ones, may occasionally be observed due to recruitment by normally contracting adjacent myocardium or to the nontransmural nature of the injury. Normal poststress wall motion in the region of a reversible defect neither confirms nor excludes an attenuation artifact.

In patients with three-vessel CAD, perfusion defects may not be seen in any or every coronary distribution, giving the false impression of absent or limited disease. The functional information obtained by GSPECT improves the detection of multivessel CAD, especially in cases of "balanced" global hypoperfusion, which may hinder the detection of segmental disease based on ungated perfusion data alone. In these patients, the ability to image poststress ischemic wall motion/thickening abnormalities significantly increases the sensitivity of myocardial perfusion imaging for the identifying multivessel and left main CAD. A reduction in poststress LVEF may also increase the sensitivity for multivessel disease and be the only indication of CAD in patients with "balanced" disease.

As a tool of differential diagnosis, GSPECT accurately distinguishes between patients with ischemic and nonischemic cardiomyopathy. Patients with nonischemic cardiomyopathy commonly present with diffuse wall motion abnormalities and globally abnormal LVEFs without the discrete perfusion defects usually noted with ischemic etiology. This differentiation has significant therapeutic implications.

Prognosis and Risk Stratification in CAD

SPECT Imaging Data. In recent years, rather than simply identifying patients with CAD, the emphasis of myocardial perfusion imaging has shifted to identifying patients with CAD who are also at risk for cardiac death and thus are in most need of revascularization. Stress myocardial perfusion imaging has been shown to be effective for assessing risk of future cardiac events in patients with known CAD. Findings on abnormal stress myocardial perfusion imaging that have been found to represent potent prognosticators of future adverse cardiac events include the following: (1) the number of reversible defects (an indicator of multivessel disease), (2) the size and severity of the reversible defects (amount of myocardium at risk), (3) the extent of fixed defects (amount of infarcted myocardium), (4) reversible defects in the left main coronary artery distribution, (5) abnormal lung accumulation of ^{201}Tl, and (6) transient left ventricular dilatation at exercise.

It should be remembered that the most severe or extensive reversible defect does not necessarily indicate the region most at risk for myocardial infarction. This correlates with the observation that mild plaques or stenosis ("vulnerable plaques") may be more subject to instability and to acute myocardial infarctions that more severe, established plaque/stenosis. Thus, the myocardial perfusion findings indicate the overall risk of adverse cardiac events for the patient, not for a particular lesion.

Ideally, to adequately express the extent and severity of perfusion abnormality present in a given patient and thus to provide maximal prognostic information, quantitative or semiquantitative assessment is optimum, such as calculating summed perfusion scores as described earlier. The risk of both cardiac death and myocardial infarction both worsens as summed stress scores (SSS) as a measure of perfusion abnormality increases. The summed difference score (SDS) as a measure of ischemic myocardium at risk is a strong predictor of future myocardial infarction. This approach also facilitates comparison of serial follow-up perfusion studies.

In terms of favorable prognoses, patients with known CAD and an unequivocally normal stress myocardial perfusion study with adequate stress have a very good prognosis, with a yearly rate of myocardial infarction or death of less than 1% to 2%.

GSPECT Functional Data. Assessment of risk in patients with CAD is enhanced by the addition of LV functional data to myocardial perfusion information. In patients with known CAD, a post-stress LVEF less than 45% or an end-systolic volume (ESV) greater than 70 mL confers a high mortality rate (≈ 8% to 9% per year), even in the presence of mild to moderate perfusion abnormalities. An LVEF greater than 45% or ESV less than 70 mL renders a low cardiac death rate (≈ 1%/year), even in the presence of severe perfusion abnormalities. When prediction of future non-fatal myocardial infarction is considered, the amount of ischemia present on the SPECT perfusion images appears to be a more accurate indicator than LVEF.

Hemodynamic Significance of Coronary Stenosis

SPECT Imaging Data. Experimental evidence indicates that coronary artery diameter narrowing greater than 50% as determined by arteriography is likely to be hemodynamically significant. In many instances, however, the exact percentage of narrowing is difficult to ascertain on routine arteriography, and stress myocardial imaging can be useful in determining the hemodynamic significance of an angiographically demonstrated stenosis. Stress-induced ischemia of the myocardium supplied by a stenotic vessel may be interpreted as strong evidence of physiologic significance of the stenosis. Because myocardial perfusion imaging is not 100% sensitive, however, a normal stress perfusion study in a particular arterial distribution is less definitive in predicting the absence of significant narrowing.

Because coronary arteriography and myocardial perfusion imaging measure different parameters (anatomy and hemodynamics, respectively), discrepancies between the two tests are not unusual. The accuracy of the estimated degree of stenosis at angiography is highly dependent on the technical aspects of the study and the method of measurement used. In addition, the significance of an angiographically determined stenosis may be increased by the presence of superimposed spasm or small-vessel disease (such as in diabetic patients) or may be mitigated by the presence of adequately functioning collateral vessels. A lesion thought to be subcritical by diameter measurement may still be hemodynamically significant if it is a long stenosis, or if it occurs in a vessel of already small diameter or in a vessel with multiple low-grade stenoses. The assessment of hemodynamic significance on stress myocardial perfusion imaging may be further complicated in patients with multivessel stenoses, in whom exercise performance may be limited by the more severe lesions, so that an exercise level sufficient to induce ischemia in the distribution of a less severe, but significant stenosis may not be reached.

These caveats aside, patients with angiographic stenoses, even left main or multivessel disease, have a relatively low risk for adverse cardiac events when no ischemia is identified on myocardial perfusion imaging.

GSPECT Functional Data. GSPECT performed within an hour or so after the completion of stress may reflect the poststress status of LV function. The induction of poststress wall motion/thickening abnormality in the region of a reversible stress-induced perfusion defect in the segment of myocardium distal to a stenosis provides independent highly specific evidence of stenosis severity. Reversible, stress-induced wall motion abnormalities confer high specificity for coronary stenoses greater than 70%.

Adequacy of Collateral Coronary Vessels

The functional significance of collateral vessels identified at coronary arteriography may be evaluated in a manner similar to that for coronary stenoses. Evidence suggests that in some patients, collaterals may maintain adequate rest perfusion to the myocardium distal to a stenosis, but may not be able to meet the oxygen demands of this tissue during exercise. Therefore, stress myocardial imaging may be able to give a clearer idea of the reserve perfusion potential of such collaterals by demonstrating the presence or absence of reversible stress-induced ischemia in the region of concern.

Evaluation of Myocardial Revascularization

SPECT Imaging Data. Chest pain after coronary revascularization procedures may or may not have a cardiac origin, but the ability to distinguish between the two is of significance. Recurrent pain from a cardiac cause may be related to occlusion of the bypass grafts or angioplastied vessel or to the progression of disease in indigenous vessels. In addition, about 25% of patients with restenosis may have no symptoms ("silent" ischemia). Postoperative exercise myocardial perfusion imaging gives information regarding the hemodynamic success of revascularization by comparing preoperative and postoperative stress images (Fig. 6–27).

After coronary artery bypass grafting, 10% to 20% of venous grafts occlude by 1 year, and up to 50% occlude by 10 years. Stress myocardial perfusion imaging is superior to both clinical findings and exercise ECG in predicting graft patency. The probability of graft occlusion increases significantly with worsening of defects that were present before surgery or with the appearance of new defects. Graft patency correlates with improved perfusion compared with presurgical scans. Reversible perfusion abnormalities not identified on the preoperative study suggest progression of disease in indigenous vessels, whereas new fixed defects may indicate perioperative myocardial injury.

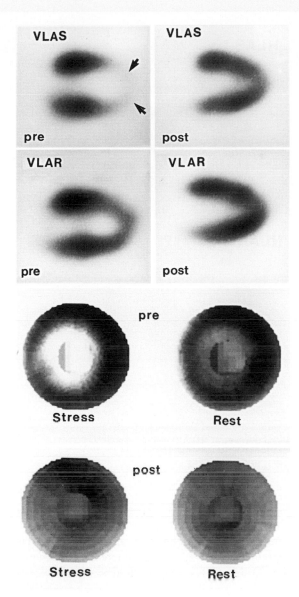

FIGURE 6–27. Pre- and postangioplasty exercise SPECT myocardial perfusion imaging. Vertical long-axis stress (VLAS) and vertical long-axis rest (VLAR) images (*left side of upper rows*) obtained before angioplasty demonstrate a large apical reversible defect (*arrows*) consistent with stress-induced ischemia in the left anterior descending artery territory. Stress and rest vertical long-axis SPECT slices obtained 6 weeks after successful angioplasty (*right side of upper rows*) show that the apical defect has significantly improved. These results are also confirmed by the pre- and postangioplasty stress and rest bull's eye plots (*lower rows*).

Percutaneous transluminal coronary angioplasty (PTCA) is associated with a 30% to 40% restenosis rate by 6 months after the procedure. Although in general, the addition of coronary stents to PTCA procedures has diminished postangioplasty restenosis compared with that of PTCA alone by about

one-third, the range of in-stent restenosis still remains about 10% to 25% at 6 months. When properly timed, stress myocardial scintigraphy can document procedural success and can diagnose restenosis, defined angiographically as a return to more than 50% stenosis. Because of post-traumatic changes at the site of coronary arterial dilatation seen early after PTCA (including elastic recoil, spasm, intramural hemorrhage, and intraluminal debris), up to half of patients show a transient reduction in coronary flow reserve immediately after PTCA, which returns to normal in days to weeks. For this reason, false-positive myocardial perfusion scans may occur during the first few weeks after PTCA. When performed 4 to 8 weeks after PTCA, scans showing reversible perfusion defects are highly predictive for coronary restenosis and the recurrence of angina, whereas the absence of such defects correlates with vessel patency.

GSPECT Functional Data. In addition to myocardial perfusion assessment, the success of revascularization can be gauged by measuring any improvement in global LV function (LVEF) or regional wall motion after the procedure. A seemingly paradoxical circumstance may be observed in many patients who have undergone coronary artery bypass surgery. In these patients, apparent septal dyskinesia may be noted with preservation of systolic wall thickening. This finding is likely related to exaggerated translational cardiac motion after surgery and does not indicate underlying pathology.

Risk Stratification after Myocardial Infarction

SPECT Imaging Data. In the post–myocardial infarction patient, myocardial perfusion imaging using submaximal exercise or pharmacologic stress provides important information regarding risk stratification. The primary strategy is to identify two distinctive groups of patients: (1) low-risk patients who require no further evaluation and may be discharged from the hospital, and (2) high-risk patients who are in need of further assessment and may benefit from revascularization therapy.

High-risk patients are identified by significant residual peri-infarct ischemia (myocardium at risk) or ischemia remote from the acute injury (multivessel disease). If the walls of the LV appear to diverge from the base toward the apex, instead of converging toward the apex, an apical ventricular aneurysm complicating a myocardial infarct should

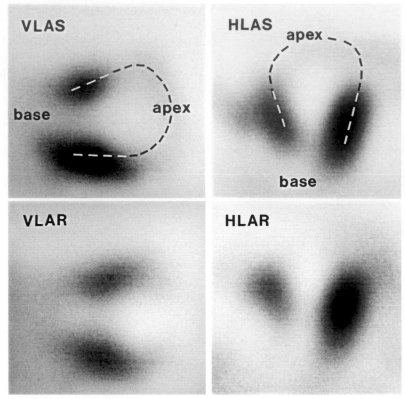

FIGURE 6–28. Left ventricular apical aneurysm. Vertical and horizontal long-axis SPECT sestamibi images at stress (VLAS, HLAS) and rest (VLAR, HLAR) demonstrate a fixed large apical defect compatible with a prior myocardial infarction with scarring. The walls of the left ventricle diverge as they go toward the apex and converge toward the base of the heart, indicating the presence of a left ventricular aneurysm at the apex.

be suspected (Fig. 6–28). Increased lung activity on thallium studies and transient ischemic dilatation are also high-risk indicators. Conversely, a normal study or a small, fixed defect in a single vascular territory allows low-risk classification, predicting about a 6% rate of cardiac events during the year after myocardial infarction.

GSPECT Functional Data. GSPECT can be used to determine residual LV function after myocardial infarction as a predictor of future adverse cardiac events. In post–myocardial infarction patients, the incidence of cardiac death or recurrent acute myocardial infarction with an LVEF less than 40% is about 40%, but the incidence is less than 10% in those with an LVEF greater than 40%.

Myocardial Viability Determination

SPECT Imaging Data. In certain circumstances, it is important to distinguish fixed perfusion defects

caused by myocardial scar from fixed defects representing viable, but non-functional salvageable myocardium. This is especially true when revascularization procedures are under consideration as a means of restoring perfusion and thereby wall motion in the affected areas, thus improving overall LV function. Revascularization procedures provide no potential for improving cardiac function in areas of scarring and are associated with significant morbidity. However, in fixed defects caused by viable but hibernating myocardium with accompanying regional wall motion abnormalities, myocardial contractile function may be restored by revascularization.

Hibernating myocardium is the result of severe coronary artery stenoses or partially reopened occlusions producing chronic hypoperfusion and ischemia. This leads to reduced cellular metabolism that is sufficient to sustain viability but inadequate to permit contractile function. Areas of hibernating myocardium usually present as segments of decreased perfusion and absent or diminished contractility, even when the patient is in a resting state. Because the myocardium is ischemic, but still viable, revascularization generally restores both perfusion and wall motion function.

Hibernating myocardium, a chronic process, should be distinguished from "stunned" myocardium, a more acute, temporary circumstance. Stunning is the result of ischemic and reperfusion injury secondary to an acute coronary artery occlusion that has reopened, either spontaneously or by thrombolytic therapy, before significant myocardial infarction can occur. Areas of stunned myocardium usually present with normal or near-normal perfusion but with absent or diminished contractility. Because the underlying myocardial cells are still viable, once blood flow has been restored, stunning generally spontaneously subsides over several weeks, with restoration of wall motion and improvement in LV function. Thus, unlike hibernating myocardium, revascularization is not needed. However, if the reopened vessel does not sufficiently restore perfusion and there is residual ischemia, chronically hibernating myocardium may result. Recently, a chronic form of so-called repetitive or cumulative stunning has been recognized in patients with CAD, which consists of multiple cycles of acute myocardial ischemia-reperfusion injury leading to chronic local contractile dysfunction. This may coexist with hibernation in ischemic heart disease to produce significant, but potentially reversible LV dysfunction.

In the presence of fixed defects on routine myocardial perfusion imaging, additional effort over and above routine myocardial imaging must be made to establish the viability of a myocardial perfusion defect when it is crucial to patient management. In this setting, reinjection, delayed, or rest-redistribution thallium imaging techniques or other imaging strategies, such as ^{18}F-FDG PET, have demonstrated that a significant number of fixed defects (up to 50%) prove to be reversible, viable, but hibernating myocardium. Such late reversibility is highly predictive of recovery of wall motion function in the involved segments after revascularization procedures, whereas irreversibility correlates with lack of recovery of myocardial function. Overall, reinjection or rest–redistribution thallium imaging has a 90% sensitivity and 50% specificity for predicting improvement in regional wall motion after revascularization.

GSPECT Functional Data. Fixed or resting perfusion defects may be classified as viable if the presence of wall motion or thickening can be confirmed (Fig. 6–29). Detectable wall motion and/or wall thickening improves the likelihood of underlying viability and can predict regional recovery of function after revascularization compared with segments with no contractile function.

Administration of the inotropic drug dobutamine in low doses can be used to stimulate and measure myocardial contractile reserve, which enhances the accuracy of predicting recovery after coronary revascularization. Improved wall motion in a hypokinetic myocardial segment after dobutamine may increase the likelihood of postprocedural success. However, the technique appears less sensitive for predicting improvement in akinetic segments compared with that of quantitative perfusion imaging. In terms of global LV function, an increase in LVEF of more than 5% (5 ejection fraction units) after low-dose dobutamine may predict LVEF improvement after revascularization.

Evaluation of Acute Chest Pain

Patients with acute chest pain can be difficult to evaluate in the emergency setting because of the low sensitivity and specificity of clinical and ECG data available at the acute presentation. Because up to 10% of patients with acute chest pain discharged from the emergency room may develop a myocardial infarction within 48 hours, a conservative admissions policy is usually adopted, which may lead to a large number of inappropriate intensive care unit admissions. Under these circumstances, less than 30% of patients admitted to the coronary care unit have acute myocardial infarction. For these reasons, it has proved cost-effective in some acute care facilities to use resting myocardial perfusion imaging for the detection of defects associated with myocardial ischemia or infarct. Immediately on arrival in the emergency room, patients are injected at rest with 10 mCi (370 MBq) of ^{99m}Tc sestamibi or tetrophosmin and imaged after initial clinical evaluation and patient stabilization. Although sensitive in this setting, the rapid redistribution of thallium renders its use less practical.

Acute myocardial infarctions present as focal perfusion defects on the myocardial perfusion images. The detection of acute myocardial infarction by this technique is highly reliable in the first 24 hours after the insult. In fact, the sooner imaging is performed after the onset of symptoms, the more

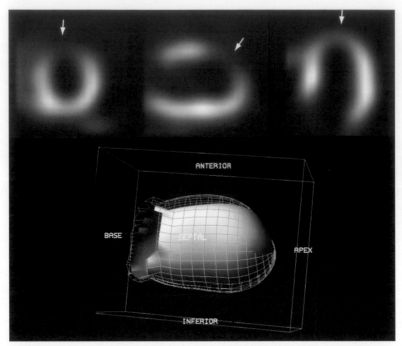

FIGURE 6–29. *Top,* **Short axis, horizontal long-axis, and vertical long-axis poststress images from a GSPECT myocardial perfusion scan reveal a distal anterior wall defect, which was noted to partially reverse on rest images with a persistent fixed component.** *Bottom,* Three-dimensional representation of the left ventricle at end-systole shows marked regional hypokinesia with mild dyskinesia in the area of the perfusion abnormality. The lack of meaningful wall motion and focal dyskinesia are consistent with scarring, indicating that revascularization would not be helpful in restoring regional myocardial function.

likely that the study will be positive. Almost all patients with myocardial infarction injected within 6 hours after onset of chest pain demonstrate perfusion defects. Sensitivity decreases thereafter with time, possibly related to the resolution of associated acute reversible ischemia in the region of infarction. However, a normal scan after this time likely confers a low risk, but does not exclude acute coronary syndromes. The tracer may be injected regardless of whether the patient is experiencing chest pain at the time of injection, although the sensitivity of the study is lower if the patient's chest pain has resolved. By using this technique, patients may be triaged and treated expeditiously with significant cost-effectiveness. Because myocardial perfusion imaging does not distinguish between old and new myocardial infarctions, it may be most effective in patients without ECG or historical evidence of previous infarction or in patients with previous baseline imaging studies. The negative predictive value of a normal study approaches 100%.

Myocardial perfusion at rest has also been used to differentiate unstable angina pectoris from acute myocardial infarction. When the study is performed during an episode of pain, about half of patients with unstable angina demonstrate perfusion defects on initial resting images. Delayed images obtained after the pain has subsided (either by using thallium redistribution or ^{99m}Tc sestamibi reinjection techniques) demonstrate that these defects are usually reversible, as opposed to those associated with completed infarction. A normal study obtained during chest pain is a strong indicator that the pain is not related to myocardial ischemia.

Preoperative Risk Assessment for Noncardiac Surgery

SPECT Imaging Data. Stress myocardial perfusion imaging can be used successfully to evaluate cardiac status before general surgical procedures. High risk for perioperative myocardial infarction is directly

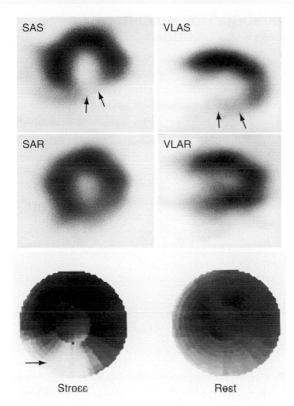

Stress   Rest

FIGURE 6–30. Inferior wall ischemia (reversible inferior wall defect). On these technetium-99m tetrophosmin SPECT images, the short-axis stress (SAS) and vertical long-axis stress (VLAS) images (*upper row*) show a defect in the inferior wall (*arrows*). There is much improved perfusion in these areas on the rest images obtained earlier the same day with a smaller dose of ^{99m}Tc-tetrophosmin. Bull's eye plots confirm the reversible stress-induced defect in the inferior wall (*arrow*). SAR, short-axis rest; VLAR, vertical long-axis rest.

related to the number and extent of reversible myocardial perfusion defects. Normal studies or those disclosing only fixed defects confer a low risk of adverse cardiac events with a negative predictive value approaching 100%. Patients with significant reversible stress-induced ischemia should be considered for coronary arteriography (Fig. 6–30). Patients with lesser findings may proceed to surgery as necessary, with appropriate steps taken to lower surgical and anesthesia risks.

GSPECT Functional Data. There is incremental prognostic value in this setting with GSPECT compared with SPECT alone. The adverse perioperative cardiac event rate has been shown to increase with decreasing LVEF values (especially <35%) and with the number of hypokinetic LV wall segments.

Noncoronary Disease States

Valvular Lesions

Exercise-induced perfusion defects may be uncommonly identified in patients with mitral valve prolapse but without angiographic evidence of CAD. The cause and significance of such defects are uncertain, but when seen, ischemia as a cause must be excluded. A normal exercise myocardial perfusion study in a patient with mitral valve prolapse, however, serves as evidence against superimposed CAD.

Patients with valvular aortic stenosis may present with angina-like symptoms in the absence of CAD. Forty percent to 50% of these patients may demonstrate reversible perfusion defects, which are thought to be related to a reduced perfusion gradient in the coronary arteries associated with tight aortic stenosis. Thus, perfusion abnormalities after exercise in patients with aortic stenosis should be interpreted with caution. Patients with aortic regurgitation, but without CAD, may exhibit stress-induced reversible defects localized to the apex of the ventricle. With defects in other regions of the ventricle, CAD must be excluded.

Left Bundle-Branch Block

Because LBBB renders ECG stress testing nondiagnostic, a noninvasive diagnosis of CAD is often sought by using radionuclide myocardial perfusion imaging. Patients with LBBB may demonstrate reversible septal or anteroseptal perfusion abnormalities during maximal exercise stress in the absence of demonstrable CAD (Fig. 6–31). Diminished septal perfusion at exercise due to asynchronous septal relaxation that is out of phase with diastolic coronary filling has been proposed as the mechanism for this phenomenon. Thus, reversible perfusion defects at exercise in the septal region of patients with LBBB are an indeterminate finding. Reversible defects elsewhere in the LV myocardium, however, retain their specificity for the diagnosis of transient ischemia. Because the frequency of stress-induced septal defects in patients with LBBB is directly related to the heart rate achieved during exercise, pharmacologic stress with adenosine or dipyridamole (which produces no significant increase in heart rate) is a useful alternative to exercise stress, producing fewer false positive studies in this setting.

Hypertensive Myocardial Hypertrophy

Because hypertension is a major risk factor for CAD, hypertensive patients are often referred for

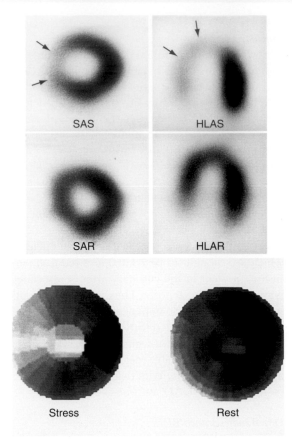

FIGURE 6–31. Left bundle-branch block (LBBB). On technetium-99m sestamibi SPECT short-axis stress (SAS) and horizontal long-axis stress (HLAS) images, there is a prominent perfusion defect in the septum (*arrows*). No discernible defect is seen on either short or horizontal long-axis rest images. These findings are also seen on the bull's eye images. Coronary angiography was normal in this patient with LBBB. SAR, short-axis rest; HLAR, horizontal long-axis rest.

myocardial perfusion scintigraphy. In patients with myocardial hypertrophy resulting from long-standing hypertension, myocardial perfusion imaging may demonstrate a relative increase in the septal wall activity on both stress and redistribution images. This increased septal count density may lead to an apparent relative decrease in activity in the lateral wall, especially on HLA SPECT images, causing a false impression of a fixed lateral wall defect (Fig. 6–32). Similar findings may occur in patients with idiopathic subaortic stenosis. Thus, a history of possible hypertension or idiopathic subaortic stenosis should be elicited in patients undergoing these studies.

RADIONUCLIDE IMAGING OF CARDIAC FUNCTION

Examinations that provide information about ventricular function play a decisive role in the detection and diagnosis of a variety of cardiac problems and in the management of patients with known heart disease. In this respect, radionuclide methods provide a noninvasive means to assess both right ventricle and LV pump performance at rest and during exercise and allow valuable insight into intracardiac and cardiopulmonary dynamics. Although these tests still have a place in clinical nuclear medicine practice, as general tools for evaluation of cardiac function, they have largely been supplanted for primary cardiac function evaluation by the widespread availability of echocardiography and the routine use of GSPECT for myocardial perfusion imaging.

Radionuclide tests of ventricular function are generally accomplished by three discrete methods:

- *GSPECT* using myocardial perfusion agents as described earlier in this chapter. This is the most frequently performed isotopic evaluation of cardiac function in clinical practice.
- *First-pass or first-transit radionuclide angiography (FP-RNA),* in which imaging is undertaken during the initial rapid transit of an intravenously administered radioactive bolus through the heart, lungs, and great vessels.
- *Equilibrium radionuclide angiography (E-RNA),* in which images of the cardiac blood pool are obtained after a radiopharmaceutical has equilibrated within the intravascular space. This procedure is also known as gated blood pool ventriculography and multigated acquisition (MUGA) study.

Although first-pass and equilibrium methods require different procedural approaches, they provide essentially identical information for qualitative and quantitative assessment of LV function. Both techniques are accurate and reproducible compared with cardiac catheterization results. Therefore, although there are specific advantages and limitations to each, either method may be used for the evaluation of ventricular function at rest or during exercise. Whichever technique is used, complete familiarity with and confidence in the procedure employed provide the best approach for successful application.

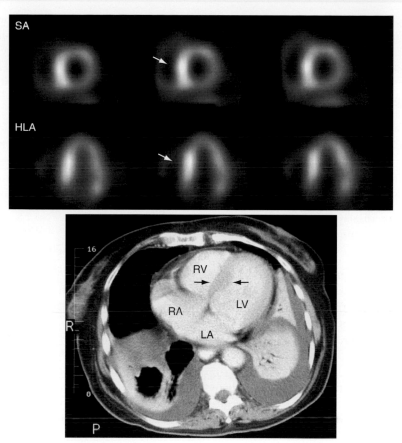

FIGURE 6–32. Asymmetric septal thickening. *Top,* Short and horizontal long-axis rest slices from a technetium-99m tetrophosmin myocardial perfusion study show relatively decreased activity in the lateral wall of the left ventricle and normal or increased activity in the septum. This pattern persisted on the poststress study suggesting a lateral wall scar. *Bottom,* A post-contrast computed tomography scan shows an asymmetrically thickened interventricular septum in this patient with hypertension. Coronary arteriography was normal. The findings on SPECT slices are due to relatively increased activity in the septum due to its hypertrophy with scaling of the images such that the normal activity in the lateral wall is suppressed, giving the false impression of a fixed perfusion abnormality.

Computer Methods

Among routine nuclear medicine procedures, those measuring cardiac function are perhaps the most dependent on computer methodology for the collection and processing of scintigraphic data. A basic knowledge of some specific computer methods is crucial to an understanding of these techniques.

Data can be acquired by a computer in *list mode* or *frame mode*. Basically, list mode involves digitizing and filing data in the time sequence in which it occurs, permitting later retrieval and manipulation of the data. In this manner, decisions concerning the sorting and formatting of the filed information and the discarding of unwanted information may be made at any time after the information is acquired. This flexibility allows the computer operator to format the data in varying time sequences, as may be dictated by the specific goals in mind. For instance, the data of a first-pass study may be formatted such that frames of several seconds' duration are generated and visual inspection of cardiac anatomy is possible. Alternatively, the data may be reformatted in frames of a fraction of a second's duration so that ventricular time-activity curves may be derived, allowing for quantification of ventricular function indices. Such flexibility necessarily has a price—the need for significant computer memory.

Frame mode acquisition requires formatting decisions to be made before the beginning of the study. After the information is collected, it cannot be reformatted to allow manipulation in varying time sequences. A major advantage is that frame mode requires substantially less computer memory.

Qualitative Data Display

When a computer system coupled with a gamma camera is used to acquire, analyze, and display the data obtained from nuclear cardiac studies, two types of information result:

- Qualitative data, displayed as images
- Quantitative data, expressed as numbers or curves

Computer-generated images of ventricular function can be processed by using computer software for edge or contrast enhancement, background subtraction, smoothing, filtering, or other manipulations to produce images of high quality. After images have been processed, they may be displayed as static images or more typically, in an endless-loop cine format that allows visual inspection of the ventricular walls during cardiac contraction and thus permits qualitative assessment of ventricular segmental wall motion.

Quantitative Data Display

Computer manipulation of the statistical information contained within digitized equilibrium or first-pass images permits the quantitation of various indices of cardiac performance. These indices are derived from changes in activity (counts) in the ventricles during the cardiac cycle and as such are free from the errors inherent in the geometric methods used in contrast ventriculography. When meticulously performed, the results, including the LVEF, are very accurate and reproducible.

The basic principle underlying this count-volume (or time-activity) approach is the assumed proportionality between measured activity and the volume of blood in which it is contained. That is, as the radioactive bolus passes through the cardiac chambers, or after the administered radioactive agent has thoroughly mixed with the blood in the cardiac chambers, any change in the count rate obtained from a region of interest defining a particular chamber reflects a proportional change in the volume of blood within that chamber.

Regions of interest over the LV and a periventricular area of background to allow for subtraction of counts from structures overlying the ventricular

area of interest are defined throughout the cardiac cycle either semiautomatically or manually, depending on operator preference. From these, a time-activity curve is generated. This curve represents changes in ventricular activity and therefore in relative ventricular volume during the cardiac cycle. It allows the calculation of perhaps the most important ventricular functional parameter: the global ejection fraction. By determining the number of counts present at end-systole and end-diastole, the difference, expressed as a percentage of the counts at end-diastole, gives the ejection fraction:

$$\text{Ejection fraction} = \frac{\text{end-diastolic counts} - \text{end-systolic counts}}{\text{end-diastolic counts} - \text{background counts}}$$

Usually the ejection fraction or changes are expressed as a percentage, although occasionally changes are expressed as ejection fraction units to avoid confusion. This solves the problem of whether a 10% decrease in a patient who previously had a 50% ejection fraction actually has a 40% or 45% ejection fraction. By stating that there is a decrease of 10 ejection fraction units, it would be clear that the resulting ejection fraction is 40%.

In most laboratories, a normal resting LVEF is at least 50%, usually in a range of 50% to 70%. The LVEF usually increases with exercise. A normal right ventricular ejection fraction is typically lower than the LVEF (by 5% to 10% [5 to 10 units]) due to the somewhat larger EDV of the right ventricle, but a stroke volume equal to the LV. A normal right ventricular ejection fraction is typically greater than 40% in normal patients. By mathematically differentiating the time-activity curves, ventricular ejection rates and filling rates may also be calculated. In addition to a global LVEF, regional ejection fractions may be derived by dividing the ventricle into segments. These ejection fractions serve a measure of segmental LV wall motion and help to quantify wall motion abnormalities.

As with any time-activity analysis of digitized images, the accuracy of the calculations depends largely on the precise selection of the regions of interest. Because it is important to determine accurately the edges of the LV and to exclude any activity in great vessels, lungs, and adjacent chambers, data processing protocols with computer algorithms for the automated detection of the LV edges as they change throughout the cardiac cycle are commonly used. These edge detection programs are accurate in most patients. It is important, however, that the physician analyzing the visual data correlate the calculated ejection fraction based on the computer selection of LV edges with his or her qualitative impression of LV function. Inaccurate definition of the aortic or mitral valve planes, with resultant inclusion of portions of either the ascending aorta or the left atrium in the LV region of interest, leads to underestimation of the LVEF. An artificially elevated LVEF may occur when a portion of the LV is excluded from the LV region of interest at end-systole. In some cases, manual selection of LV edges must be performed to ensure accurate ejection fraction determination.

Selection of the background region of interest is also of considerable importance so that the ejection fraction is not underestimated or overestimated. Overestimation and thus oversubtraction of background artificially elevates ejection fraction, whereas underestimation erroneously reduces ejection fraction values. There are various standard areas for placement of background regions of interest (usually periventricular), which should be consistently used for all such determinations to ensure the validity of technique.

Functional Images

By using various computer algorithms, functional or parametric images may also be generated. Rather than emphasizing spatial resolution, these images display global or regional changes in radioactivity, reflecting ventricular function. The images may be produced from data obtained by either gated equilibrium or first-pass techniques. Although a number of functional images may be derived, those in common use include stroke volume, ejection fraction, phase, paradox, and amplitude images.

Stroke Volume Image

The *stroke volume* image may be obtained by subtracting the end-systolic frame of the ventriculogram from the end-diastolic frame and displaying the resultant distribution of activity in a gray-scale or color format (Fig. 6–33). This image presents the distribution of relative regional volume changes in each ventricle, reflecting the amount of blood ejected from each region of the ventricle during systole.

Ejection Fraction Image

The *ejection fraction image* is obtained through computer manipulation of the end-systolic and end-

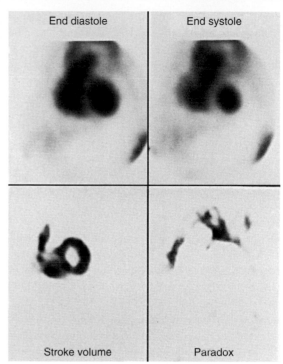

FIGURE 6–33. Normal gated equilibrium radionuclide angiogram (E-RNA) with functional images. End-diastolic and end-systolic images of the heart in the 45-degree left anterior oblique projection are shown, with subsequent computer manipulation of the data to produce functional images. The *stroke volume image* demonstrates a darkened, circular shell, corresponding to left ventricular wall motion obtained by subtracting the end-systolic from the end-diastolic image. This shell corresponds to the amount of blood ejected from the left ventricle during systole (the stroke volume). The *paradox image* displays activity only in the regions of the atria that are contracting as the ventricles fill. No focal darkened area in the region of the left ventricular wall is seen to suggest the presence of localized dyskinesia (paradoxical wall motion).

diastolic images to provide a static representation of the ejection fraction equation, that is, the stroke volume image divided by the end-diastolic image.

Typically, the ejection fraction and the stroke volume images obtained in the 45-degree left anterior oblique projection are similar. Both images allow qualitative assessment of regional ventricular function, including ejection fraction values as relative measures of local wall motion. The images frequently resemble a horseshoe or incomplete doughnut because most of the volume and ejection fraction changes occur at the apex, posterior wall, and distal septal walls in this projection. The basal portion of the heart, which constitutes the membranous portion of the interventricular septum and the aortic outflow tract, contributes little to ventricular function and may therefore present as a relative defect in the activity distribution. The central portion of the LV chamber also appears as an area of decreased activity because the relative count changes in the center of the ventricle are small during systole. Defects in the horseshoe or doughnut distribution of the "ejection shell" indicate areas of diminished stroke volume or ejection fraction, as may be found in regional hypokinesis or akinesis. Dyskinetic segments are not evaluated in these images because negative changes are given a zero value by the functional image program.

Paradox Image

Dyskinetic segments, which may be associated with LV aneurysms, can be identified by using another type of functional image called the *paradox image,* in which the diastolic frame of the ventriculogram is subtracted from the systolic frame (Fig. 6–34). With normal LV contraction, no areas of focally increased activity should be identified in the region of the LV wall. Thus, in normal images, only the atria and the great vessels are seen. In the presence of regional dyskinesia, however, a focal area of increased activity appears in the image because the ESV in the region of paradoxical motion bulges beyond and thus exceeds the distribution of EDV. Thus, subtraction of the two volume distributions leaves a focus of net increased activity at the site of dyskinesia.

Phase and Amplitude Analysis

These are examples of parametric functional images that display the sequence and degree of contraction of the cardiac chambers as well as individual wall segments of the left or right ventricle (Fig. 6–35). Such analysis permits sensitive evaluation of regional wall motion, as well as more precise differentiation between atrial and ventricular contraction. In this method, a summary of the characteristics of heart motion is derived through Fourier analysis of the digital data. The derived parameters of phase and amplitude are then displayed as functional images that allow the evaluation of the sequence of regional contraction and magnitude of segmental wall motion, respectively.

With phase analysis, each myocardial segment in the left anterior oblique projection is assigned a phase angle that categorizes the temporal motion of that segment of myocardium. The phase image represents only the information related to *synchrony* or *asynchrony* of wall motion and is independent of the magnitude of that motion. Further, each

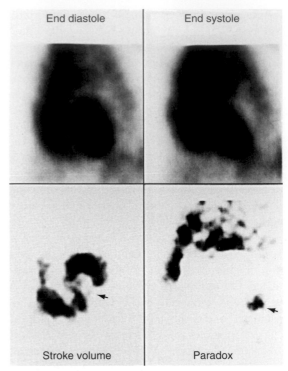

FIGURE 6–34. Left ventricular aneurysm. The end-diastolic and end-systolic frames from a gated equilibrium radionuclide angiogram (E-RNA) are displayed with the functional paradox and stroke volume images. The stroke volume image demonstrates a break in the stroke volume shell seen in the region of the left ventricular apex (*arrow*), which could be interpreted as akinesia in this patient. However, the paradox image shows a focal darkened area in the same region (*arrow*), compatible with focal dyskinesia (paradoxical wall motion) and consistent with a left ventricular apical aneurysm.

myocardial segment is assigned a value describing the magnitude of its wall excursion. The amplitude image thus derived represents the extent of regional wall motion regardless of the time of occurrence within the cardiac cycle. Different formats may be used for phase and amplitude image display, including static gray or color scales or histograms showing the regional distribution of phase and amplitude within the heart. In addition, a functional cine of the entire gated study played frame by frame may be used to display a dynamic wave of contraction sweeping across the heart, characterizing any conduction abnormalities and/or segmental wall motion abnormalities.

In a normal phase analysis, the contraction pattern is expected to follow a standard sequence: atrial contraction fills the ventricular chambers, followed by contraction of the ventricles. Because the

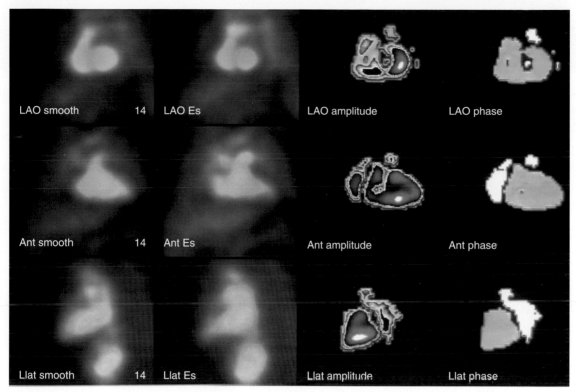

FIGURE 6–35. Normal gated equilibrium radionuclide angiography (E-RNA). Gated images of the cardiac blood pool are noted in the first two columns in static display of end-diastole and end-systole (from left to right). Left anterior oblique (LAO), anterior (Ant);, and left lateral (Llat) standard projections are presented. The amplitude and phase images give a static representation of the dynamic characteristics of the cardiac chambers, include sequence of contraction (*phase*) and degree of contraction (*amplitude*). The atria clearly show decreased contraction magnitude (less red) on the amplitude images compared with the ventricles. The phase images clearly separate the atria from the ventricles due to the normal alternating nature of their times of contraction (systole).

atria are filling when the ventricles are emptying and vice versa, they can be thought of as contracting with the phase difference of 180 degrees apart. Thus, the normal phase pattern, as seen in the functional image, shows the ventricles at one value of phase and the atria at 180-degree phase difference relative to the ventricles. A normal phase analysis is shown in Figure 6–36. Similarly, a dyskinetic, paradoxical myocardial segment would also be assigned a phase angle of about 180 degrees out of phase with the normal motion of the surrounding myocardium.

Abnormal phase patterns may be found in patients with CAD, cardiac pacemakers, right or LBBB, Wolff-Parkinson-White syndrome, and ventricular tachycardia. Thus, the information obtained from phase analysis gives a demonstration of the mechanical (wall motion) manifestations of underlying conduction abnormalities, showing clearly the relations between the electrical and mechanical sequences. Isolated regional phase

abnormalities are commonly produced by scars, seen as areas of hypokinesia (Fig. 6–37), or by ventricular aneurysms producing focal areas of dyskinetic wall motion, which contract out of phase with the remainder of the ventricular wall (Fig. 6–38).

First-Pass Studies

Principle

In first-pass or first-transit radionuclide angiocardiography (FP-RNA), a bolus of radioactivity is injected into a large peripheral vein, and the initial rapid transit of the bolus through the heart, lungs, and great vessels is imaged in rapid sequence using a gamma camera. The data are processed by a computer, from which subsequent anatomic images can be obtained for visual interpretation, including ventricular wall motion. In addition, the quantitative analysis of the images can provide a number of hemodynamic indices, the most notable of which are left and right ventricular ejection

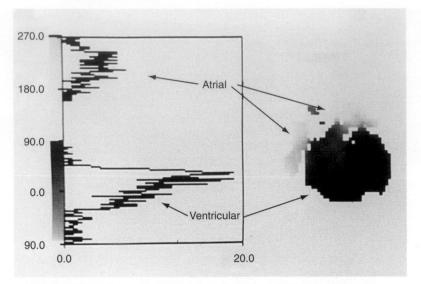

FIGURE 6–36. Phase analysis of a normal gated equilibrium radionuclide angiogram (E-RNA) in the left anterior oblique projection. The phase information is displayed as a histogram on the *left* and as a gray-scale image on the *right*. Clearly separated are the ventricular and atrial contraction peaks, with differentiation of the temporal sequence of atrial and ventricular contraction on the gray-scale image.

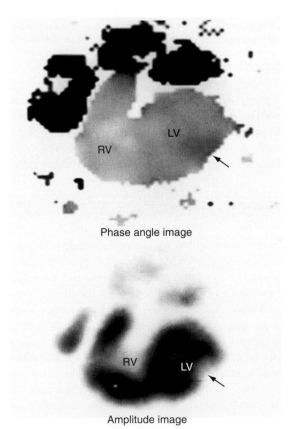

Phase angle image

Amplitude image

FIGURE 6–37. Left ventricular regional hypokinesia. In the phase and amplitude images, the arrows indicate an area of late (tardokinesia) or diminished (hypokiniesia) contraction inferolaterally compatible with segmental myocardial scarring. The amplitude image demonstrates a defect compatible with severe hypokinesia or akinesia. The phase image indicates an abnormality in the timing of minimal wall motion, likely related to recruitment of the scarred area by adjacent viable myocardium. RV, right ventricle; LV, left ventricle.

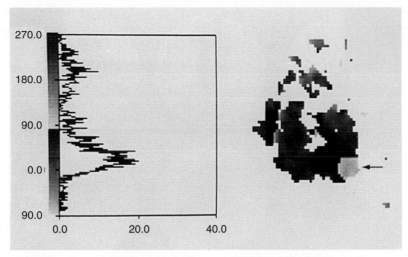

FIGURE 6–38. Phase analysis of a gated equilibrium radionuclide angiogram (E-RNA) demonstrating a left ventricular apical aneurysm. The phase information is displayed as a histogram on the *left* and as a gray-scale image on the *right*. On the histogram, a discrete peak for the ventricular contraction is seen, but there is significant broadening of the atrial peak compatible with a dyskinetic (out-of-phase) segment of left ventricular myocardium appearing during atrial contraction (*arrow*). The gray-scale image on the *right* clearly depicts the focal aneurysm (contracting paradoxically and "out of phase" with the remainder of the left ventricle) as a lighter shade of gray.

fractions. The technique can be used in patients both at rest and during stress.

Radiopharmaceutical

Because the time for imaging of the first-pass study is necessarily limited, images of adequate statistical quality can be obtained only by administering a sufficient bolus of radioactivity, usually a minimum of 10 mCi (370 MBq). In addition, because each study requires a separate injection of radioisotope, a radiopharmaceutical that clears rapidly from the blood is necessary if multiple determinations are to be performed. Because of their rapid clearance by the liver and kidneys, respectively, ^{99m}Tc-labeled sulfur colloid and ^{99m}Tc-labeled diethylene triamine pentaacetic acid (DTPA) are frequently used. Any ^{99m}Tc-labeled pharmaceutical may be used, however, if a repeat determination is not immediately contemplated. In fact, ^{99m}Tc blood pool agents may be used to obtain a first-pass study immediately before gated equilibrium imaging, so that both examinations are performed with only one radionuclide injection, allowing accurate determinations of both left and right ventricular ejection fractions.

Technique

The uniqueness of the first-pass examination is that the radioactive bolus progresses through the heart in such a manner that each chamber is visualized separately in temporal sequence, and problems with interfering activity in overlapping chambers, such as may be encountered with equilibrium imaging, are avoided (Fig. 6–39). A high sensitivity or general all-purpose collimator provides adequate statistical data collection. The examination may be performed in any view that places the cardiac ventricles reasonably near the camera face. The 30-degree RAO projection is most frequently used because it best allows separation of ventricular activity from atrial or aortic activity. Other projections may be used, depending on the particular aim of the study. Because only one projection can be obtained with each radionuclide bolus injection, multiple injections may be needed if several projections are required.

The collection of data in first-pass studies begins just before the injection of the radioactive bolus and is terminated after the activity traverses the left heart and is seen in the great arterial vessels. The entire study is normally completed in 30 to 60 seconds, over 5 to 10 cardiac cycles. Data are usually acquired by the computer in standard list mode as a sequence of images. Gated acquisition may also be used in synchrony with the patient's ECG, which allows better definition of the ventricular wall contours and evaluation of regional wall motion by the cine display of gated images. After

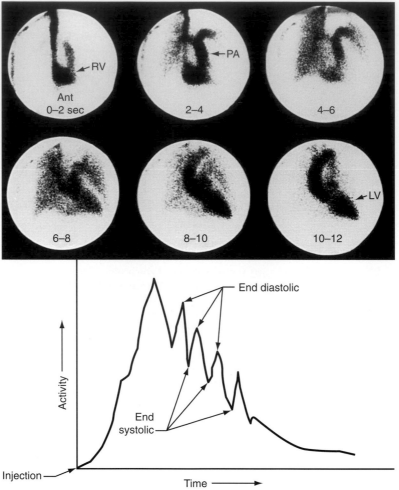

FIGURE 6–39. Normal first-pass radionuclide angiogram (FP-RNA). *Top,*
Selected images from a normal FP-RNA demonstrate the sequential identification of right
ventricle (RV), pulmonary artery (PA), lungs, and left ventricle (LV). Such temporal
separation of chamber activity allows selective evaluation of both RV and LV function.
Bottom, Time-activity curve obtained by using a region of interest over the RV displays the
passage of the radionuclide bolus propelled by multiple cardiac cycles (usually 5 to 10),
seen as peaks and valleys corresponding to sequential heart beats. RV ejection fraction can
be derived from this curve.

the study has been acquired and processed, the data
may be replayed and analyzed at the workstation.

Image Interpretation

First-pass radionuclide angiography is particularly
well-suited to obtain the following functional
information:

- Measurement of right ventricle function
  (ejection fraction)
- Assessment of ventricular function at peak
  exercise

- Quantification of left-to-right intracardiac
  shunts

Because the first pass of the radioactive bolus
through the heart and lungs takes place over multiple cardiac cycles, the data from several of these
cycles can be analyzed or summed to form a single
cycle of sufficient statistical nature for detailed
visual and quantitative inspection. When viewed
in endless-loop cine display, visual assessment of
regional ventricular wall motion is possible.
Although first-pass images of ventricular contrac-

tion are not of the statistical quality of equilibrium blood pool images and are usually limited to only one projection, the results are similar.

Cardiac Function

Quantitative assessment of the data presented in the digital images provides information regarding ventricular ejection fractions, ejection rates, cardiac output, and stroke volume as well as end-diastolic and end-systolic volumes. These parameters are usually acquired at rest. Uncommonly, the procedure may be performed at peak stress to assess ventricular contractile reserve and provides significant prognostic information in the setting of CAD. A significant fall in LVEF at peak exercise or an exercise LVEF of less than 40% confers a worse prognosis in patients with known CAD. Information concerning intracardiac and cardiopulmonary circulations can also be derived, including the calculation of pulmonary transit times.

Right Ventricular Function. Because of better separation of the right ventricle from the right atrium and left ventricle, first-pass determinations of right ventricular ejection fractions are in general more accurate than those obtained by using gated equilibrium technique, whereas LVEFs are comparable using the two techniques.

Intracardiac Shunts

In general, two-dimensional Doppler echocardiography is the initial procedure of choice in evaluating congenital heart disease and intracardiac shunts. However, in certain institutions offering expertise and experience in radionuclide techniques, FP RNA can offer accurate assessment.

Left-to-Right Intracardiac Shunts. First-pass studies can provide information needed to diagnose and quantify left-to-right intracardiac shunts. This is made possible by analysis of time-activity curves obtained from a region of interest placed over a lung at a distance from the heart. A compact bolus of activity is essential to an accurate study. Early pulmonary recirculation of the radiopharmaceutical through a left-to-right shunt may be detected as an alteration in the normal curve, evidenced by a small second peak proportional to the size of the shunt. Various methods of analysis of FP-RNA data allow for shunt quantification, with accuracy equal to that of contrast arteriography. Although various mathematic approaches are available for the calculation of shunt size, the gamma variate

function method provides the most accurate and reproducible technique. When using this method, pulmonary-to-systemic flow ratios of 1.2 : 1 or greater are considered evidence of left-to-right shunting.

Right-to-Left Intracardiac Shunts. Although right-to-left shunts may occasionally be defined on first-pass studies by early appearance of the radioactive bolus in the left heart or aorta through the intracardiac shunt before appearance of the bolus in the lungs, this method is not sensitive for the detection of such shunts, nor does it allow for accurate quantitation.

The magnitude of right-to-left shunts can be estimated by using an intravenous injection of the pulmonary perfusion radiopharmaceutical, ^{99m}Tc–macroaggregated albumin (MAA). In most patients only about 4% to 6% of the injected ^{99m}Tc-MAA will bypass the lungs to localize in the capillaries of the systemic circulation. A whole-body scan, using regions of interest over the entire body and the lungs, allows an estimation of systemic activity, which is proportional to the size of the right-to-left shunt.

Equilibrium Radionuclide Angiography (Gated Blood Pool Ventriculography)
Principle

Equilibrium radionuclide angiography (E-RNA) or gated blood pool ventriculography consists of imaging the cardiac blood pool after the injected tracer has mixed thoroughly with the intravascular space. Images are typically obtained by synchronizing the gamma camera collection of data with the ECG signals from the patient at rest, but less commonly may be acquired during exercise or pharmacologic stress. Sophisticated, semi-automated computer software is used to process the data, producing high quality cine images of the beating heart as well as a reproducible left ventricular volume curve from which ventricular functional parameters are derived. This output permits qualitative visual analysis of the size, configuration, and wall motion of the cardiac chambers and correlation with quantitative functional parameters of global and regional ventricular performance. Because the LV volume curve is based solely on LV blood pool count changes over the cardiac cycle, the LVEF derived is free of confounding geometric assumptions regarding LV shape and size and thus permits highly accurate, reproducible results.

Although E-RNA remains a valuable clinical technique, its use has significantly declined in recent years because of the widespread availability of echocardiography and the use of gated-SPECT myocardial perfusion imaging. However, when an accurate non-invasive determination of LVEF is desired, such as in patients in which echocardiography may be technically difficult, or when serial studies are needed to precisely monitor changes in LVEF, such as during cardiotoxic chemotherapy, gated blood pool ventriculography can be quite useful.

Radiopharmaceutical

Basically, any radiopharmaceutical that is compartmentalized to the intravascular space for the time period required to obtain the study may be used. Technetium-99m labeled autologous red blood cells are the agent of choice.

Various methods of labeling autologous red blood cells with ^{99m}Tc have been described (see Appendix E–1), including in vivo, modified in vivo, and in vitro techniques. All methods use the initial introduction of stannous (tin) ion, which enters the red blood cells. The intracellular stannous ion then acts as a reducing agent, which permits the binding of subsequently introduced ^{99m}Tc-pertechnetate to the β-chain of the hemoglobin molecule. Superior labeling efficiency is obtained by using in vitro methods (such as the UltraTag method), in which the patient's blood sample is labeled externally and then reinjected, although under most circumstances, adequate tagging of the red blood cells can be obtained by using in vivo methods.

The in vivo labeling procedure consists of intravenous injection of 0.5 to 1.0 mg of stannous ion, frequently as stannous pyrophosphate. After allowing the tin ion to equilibrate in the blood for 20 minutes, about 20 mCi (740 MBq) of ^{99m}Tc-pertechnetate is injected. With the tin acting as a complexing agent, a sufficient number of red blood cells are tagged in vivo to allow for labeling of the intravascular space. Although this technique provides sufficient tagging in most patients, a certain amount of injected ^{99m}Tc is rapidly lost from the intravascular space and does not participate in the labeling process. The percentage of injected technetium that remains intravascular and labels red blood cells is difficult to quantify but probably is about 75%. The percentage of radioisotope lost to the extravascular space contributes to longer imaging times as well as to background and thus to the degradation of images.

A modified in vivo technique provides for a combination of both in vivo and in vitro labeling procedures, giving a labeling efficiency of about 90%. This results in an increased intravascular concentration of ^{99m}Tc, with subsequent improvement in the quality of radionuclide images.

Because the technetium red blood cell bond lasts considerably longer than does the 6-hour half-life of ^{99m}Tc, the physical half-life of the radiopharmaceutical determines the length of time over which serial imaging is possible. With the use of 20 to 30 mCi (740 MBq to 1.11 GBq) of ^{99m}Tc-pertechnetate, delayed imaging is possible for up to 10 to 12 hours after injection.

Gated Technique

Widespread use of cardiac ECG-gating was initially achieved in conjunction with equilibrium radionuclide angiography. The general principles involved have also been applied to gated-SPECT myocardial perfusion imaging as well.

After the cardiac blood pool has been labeled, gated images of the heart are obtained. Gating is performed by using a computer coupled with an R wave trigger or physiologic "gate" that signals the computer to begin recording data in the computer memory at the onset of the ECG R wave. This synchronizes the collection of data from the gamma camera with the onset of each cardiac cycle within the patient. The computer divides the R-R interval of each cardiac cycle into equal subdivisions, numbering from 16 to 32. Data collected from the scintillation camera are sorted during each cardiac contraction so that corresponding statistical information is filed temporally into one of the R-R interval segments, depending on its displacement in time from the initial R wave (Fig. 6–40). Such sorting of data over numerous cardiac cycles allows for the accumulation of enough statistical data in each interval subdivision to allow for creation of a series of single composite images, each representing one point of cardiac contraction.

When the sequence of individual images is subsequently played in cine format, an image of the blood in the chambers of the beating heart is produced, which represents a summation of the several hundred cardiac cycles needed to collect sufficient data. Images may be acquired for a certain number of counts ($\approx$ 3 to 6 million total counts) or, less frequently, for a set number of cardiac cycles. This gating process is the basis of all E-RNA and may be used in the collection of data from first-pass examinations as well.

Image sequence

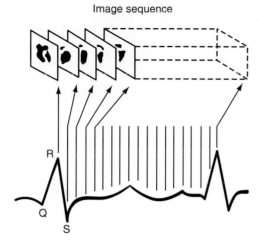

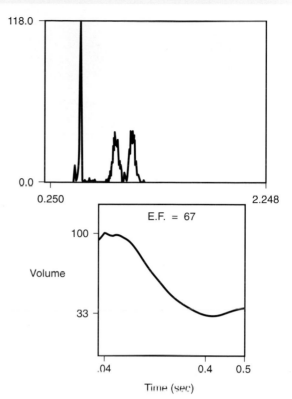

FIGURE 6–40. Gated technique for equilibrium radionuclide angiogram (E-RNA). Data collection is triggered by the R wave, with the cardiac cycle divided temporally into discrete frames. Counts arriving during any division are placed in the computer matrix relevant to that division. After several hundred cardiac cycles, there is enough information in each frame to form a useful image. These frames (images) can be sequentially viewed in a dynamic cine format as an endless loop of the same composite (summed) cardiac cycle replayed over and over.

FIGURE 6–41. Cardiac arrhythmia. *Top,* The R-R histogram gives an indication of the number of normal and abnormal cardiac beats collected during gated equilibrium radionuclide angiography (E-RNA) based on variation of the lengths of their R-R intervals. The tall, thin peak is from the normal sinus rhythm. The lower, broader peaks correspond to aberrant beats with abnormally long R-R intervals. *Bottom,* A time-activity curve (left ventricular counts/volume curve) derived from this data is abnormal and does not return to baseline. This finding should raise the suspicion of a cardiac arrhythmia.

Because of the inherent reliance of gated methodology on ECG input, the success of the technique is necessarily related to the consistency of cardiac rate and rhythm in a given patient. Ordinarily, because the length of systole does not change proportionally as the length of the cardiac cycle increases or decreases, minimal variations in heart rate during acquisition do not significantly affect the study. Severe disturbances in rhythm, however, cause distortion of the data obtained. Although a small number of aberrant cardiac cycles may be tolerated (<10%), as the number of such beats increases, there is a progressive degradation of the recorded data, which may give false information regarding such measurements as regional wall motion and LVEF. Computer software to access the quality of the data provides the operator with a histogram of distribution of the lengths of R-R intervals over the acquisition time of the study. These histograms allow for easy recognition of aberrant beats (Fig. 6–41). In a patient with normal rhythm, the histogram demonstrates a single, well-defined peak. With aberrant beats, there are additional, smaller peaks.

In patients with occasional aberrant beats, the validity of the data may be preserved by *arrhythmia filtering*. This process allows for the rejection of cardiac cycles that do not conform to the average length of a cardiac cycle in a particular patient. However, because such arrhythmic information is excluded from the study, the time of acquisition for the examination increases. The most convenient method of arrhythmia filtering involves the use of real-time list mode to hold the data briefly in a buffer while the R-R interval of a beat is measured. If the R-R interval is outside accepted limits (usually by about 10% variation), the counts associated with the beat are rejected and thus do not contribute to the final image data set.

A high-resolution parallel-hole collimator may be used when performing planar E-RNA, provided that the count-rates are adequate. This method provides the best spatial resolution for evaluation of regional wall motion. General low-energy, all-

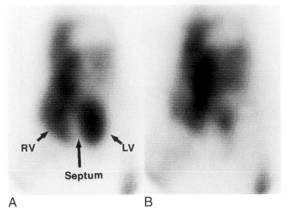

A　　　　　　B

FIGURE 6–42. Normal gated equilibrium radionuclide angiogram (E-RNA). The views obtained in the left anterior oblique projection ("best septal view") depict end-diastole (*A*) and end-systole (*B*). The right ventricle (RV), left ventricle (LV), and septum are easily identified.

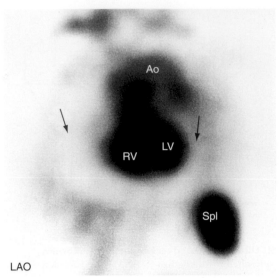

LAO

FIGURE 6–43. Pericardial effusion. A gated blood pool image clearly demonstrates the right (RV) and left ventricles (LV), the aorta (Ao), and the spleen (Spl). There is a photopenic "halo" around the ventricles (*arrows*) due to a large pericardial effusion. LAO, left anterior oblique view.

purpose, parallel-hole collimators may also be used at rest and provide a good compromise between sensitivity and resolution. General all-purpose and high-sensitivity collimators are often desirable for exercise studies because they provide increased sensitivity for the collection of images during the necessarily short intervals of exercise.

After the intravascular space has been labeled, resting studies usually require about 5 to 10 minutes per view, whereas exercise images are generally collected over several minutes. In resting studies, three views are normally obtained to allow for adequate visualization of the cardiac chambers and great vessels. These include (1) an anterior view, (2) a left anterior oblique ("best septal") view at about 45 degrees to visualize the septum and allow separation of the left and right ventricles (Fig. 6–42), and (3) a left lateral or 70-degree left anterior oblique view. A caudal tilt of the camera detector of about 10 degrees is recommended for acquisition of the 45-degree left anterior oblique view to maximize separation of the left ventricle from the left atrium. During exercise, usually only the 45-degree left anterior oblique view is imaged, to permit calculation of LVEF changes at various levels of stress.

In addition to the routine planar imaging of the cardiac blood pool, gated-SPECT acquisition may be performed and the LV displayed as short- or long-axis tomographic slices or three-dimensional volumetric images. Although not commonly employed, it may be used to improve assessment of regional wall motion and to calculate absolute LV volumes as well as LVEF. LVEFs obtained by this technique are usually somewhat higher than routine planar studies.

Image Interpretation

When E-RNA images are viewed cinematically in an endless-loop display, they present the image of the blood pool in a beating heart, which can then be qualitatively and quantitatively analyzed by using various computer programs.

Qualitative Data. Cinematic computer display of gated images allows for the visual assessment of regional wall motion of both the left and right ventricles. In addition to ventricular wall excursion, relative sizes of the cardiac chambers, the size and position of the great vessels, the relative thicknesses of ventricular walls (particularly the septum) and the pericardial space (Fig. 6–43), and any filling defects within the cardiac blood pool should be noted (Table 6–3).

Ventricular wall excursion is inferred by the impact of wall motion on the immediately adjacent portion of the blood-filled cavity. Once contraction begins, all ventricular wall segments should contract simultaneously, although some walls demonstrate greater absolute excursion than others. Generally, the anterior, posterior, and lateral walls appear to move to a greater degree than the septum, apex, and frequently the inferior wall.

TABLE 6–3.	Gated Cardiac Equilibrium Blood Pool Imaging Visual Data Analysis

Quality of red blood cell labeling
Overall distribution of labeled red blood cells
Course and caliber of great vessels
Relative pulmonary blood pool activity
Thickness of pericardial–myocardial space
Shape and thickness of interventricular septum
Clot or mass within the cardiac chambers
Size of each chamber
Chamber wall motion
Sequence of chamber contraction

Segmental wall motion abnormalities are usually described as *hypokinesis* (relatively diminished wall motion), *akinesis* (no wall motion), and *dyskinesis* (paradoxical wall motion). Areas of injured or scarred myocardium usually present as regions of hypokinesis or akinesis, whereas ventricular aneurysms appear as focal areas of dyskinesis. Lesions are localized as nearly as possible to particular segments of the LV wall by correlating the multiple views obtained. The evaluation of septal wall motion frequently presents a problem. Normally, the septum shortens or thickens and moves slightly toward the LV cavity during systole. Paradoxical septal motion (toward the right ventricle during systole) should be considered abnormal and is frequently associated with previous coronary artery bypass surgery or septal infarction.

Although wall motion abnormalities are almost always evident on visual inspection of cine images, the already described functional images generated by computer software may aid in the evaluation of regional wall motion.

Quantitative Data

Systolic Function. By using a region of interest over the LV blood pool, a time activity curve is generated depicting the change in LV volume during the summed cardiac cycle. From this LV volume curve, LV functional parameters are derived. These include both systolic and diastolic indices, the most important of which is the LVEF.

In addition to LVEF and ejection rates, various other indices of LV function may be calculated as needed, including LV volumes and regional ejection fractions.

Because the LV is not temporally segregated from the other cardiac chambers, as in first-transit studies, a common problem for LVEF determination is the inclusion of a small amount of left atrium or left atrial appendage in the selected region of interest. Normally, the left atrium lies sufficiently posterior to the LV, so that counts within this chamber do not contribute significantly to LV activity. When the left atrium is enlarged, however, a portion of this structure may be included in the determination and falsely lower the ejection fraction. Differentiation of the LV from the atrium using phase analysis may aid in excluding any left atrial activity from the desired region of interest.

Unlike first-transit studies, right ventricular ejection fractions are often not reliably calculated from the equilibrium study because the right ventricle is not easily separated from the right atrium or an enlarged LV. If an accurate right ventricular ejection fraction is desired, it may be better obtained by performing a first-pass examination during the initial transit of the bolus at the beginning of the study. Furthermore, because data are obtained at equilibrium of the injected dose, shunt quantification is not possible with the gated blood pool technique.

Diastolic Function. Because diastolic dysfunction may precede abnormalities of systolic function (i.e., ejection fraction) in a variety of cardiac disease states, including CAD, quantitation of diastolic parameters may permit the early detection of LV functional impairment. The diastolic parameters available from the LV time-activity (volume) curve include ventricular filling and ejection rates. The most frequently derived LV diastolic parameter, peak filling rate (PFR), reflects the early, rapid-filling phase of diastole and is commonly seen as a measure of LV compliance. A normal PFR is usually greater than 2.5 end-diastolic volumes per second in young adults. Unlike LVEF, which remains relatively constant during aging, the PFR declines with age as compliance of the LV diminishes.

Diastolic dysfunction, as defined by parameters such as subnormal PFR, has been shown to occur in patients with CAD who have preserved systolic function (LVEF) and no evidence of active ischemia or previous infarction. Assessment of diastolic function parameters may also play an important role in the evaluation of congestive heart failure. About 40% of patients with a diagnosis of congestive heart failure demonstrate normal LV systolic function but impaired diastolic filling. Filling rate indices may be influenced by unrelated parameters, such as systolic ejection fraction and

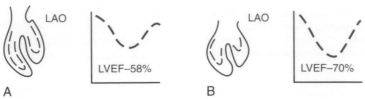

FIGURE 6–44. Effect of exercise on the left ventricular ejection fraction (LVEF) in a normal patient. With maximal exercise, the ejection fraction normally rises at least 5% (5 ejection fraction units). The schematic cardiac diagram is shown for both rest (*A*) and exercise (*B*) in the left anterior oblique (LAO) projection, with both the systolic (*broken lines*) and diastolic (*solid lines*) ventricular wall outlines. The computer-generated time-activity curve represents volume changes in the left ventricle over the cardiac cycle. The curve begins with diastole and shows that at end-systole (represented by the lowest portion of the curve), there is relatively less residual activity (end-systolic volume) in the left ventricle in the exercise state as the stroke volume and ejection fraction rise.

length of cardiac cycle, as well as by noncoronary diseases of the heart, including systemic hypertension, "normal" age-related decline in PFR, and anti-ischemic therapy.

Clinical Applications

Coronary Artery Disease

With the ascendancy of GSPECT myocardial perfusion imaging as the preferred radionuclide method for the diagnosis of suspected CAD and the risk stratification of patients with known CAD, the use of E-RNA in these settings has significantly declined, because LV perfusion and function are now available in a single test.

However, true resting LVEF in patients with known CAD obtained by either method remains a significant indicator of long-term prognosis in patients with stable CAD. Prognosis deteriorates as the LVEF at rest falls below 45% to 50%. Conversely, event rates are low in patients with normal resting LVEF.

Exercise or pharmacologic stress RNA may still be uncommonly employed, using either first-pass or equilibrium technique, to obtain prognostic information in patients with known CAD. Most protocols involve an initial resting baseline determination of ventricular wall motion and ejection fraction, with subsequent serial images obtained over a period of stepwise increases in stress. The two principal criteria for evaluating LV functional response to exercise are assessment of LVEF and regional wall motion. The physiologic basis underlying exercise-induced abnormalities assumes that the hypoperfused, ischemic areas of myocardium distal to significant stenotic lesions do not respond with effective contraction under stress, thereby giving rise to regional wall motion abnormalities

and regionally or globally decreased ejection fractions. In normal subjects, the LVEF increases during maximal exercise, usually by more than five percentage points (ejection fraction units) above resting levels (Fig. 6–44). Failure of the LVEF to rise by 5%, or a decrease during peak exercise, is considered abnormal. A decline in LVEF in response to stress or an abnormal peak exercise LVEF is an important indication of the severity of CAD and confers a worse prognosis. Further, a peak exercise LVEF of less that 30% indicates a high risk of future adverse cardiac events and reduced survival.

Myocardial Infarction

Prognosis after myocardial infarction is related to infarct size as reflected by global LVEF and extent and degree of wall motion abnormalities. Large infarcts may produce extensive wall motion abnormalities with significantly decreased LVEFs, whereas smaller injuries may produce only focal wall motion impairment with a normal or slightly decreased LVEF or no abnormality at all. Anterior infarcts generally lower LVEF to a greater degree than do inferior wall lesions.

Both ejection fraction and wall motion abnormalities may change significantly in the acute phase of the insult, especially in the first week after infarction, and then generally stabilize by 2 weeks. After about 12 weeks, the findings are fully evolved. Any improvement in ejection fraction or wall motion over the evolutionary course of the myocardial infarction may result from recovery of initially stunned myocardium, or from therapeutic or spontaneous reperfusion that rescues local tissue and hence myocardial function.

The resting LVEF as determined by gated radionuclide ventriculography has proved to be a

TABLE 6–4.	Characteristic Findings on Gated Blood Pool Imaging in Patients with Noncoronary Heart Disease	

LESIONS	FINDINGS
VALVULAR	
Aortic regurgitation	Dilated LV cavity with hypertrophy; normal or decreased LVEF
Aortic stenosis	Normal LV cavity and LVEF; LV hypertrophy; dilated LA
Mitral regurgitation	Dilated LV cavity and normal or decreased LVEF; normal LV wall thickness; dilated LA
Tricuspid regurgitation	Dilated RV cavity and decreased RVEF; dilated RA
HYPERTENSIVE	LV concentric hypertrophy; normal or supranormal LVEF; diastolic dysfunction
CARDIOMYOPATHY	
Dilated (congestive)	Dilatation of all four chambers; decreased LVEF and RVEF; decreased LV wall thickness
Ischemic	Normal or dilated LV cavity and decreased LVEF; decreased LV wall thickness; normal or dilated LA
Hypertrophic	Normal or small LV cavity; normal or supranormal LVEF; severe LV hypertrophy; normal or dilated LA
Restrictive	Normal LV cavity and normal or decreased LVEF; normal or increased RV cavity and normal or decreased RVEF
SEPTAL DEFECT	
Atrial	Dilated RV cavity and decreased RVEF; dilated RA with normal or dilated LA
Ventricular	Normal or increased LV cavity and normal or increased LVEF; dilated RV and normal or decreased RVEF; dilated LA

LV, left ventricle; RV, right ventricle; LA, left atrium; RA, right atrium; EF, ejection fraction.
Adapted from Dilsizian V, Rocco TP, Bonow RO, et al: Cardiac blood-pool imaging II: applications in noncoronary heart disease. J Nucl Med 31:10–22, 1990.

reliable measure of the impact of coronary occlusion on LV function in early myocardial infarction and, as such, has shown to be an important predictor of prognosis. In this setting, an ejection fraction of 0.30 during the first 24 hours after infarction appears to represent a watershed, with about 50% of the patients with values at or below this level succumbing to LV failure or death. This represents a nearly ninefold higher mortality rate than is seen in patients with a LVEF of greater than 30%. Conversely, only about 2% of patients with higher ejection fractions die acutely. During early recovery from the initial insult, a predischarge resting LVEF of 40% or less remains a potent predictor of future events and death, with the 1-year mortality rate increasing exponentially as the resting LVEF falls below 0.40.

Noncoronary Disease

Characteristic findings on gated blood pool imaging in patients with noncoronary heart disease are shown in Table 6–4. Radionuclide ventriculography may aid in the differential diagnosis of cardiopulmonary disease by helping distinguish dyspnea related to primary LV failure from that caused by chronic pulmonary disease, when differentiation on clinical grounds is not possible. Right ventricular dysfunction and cardiac chamber dilatation with a normal left ventricle are usually associated with chronic obstructive pulmonary disease, whereas pulmonary vascular congestion related to LV failure is accompanied by LV enlargement or functional abnormalities. In patients with known chronic obstructive pulmonary disease, a resting right ventricular ejection fraction of less than 0.35 is a relatively sensitive predictor of pulmonary artery hypertension.

Chemotherapeutic Cardiotoxicity. E-RNA is used in monitoring LV function in patients receiving cardiotoxic chemotherapy agents, principally because the technique is capable of detecting small serial reductions in LVEF with reproducible results.

The most common setting in this regard is the serial assessment of LVEFs to monitor the dose-related cardiotoxicity of anthracyclines, such as doxorubicin, during the course of treatment. The study is of use in selecting patients who may best tolerate the medication and in monitoring those who receive it to determine the onset of cardiac toxicity. Patients receiving doxorubicin usually do not have toxic cardiac responses below cumulative doses of about 400 mg/m². With increasing dose, however, a largely irreversible dilated cardiomyopathy may result with diminished LV function, ultimately leading to congestive cardiac failure. Because administration of doxorubicin produces an acute transient reduction of LVEF, in addition to long-term toxicity, serial measurements should be taken about 2 weeks after the last dose to allow recovery to occur and to determine the new baseline value.

LVEF should be obtained in patients before doxorubicin therapy is begun to obtain a baseline value. This is especially important in patients with suspected or known cardiac dysfunction who are at greater risk of developing CHF. Doxorubicin therapy is initiated with special caution in patients with ejection fractions below the normal range. Parameters predictive of developing cardiotoxic CHF include a baseline LVEF less than 60%; a drop from baseline LVEF to 50% or less, and advancing age. A reduction from baseline LVEF of 10 ejection fraction units or to below 45% is usually considered significant. Frank congestive heart failure is preceded by a progressive fall in LVEF. Serial radionuclide studies permit the withdrawal of doxorubicin therapy in these patients, thereby preventing life-threatening cardiac complications.

Cardiomyopathy. Cardiomyopathies constitute a group of heterogeneous primary myocardial diseases usually classified as dilated, hypertrophic, or restrictive. Gated blood pool imaging has proved useful not only in detecting cardiomyopathies but also in evaluating the degree of systolic or diastolic functional impairment and assessing the effects of medical therapy. Hypertrophic cardiomyopathy typically presents with a normal or elevated LVEF and hyperdynamic systolic function, with evidence of ventricular wall thickening, especially in the basal interventricular septum, and a concomitantly small LV cavity. Eighty percent or more of these patients exhibit impaired diastolic function (Fig. 6–45). Dilated cardiomyopathies typically present with LV chamber dilatation and diffuse hypokinesis, with a reduced LVEF of less than 40%. Right ventricular dysfunction and dilatation may also be present. Generally, marked biventricular enlargement with global dysfunction is more likely to be of nonischemic origin, whereas the presence of focal left ventricular wall motion abnormalities and relatively preserved right ventricular function favor a diagnosis of ischemic cardiomyopathy.

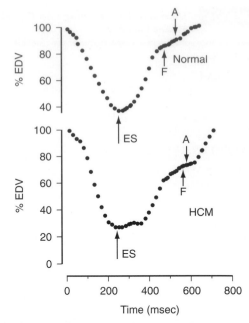

FIGURE 6–45. Left ventricular time-activity curves from a normal subject and a patient with hypertrophic cardiomyopathy (HCM). Despite normal systolic function, the patient with HCM has impaired left ventricular diastolic as evidenced by the flattened slope of the diastolic portion of the curve. Derived diastolic parameters reveal reduced peak filling rate, prolongation of the time to peak filling rate, and increased contribution of atrial systole to total left ventricular filling. EDV, end-diastolic volume; ES, end-systole; F, end of rapid filling; A, onset of atrial systole. (From Dilsizian V, Rocco TP, Bonow RO, et al: Cardiac blood pool imaging II: applications in noncoronary heart disease. J Nucl Med 31:10–22, 1990.)

Congestive Heart Failure. Although echocardiography is the initial procedure of choice in the evaluation of cardiac function in the setting of CHF, when E-RNA is performed, both LVEF and LV diastolic function should be assessed. Approximately 30% of patients presenting with congestive heart failure have isolated or predominant diastolic dysfunction, with hypertensive hypertrophic cardiomyopathy being the underlying cause in a large number. The E-RNA findings include a normal LV cavity, normal LVEF, and impaired LV filing as measured by a reduced PFR and exaggerated time to peak filling. Because the treatment for diastolic LV failure is different from primary systolic failure, this distinction has important therapeutic implications.

Cardiac Valvular Disease. In general, two-dimensional Doppler echocardiography is the procedure of choice in noninvasive evaluation of suspected valvular cardiac disease, although nuclear methods may be useful in some settings. In practice, E-RNA is not commonly used to evaluate valvular stenosis but may play a role in the assessment of valvular insufficiency. In patients with aortic regurgitation, quantification of aortic regurgitant fraction, indicating the severity of disease, and LVEF are important clinical parameters. As the resting LVEF declines below about 55%, patient prognosis worsens. Evaluation of patients with known aortic regurgitation during exercise has been used to predict the appropriateness and timing of valvular surgery by determining whether LVEF fails to rise or actually falls during exercise, as a measure of reduced LV contractile reserve. However, in practice, this is uncommonly performed.

In the preoperative evaluation mitral regurgitation, declining LV dysfunction as measured by LVEF correlates with a poor prognosis. As LVEF falls below about 60%, prognosis becomes unfa-

vorable. Further, patients with combined LV and RV dysfunction have an even worse prognosis.

In patients with idiopathic hypertrophic subaortic stenosis, radionuclide findings include a markedly elevated LVEF and small LV cavity, with asymmetric thickening of the upper portion of the ventricular septum.

Myocardial Infarct-Avid Imaging

Although the use of infarct-avid radiopharmaceuticals such as ^{99m}Tc-stannous pyrophosphate and ^{111}In-labeled antimyocin antibody for the imaging of acute myocardial infarcts has played a role in the diagnosis of acute myocardial infarction, advances in enzymatic diagnosis have rendered such imaging obsolete in almost all clinical settings.

POSITRON EMISSION TOMOGRAPHY

The cardiac applications of PET are discussed in detail in Chapter 13.

PEARLS & PITFALLS

Myocardial Perfusion Studies

The common indication for myocardial perfusion studies is to determine whether there is normal perfusion, ischemia, or infarction. The images obtained represent relative, not absolute blood flow.

Technetium 99m sestamibi and tetrophosmin have a higher photon energy (140 keV) than do the mercury daughter x-rays (69 to 81 keV) from ^{201}Tl. As a result there is less soft-tissue attenuation with ^{99m}Tc-labeled radiopharmceuticals than with thallium.

Myocardial uptake of ^{201}Tl-chloride and ^{99m}Tc-sestamibi or tetrophosmin is proportional to regional blood flow and requires cell viability.

Thallium is actively taken up by the Na^+-K^+ pump in the cells, whereas ^{99m}Tc sestamibi and tetrophosmin passively diffuse across the membrane and localize primarily in cytoplasmic mitochondria.

Thallium redistributes over time, so post-stress images must be obtained immediately after injection. Technetium-99m sestamibi and tetrophosmin do not redistribute, and the best

images are made 30 to 90 minutes after injection to allow for clearance of interfering background activity from the liver but before the activity reaches the transverse colon.

Infarcts and hibernating myocardium produce perfusion defects on the rest images.

Stress images are needed to elucidate ischemia with lesser degrees of stenosis (50% to 90%). Stenoses less than 50% in diameter are not detected at rest and are variably diagnosed with exercise imaging.

Stress may be physical or pharmacologic. Physical stress should be discontinued with patient exhaustion, claudication, severe angina or hypotension, arrhythmia or severe ECG changes, or attainment of more than 85% of maximal predicted heart rate (220 minus the patient's age in years).

Dipyridamole and adenosine are used instead of physical stress to dilate normal coronary arteries. Vessels in ischemic areas are already maximally dilated and do not dilate further.

PEARLS & PITFALLS—cont'd

The adverse effects of dipyridamole are reversed with 100 to 200 mg of intravenous aminophylline. Dipyridamole and adenosine should not be used in patients with asthma or reactive airway diseases.

Dobutamine is inotropic and chronotropic and is used as a form of pharmacologic stress. Adverse effects may be reversed by using short-acting β-blockers.

The most common cause of false-negative examinations is submaximal stress. The most common cause of false-positive examinations is artifacts.

The myocardium normally thins at the cardiac apex, in the membranous septum, and near the base of the inferior wall.

On thallium scans, the degree of stress can be inferred from splanchnic activity. The more activity, the less adequate the stress.

A high degree of lung activity on exercise thallium images (>50% of peak myocardial activity) is related to poor prognosis, more extensive disease, and LV dysfunction at exercise. On ^{99m}Tc sestamibi scans, lung activity is uncommon. When seen, its significance is unknown.

Transient LV dilatation with exercise may be related primarily to subendocardial ischemia and less often to real LV dilatation. It is a sign of a poor prognosis.

With adequate exercise, the sensitivity and specificity of myocardial SPECT are each about 85%.

An occluded coronary artery with adequate collaterals or balanced three-vessel disease can produce an apparently normal scan.

Real defects on myocardial perfusion images should be seen on at least two views (e.g., short and vertical or horizontal long axes).

Defects seen at stress but not at rest are usually (but not always) ischemia. LBBB may produce myocardial perfusion findings indistinguishable from stress-induced reversible septal ischemia.

A defect seen at the base of the heart is frequently artifactual unless it extends to the apex.

Not all fixed defects (seen both at rest and post-stress) are infarcts. They may also be soft-tissue attenuation artifacts or hibernating or repetitively stunned myocardium.

Hibernating myocardium is a chronically hypoperfused area that has reduced cellular metabolism. This area has decreased contractility. Revascularization is usually needed.

Stunned myocardium is due to an acute occlusion with relatively rapid perfusion return. These areas have normal or near-normal perfusion and decreased contractility. Revascularization is not usually needed.

Defects seen on rest (redistribution) images but not on post-stress images (reverse redistribution) are real but are of uncertain cause and significance. They frequently are associated with prior myocardial injury or revascularization procedures.

LV walls that diverge toward the apex should raise suspicion of a LV aneurysm.

Diaphragmatic attenuation looks like an inferior wall defect. It often goes away on prone images.

Diaphragmatic (cardiac) creep presents as a reversible inferior wall defect.

Relatively intense gastrointestinal activity adjacent to the inferior wall can cause an apparent inferior myocardial defect on SPECT studies as a result of a reconstruction artifact.

Breast attenuation usually causes an apparent defect in the anterior or lateral LV wall.

Bull's eye plots underestimate apical defects and overestimate basal defects.

GSPECT markers of high-risk CAD include the following: multiple perfusion defects indicative of multivessel disease; large, severe perfusion defects; transient LV dilatation; increased thallium lung/heart ratio; end-systolic volume (ESV) (>70 mL); and a post-stress LVEF less than 40%.

Equilibrium Radionuclide Angiography

Gated equilibrium radionuclide angiograms (MUGA scans) are performed with ^{99m}Tc red blood cells. Common indications include assessment of LVEF and regional wall motion.

The normal LVEF is 50% to 65%. The lower limit is 50% in older people. Ejection fractions higher than 70% may reflect hypertrophy, valvular regurgitation or idiopathic hypertrophic subaortic stenosis (IHSS).

The normal right ventricular ejection fraction is 40% to 50%.

PEARLS & PITFALLS—cont'd

A time-activity (gated E-RNA LV volume) curve that does not come back to baseline may be due to a cardiac arrhythmia. Inspection of the R-R histogram reveals multiple peaks. More than 10% rejected beats will result in an inaccurate LVEF calculation.

If the left anterior oblique view (best septal view) is not precise, overlap of the left ventricle with the left atrial appendage, right ventricle, or the great vessels may cause a falsely low LVEF. Oversubtraction of background will cause a falsely high LVEF.

Regional wall motion abnormalities on a resting MUGA scan are usually due to myocardial infarction but may be seen in stunned or hibernating myocardium.

A photopenic halo around the cardiac blood pool activity is usually due to a pericardial effusion.

SUGGESTED READINGS

Elhendy A, Ba JJ, Poldermans D: Dobutamine Stress Myocardial Perfusion Imaging in Coronary Artery Disease. J Nucl Med 43:1634–1646, 2002.

Go V, Bhatt MR, Hendel RC: The diagnostic and prognostic value of ECG-Gated SPECT myocardial perfusion imaging. J Nucl Med 45:912–921, 2004.

Hachamovitch R, Berman DS: The use of nuclear cardiology in clinical decision making. Semin Nucl Med 35:62–72, 2005.

Jadvar H, Strauss HW, Segall GM: SPECT and PET in the Evaluation of Coronary Artery Disease. RadioGraphics 19:915–926, 1999.

Machac J: Cardiac positron emission tomography imaging. Semin Nucl Med 3517–3536, 2005.

Meine TJ, Hanson MW, Borges-Neto S: The Additive Value of Combined Assessment of Myocardial Perfusion and Ventricular Function Studies. J Nucl Med 45:1721–1724, 2004.

Paul AK, Nabi HA: Gated myocardial perfusion SPECT: basic principles, technical aspects, and clinical applications. J Nucl Med Tech 32:179–187, 2004.

Travin MI, Bergmann SR: Assessment of myocardial viability. Semin Nucl Med 35.2–16, 2005

Respiratory System

7

INTRODUCTION

Radionuclide lung imaging most commonly involves the demonstration of pulmonary perfusion using limited capillary blockade, as well as the assessment of ventilation using inspired inert gas, usually xenon, or radiolabeled aerosols. Although these studies are essentially qualitative, they have an advantage over most quantitative tests of global lung function in distinguishing between diffuse and regional pulmonary disease. Most significantly, the ability to display both regional airway and vascular integrity forms the basis for the noninvasive diagnosis of pulmonary emboli. Ventilation (V) and perfusion (Q) scans are often referred to as V/Q scans. Evaluation of lung cancer and staging are discussed in Chapter 13 on positron-emission tomography (PET) scanning. Some aspects of pulmonary infection and inflammation imaging are presented in Chapter 12.

ANATOMY AND PHYSIOLOGY

The trachea divides into the right and left mainstem bronchi, and these in turn divide to form lobar bronchi. The lobar divisions on the right are the upper-, middle-, and lower-lobe bronchi; on the left, there are just upper- and lower-lobe bronchi. The lobes are further divided into segments based on bronchopulmonary anatomy, which are shown in Figure 7–1. Knowledge of the anatomy of the lobes and segments of the lungs is essential for accurate interpretation of radionuclide pulmonary images.

Inspiration produces a negative intrapleural pressure, which is generated by action of the thoracic cage musculature and the diaphragm. Each terminal respiratory unit or alveolus is elastic, and this elasticity provides the major impetus for expiration. Adults have about 250 to 300 million alveoli, with an average diameter of 150 μm per alveolus. It is important to remember that the direct anatomic pathway is not the only means by which air can enter the alveoli. If a bronchiole is blocked, air may get into the distal alveoli through the pores of Kohn, which provide direct communication between neighboring alveoli. In addition, the canals of Lambert connect the respiratory bronchioles and alveolar ducts. Both of these indirect pathways allow collateral ventilation in the peripheral lung and often prevent collapse of an obstructed pulmonary segment or segments.

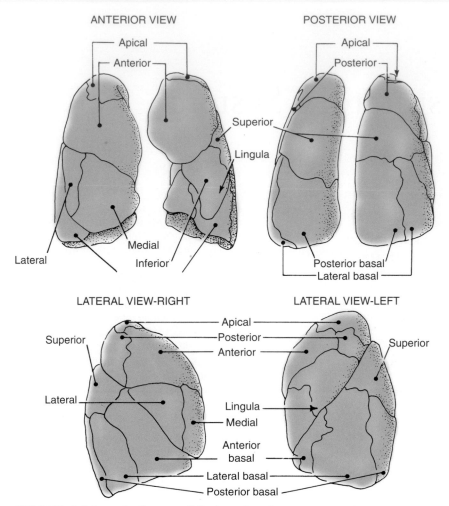

ANTERIOR VIEW

POSTERIOR VIEW

LATERAL VIEW-RIGHT

LATERAL VIEW-LEFT

FIGURE 7–1. Schematic diagram of the bronchopulmonary segments.

The main pulmonary arteries divide in each lung to follow the divisions of the bronchi and bronchioles to the level of the alveoli. Each alveolus is supplied by a terminal pulmonary arteriole, which in turn gives rise to capillaries. The capillaries that surround the alveoli are between 7 and 10 μm in diameter. The lungs also receive blood from the aorta via the bronchial arteries, which follow the bronchial tree as far as the respiratory bronchioles. The bronchial arteries anastomose at the capillary level with the pulmonary circulation, and most of the blood from the bronchial arteries returns to the left atrium via the pulmonary veins. The bronchial circulation supplies about 5% of the blood flow to the lung under normal circumstances.

Gravity and patient position have a significant impact on both ventilation and perfusion. However, the alteration of blood flow throughout the lungs with positional change is much more marked than accompanying changes in ventilation. In the upright position, intrapleural pressure is significantly more negative at the apices than at the lung bases. As a result of this negative pressure difference, the upper lung zone alveoli are held more open in expiration than are the lower lung alveoli, which are relatively collapsed. The increased potential volume in the lung bases provides a greater change in alveolus size during inspiration than at the apices, with the net effect that ventilation (air exchange) is greater in the lower lungs. Normally, ventilation in the lower portion of the lung is about 150% of that in the apex.

Pulmonary perfusion is also unevenly distributed throughout the lungs. Maximal pulmonary blood flow normally occurs in the lung zone bracketing the junction of the lower third and upper two thirds of the lungs. In the upright position, the apex receives only about one third of the blood flow per unit volume as compared with the bases. In the supine position, however, perfusion is more uniform, although again there is relatively increased blood flow in the dependent portions of the lung. In patients who demonstrate more flow to the upper lobes, congestive failure with increased left atrial pressure or α_1-antitrypsin deficiency should be considered.

Thus, in the normal, upright patient, both ventilation and perfusion increase progressively from the lung apex to the bases, although this gradient is more pronounced for perfusion. Because ventilation increases much less rapidly from apex to base, the ventilation-perfusion ratio changes in the reverse direction, increasing from base to apex. In the supine position, both ventilation and perfusion gradients are less pronounced, resulting in more even ventilation and perfusion throughout the lungs.

Uncommonly, acute changes in perfusion affect ventilation; local ischemia and hypoxia can cause reflex bronchoconstriction, with a resulting shift of ventilation away from the hypoperfused areas. However, this phenomenon appears to be transient and is uncommonly demonstrated in humans. Conversely, abnormalities of ventilation commonly cause redistribution of pulmonary perfusion; hypoventilation leads to regional hypoxia and reflex vasoconstriction with redistribution of perfusion away from the hypoventilated regions.

RADIOPHARMACEUTICALS

Perfusion Imaging Agents

Technetium-99m (^{99m}Tc) macroaggregated albumin (MAA) is the radiopharmaceutical used for pulmonary perfusion imaging. It localizes by the mechanism of capillary blockade. In general, fewer than 1 in 1000 (<0.1%) of the capillaries are blocked. In the absence of shunts, 95% of the particles are removed from the circulation on the first pass through the pulmonary capillary bed. About 5% of particles measure less than 5 μm in diameter and pass through the capillary system. For purposes of pulmonary perfusion imaging, it is important to use a sufficient number of particles to allow for good statistical distribution. In general, injection of a minimum of 100,000 particles, and optimally between 200,000 and 600,000 particles, is required.

The production of ^{99m}Tc-MAA entails aggregation of human serum albumin using heat and a reducing agent to form the particles. Visual inspection of the preparations through the use of a microscope and hemocytometer demonstrate whether the MAA particles are too large or have clumped. The particle size of ^{99m}Tc-MAA generally ranges from 5 to 100 μm, with most in the range of 10 to 30 μm. MAA has a biologic half-life in the lung of 2 to 4 hours, depending on the kit manufacturer and preparation. Some preparations begin to break down as early as 30 minutes after injection. The particle fragments enter the general circulation as smaller particles, which are usually removed from the circulation by the liver and spleen. The normal administered activity in adults is 3 to 5 mCi (111 to 185 MBq); in children, 25 to 50 μCi (0.9–1.85 MBq)/kg. The lung is the critical organ. The absorbed dose to the lung is variable but is about 0.5 rad (5 mGy) for a 3-mCi (111-MBq) dose.

Technetium-99m MAA should be injected during quiet respiration, with the patient supine to minimize the normal perfusion gradient between the apex and lung base. Because the MAA particles tend to settle out in solution, the syringe should be gently agitated before injection to ensure even mixing. A peripheral vein is preferred, and administration through a Swan-Ganz catheter or any indwelling catheter port containing a filter generally should be avoided. To assist in homogeneous pulmonary distribution of the particles, injection should be made slowly, usually over three to five or more respiratory cycles, and the injected volume should be at least 1 to 2 mL. If blood is drawn into the syringe to confirm an intravascular needle location, it is important not to let the blood sit long in the syringe because this may allow the formation of small, clinically insignificant, labeled blood clots, which, when injected, result in focal hot spots on the perfusion scan (Fig. 7–2).

A relative contraindication to performing particulate perfusion lung scans is severe pulmonary hypertension because the blockade of additional lung capillaries may acutely exacerbate the condition and its cardiac complications. Care should also be taken in patients with known right-to-left shunts, although adverse effects on the coronary or cerebral circulations have rarely been observed. In these patients, however, as well as in infants and children, it is probably prudent to reduce the number of injected particles to 100,000 to 200,000. The presence of a right-to-left shunt can be easily recognized on posterior images by the immediate presence of renal activity, usually best seen on the posterior or lateral views, and can be confirmed by

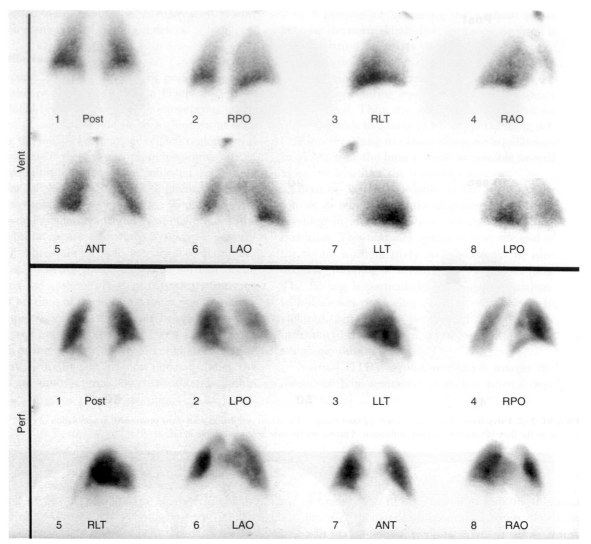

FIGURE 7–8. Normal ^{99m}Tc-DTPA aerosol ventilation scan (*top*) with accompanying ^{99m}Tc-MAA perfusion scans (*bottom*).

can clinically mimic pulmonary emboli and is an important component of the interpretation of ventilation-perfusion lung scans. Clinical presentations are frequently vague and may be mimicked by a variety of thoracic and abdominal disorders. Although multislice spiral computed tomography (CT) may be the initial test of choice to diagnose pulmonary embolism in many institutions, radionuclide ventilation-perfusion imaging, when properly performed and interpreted, is an effective noninvasive procedure for the detection of pulmonary embolus. In addition, a normal scan essentially excludes the diagnosis. Even in the small percent-

age of patients in whom the studies are nondiagnostic, radionuclide imaging may be used to guide CT-arteriography thereby increasing the sensitivity of the examination. V/Q scans are often perferred over CT-angiography for patients who have contrast allergies, are in renal failure, or who are too large for the CT-scanner gantry.

Diagnostic Principle

The diagnosis of pulmonary thromboembolism by ventilation-perfusion imaging is based on the disassociation between ventilation and perfusion as a result of the obstruction of pulmonary segmental arterial blood flow by the embolus. With ^{99m}Tc-MAA imaging, the MAA particles are unable to enter the capillary bed distal to the arterial occlusion, so that the portion of lung supplied by the involved artery appears as a perfusion defect outlined by the normally perfused adjacent lung parenchyma. Because ventilation is generally unaffected, the xenon or aerosol images remain normal in the same distribution. Thus, the most typical manifestation of the pulmonary emboli is as a wedge-shaped perfusion defect with preserved ventilation: the segmental ventilation-perfusion mismatch (Fig. 7–9).

Although this principle is simple, its practical application in various clinical settings can present one of most difficult challenges confronting the nuclear imaging physician. For this reason, much effort has been directed toward defining the language used to describe the findings on ventilation-perfusion imaging as well as the criteria used to translate them into diagnostic conclusions. In this regard, a thorough understanding of basic definitions and concepts is imperative.

Basic Concepts

A *perfusion defect* is a focus of absent or diminished pulmonary activity on perfusion images. Perfusion

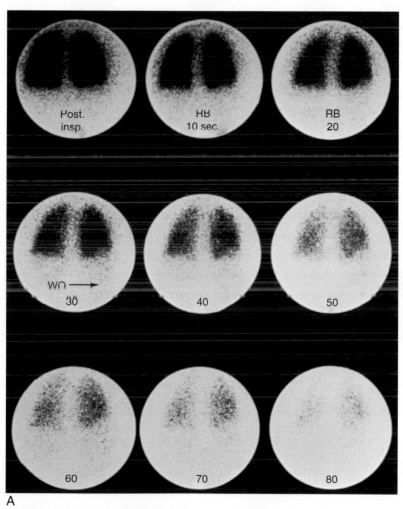

A

FIGURE 7–9. Multiple pulmonary emboli. *A,* The posterior images from a xenon-133 ventilation scan demonstrate normal ventilation bilaterally, with good washout (wo) and no areas of trapping. *B,* Technetium-99m macroaggregated albumin perfusion images demonstrate multiple unmatched wedge-shaped peripheral large segmental defects (*arrows*) in both the right and left lungs.

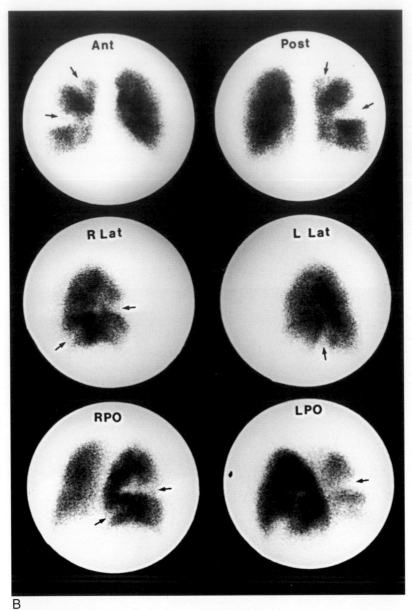

B

FIGURE 7–9, cont'd

For legend see p. 169

defects are nonspecific, and a list of differential diagnoses is given in Table 7–1. With a pulmonary embolism, perfusion does not have to be completely absent in the region of the defect because partially occluding pulmonary emboli are possible. Perfusion defects are classified as segmental or nonsegmental.

Segmental perfusion defects may involve all or part of a bronchopulmonary anatomic segment. Classically, these defects are pleural based and wedge shaped. They are best described by the particular bronchopulmonary segment that they occupy. Because segmental defects are the hallmark of pulmonary emboli and nonsegmental defects are not, the ability to distinguish between them is crucial to lung scan interpretation. This requires both careful characterization of defect configuration and an appreciation of the pulmonary segmental anatomy as it appears on perfusion lung images. Figure 7–10 shows the individual pulmonary segments in the projection that best visualizes each segment.

TABLE 7–1.	Causes of Defects on Perfusion Lung Scans

Pulmonary embolism (thrombotic, septic, marrow, or air)*
Bulla or cyst
Localized hypoxia due to asthma, bronchitis, emphysema
Surgery (e.g., pneumonectomy)
Pleural effusion*
Tumor (hilar or mediastinal)*
Metastases (hematogenous or lymphangitic)
Hilar adenopathy (lymphoma, sarcoidosis)
Pulmonary artery atresia or hypoplasia*
Fibrosing mediastinitis*
Radiation therapy*
Pneumonia
Pulmonary edema
Atelectasis
Fibrosis (postinflammatory, postradiation, pleural thickening)
Vasculitis*

*Entity may cause a ventilation–perfusion mismatch.

TABLE 7–2.	Causes of Decreased Perfusion to One Lung

Pulmonary agenesis or stenosis
Swyer-James syndrome
Embolus
Pneumothorax
Massive effusion
Mediastinal fibrosis
Tumor
Aortic dissection

Segmental defects are further characterized by size, with a large segmental defect occupying 75% or more of a lung segment, a moderate segmental defect occupying 25% to 75% of the segment, and a small segmental defect occupying less than 25% of the segment. The significance of a defect with respect to the likelihood that it is caused by a pulmonary embolus is directly related to defect size and the number of defects present; larger segmental defects are more significant, and the probability of pulmonary emboli increases as the number of identifiable large defects increases. When assessing a pulmonary perfusion study for the number and size of defects, the concept of segmental defect equivalence allows two moderate segmental defects to be summed so that they have the same diagnostic implication as one large segmental defect. Small defects, however, are not summed to form larger equivalents. Thus, it is possible to assemble combinations of moderate and large segments to determine the total number of segments involved for assessment of the probability of the presence of pulmonary emboli. An exception to the concept of defect size and significance is that solitary perfusion defects involving an entire lung (Table 7–2) or lobe of a lung represent uncommon presentations of pulmonary emboli. Both current and retrospective literature indicate that small segmental defects are uncommonly associated with pulmonary emboli.

Nonsegmental perfusion defects are those that do not correspond to bronchopulmonary anatomic segments and are generally not wedged shaped, but they may or may not be pleural based. In some instances, they are caused by nonpulmonary abnormalities, including hilar structures, pleural effusions, alterations in diaphragmatic contour or position, cardiomegaly, or normal variants or pathology of hilar or mediastinal structures. Primary intrapulmonary abnormalities may also cause nonsegmental defects, including those produced by neoplasms, bullae, pneumonia, hemorrhage, edema, or other infiltrates. The significance of nonsegmental defects is that they are not associated with pulmonary emboli.

Perfusion defects, particularly segmental defects, are further classified with respect to whether they exhibit ventilation. A *mismatch* refers to the circumstance in which a perfusion defect is seen to ventilate normally. Segmental mismatches are a hallmark of pulmonary emboli. Classically, a mismatch requires that the chest radiograph be normal in the same region. When a ventilation abnormality occurs in the same region as a perfusion defect, this constitutes a ventilation-perfusion *match*. Such ventilation abnormalities may occur as wash-in defects on aerosol or xenon studies, as washout abnormalities (focal trapping) on xenon images, or as both. Ventilation perfusion matches may have significance in the diagnostic schema for the diagnosis of pulmonary emboli, depending on their size, number, and location in the lungs. The term *triple match* is often used to refer to a ventilation-perfusion match accompanied by a corresponding chest radiographic abnormality of the same size, usually, but not always, an airspace opacity.

For purposes of regional localization of lung scan abnormalities, it is useful to divide the lungs into upper, middle, and lower zones of equal height, obtained by dividing the lungs into thirds

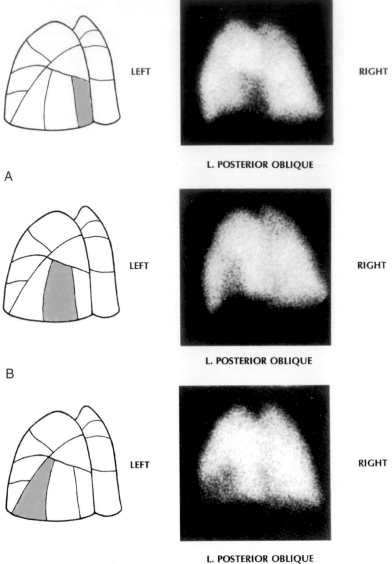

A

B

C

FIGURE 7–10. Segmental perfusion defects. Each is shown diagrammatically and in the position that best demonstrates the defect on the perfusion scan. Right, left, posterior, and anterior refer to the scintigrams. (From Mandell CH: Scintillation Camera Lung Imaging. New York, Grune & Stratton, 1976, pp 10–17, 20–27, 30–38, 42–51.). *A*, Left lower-lobe posterior basal segment. *B*, Left lower-lobe lateral basal segment. *C*, Left lower-lobe anterior medial basal segment. *D*, Left lower-lobe superior segment. *E*, Left upper-lobe posterior apical segment. (*F*, Left upper-lobe superior lingular segment. The lingular segment is often difficult to identify because of the normal cardiac defect. *G*, Left upper-lobe inferior lingular segment. The lingular segment is often difficult to identify because of the normal cardiac defect. *H*, Left upper-lobe anterior segment. *I*, Right lower-lobe posterior basal segment. *J*, Right lower-lobe superior segment. *K*, Right lower-lobe anterior basal segment. *L*, Right lower-lobe lateral basal segment. *M*, Right middle-lobe medial segment. *N*, Right middle-lobe lateral segment. *O*, Right upper-lobe posterior segment. *P*, Right upper-lobe anterior segment. *Q*, Right upper-lobe apical segment.

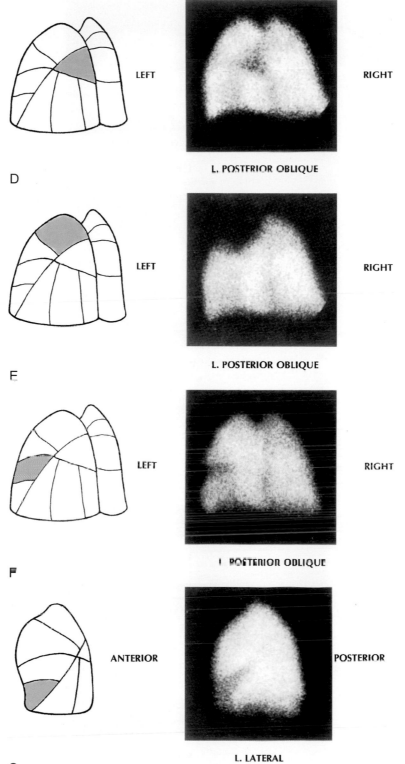

D

LEFT   RIGHT

L. POSTERIOR OBLIQUE

E

LEFT   RIGHT

L. POSTERIOR OBLIQUE

F

LEFT   RIGHT

L. POSTERIOR OBLIQUE

G

ANTERIOR   POSTERIOR

L. LATERAL

FIGURE 7–10, cont'd
For legend see opposite page

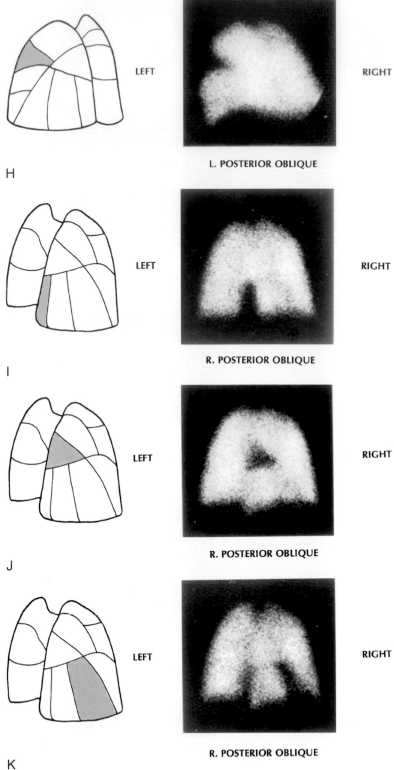

LEFT   L. POSTERIOR OBLIQUE   RIGHT

H

LEFT   R. POSTERIOR OBLIQUE   RIGHT

I

LEFT   R. POSTERIOR OBLIQUE   RIGHT

J

LEFT   R. POSTERIOR OBLIQUE   RIGHT

K

FIGURE 7–10, cont'd

For legend see p. 172

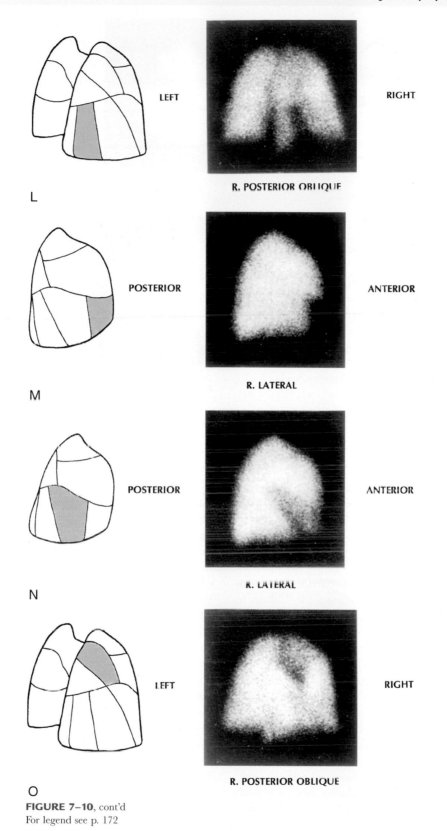

L   LEFT / RIGHT
R. POSTERIOR OBLIQUE

M   POSTERIOR / ANTERIOR
R. LATERAL

N   POSTERIOR / ANTERIOR
R. LATERAL

O   LEFT / RIGHT
R. POSTERIOR OBLIQUE

FIGURE 7–10, cont'd
For legend see p. 172

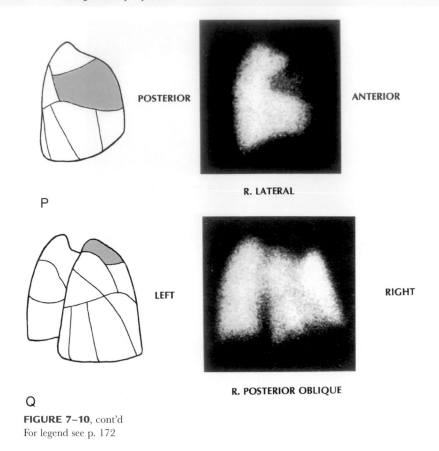

POSTERIOR

ANTERIOR

R. LATERAL

P

LEFT

RIGHT

Q

R. POSTERIOR OBLIQUE

FIGURE 7–10, cont'd
For legend see p. 172

from apex to base. The position of an abnormality, especially a single ventilation-perfusion match, with respect to these zones may add to its significance.

Analysis of Images

An orderly and consistent approach to lung scan analysis aids greatly in determining the findings to which interpretive criteria are to be applied. Analysis requires meticulous review and comparison of three separate sets of images: the perfusion images, the ventilation images, and the chest radiograph. Analysis of the perfusion scans first entails the identification and classification of any defects according to their appearance. Defects corresponding to anatomic divisions should be classified as lobar or segmental. If the defect is segmental, then further evaluation of its size as large, moderate, or small is required. Those defects that are not anatomic or do not respect segmental boundaries may be considered nonsegmental and unlikely to represent pulmonary emboli. Segmental defects, especially those of large or moderate size, should then be compared with the identical region on the ventilation scan to

determine whether a corresponding ventilatory abnormality is present. This allows characterization of the defect as matched or mismatched. Perfusion defects are then compared with findings on a recent chest radiograph to assess the presence of any correlative abnormalities, including infiltrates, pleural effusions, masses, or bullae. If available, any prior ventilation-perfusion lung scans should be reviewed as part of image analysis because persistent defects from previous pulmonary emboli are a common cause of false-positive findings for acute emboli.

Although lung scan interpretation is easiest in the presence of a clear chest radiograph, the presence of either a localized infiltrate or diffuse lung disease should not be seen as an insurmountable problem. Any approach that does not attempt to interpret pulmonary emboli in the presence of infiltrates or diffuse lung disease will result in a large number of scans being read as indeterminate and will unnecessarily subject a large number of patients to further studies. One of the most common situations involves the presence of one or more localized pulmonary infiltrates on the chest radiograph of a patient suspected of having pulmonary emboli. Certainly, the infiltrate or infiltrates could represent either inflammatory disease or pulmonary emboli with infarction. Because pulmonary emboli are generally multiple, however, and because only about 25% of such lesions progress to infarction, the likelihood is excellent that ventilation-perfusion mismatches suggesting pulmonary embolus may be found elsewhere, in areas of otherwise radiographically normal lung. In the absence of such findings, some diagnostic probability information can nevertheless be obtained by comparing the size of the radiographic infiltrate with the size of the corresponding perfusion deficit. When a perfusion defect is substantially smaller than the corresponding radiographic abnormality, the probability of pulmonary embolus is low. Conversely, when the perfusion defect is substantially larger than the radiographic infiltrate, the probability of such an occurrence is high (Table 7–3). A perfusion defect that corresponds closely in size to an infiltrate carries an intermediate probability of embolus. In this latter case, if clinical suspicion is high, CT-angiography may be indicated.

Normal or near-normal perfusion lung scans may occur in a large percentage of patients with a diffusely abnormal chest radiograph, such as in the setting of pulmonary edema. Although the presence of perfusion abnormalities in such patients may cause difficulty in interpretation, the surprising number of normal or near-normal scans obtained indicates that pulmonary emboli can be effectively excluded in many patients with underlying lung diseases. As stated earlier, a normal ventilation-perfusion lung scan in any patient essentially excludes the possibility of recent significant pulmonary embolization.

With or without a normal chest radiograph, careful correlation of any perfusion abnormalities with the corresponding regions on the ventilation study should be undertaken to exclude airway disease as a cause for a perfusion defect. Multiple matched small ventilation-perfusion abnormalities with a clear chest radiograph demonstrate a low probability of pulmonary embolus. Because the ventilation examination is usually performed in the posterior position, it is best compared with the posterior perfusion image. If perfusion defects are best seen or seen only on another projection, a repeat ventilation study in the view that best demonstrates the lesion may be undertaken to evaluate airway patency in that region. If the perfusion defect corresponds to a prominent chest radiograph infiltrate, however, a ventilation defect is to be expected, and a repeat study usually is not of value.

LUNG SCAN INTERPRETATION

The interpretation of ventilation-perfusion images in the setting of suspected pulmonary emboli involves the determination of the probability of pulmonary emboli based on a set of specific interpretive criteria. These criteria have evolved over many years as experience with ventilation-perfusion lung imaging has increased. Criteria have been defined by an extensive and ambitious project known as the Prospective Investigation Of Pulmonary Embolism Diagnosis (PIOPED). PIOPED is a multi-institutional study involving tertiary care hospitals designed to evaluate the efficacy of

TABLE 7–3.	Angiographic Findings in Regions with Scintigraphic Perfusion Defects and Radiographic Abnormalities	
SIZE OF PERFUSION DEFECT COMPARED WITH RADIOGRAPHIC ABNORMALITY	**PULMONARY EMBOLISM (%)**
Smaller	7
Equal	26
Larger	
V/Q mismatch	89
V/Q match	<5

Reprinted with modifications from Biello DR, Mattar AG, Osei-Wusu A, et al: Interpretation of indeterminate lung scintigrams. Radiology 133:189–194, 1979.

various means of diagnosing acute pulmonary embolism. More specifically, the goal of PIOPED is to determine the sensitivity and specificity of ventilation-perfusion lung scanning by using a specific set of diagnostic criteria.

Assigning Probability

After applying a set of diagnostic criteria to a lung scan, a determination of the probability or likelihood that pulmonary emboli are the cause of the observed ventilation-perfusion pattern is made. The categories of probability assigned are traditionally those of high, intermediate, or low probability. A *high probability* ventilation-perfusion pattern indicates a greater than 80% likelihood that pulmonary emboli are present, and a *low probability* pattern confers a less than 20% likelihood. Scans that are not deemed to be within the high or low categories are assigned an *intermediate probability*, which encompasses the wide range of likelihood between 20% and 80%. By using clinical and laboratory findings as well as pretest probability, some authors have suggested that interpreters assign a more specific percentage of probability within this range when possible. Reanalysis of the original PIOPED database has allowed the assignment of a *very low probability* to a lung scan indicating a less than 10% probability that pulmonary emboli are present. A lung scan with a very low probability interpretation has a similar diagnostic reliability as a high probability interpretation. A lung scan given a normal designation indicates a probability of pulmonary emboli approaching zero. Although the term *indeterminate* has been used synonymously with that of *intermediate* probability, the former term should ideally be reserved for studies in which an estimate of probability cannot be given because of technical limitations. When a combination of criteria is present on a single lung scan, the criterion producing the highest level of probability is that which should be assigned to the scan being interpreted.

PIOPED Interpretive Criteria

The PIOPED II criteria are perhaps the most widely used interpretive scheme for assigning a probability of pulmonary emboli to a ventilation-perfusion lung scan. The data from the PIOPED study are constantly being refined so that minor adjustments to the original set of criteria have been made. These PIOPED II criteria are given in Table 7–4. Another way of approaching the same data is given in Table 7–5. A thorough familiarity with

| **TABLE 7–4.** | **PIOPED II Criteria for Combined Ventilation-Perfusion Scan Interpretation** |

HIGH PROBABILITY

Two or more large mismatched segmental defects without a radiographic abnormality or the equivalent in moderate defects (two moderate defects equals one large defect)

INTERMEDIATE PROBABILITY

One moderate to less than two large segmented mismatched defects

Difficult to categorize as high or low

Solitary moderate or large segmental size triple match in lower lobe (zone)

LOW PROBABILITY

A single large or moderate matched ventilation-perfusion defect

More than three small segmental lesions

Absent perfusion in an entire lung

Solitary lobar mismatch

Moderate sized pleural effusion (greater than costophrenic angle but less than one-third of pleural cavity with no other perfusion defect in either lung

Heterogeneous perfusion

VERY LOW PROBABILITY

Nonsegmental lesion (e.g. prominent hilum, cardiomegaly, elevated hemidiaphragm, linear atelectasis, costophrenic angle effusion) with no other perfusion defect in either lung

Perfusion defect smaller than radiographic lesion

Two or more ventilation-perfusion matched defects with regionally normal chest x-ray and some areas of normal perfusion elsewhere in the lungs

One to three small segmental perfusion defects

A solitary triple matched defect in the mid or upper lung zone confined to a single segment

Stripe sign around the perfusion defect (best tangential view)

Pleural effusion of one-third or more of the pleural cavity with no other perfusion defect in either lung

NORMAL

No perfusion defects. Perfusion scan must outline the shape of the lungs seen on chest x-ray (which could be abnormal; e.g., scoliosis or pneumonectomy)

these criteria is crucial to the consistent and reliable interpretation of lung scans in the setting of suspected pulmonary embolism. To maintain a high specificity for the patterns described, especially high probability, some sensitivity is unavoidably lost.

It should be apparent from perusing the specific PIOPED II criteria in Table 7–4 that only the

TABLE 7–5.	Probability of Pulmonary Emboli by Ventilation-Perfusion Scan Findings			
PERFUSION DEFECTS	**VENTILATION**	**VENTILATION-PERFUSION**	**CHEST X-RAY**	**PROBABILITY OF PULMONARY EMBOLISM**
≥2 large segmental	Normal	Mismatch	Normal	High
≥2 moderate + 1 large segmental	Normal	Mismatch	Normal	High
≥4 moderate segmental	Normal	Mismatch	Normal	High
1 moderate to <2 large segmental	Normal	Mismatch	Normal	Intermediate
1 moderate segmental	Abnormal	Match	Normal	Intermediate
>3 small segmental	Irrelevant		Normal	Low
<3 small segmental	Irrelevant	—	Normal	Very low
Large: related to pleural effusion	Abnormal	Match	Large effusion	Low
Small: related to pleural effusion	Abnormal	Match	Small effusion	Intermediate
Any size: multiple	Abnormal	Match	Normal	Low
Any size: lower lung zone	Abnormal	Match	Opacity	Intermediate
Any size: upper or middle lung zone	Abnormal	Match	Opacity	Very low
Any size: considerably smaller than chest x-ray abnormality	Irrelevant	—	Opacity	Very low
Any size: considerably larger than chest x-ray abnormality	Irrelevant	—	Opacity	High
Any size: with stripe sign	Irrelevant	—	Irrelevant	Very low
Nonsegmental	Irrelevant	—	Irrelevant	Very low
No defects	Irrelevant	—	Irrelevant	Normal

classic pattern of ventilation-perfusion mismatch is indicative of a high probability of pulmonary emboli, with a minimum equivalent of two large mismatched defects required to make such a diagnosis (Figs. 7–11 and 7–12). This requirement seems reasonable because pulmonary emboli are multiple in 90% of cases and bilateral in 85%. Fewer than two large mismatches or single smaller mismatches (down to one moderate size) are essentially nondiagnostic, rendering an intermediate probability of pulmonary embolism. Various other criteria for intermediate, low, and very low probability primarily involve combinations of matched ventilation-perfusion defects with and without radiographic abnormalities, and perfusion defects, including small defects, compared with the radiographic findings. Nonsegmental defects alone are always associated with a very low probability of pulmonary embolism.

The significance of the categories of probability as defined by the PIOPED criteria is perhaps best placed in perspective by briefly considering the data underlying the derived categories. It is the responsibility of the interpreting physician to communicate effectively the meaning of a reported probability to referring clinicians, so that patient management is optimized.

High Probability Lung Scans

The specificity of a high probability scan is 97%, with a positive predictive value of 88%. However, although very specific, high probability lung scans have a sensitivity of only 40% and fail to identify 60% of patients with pulmonary emboli. Thus, a high probability scan usually indicates pulmonary embolism, but only a minority of patients with pulmonary embolism have a high probability scan.

Intermediate Probability Lung Scans

An intermediate probability scan is not helpful in establishing a diagnosis. However, when combined

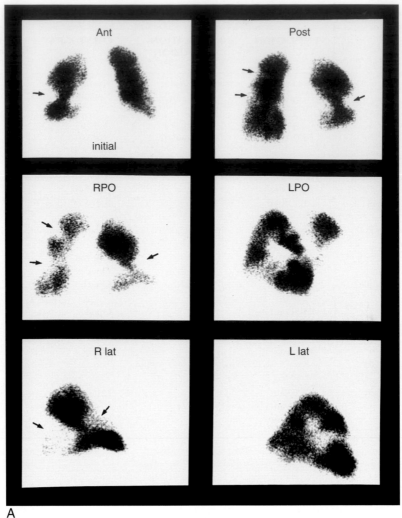

FIGURE 7–11. Resolution of multiple pulmonary emboli. *A,* An initial perfusion scan done on a young patient with a normal chest radiograph and a normal ventilation scan demonstrates multiple peripheral wedge-shaped defects (*arrows*). *B,* A follow-up perfusion scan performed 8 weeks later shows complete resolution of the defects.

with the level of clinical suspicion of pulmonary embolism, further evaluation with noninvasive peripheral venous studies, pulmonary CT angiography, or, in some very rare instances, selective pulmonary arteriography may be indicated.

Low and Very Low Probability Lung Scans

In PIOPED, the negative predictive value of a low probability scan is 84%. The frequency of pulmonary emboli in patients with lung scans in the low probability category is still about 15%. Thus, low probability scans should not be misinterpreted by referring physicians as completely ruling out pulmonary emboli. Because of the possibly misleading nature of a low probability scan, continued analy-

ses of the PIOPED data have allowed development of additional criteria, permitting identification of lung scans with a very low probability of pulmonary emboli. These scans have a positive predictive value of pulmonary emboli of less than 10%. These criteria include

- Nonsegmental perfusion abnormalities (positive predictive value [PPV], 8%)
- Perfusion defects smaller than corresponding chest radiographic opacities (PPV, 8%)
- A perfusion defect with a stripe sign (PPV, 7%)
- Triple-matched defects in an upper or middle lung zone (PPV, 4%)
- Matched V/Q abnormalities in two or three zones of a single lung (PPV, 3%)

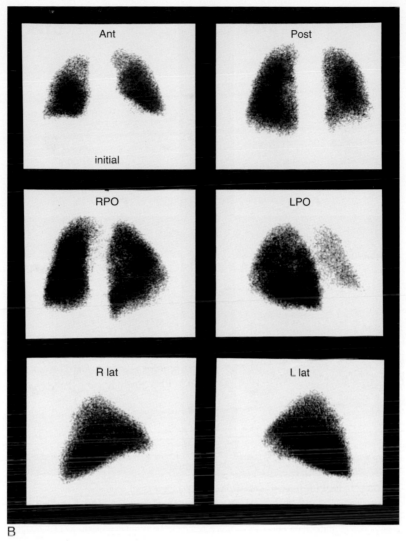

B

FIGURE 7–11, cont'd
For legend see opposite page

■ One to three small segmental perfusion defects
(PPV, 1%)

Normal Lung Scans

The negative predictive value of a near-normal or
normal scan is more than 90%. A normal ventilation-perfusion lung scan interpretation excludes
clinically significant pulmonary emboli.

Gestalt Interpretation

Gestalt, or overall pattern, interpretation of ventilation-perfusion scans by some physicians may add
to the accuracy of lung scan assessment and is often
used adjunctively in combination with specific

PIOPED criteria. This approach should be
reserved for the very experienced interpreter
because the basis for interpretation may be difficult
to explain in a potential legal setting.

Optimizing Interpretation

Incorporation of Clinical Information

Interpretation of ventilation-perfusion images
correlates well with the likelihood of finding
pulmonary emboli with selective pulmonary
angiography (Table 7–6). Even though the clinical
presentation of pulmonary emboli is nonspecific,
risk factors and clinical findings suggestive of pulmonary emboli may be used to formulate a clinical

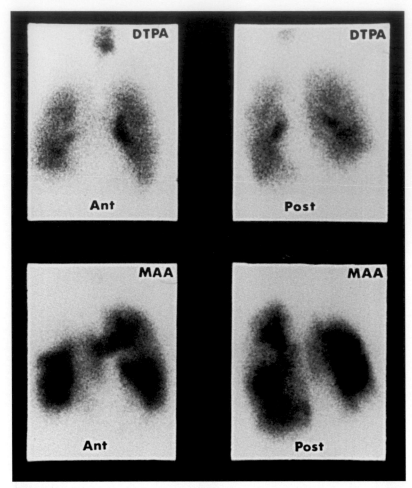

FIGURE 7–12. Pulmonary emboli. A ^{99m}Tc-DTPA aerosol ventilation scan (*top*) and ^{99m}Tc-macroaggregated albumin (MAA) perfusion scan (*bottom*) were used to evaluate this patient who could not be moved from an intensive care unit. The perfusion images show a large defect in the right upper lobe, which is seen to be ventilated on the DTPA images.

pretest likelihood of pulmonary emboli that may be combined with the ventilation-perfusion scan results to determine an overall likelihood of the presence of the disease. The predictive value of both high and low probability lung scans is optimized when supported by clinical impressions suggesting either the presence or absence of emboli. Such information can be especially useful when assessing the significance of low probability scans. Although patients with low or very low probability scans without significant risk factors have a combined prevalence of pulmonary embolism of only

TABLE 7–6.	Comparison of Scan Category Sensitivity and Specificity	
SCAN CATEGORY	**SENSITIVITY (%)**	**SPECIFICITY (%)**
High probability	41	97
High or intermediate probability	82	52
High, intermediate or low probability	98	10

Adapted from The PIOPED Investigation: Value of ventilation/perfusion scan in acute pulmonary embolism: Results of the Prospective Investigation of Pulmonary Embolism Diagnosis (PIOPED). JAMA 263:2753-2759, 1990.

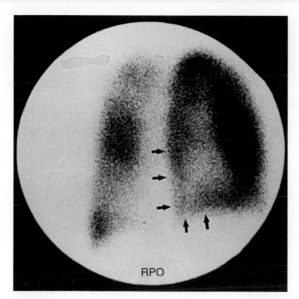

FIGURE 7–13. Stripe sign. A single view from a perfusion lung scan in a patient with chronic obstructive pulmonary disease shows a perfusion defect in the right lower lobe, but this does not extend all the way to the periphery of the lung. The rim of activity near the pleura (*arrows*) indicates a low probability of pulmonary embolus.

4%, with one or more than one significant risk factors, the prevalence values are increased to 12% and 21%, respectively. Thus, in patients with low probability lung scans and important risk factors, further investigation, including lower-extremity noninvasive venous studies and/or pulmonary CT angiography, may be warranted. Further, a low probability scan with a strong pretest clinical impression of the absence of pulmonary emboli makes the probability of pulmonary emboli remote. The presence of associated risk factors does not change the significance of a normal lung scan in essentially excluding a diagnosis of pulmonary embolism.

Ancillary Signs

The *stripe sign* consists of a thin line or stripe of activity representing perfused lung tissue between a perfusion defect and the adjacent pleural surface. Perfusion defects presenting with a stripe sign are very unlikely to represent pulmonary emboli based on the assumption that non–pleural-based lesions are not emboli. These defects should be interpreted as having a very low probability of being pulmonary emboli in the absence of perfusion abnormalities elsewhere in the lungs (Fig. 7–13).

The *fissure sign* refers to linear perfusion deficits corresponding to the interlobar pulmonary fissures, both major and minor. This sign is commonly seen in the presence of pleural fluid in the fissures but may also be seen in the presence of fissural pleural thickening and is frequently observed in patients with COPD (see Fig. 7–5).

Special Situations

Pleural Effusions

Pleural effusions may produce perfusion defects by loculation or compression of lung parenchyma. There are conflicting reports regarding the significance of matched ventilation-perfusion defects corresponding to radiographic pleural effusions of similar size. Analysis of the PIOPED data suggests that matched defects caused by small pleural effusions (those producing only costophrenic angle blunting) should be classified as intermediate probability, whereas defects caused by larger effusions should be classified as low probability. Still, recent information indicates that pulmonary emboli are associated with pleural effusions of all sizes, and thus, all pleural effusion–related matched ventilation-perfusion abnormalities should be assigned an intermediate probability of pulmonary emboli regardless of size. In general, pleural effusions that do not produce perfusion defects are irrelevant to the interpretation of a V/Q lung scan.

Diffuse Lung Disease

The overwhelming majority (75%) of patients with diffuse lung disease, such as relatively homogeneous infiltrates produced by pulmonary edema, have normal or near-normal perfusion lungs scans in the absence of pulmonary emboli (Fig. 7–14). Thus, such abnormalities on chest radiographs should not discourage the use of ventilation-perfusion lung imaging because pulmonary emboli may be successfully excluded in the presence of a normal perfusion pattern.

Airway Disease (Chronic Obstructive Pulmonary Disease)

Severe diffuse COPD may significantly lower the sensitivity and specificity of lung scans in diagnosing pulmonary embolism. In COPD, both nonsegmental and segmental perfusion defects may occur, making differentiation from superimposed pulmonary emboli impossible without an accompanying ventilation study. When COPD is severe and diffuse, even the combined ventilation-perfusion

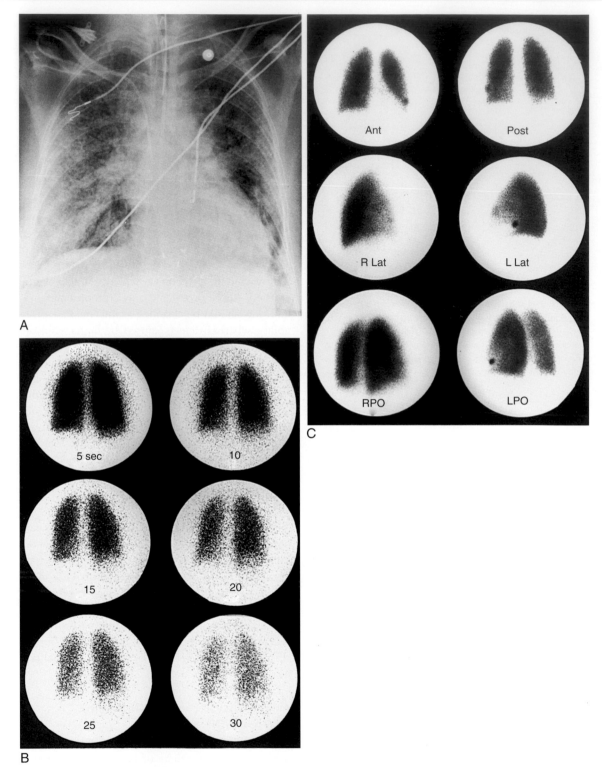

FIGURE 7–14. The chest radiograph (A) in this patient with adult respiratory distress syndrome demonstrates extensive bilateral alveolar infiltrates. Ventilation (B) and perfusion (C) lung scans were performed to evaluate sudden hypoxemia. Even though the chest radiograph has marked infiltrates, both scans are normal, excluding pulmonary emboli. Incidental note is made of a hot spot in the left lingula. The injection was made through a right subclavian catheter, and the activity is due to a tiny labeled clot that came off the end of the catheter during the injection.

study may not provide an answer. In fact, in patients with matched ventilation-perfusion defects accompanied by extensive ventilation abnormalities involving greater than 50% of the lung fields, interpretation may be so difficult as to warrant an intermediate probability or even an indeterminate reading, especially when matched defects of a segmental nature are present. CT-angiography may be indicated if emboli are strongly suspected clinically. In the presence of severe COPD, however, even CT-angiography may be fraught with interpretive error.

Location of Triple Matches

There is some evidence that pulmonary embolism is significantly more common in the presence of triple matches located in lower lung zones, where blood flow is greater, than with triple matches in the upper and middle lung zones. Thus, matching ventilation-perfusion defects corresponding to chest radiographic opacities isolated to the upper and middle lung zones imply a very low probability of pulmonary emboli, whereas similar findings in the lower lung zones represent an intermediate probability of pulmonary emboli. There appears to be no differences in the prevalence of pulmonary emboli among various sizes of triple matches.

Lobar or Whole-Lung Defects

Solitary lobar or solitary whole-lung perfusion defects are unusual presentations for pulmonary emboli. Other possibilities, including hilar masses, mediastinal fibrosis, and hypoplastic pulmonary artery (Fig. 7–15), should be considered.

Incorporation of Noninvasive Deep Venous Testing

Because pulmonary emboli are a complication of deep venous thrombosis, noninvasive evaluation of the veins of the lower extremity, including ultrasound, has become an important diagnostic tool in patients with suspected pulmonary emboli. In patients with nondiagnostic (intermediate or low probability) lung scans and low clinical suspicion of pulmonary emboli, normal lower extremity noninvasive venous ultrasound may obviate further testing and allow conservative patient management. Positive noninvasive testing renders a patient a candidate for anticoagulation therapy. A combination of lower extremity ultrasound and plasma D-dimer assessment, a specific breakdown product of clot fibrinolysis, may provide even more infor-

mation to direct patient management and may reduce the need for further imaging when both are negative.

Computed Tomography and Pulmonary Arteriography

In many health care institutions, CT angiography is the preferred initial imaging study for suspected pulmonary embolus, and some recent clinical algorithms do not include radionuclide ventilation perfusion imaging. To some extent, this may be the result of the high number of indeterminate or intermediate probability scan interpretations and the generally perceived higher interobserver interpretive variance for V/Q imaging compared to spiral CT angiography. With the advent of 16 and higher detector row CT scanners, coverage of the entire chest in 1 mm or submillimeter resolution can be achieved in one short breath hold or in less than 10 seconds. Very high resolution axial images of the pulmonary arteries with three-dimensional reconstruction are possible. CT scanning is often definitive when intermediate V/Q scan results are obtained (Figs. 7–16 and 7–17). The specificity for

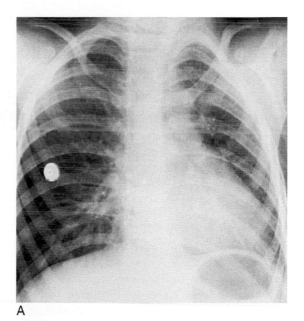

A

FIGURE 7–15. Hypoplastic or absent left pulmonary artery. *A*, The chest radiograph demonstrates the classic findings compatible with this entity, including volume loss and bronchial vascularity. *B*, The ventilation scan demonstrates good ventilation in both lungs, with slightly more rapid washout (wo) on the *left*. *C*, The perfusion scan demonstrates completely absent perfusion to the left lung.

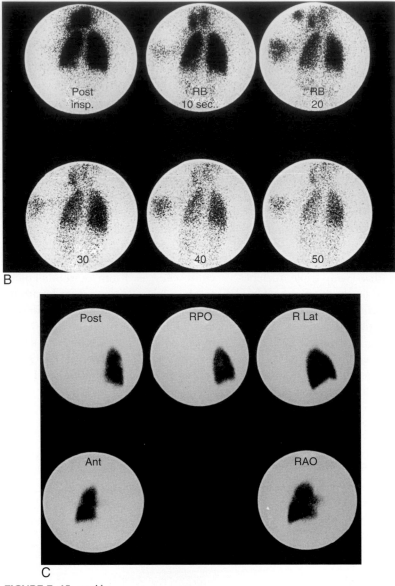

FIGURE 7–15, cont'd
For legend see p. 185

pulmonary emboli detection with multidector CT is greater than that of V/Q scanning, and the familiarity of most radiologists and referring physicians with CT will undoubtedly increase the frequency of this methodology. Some difficulties with spiral CT protocols are the need for very precise timing of the contrast bolus to produce a diagnostic examination, and the clinical quandary presented by the detection of small peripheral emboli in normal persons or patients with minor symptoms.

Despite the advantages of spiral CT, V/Q scanning will likely continue to play a role in evaluation of pulmonary emboli, right-to-left shunts, and regional pulmonary function. Pulmonary arteriography, which has been the gold standard for diagnosis of pulmonary emboli, is now uncommonly performed.

Lung Scan Follow-up of Pulmonary Emboli

Once the diagnosis of pulmonary embolism has been established, perfusion imaging may be used to follow the course of the disease. Typically, there is some evidence of change in the pattern of perfusion defects in the first few days after the

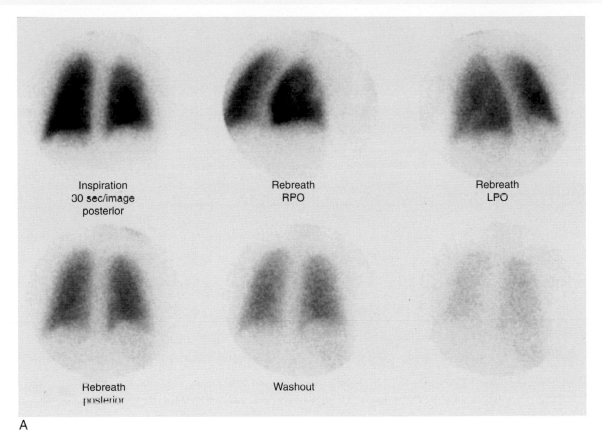

Inspiration
30 sec/image
posterior

Rebreath
RPO

Rebreath
LPO

Rebreath
posterior

Washout

A

FIGURE 7–16. Large central partially occluding pulmonary embolism. *A*, Xenon ventilation perfusion images are normal, whereas the perfusion images (*B*) show substantially reduced blood flow to the right lung. *C*, A contrasted CT scan clearly shows a large filling defect (*arrow*) in the right main pulmonary artery.

embolism. Defects may become smaller or disappear altogether, and new defects may appear. New defects may result from fragmentation of larger, centrally placed clots that pass to the lung periphery or from altered regional perfusion pressure in the lung, which may convert a partially obstructing clot to a complete obstruction. Of course, recurrent emboli also produce new defects, but the mere presence of new defects per se cannot be used to establish recurrent embolization during this period.

The ultimate fate of pulmonary emboli is variable and depends to some extent on the size of the emboli and the age of the patient. The larger the initial defect and the older the patient, the less likely is the pulmonary perfusion scan to return to normal. Emboli occurring in the presence of underlying diffuse diseases are also less likely to show complete resolution, as are those that produce actual infarction of lung.

Because persistent defects may be mistaken for acute pulmonary emboli on subsequent ventilation-perfusion scans, it is strongly recommended that patients with high probability scans or those with intermediate probability scans who are treated for pulmonary emboli be followed with a 3-month baseline study for future reference if symptoms suggestive of new pulmonary emboli occur. Thromboembolic perfusion defects persisting at 3 months are likely to remain unresolved.

Nonembolic Diseases

Chronic Obstructive Pulmonary Disease

Emphysema and chronic bronchitis are the most common forms of COPD. Both diseases are associated with patchy, uneven ventilation, reduced lung compliance, and increased peripheral resistance. In emphysema, there is parenchymal destruction distal to the terminal bronchioles, causing

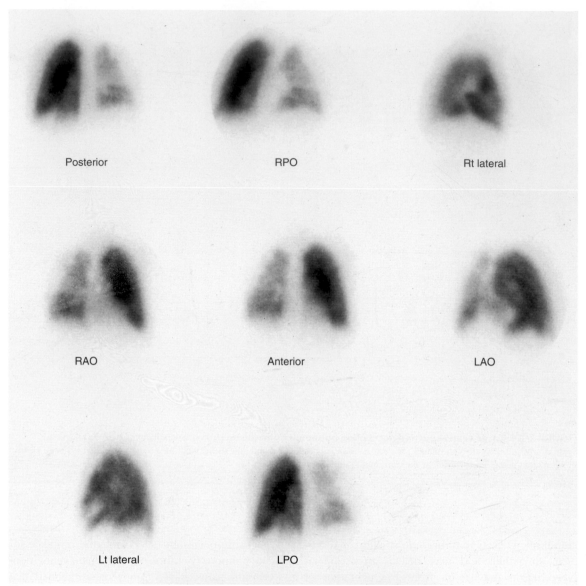

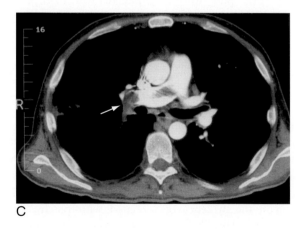

B

C

FIGURE 7–16, cont'd
For legend see p. 187

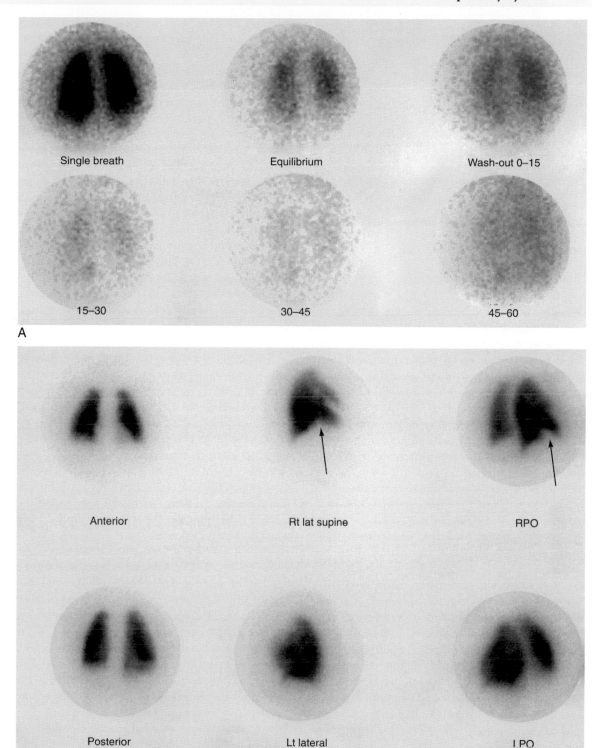

FIGURE 7–17. Small pulmonary embolism. *A,* Xenon ventilation images are normal, whereas the perfusion images (*B*) shows a moderate segmental defect in the right lower lobe corresponding to an intermediate probability for pulmonary embolism. The CT scan (*C*) however clearly shows a small pulmonary embolism (*arrow*) in the vessels of the right lower lobe.

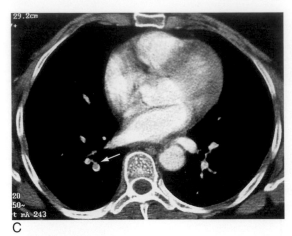

FIGURE 7–17, cont'd
For legend see p. 189

damage in the secondary pulmonary lobules; this includes damage to the alveoli as well as to the pulmonary capillaries. Extensive destruction may result in the formation of bullae. On ventilation-perfusion lung scans, these changes result in matched ventilation-perfusion abnormalities that typify airway disease.

Pulmonary ventilation imaging is most helpful in characterizing the regional distribution of airway abnormalities and, to a lesser extent, in delineating the clinical severity of the disease. It is not uncommon for a patient to have marked changes on the ventilation scan but a relatively normal chest radiograph because the typical radiographic changes are often late manifestations of emphysema.

In patients with early or mild COPD, the perfusion scan may be normal or near normal. As the destruction of lung parenchyma progresses, however, it characteristically produces multiple subsegmental or nonsegmental perfusion defects, which may be relatively focal and discrete or diffusely scattered throughout the lungs, giving a coarsely mottled pattern. Perfusion defects may also be caused by regional hypoxia producing reflex vasoconstriction and by bullae themselves or their compression of adjacent lung. Large apical bullae may render strikingly reduced or absent perfusion to the upper lung zones.

In the presence of COPD, the perfusion scan is nonspecific unless accompanied by a ventilation study. Ventilation scans performed with ^{133}Xe characteristically reveal abnormalities in the involved areas on the single-breath images and less frequently on the equilibrium views. Washout images usually demonstrate areas of delayed clearance

(trapping) that may correspond to the initial defects seen on the single-breath views. Ventilation abnormalities that correlate with defects seen on the perfusion scan constitute a ventilation-perfusion match, a hallmark of primary airway disease (Fig. 7–18). This finding may be of great value in distinguishing between COPD and superimposed pulmonary emboli when the latter are suspected. Many patients who present for ventilation-perfusion imaging for evaluation of pulmonary emboli have COPD. Thus, it is important to correlate carefully the ventilation and perfusion scans. If all the defects are small and subsegmental and have matched ventilation defects, emphysema is likely. The diagnosis of pulmonary embolism is not made unless there are at least two superimposed mismatched large segmental defects (Fig. 7–19).

The sensitivity of the ventilation scan for detection of chronic obstructive airway disease varies with the imaging phase of the examination. The ^{133}Xe single-breath image detects about 70% of matched ventilation-perfusion abnormalities, whereas the equilibrium images detect only 20% of such defects. In fact, the equilibrium images may well be normal if rebreathing of xenon is sufficient to allow collateral pathway filling of postobstructive lung. The washout or clearance phase, however, is much more sensitive, detecting more than 90% of matched ventilation-perfusion lesions as regional trapping of xenon. Because the late phase is most sensitive, particular care should be given to this part of the examination. A ^{133}Xe washout study in patients with suspected COPD should continue for at least 3 to 5 minutes because single-breath and equilibrium images may be normal in these patients. Because they do not permit washout imaging, short-lived isotopes, such as ^{81m}Kr, are of less value than is ^{133}Xe in assessing subtle obstructive changes. When using ^{99m}Tc-DTPA aerosol ventilation imaging in patients with COPD, little or no peripheral activity may be seen in the lungs because increased turbulence in the large airways causes marked deposition in the trachea and bronchi (Fig. 7–20).

Ventilation-perfusion scintigraphy has also been used to investigate less common forms of COPD, such as α_1-antitrypsin deficiency and cystic fibrosis. α_1-Antitrypsin deficiency is a recessive inherited form of panlobular emphysema in which homozygotes demonstrate marked abnormalities of ventilation and perfusion predominating in the lower lungs, and even heterozygotes may show delayed clearance of xenon from these zones. Ventilation-

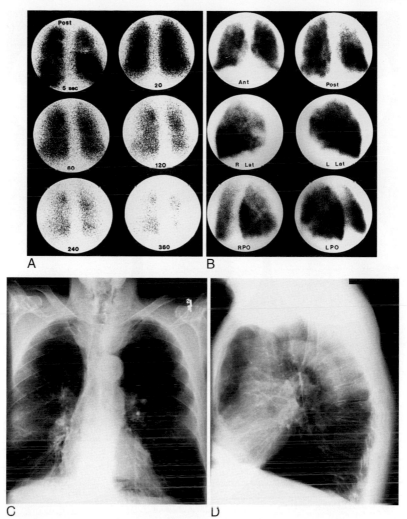

FIGURE 7–18. Chronic obstructive pulmonary disease. The xenon ventilation scan (*A*) shows areas of decreased activity on the initial image. The washout images demonstrate markedly delayed washout with focal areas of trapping remaining at 6 minutes. *B*, The perfusion images show patchy distribution but no wedge-shaped segmental defects. The posteroanterior (*C*) and lateral (*D*) chest radiographs show the expected lung hyperinflation, increased anteroposterior chest diameter, and flattened hemidiaphragms.

perfusion studies performed in patients with cystic fibrosis demonstrate patchy segmental defects in perfusion and markedly disturbed ventilation, particularly in the washout phase.

Mucous Plugs

Mucous plugging of one or more airways is a common cause of hypoxia and may produce matched segmental ventilation-perfusion defects on lung scans. The ventilation scan demonstrates little or no activity in the involved lung segment on inspiration images and may demonstrate significant trapping on the washout images where there is col-

lateral air drift (Fig. 7–21). Perfusion in the affected area is usually reduced, owing to reflex arteriolar constriction induced by local hypoxia. The chest radiograph may be normal or may show some volume loss associated with postobstructive atelectasis.

Asthma, Bronchiectasis, and Bronchitis

Asthma, bronchiectasis, and bronchitis all cause airway obstruction by different but often overlapping mechanisms. Asthma is primarily related to acute spastic narrowing of the bronchi. Bronchiectasis destroys the elastic and muscular

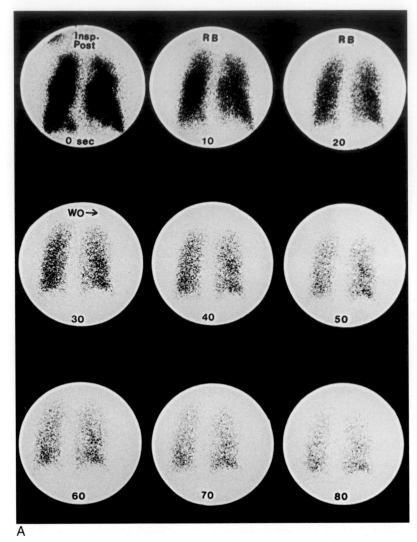

FIGURE 7–19. Pulmonary embolism in a patient with chronic obstructive pulmonary disease. *A,* The ventilation scan demonstrates areas of marked abnormality with trapping at both bases. *B,* The perfusion scan shows several additional large unmatched segmental defects (*arrows*) that do not have a rim of peripheral activity. In this case, even though the patient has chronic obstructive pulmonary disease, there is a high probability of pulmonary emboli.

tissue in the bronchial walls, causing dilation and sometimes collapse, usually with associated infection. Bronchitis results in large amounts of viscous mucus in the bronchi. Often, all three disorders are present in the same patient (frequently a smoker) and may ultimately lead to emphysema. These diseases are characterized by acute episodic exacerbation, during which significant ventilation and accompanying perfusion abnormalities are found on pulmonary ventilation-perfusion scans. Despite the clinical symptoms, chest radiographs are often negative, and excluding the presence of superim-

posed diseases such as pulmonary emboli may be difficult.

Scattered matched segmental perfusion defects are generally present during an acute asthma attack, related to reflex vasoconstriction secondary to regional hypoxia. Corresponding ventilation defects are frequently noted during the single-breath xenon study but may become less apparent with rebreathing, and regional areas of delayed wash-out are also usually identified. The geographic location of these abnormalities within the lungs may characteristically change during the

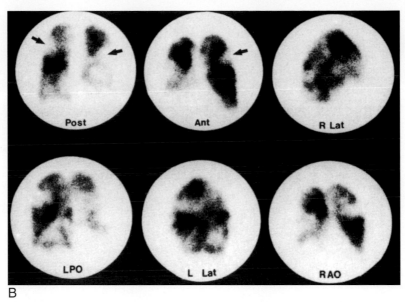

B

FIGURE 7–19, cont'd
For legend see p. 192

same or subsequent attacks, giving an altered pattern of ventilation-perfusion abnormalities on serial lung scans (Fig. 7–22). This provides a scintigraphic distinction from chronic emphysema, which results in a fixed location of the abnormalities. In asthmatic patients who do not have COPD, ventilation-perfusion scans frequently return to normal within 24 hours after treatment with bronchodilators. This may be used to distinguish between pulmonary emboli and asthma if they cannot be differentiated on the basis of initial clinical and scintigraphic assessment. The detection of wheezing or ascertainment of a prior history of asthma in a patient undergoing imaging for suspected pulmonary emboli may greatly aid in the interpretation of the images and in determining the need for repeat imaging after bronchodilator administration.

Unlike asthma, the perfusion defects produced by bronchiectasis are constant in location (generally restricted to the lung bases) and are in large part related to reflex vasoconstriction secondary to local hypoxia. Regional ventilation defects with or without associated trapping are the expected findings on the xenon study.

Lung Neoplasms

If large enough, any lung neoplasm, whether benign, malignant, or metastatic, may produce

localized ventilation-perfusion defects corresponding to the lesion on a lung scan. If there is secondary pulmonary arterial or bronchial obstruction, then larger ventilation-perfusion abnormalities in the lung distal to the lesion may occur, with possible delayed washout of xenon. If the lesion is bronchial (such as an adenoma), there may be distal hypoxia with a reflex decrease in perfusion. With lesions that cause arterial compression, the perfusion abnormality is generally more striking than is the ventilatory impairment (Fig 7–23).

The use of ventilation-perfusion imaging in staging and evaluating the extent of local tumor invasion has been supplanted by CT. PET and PET/CT scanning are being used to stage and evaluate response to therapy of non–small-cell lung cancers and to evaluate solitary pulmonary nodules (Chapter 13). Preoperative radionuclide lung imaging, however, may still play a role in the assessment of regional lung function to predict expected residual function after surgical resection of a lobe or entire lung. This is usually done in conjunction with standard spirometry. These evaluations are particularly important because coexistent chronic lung disease is common in these patients.

In patients with multiple tumor microemboli or lymphangitic carcinomatosis, there may be multiple small linear perfusion defects that outline the

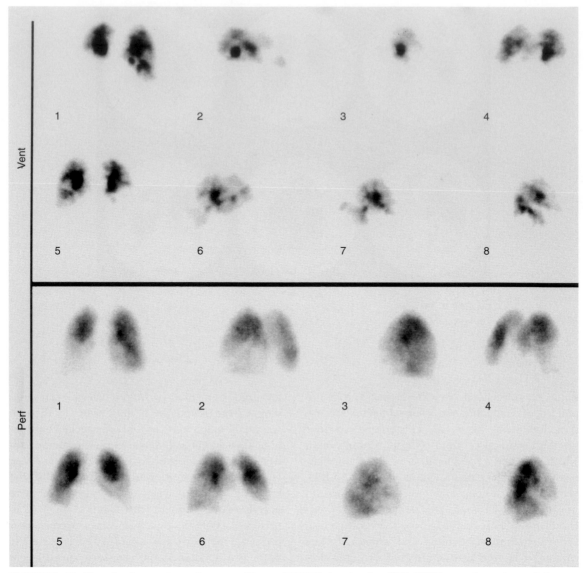

FIGURE 7–20. Chronic obstructive pulmonary disease (COPD). A technetium ⁹⁹ᵐTc-DTPA aerosol scan (*upper set*) shows marked central deposition of the aerosol due to COPD which limits interpretation for pulmonary embolism significantly. The ⁹⁹ᵐTc-MAA perfusion images (*lower set*) are more normal but still inhomogeneous.

bronchopulmonary segments, a finding known as *contour mapping* (Fig. 7–24). Segmental contour mapping may be present even when the chest radiograph and ventilation scans are normal. The sign may be of value in differentiating these conditions from suspected pulmonary embolism, in which the perfusion defects usually occupy all or parts of segments. This finding is usually seen incidental to imaging for other reasons because routine ventilation-perfusion lung scanning is of no real value in the detection or assessment of pulmonary metastases.

Inflammatory Disease

When a localized infiltrate is identified on the chest radiograph of a patient with thoracic symptoms, pneumonitis is the foremost consideration, although in certain patients other causes, such as pulmonary emboli, may need to be excluded. In the presence of any radiographic infiltrate, regardless of cause, both ventilation and perfusion are expected to be markedly decreased or absent in the involved area on lung imaging. The areas of infiltration usually do not ventilate on the initial or

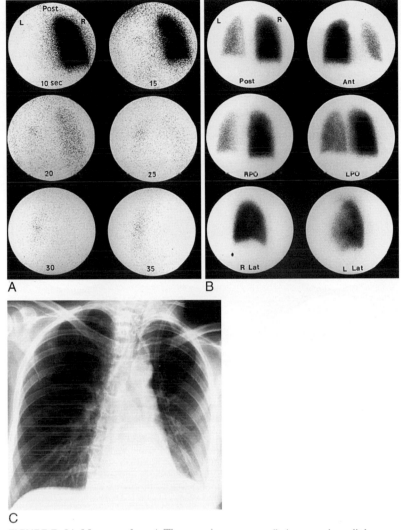

FIGURE 7–21. Mucous plug. *A,* The posterior xenon ventilation scan shows little or no activity in the left lung initially and a little trapping at 35 seconds. *B,* The perfusion scan shows a small left lung with generally diminished perfusion. *C,* An anteroposterior chest radiograph shows volume loss on the left due to postobstructive atelectasis. The findings were due to a mucous plug in the left mainstem bronchus.

rebreathing studies and do not retain xenon during the washout procedure unless there is associated obstruction. With pneumonic infiltrates, the ventilation defects are normally larger than are the perfusion defects (Fig. 7–25), and ventilation and perfusion abnormalities often persist for some time after an infiltrate has resolved on the chest radiograph. For this reason, if a perfusion defect appears significantly larger than is the corresponding radiographic infiltrate in a patient with presumed pneumonia, then a series of recent chest radiographs, if available, should be reviewed

because a partially resolved pneumonia may be the cause of the discrepancy.

When the cause of an infiltrate is in doubt, the size of the perfusion defect in relation to that of the radiographic infiltrate may provide a clue to its etiology. In small or early pneumonias, there is almost always a perfusion defect that is smaller than or equal in size to the corresponding radiographic infiltrate. With large pneumonias (such as lobar pneumonia), the perfusion deficit is usually the same size as the radiographic infiltrate. Perfusion defects that appear significantly larger than the

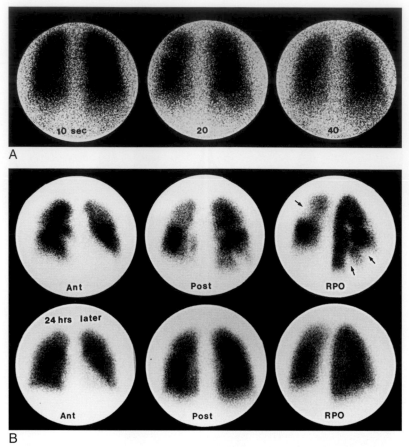

FIGURE 7–22. Asthma. *A,* Posterior images from the washout portion of a xenon ventilation scan show poor washout with little decrease in activity on the sequential 20-second images. *B,* A perfusion scan (*top*) shows multiple large and small segmental defects (*arrows*) that cleared within 24 hours after bronchodilator therapy (*bottom*).

radiographic abnormality or that are out of proportion to the ventilatory defect may raise a suspicion of pulmonary embolus in the appropriate clinical setting. Frequently, such a suspicion may be substantiated by the presence of segmental ventilation-perfusion mismatches in other areas of radiographically normal lung. In the absence of corroborating perfusion defects elsewhere in the lungs, CT-angiography may be needed to exclude the diagnosis. Matched apical abnormalities may be seen with old tuberculosis (Fig. 7–26).

Cardiovascular Abnormalities

Normal cardiovascular structures commonly cause significant defects on the ventilation-perfusion images, which may be accentuated in disease. These defects are typically nonsegmental and usually conform to the radiographic appearance of the structures producing them. Thus, it is important to examine the chest radiograph for cardiovascular abnormalities, particularly structural enlargement, abnormal contours, aneurysmal dilations, and changes due to either congestive failure or pulmonary hypertension.

Uncomplicated congestive heart failure is typically characterized by nonsegmental perfusion defects, which are usually diffuse and scattered throughout both lungs but may occasionally be focal. Fissure signs may be present, as well as other abnormalities due to pleural effusions, cardiac enlargement, redistribution of pulmonary blood flow to the upper lung zones, or pulmonary edema. Occasionally, superimposed pulmonary emboli may be suspected in patients with conges-

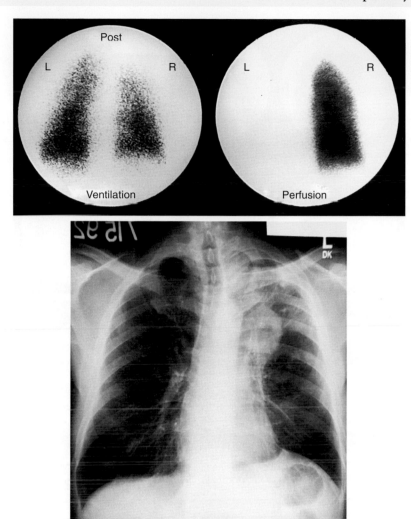

FIGURE 7–23. Lung cancer. *Top,* Posterior images from a ventilation-perfusion scan show ventilation of the left lung but no perfusion. *Bottom,* The chest radiograph shows a large left hilar mass that has constricted the left pulmonary artery.

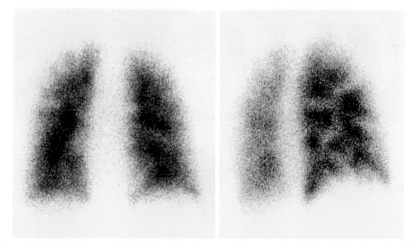

FIGURE 7–24. Lymphangitic tumor spread. The pattern seen on these anterior (*left*) and right posterior oblique (*right*) lung perfusion images is referred to as contour mapping. Thickening of the intersegmental interstitium at the periphery of the pulmonary segments has resulted in perfusion defects (lines) that outline the segments.

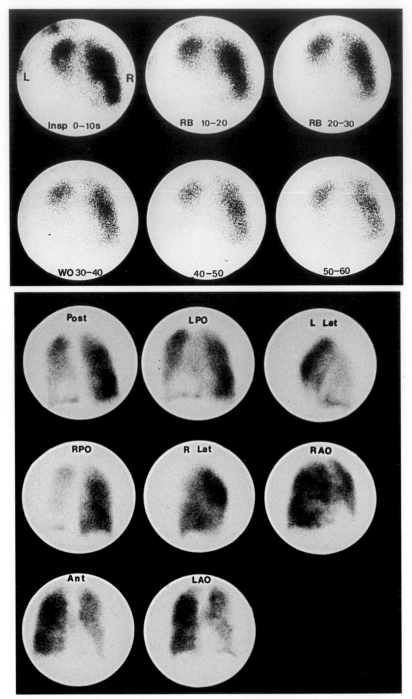

FIGURE 7–25. Pneumonia. *Top,* The ventilation scan demonstrates a marked area of nonventilation in the left lung base. *Bottom,* The perfusion scan shows a defect that is smaller than the ventilation defect, in the area where an infiltrate was identified on a chest radiograph. Note the presence of the stripe sign particularly on the posterior perfusion image.

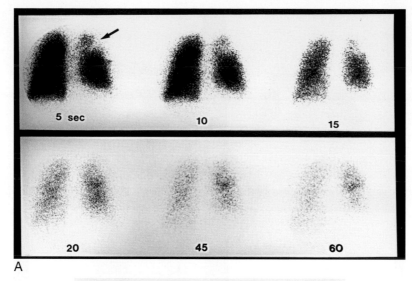

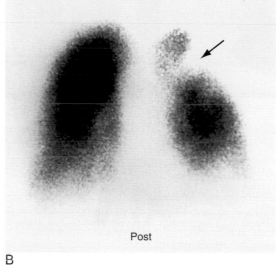

FIGURE 7–26. Tuberculosis. *A,* Posterior xenon ventilation scan shows an area
of initially decreased ventilation (*arrow*), with trapping seen later in the same area.
B, Posterior image from the perfusion lung scan shows decreased perfusion (*arrow*)
in the same area (a matched defect).

tive heart failure, and differentiation of the two
entities by scintigraphic techniques may be difficult,
especially when congestive heart failure is manifested by pulmonary edema or pleural effusions.
Diffuse interstitial edema is frequently not a
problem because a relatively normal perfusion scan
may be obtained in the absence of emboli. When
patchy alveolar edema is present, however, focal
perfusion defects may result, usually corresponding
to localized alveolar densities seen on the chest radiographs. In these cases, a high probability of superimposed pulmonary emboli may be assessed if
segmental ventilation-perfusion mismatches are
identified in areas of relatively normal lung. If a
distinction cannot be made, CT-angiography may
be necessary to establish the diagnosis.

Loculated pleural effusions accompanying congestive heart failure may cause peripheral defects in

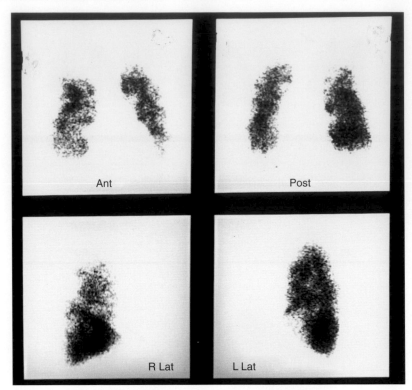

FIGURE 7–27. Vasculitis. Perfusion scan images show bilateral patchy small segmental defects. This pattern could also be seen in a variety of abnormalities, including multiple small emboli.

the lungs, but these are usually easily discernible on the chest radiograph and rarely appear segmental or multiple on upright views. To minimize the imaging problems, patients with pleural effusions are normally injected in the supine position and imaged in the upright position.

Pulmonary hypertension results in a reversal of the perfusion gradient in the lungs, producing a redistribution of pulmonary blood flow to the upper lung zones. Because of accompanying perivascular fibrosis in patients with chronic pulmonary hypertension from various causes, the lung bases generally remain poorly perfused, regardless of the position in which the patient is injected. In addition, focal and segmental basilar perfusion defects may also be present.

A multitude of other diseases related to the cardiovascular system can cause abnormalities on the ventilation-perfusion scans. However, these scan abnormalities can frequently be sorted out when reviewed with the benefit of clinical history and recent chest radiographs. Numerous bilateral, very small perfusion defects with normal ventilation should raise the possibility of either vasculitis (Fig. 7–27) or fat emboli (Fig. 7–28).

DEEP VENOUS IMAGING AND THROMBUS DETECTION

The introduction of radiolabeled monoclonal antibodies that recognize specific sites on activated components of clotted blood represents a new approach to the diagnosis of deep venous thrombosis, however such techniques have not been clinically useful to date. One Food and Drug Administration–approved radiopharmaceutical is ^{99m}Tc apcitide, which binds to receptors on activated platelets and to a lesser extent to endothelial cells. There is normally activity present in the liver and kidneys and excretion via the urinary tract and biliary system. Diagnosis is based upon significant asymmetry in activity between the two lower extremities. The agreement rate between this technique and the "gold standard" of contrast venography is only 50% to 75%.

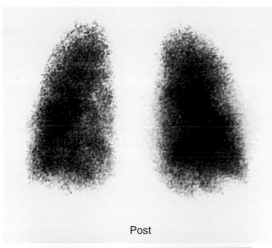

Post

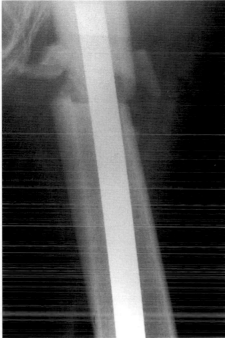

FIGURE 7–28. Fat emboli. Posterior image from a perfusion lung scan (*top*) demonstrates a fine, mottled pattern due to fat emboli occurring after this patient had an intramedullary femoral rod (*bottom*) placed for a fracture.

PEARLS & PITFALLS

Unless it is completely and absolutely normal, never interpret a ventilation-perfusion scan without a recent chest radiograph.

A normal perfusion lung scan essentially excludes clinically significant pulmonary emboli. An abnormal ventilation scan or chest radiograph will not change this assessment.

PEARLS & PITFALLS—cont'd

In addition to pulmonary embolism, other causes of perfusion defects are COPD, pneumonia, asthma, tumor, mediastinitis, mucous plug, fat emboli, and vasculitis.

Most perfusion defects caused by pulmonary emboli are wedge-shaped and extend to the periphery. They are usually bilateral and multiple.

In the interpretation of V/Q lung scans, an *unmatched defect* refers to one that is seen on the perfusion scan without an accompanying ventilation abnormality. It does not refer to a defect on the ventilation scan when the perfusion scan is normal. Similarly, it does not refer to comparison of the perfusion scan to the chest radiograph, or to comparison of the ventilation scan to the chest radiograph.

Become thoroughly acquainted with the PIOPED criteria for evaluating the likelihood of pulmonary embolism on ventilation-perfusion scans.

Even a low probability scan has a 15% to 20% probability of pulmonary embolism. A very low probability scan has a positive predictive value of less than 10%.

A scan with a combination of findings that does not clearly fit a defined category is most likely an intermediate probability scan.

Asthma, mucous plugs, and COPD can cause segmental perfusion defects, but they should not have normal ventilation scans.

A stripe sign of peripheral activity around a perfusion defect is frequently seen with COPD and indicates a very low probability defect.

When there is an infiltrate on the chest radiograph and a smaller perfusion defect, pneumonia is a common cause. When there is a small infiltrate and a relatively larger perfusion defect, pulmonary emboli should be considered.

If there is ventilation of one whole lung but no perfusion, the differential diagnosis includes congenital absence of the pulmonary artery, massive central pulmonary embolus, mediastinal fibrosis, or hilar neoplasm.

A focal hot spot in the lung is due to an injected labeled clot that was either formed in the syringe or dislodged from the end of the central line through which ^{99m}Tc-MAA was injected.

PEARLS & PITFALLS—cont'd

On an aerosol ventilation scan, collection of activity in the central bronchi is an indication of COPD.

Poor perfusion to the lung apices may be normal after lung transplantation.

Large segmental ventilation-perfusion mismatches are more likely to represent pulmonary emboli than are small ones.

Multiple irregular tiny perfusion defects can be due to COPD but also to fat emboli and vasculitis.

Parenchymal renal activity on a ^{99m}Tc-MAA scan indicates a possible right-to-left shunt. This can be confirmed by noting activity in the brain.

While over 90% of pulmonary embolism studies are now performed by CT-angiography, V/Q scans remain useful in patients with renal failure, contrast allergies, or other situations in which CT is difficult or not available.

SUGGESTED READINGS

Gottschalk A: New Criteria for Ventilation-Perfusion Lung Scan Interpretation: A Basis for Optimal Interaction with Helical CT Angiography. RadioGraphics 20:1206–1210, 2000.

Gottschalk A, Stein PD, Goodman LR, et al.: Overview of prospective investigation of pulmonary embolism diagnosis. Semin Nucl Med 32:173–182, 2002.

Hatabu H, Uematsu H, Nguyen B, et al.: CT and MR in pulmonary embolism: a changing role for nuclear medicine in diagnostic strategy. Semin Nucl Med 32:183–192, 2002.

Line BR: Scintigraphic studies of non-embolic lung disease. In Sandler MP, Coleman RE, Patton JA et al. (eds): Diagnostic Nuclear Medicine, 4th ed. New York, Lippincott, Williams and Wilkins, 2003, pp 377–412.

Sostman HD, Gottschalk A: Evaluation of patients with suspected venous thromboembolism. In Sandler MP, Coleman RE, Patton JA et al. (eds): Diagnostic Nuclear Medicine, 4th ed. New York, Lippincott, Williams and Wilkins, 2003, pp 345–366.

Stein PD, Gottschalk A: Review of criteria appropriate for a very low probability of pulmonary embolism on ventilation-perfusion lung scans: a position paper. RadioGraphics 20:99–105, 2000.

Worsley DF, Alavi A: Radionuclide imaging of acute pulmonary embolism. Semin Nucl Med 33:259–278, 2003.

Gastrointestinal Tract

8

LIVER–SPLEEN IMAGING

Computed tomography (CT) and ultrasound offer better anatomic display of liver and spleen architecture than does radionuclide liver–spleen imaging, which is seldom performed. However, there remain some indications for technetium colloid liver–spleen scanning, such as the confirmation or evaluation of suspected hepatocellular diseases, hepatomegaly or splenomegaly, and the confirmation of specific space-occupying lesions such as hepatic focal nodular hyperplasia. Although this section is primarily directed toward these applications, as with the interpretation of any examination, it is prudent to have an understanding of other important entities that may be present incidentally, as well as their scintigraphic appearance.

Radiopharmaceuticals

The liver and spleen are organs of widely differing functions, but radionuclide colloid imaging capitalizes on a function common to both: phagocytosis. The most commonly used agent is Technetium-99m (^{99m}Tc) sulfur colloid, with an average particle size of 0.3 to 1.0 μm, which is larger than a true colloid. The uptake and distribution of ^{99m}Tc colloid in the liver reflect both the distribution of functioning reticuloendothelial cells and the distribution of hepatic perfusion. In normal patients, most particles are rapidly accumulated by the phagocytes of the reticuloendothelial system of both the liver (Kupffer cells) and the spleen, allowing simultaneous imaging of both organs. Technetium colloid agents are cleared from the bloodstream with a half-time of 2 to 3 minutes. Under usual circumstances, 80% to 90% of the injected particles are sequestered by the liver, and 5% to 10% localize in the spleen. A small percentage of particles appears in other reticuloendothelial sites, particularly the bone marrow, but usually in amounts insufficient to permit imaging. In theory, there is some correlation between particle size and organ avidity for colloid: the larger particles are favored by the spleen, smaller particles go to the liver, and the smallest particles are sequestered by the bone marrow. As discussed later, visualization of uptake in the bone marrow on a technically satisfactory colloid liver–spleen scan is an abnormal finding. However, when amounts of ^{99m}Tc colloid significantly higher than the usual liver–spleen scanning dose are used, routine bone marrow imaging is possible.

Planar Imaging and Single-Photon Emission Computed Tomography

Sample imaging protocols for both planar and single-photon emission computed tomography (SPECT) imaging techniques as well as dosimetry are presented in Appendix E–1.

Imaging is performed using 4 to 6 mCi (148 to 222 MBq) of ^{99m}Tc sulfur colloid. Adequate accumulation of ^{99m}Tc sulfur colloid in the liver requires about 5 to 10 minutes in normal patients. This allows for an optimal target (liver–spleen)-to-background (blood pool) ratio. In patients with compromised hepatic function and/or portal hypertension, optimal liver concentration of the radiopharmaceutical may take considerably longer. In such patients, it is wise to wait 20 to 30 minutes before imaging.

Routine gamma camera images for liver–spleen scanning consist of anterior and posterior views as well as both lateral views. Each image is obtained for 500 to 1000 k counts by using a low-energy parallel-hole collimator. Various oblique images may be routinely obtained or performed as needed for further evaluation of a suspected abnormality in either organ. One anterior view with a lead marker identifying the right inferior costal margin is usually obtained as well. The marker should be of a known size so that hepatic and splenic measurements may be obtained. SPECT scanning of the liver occasionally adds additional information, although focal areas of decreased activity due to normal biliary and vascular structures often make interpretation difficult.

Tomographic imaging using ^{99m}Tc colloid requires a fundamental knowledge of cross-sectional anatomy of the liver and spleen as well as of surrounding unimaged structures. Transaxial images are displayed in the conventional CT format along with coronal and sagittal reconstructions. In general, defects thought to represent significant pathology should be seen in at least two orthogonal planes to be described with confidence. SPECT is most frequently used to evaluate known or suspected focal or multifocal space-occupying disease. In this setting, SPECT sensitivity and accuracy of localization have been shown to be superior to planar imaging. SPECT has proved especially useful in ^{99m}Tc red blood cell blood pool imaging for suspected liver hemangiomas using the same technical parameters as for ^{99m}Tc colloid. Vascular structures appearing as characteristic defects on colloid SPECT images are usually identifiable as areas of increased activity on the labeled red blood cell images. Accuracy of interpretation may be improved by use of SPECT-CT fusion imaging.

Normal Liver Scan

In the normal liver, there is a homogeneous distribution of ^{99m}Tc sulfur colloid throughout the organ. The liver usually consists of a dominant right and a smaller left lobe (Fig. 8–1), which may occasion-

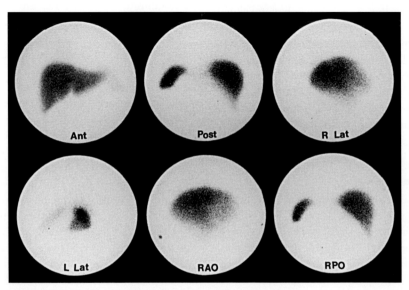

FIGURE 8–1. Normal sulfur colloid liver–spleen scan.

ally be absent. Numerous variant liver shapes have been described, the most notable of which are a long, thin right lobe (Riedel's lobe) and a prominent quadrate lobe. The porta hepatis is frequently identifiable as an area of decreased activity in the inferomedial aspect of the right lobe; this should not be mistaken for a lesion. Peripheral marginal indentations in the liver may normally be produced by the lateral rib margins, the xiphoid, the gallbladder, the right kidney, the suprahepatic veins, the heart, and intrathoracic abnormalities that affect the diaphragmatic configuration. A right lobe defect is commonly seen in many anterior views, owing to attenuation of the photons by overlying breast tissue (Fig. 8–2).

The normal liver is pliable and changes shape from deep inspiration to expiration as well as from upright to supine position. Normal length of the right lobe of the liver is generally 17 to 18 cm on the anterior view, measured from the highest point to the inferior tip of the right lobe. Evaluation of a liver–spleen scan should include (1) the size, shape, and position of the liver and spleen; (2) the homogeneity of activity within the organs; (3) the presence of any focal defects in activity; and (4) the relative distribution of colloid among the liver, spleen, and bone marrow.

Abnormal Liver Scan

Any localized space-occupying process in the liver may present as a focal area of decreased activity (commonly referred to as a *defect*) on a technetium colloid scan, provided that it is of sufficient size to be detected. Radionuclide imaging simply confirms the presence or anatomic location of focal lesions

TABLE 8–1.	Differential of Focal Hepatic Lesions on Technetium 99m Colloid Scans

DECREASED UPTAKE
Metastasis (especially colon)
Cyst
Hepatoma (especially in cirrhosis)
Adenoma
Hematoma
Hemangioma
Abscess
Pseudotumor (cirrhosis)

INCREASED UPTAKE
Focal nodular hyperplasia
Cirrhosis with regenerating nodule
Budd-Chiari syndrome (caudate lobe)
Superior vena caval obstruction (arm injection, quadrate lobe)

in the liver rather than providing a definitive histologic diagnosis. The size and location of a lesion are of paramount importance in determining whether it will be detected by gamma camera techniques. By using present technology, lesions as small as 8 mm may be identified, and those 2 to 2.5 cm in size are routinely imaged. The nearer these lesions are to the surface of the organ, and therefore to the camera collimator surface, the more readily they may be detected.

Defects in the hepatic parenchyma are nonspecific. Solitary intrahepatic defects may be produced by various lesions, any of which may also be multiple (Tables 8–1 and 8–2). In any patient with several liver defects, however, metastatic

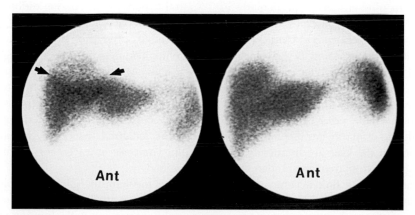

FIGURE 8–2. Normal anterior liver–spleen scan. *Left,* A defect (*arrows*) is seen in the upper aspect of the right lobe due to attenuation by overlying breast tissue. *Right,* The breast has been raised eliminating the artifact.

TABLE 8–2.	Nuclear Imaging Appearances of Liver Lesions on ^{99m}Tc Colloid and Other Scans
LESIONS	**APPEARANCE**
Hepatic adenoma	Usually photopenic defect
	Rarely normal activity
	^{99m}Tc RBCs—normal
	^{99m}Tc hepatobiliary:
	perfusion—normal,
	parenchymal—decreased,
	washout—delayed
Focal nodular hyperplasia	30% photopenic defect
	30% normal activity
	40% increased activity
	^{99m}Tc hepatobiliary:
	perfusion—increased,
	parenchymal—normal,
	washout—delayed
Cavernous hemangioma	Photopenic defect
	^{99m}Tc RBCs:
	perfusion—decreased,
	blood pool—increased
Hepatocellular carcinoma	Photopenic defect
	^{67}Ga—avidly increased
	^{99m}Tc RBCs—rarely increased
	^{99m}Tc hepatobiliary:
	perfusion—decreased,
	parenchymal—normal or
	decreased,
	washout—delayed
Cholangiocarcinoma	Photopenic defect
Metastases	Photopenic defect, early hyperperfusion
Liver abscess	Photopenic defect
	^{67}Ga—80% increased
Focal fatty infiltration	Photopenic defect
	^{133}Xe—increased

^{99m}Tc, technetium-99m; RBCs, red blood cells; ^{67}Ga, gallium-67; ^{133}Xe, xenon-133.

disease must be a prime consideration, particularly when accompanied by hepatomegaly or a known primary lesion. In most instances, particularly in cases of equivocal liver scan findings, ultrasonography or CT should be performed. A large area of decreased activity in the liver may be produced by the inclusion of part of that organ in a radiation therapy portal. This type of defect, however, is usually readily recognized by its sharp linear edges, which correspond to the sides of the treatment portal. In addition to primarily intrahepatic lesions, peripheral defects in the liver are frequently produced by adjacent extraparenchymal pathology, including subdiaphragmatic fluid accumulations or renal tumors, or by peripheral lesions of a primary hepatic origin, including subcapsular hematoma.

Increased radiocolloid concentration by the spleen and bone marrow compared with the liver (colloid shift) may be found in patients with diseases that cause derangement of hepatic function and/or portal hypertension. Among diffuse hepatocellular diseases, hepatic cirrhosis is the most common abnormality presenting in this fashion. Colloid shift accompanied by other typical scintigraphic findings is a hallmark of this disease. Even patients with diffuse hepatic metastases may show colloid shift. The distribution of colloid in the bone marrow should be carefully examined in such patients because localized defects in colloid activity indicating marrow involvement by tumor may be identified.

The mechanisms governing colloid shift have variously been attributed to (1) the consequences of portal hypertension with shunting of colloid-laden blood away from the liver to the spleen and bone marrow, or (2) a decrease in the number or func-

TABLE 8–3.	Diffuse Pulmonary Uptake of Technetium 99m Sulfur Colloid

Hepatic cirrhosis
Chronic obstructive pulmonary disease with
  superimposed infection
Bacterial endotoxin
Estrogen therapy
Neoplasms (various primary tumors and metastases,
  including hepatoma)
Disseminated intravascular coagulopathy
Mucopolysaccharidosis type II (Hunter's syndrome)
Histiocytosis X
Faulty colloid preparation (excess aluminum)
High serum aluminum level (antacids)
Children (normal minimal uptake)
Transplant recipients
Pulmonary trauma

tional capability of hepatic Kupffer cells, thereby decreasing liver clearance of sulfur colloid. In various liver diseases, either or both of these principles may play a role. The observation that alleviation of portal hypertension does not necessarily result in a return to a normal radiocolloid distribution has led some investigators to postulate that intrahepatic shunting, not portal hypertension per se, plays the major role in producing the phenomenon of colloid shift, especially in cirrhotic patients. Such shunting would allow portal blood to bypass hepatic sinusoids, making more colloid available to the spleen and bone marrow. Indeed, there is good experimental evidence for such a mechanism.

Other abnormal distributions of colloid include activity in renal transplants, diffuse lung activity, and focal hot spots in the liver (see Table 8–1). In patients with renal transplants undergoing rejection, the transplant may be visualized. This may occur long after the episode of rejection and does not necessarily indicate acute rejection. Diffuse pulmonary activity may be noted occasionally in cirrhosis, infection, and many other entities (Table 8–3). For patients with cirrhosis, the mechanisms postulated involve increased pulmonary phagocytosis or altered pulmonary endothelium.

In the presence of superior vena cava or innominate venous obstruction, a bolus of activity injected into an ipsilateral arm vein can travel via the collaterals to a recanalized umbilical vessel, delivering a large amount of activity to the anterior mid-portion of the liver (quadrate lobe), which causes a focal hot spot. Other entities that may cause apparent focal areas of increased hepatic

activity are Budd-Chiari syndrome (hepatic vein obstruction), focal nodular hyperplasia, and cirrhosis (regenerating nodules).

Alcoholic Liver Disease

A spectrum of technetium colloid scan findings is presented by alcoholic liver disease. In its early phases, alcoholic hepatitis or fatty infiltration may present as a normal-sized or enlarged liver with diffusely diminished or inhomogeneous activity. As the disease progresses and parenchymal scarring becomes more prevalent, the liver may become smaller than normal. An oddity of this disease is that the right lobe is frequently more affected, giving a typical pattern of a small right lobe and a relatively enlarged left lobe. This probably occurs because the portal vein delivers more blood flow (and alcohol) to the right lobe of the liver.

Fatty infiltration of the liver may be focal or diffuse. Focal fatty infiltration is seen on CT as an area of low attenuation and can be confused with a neoplastic process. Usually, it can be differentiated from a true mass on CT by noting that there is no mass effect and that portal vessels run through the low-density area. If a technetium colloid scan is performed, the area typically shows normal reticuloendothelial activity. Fatty infiltration can also be noted as an incidental finding on a xenon ventilation lung scan by noting xenon retention in the liver, either focally or diffusely.

As the process of injury, scarring, and regeneration continues, activity within the organ becomes less homogeneous and is sometimes so coarsely mottled as to be confused with space-occupying lesions. In cirrhotic patients with this mottled pattern or with a large dominant defect, especially those who have demonstrated sudden unexplained clinical decompensation, superimposed hepatoma must be considered.

Colloid shift to the spleen and bone marrow is another prominent feature of all phases of alcoholic liver disease. When hepatocyte function is severely depressed, persistence of technetium colloid in the blood pool may also be identified on static images, especially in the cardiac area. In the advanced stages of disease, the spleen is frequently enlarged, a finding that may correlate with portal hypertension. In some patients, ascites may be imaged on the anterior view as medial displacement of the right lobe of the liver from the ribs and lateral abdominal wall (Fig. 8–3).

Irrespective of its cause, hepatic cirrhosis may present with any of the findings described for

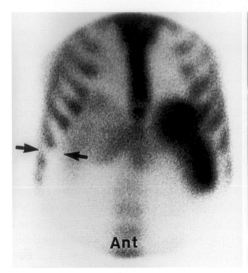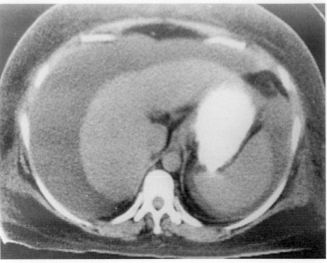

FIGURE 8–3. Cirrhosis with ascites. *Left,* Marked hepatocellular dysfunction and colloid shift are shown, with bone marrow activity, increased splenic activity, and some pulmonary parenchymal activity. The liver is small and displaced medially by ascites (*arrows*). *Right,* The ascites and small liver are easily appreciated on computed tomography scan.

alcohol-induced disease. The particular scintigraphic appearance of the organ depends primarily on the stage and severity of the disease.

Diffuse and Infiltrative Disorders

Any disease that secondarily invades the liver may produce a pattern of hepatomegaly, with or without focal defects, and commonly with diffusely diminished activity. Disease entities that may produce this pattern are listed in Table 8–4. Hepatitis may present in this manner, reflecting

TABLE 8–4.	Causes of Hepatomegaly with Slightly Decreased Activity on Technetium-99m Sulfur Colloid Scans

Normal variant (i.e., large patient with soft tissue attenuation)
Diffuse hepatocellular disease (e.g., hepatitis)
Metastases
Diabetes mellitus
Fatty infiltration
Hemochromatosis
Amyloidosis
Lymphoma
Leukemia
Sarcoidosis
Lipid storage disorders
Passive congestion

diffuse parenchymal edema. If hepatic function is compromised, colloid shift may also be seen (Fig. 8–4).

Metastatic Disease

CT scanning is the initial test of choice if a hepatic tumor or metastasis is suspected. Radionuclide liver–spleen scanning usually detects these as serendipitous findings when the examination is performed for some other reason. Applications of tumor-specific radiopharmaceuticals are discussed in Chapter 11.

The most characteristic presentation of liver metastasis on a technetium colloid scan is as multiple focal defects (Fig. 8–5), although the lesions may present as coarsely inhomogeneous activity or simply as hepatomegaly. By using discrete hepatic defects as the diagnostic criterion for metastatic disease, the liver scan demonstrates a detection sensitivity of about 75% to 80% for all types of primary tumors, especially when scintigraphic data are integrated with available clinical information. Individual sensitivity varies with the particular primary lesion.

Systemic chemotherapy for primary hepatic tumors and intrahepatic metastases generally has poor results. This has prompted use of direct infusion of the chemotherapeutic agents into the hepatic artery. Evaluation of the catheter placement and distribution of blood flow can be done either with contrast angiography or by administra-

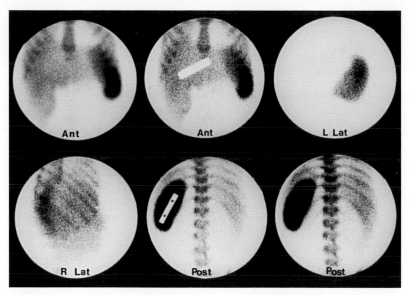

FIGURE 8–4. Hepatitis. This picture is similar to that of fatty infiltration of the liver, although in this case, there is splenomegaly as well. The basic findings are marked colloid shift, splenomegaly, and an enlarged liver with diffusely decreased activity.

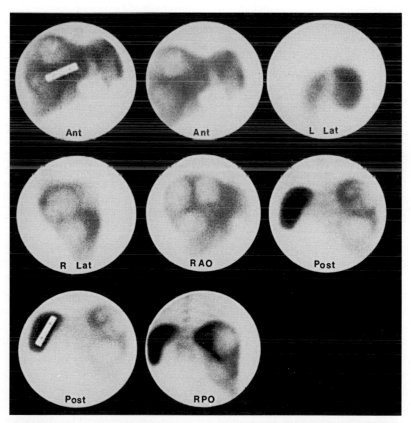

FIGURE 8–5. Metastatic colon carcinoma. Multiple large focal defects are identified throughout the liver. In this particular case, the metastatic disease is extensive enough that some colloid shift can be identified on the right posterior oblique view.

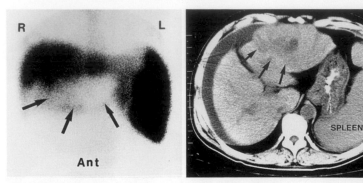

FIGURE 8–6. Hepatoma in a patient with cirrhosis. *Left,* The liver–spleen scan reveals a small liver and large spleen. There is a large cold defect (*arrows*) in the inferior aspect of the left lobe of the liver. *Right,* Computed tomography scan shows a bulging, poorly defined, low-density lesion in the left lobe (*arrows*), as well as ascites and splenomegaly.

tion of 1 to 4 mCi (37 to 148 MBq) of ^{99m}Tc macroaggregated albumin (MAA) (not colloid). The MAA lodges in the capillaries served by the catheter.

Primary Liver Neoplasms

Hepatoma

Hepatoma usually presents as a focal defect on sulfur colloid images (Fig. 8–6), although uncommon multifocal forms exist. The lesions frequently occur in association with pre-existing diffuse hepatic diseases, most notably alcoholic or postnecrotic cirrhosis. The appearance of a prominent localized colloid deficit in a patient with one of these associations should alert the physician to the possibility of hepatoma. Hepatomas are also noted to be generally gallium-67 (^{67}Ga)–avid.

Focal Nodular Hyperplasia

The benign neoplasm of focal nodular hyperplasia generally occurs as an asymptomatic mass or as a serendipitously discovered lesion found predominantly in women. The lesions are unique as they contain adequate numbers of Kupffer cells, so that they normally concentrate and occasionally hyperconcentrate radiocolloid. Thus, in most cases, they appear indistinguishable from normal hepatic parenchyma (Fig. 8–7); infrequently, they present as regions of increased activity on liver scans. When lesions discovered by other imaging modalities are of sufficient size to be detected by liver scintigraphy but appear normal on the liver scan, the diagnosis of focal nodular hyperplasia may be presumed in the proper clinical setting. In a minority of cases, insufficient colloid is concentrated by the lesions, so that they are perceived as photopenic

areas on the scan. When this occurs, the mass cannot be differentiated from other causes of parenchymal defects.

Hepatic Cell Adenomas

Hepatic cell adenomas are usually encountered in young women who have used birth control pills. Although the disease usually is asymptomatic, hemorrhage, often of massive degree, occasionally occurs. Because Kupffer cells are not a prominent feature of these lesions, adenomas present as focal defects on technetium colloid images. When birth control pills are withheld, these lesions may rapidly regress.

Miscellaneous Focal Lesions

Abscess

Abscess commonly presents as a nonspecific solitary focal defect on liver scans, although multiple lesions may occur. The diagnosis is frequently suggested by history.

Budd-Chiari Syndrome (Hepatic Vein Thrombosis)

Hepatic vein thrombosis may occur secondary to tumor invasion or hypercoagulation syndromes, but frequently no underlying cause is identified. The disease usually presents as an enlarged, congested tender liver accompanied by ascites. With early or partial hepatic vein obstruction, technetium colloid activity in the liver becomes diffusely mottled. As thrombosis progresses, activity in both lobes steadily decreases. Typically, the caudate lobe simultaneously enlarges and shows relatively increased activity. This latter phenomenon has been explained by the presence of separate venous drainage directly into the vena cava for the caudate

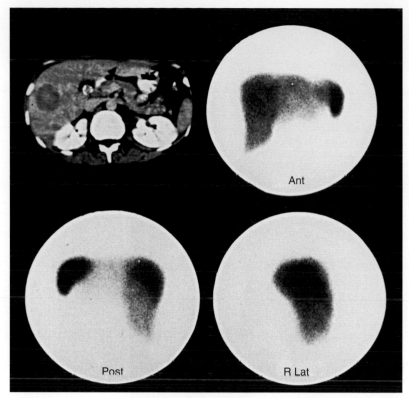

FIGURE 8–7. Focal nodular hyperplasia. A postcontrast abdominal computed tomography scan of the liver in a young woman with right upper quadrant pain demonstrates a well-defined, focal, low-density lesion in the right lobe of the liver. A liver–spleen scan obtained in the same patient demonstrates a normal technetium-99m sulfur colloid distribution in the region of the lesion. When this discrepancy occurs, focal nodular hyperplasia is the prime consideration.

lobe, which is unaffected by thrombosis of the major hepatic veins.

HEPATIC BLOOD POOL IMAGING

Although hemangiomas and cysts are usually occult, asymptomatic lesions, ultrasound can reliably distinguish between cysts (which are hypoechoic) and hemangiomas (which are hyperechoic). CT with intravenous contrast is more specific, usually demonstrating characteristic progressive enhancement toward the center of a hemangioma. Cavernous hemangioma is highly likely when a defect seen with ^{99m}Tc sulfur colloid imaging shows increased activity after administration of a ^{99m}Tc blood pool agent, such as ^{99m}Tc red blood cells, owing to labeling of the blood pool in the lesion. To allow equilibration of the hemangioma blood pool with the labeled red blood cells, delayed imaging (sometimes over several hours) may be necessary when planar imaging is used. Dynamic or

blood flow images frequently show normal or decreased perfusion of the lesions. Use of SPECT in the setting of suspected hepatic hemangioma increases the sensitivity of the study, especially when lesions are deep or less than 5 cm in diameter (Fig. 8–8). SPECT provides nearly 100% sensitivity for detection of hemangiomas larger than 1.5 cm in diameter; sensitivity is 50% or less for lesions smaller than 1.0 cm in diameter.

Normal Spleen Scan

On the posterior and anterior views of a technetium colloid scan, the normal spleen exhibits homogeneous activity equal to or less than that of the liver. The organ is ovoid in configuration, with occasional thinning of the anterior aspect. The normal length of the spleen on a posterior scan is about 10 ± 1.5 cm and should not exceed 13 cm. In children up to 18 years of age, the normal size in centimeters can be estimated by using the following formula:

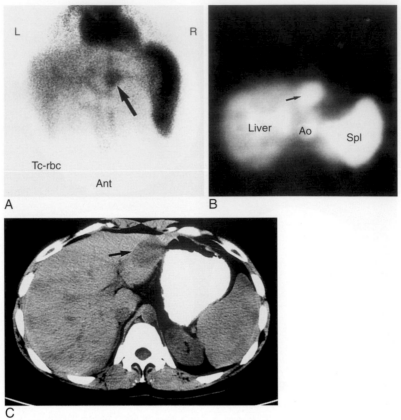

FIGURE 8–8. Hepatic hemangioma. *A,* A planar anterior view of the abdomen on a technetium-99m-labeled red blood cell scan shows marked blood pooling in the heart and spleen. A focal lesion with similar activity (*arrow*) also is seen in the left lobe of the liver. *B,* A transaxial SPECT image of the abdomen shows the liver, aorta, spleen, and hypervascular lesion (*arrow*). *C,* A CT scan without intravenous contrast shows the hemangioma (*arrow*) to be hypodense relative to the liver. Cavernous hemangiomas characteristically become isodense on CT if intravenous contrast is used and delayed images are obtained.

$$5.7 + (0.31 \times \text{age in years})$$

Routine imaging of the spleen and liver uses ^{99m}Tc sulfur colloid. Isolated imaging of the spleen is also possible with ^{99m}Tc-labeled heat-damaged red blood cells, which are sequestered by the spleen; however, such scans are rarely necessary for clinical diagnosis. When imaging the spleen with colloid, routine anterior, posterior, and lateral liver–spleen scan views are obtained. Left anterior oblique and left posterior oblique views at varying degrees of obliquity also may be useful. Occasionally, a right posterior oblique view may be needed to separate the left lobe of the liver from the spleen. After surgery or trauma, there may be questions about splenic remnants or accessory spleens. Historically, these were imaged with heat-damaged red blood cells; however, for most purposes, use of ^{99m}Tc colloid is adequate (Fig 8–9).

Abnormal Spleen Scan
Focal Lesions

Solitary or multiple splenic defects are nonspecific and may be produced by a number of abnormalities. Careful correlation with pertinent clinical history is necessary to distinguish among these. More common abnormalities that may present as defects within the organ are cysts, hematomas, abscesses (Fig. 8–10), infarctions, and neoplasms. Peripheral wedge-shaped defects may often be correlated with infarcts (Fig. 8–11), especially when a pertinent history, such as of hemoglobinopathy, is obtained.

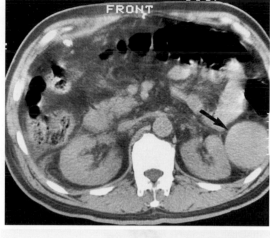

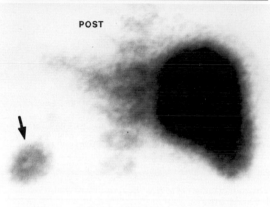

FIGURE 8–9. Accessory spleen. *Top,* In this patient who had a previous splenectomy, a computed tomography scan revealed a soft-tissue mass (*arrow*) lateral to the left kidney. *Bottom,* A posterior image from a technetium-99m colloid scan in the same patient demonstrates functioning tissue (*arrow*), which represents an accessory spleen or splenic remnant.

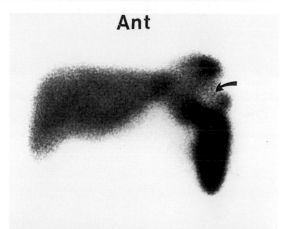

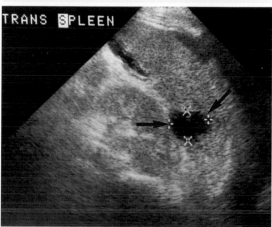

FIGURE 8–10. Splenic abscess. *Top,* In this drug abuser with a fever, an anterior view from a Technetium-99m colloid liver–spleen scan reveals a cold defect (*arrow*). *Bottom,* A transverse image from a left upper quadrant ultrasound shows a hypoechoic lesion (*arrows*). The low-level internal echoes and lack of enhanced transmission exclude a splenic cyst.

Metastatic lesions to the spleen are uncommon, although tumors such as lymphoma (Fig. 8–12), melanoma, chorioepithelioma, or soft-tissue sarcoma may present with splenic lesions. Primary splenic neoplasms are extremely rare. Focal areas of decreased activity in the spleen occur in less than 1% of liver–spleen scans. If trauma is excluded as a cause, one third of such defects are due to splenic infarcts, one third to lymphoma, and one third to metastatic disease. A history of immunosuppression or drug abuse increases the likelihood of abscess.

Splenomegaly

Liver–spleen scans may be ordered to confirm clinical suspicion of splenomegaly, although ultrasound is usually less expensive. The causes of splenomegaly are numerous (Table 8–5), and unless focal space-occupying disease is identified, scans are generally unhelpful in determining the cause. Infiltrative disorders produce varying degrees of splenomegaly, with or without alterations in splenic activity. The findings are largely nonspecific and are best interpreted in light of clinical observations. Perhaps the one exception to this is massive splenomegaly, which is most often caused by chronic lymphocytic leukemia.

Trauma

CT is the imaging method of choice for acute splenic trauma. The role of radiocolloid spleen imaging is usually very limited. After abdominal trauma, splenic tissue may seed to other locations (splenosis), such as the lung and peritoneal cavity.

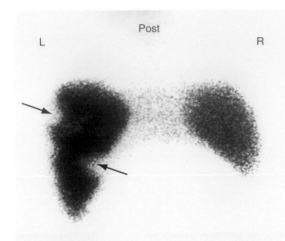

FIGURE 8–11. Splenic infarcts. A posterior image from a technetium-99m colloid liver–spleen scan shows an enlarged spleen with multiple peripheral wedge-shaped defects (*arrows*), which are characteristic of infarcts.

TABLE 8–5.	Diseases Affecting Splenic Size and Activity

MASSIVE ENLARGEMENT
Chronic leukemia
Myelofibrosis
Glycogen storage diseases
Thalassemia major

MODERATE ENLARGEMENT
Cirrhosis with portal hypertension
Hepatitis, acute or chronic
Hemolytic anemia
Mononucleosis
Lymphoma*

MINIMAL ENLARGEMENT
Congestive heart failure
Metastatic disease*
Collagen disease
Infections
Increased activity
Portal hypertension
Anemia
Leukemia
Lymphoma*
Sepsis
Melanoma*
Stress (recent surgery or chemotherapy)
Hepatocellular dysfunction (colloid shift)

*Depending on disease stage, these entities may also cause decreased activity.

Such tissue fragments usually accumulate radiocolloid and, when identified on ultrasound or CT imaging, can be substantiated as splenic tissue by using ^{99m}Tc sulfur colloid imaging.

Nonvisualization of the Spleen

In certain cases, the spleen may not be visualized on a ^{99m}Tc colloid scan even in the absence of a history of splenectomy (Table 8–6). Congenital asplenia may be associated with a number of cardiovascular, pulmonary, and abdominal anomalies. In sickle cell anemia, the spleen may not be seen because of atrophy related to repeated infarctions (autosplenectomy); in some of these patients, the spleen remains anatomically intact but with depressed or absent reticuloendothelial function, owing to reversible mechanical obstruction of blood flow by the abnormal configuration of the red blood cells (functional asplenia).

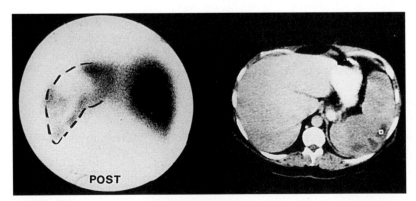

FIGURE 8–12. Lymphoma of the spleen. *Left,* A left anterior oblique technetium-99m colloid view demonstrates massive replacement of the spleen with little remaining reticuloendothelial activity. The spleen has been outlined. *Right,* The amount of replacement is much greater than is suggested by the computed tomography scan.

TABLE 8–6.	Causes of Splenic Defects on Technetium-99m Colloid Scan

FOCAL DEFECTS
Infarct
Lymphoma
Metastasis
Cyst
Abscess
Hematoma or splenic artery aneurysm
Anatomic variation
Artifact

NONVISUALIZATION
Splenectomy
Sickle cell disease (functional or autosplenectomy)
Congenital absence of spleen (isolated or Ivemark's
  syndrome)
Tumor replacement
Infarction
Traumatic avulsion or volvulus
Functional asplenia

GASTROINTESTINAL BLEEDING STUDIES

Both ^{99m}Tc red blood cells and ^{99m}Tc colloid can effectively be used to localize gastrointestinal (GI) bleeding; however, labeled red blood cells are almost always used and have greater specificity. Both radiopharmaceuticals provide similar information, and sensitivity with both is significantly greater than with angiography for the detection of lower GI bleeding, with the added advantage of being noninvasive. Because of significant background activity in the upper abdomen and the diagnostic efficacy of endoscopy in the GI tract, nuclear imaging techniques are most advantageous in evaluating lower GI bleeding, although active small-bowel, duodenal, and distal gastric hemorrhage are routinely detected when proper timing and technique for imaging are used. The accuracy of endoscopy in making the diagnosis of upper GI bleeding exceeds 90%.

The common causes of lower GI bleeding in adults are diverticular disease, angiodysplasia, neoplasms, and inflammatory bowel disease. Preoperative localization of a bleeding site permits a more rational, tailored approach to angiography and surgical intervention. Because bleeding from these causes frequently is intermittent, chances of detecting the site of hemorrhage are enhanced by a radiopharmaceutical with a long intravascular half-life, such as labeled red blood cells. Angiography

may be negative in patients with intermittent bleeding or bleeding rates below 1.0 mL/minute. With radionuclide techniques, bleeding rates on the order of 0.2 mL/ minute are reliably detected, and the sensitivity has been reported to be good even for bleeding rates as low as 0.04 mL/minute, although a total volume of 2 to 3 mL of blood is necessary. These techniques are best applied to patients who are bleeding acutely. Patients with chronic, low-volume blood loss presenting with guaiac-positive stools or chronic anemias seldom benefit from the examination.

Intravascular blood pool agents, such as ^{99m}Tc red blood cells, are the agents of choice in the investigation of GI hemorrhage, especially in cases of intermittent or slow bleeding, with a sensitivity greater than 90%. Because the agent remains in the intravascular space, imaging may be performed over a period of 24 hours. Any free technetium that is not bound to red blood cells is excreted by the kidneys and gastric mucosa and passes into the bladder, small bowel, and colon. This latter problem is obviated somewhat by use of in vitro or modified in vivo labeling techniques, which allow for a higher degree of red blood cell tagging and therefore a lower percentage of free technetium. With red blood cells, most bleeding sites show an initial focus of activity, which increases and changes position and/or configuration with time. If the activity remains in the same location, static vascular abnormalities, such as an aneurysm or angiodysplasia, should be suspected. When delayed imaging is necessary to identify a bleeding site, there may be uncertainty with respect to the site of origin. If the extravasated intraluminal agent is not identified shortly after its deposition, it may move to a more proximal or distal site during any prolonged intervals between images, especially with the increased peristalsis present in most patients with GI bleeding. However, establishing the mere presence of slow bleeding into the bowel remains possible, and therefore, the study is undoubtedly of value in many patients.

Technetium-99m sulfur is uncommonly used as a GI hemorrhage imaging agent but has a few advantages for the investigation of acute bleeding. Technetium-99m sulfur colloid is readily available, inexpensive, and easy to prepare. The colloid clears rapidly from the intravascular space via the reticuloendothelial system, providing excellent contrast between background and extravasated isotope at the bleeding site. The rapid blood clearance of radiocolloids is also a disadvantage in that the patient must be actively bleeding during the short time that the colloid is intravascular (vascular half-time, 2.5 to 3.5 minutes); thus, significant intermittent hemorrhage may be missed. In addition, liver and spleen activity may interfere with detection of bleeding sites in the upper abdomen. These factors lead to a relatively lower overall sensitivity for bleeding detection with labeled sulfur colloid than with labeled red blood cells.

Technique

In vitro methods have the highest red blood cell labeling efficiency, and are thus preferred for GI bleeding scans. The procedure is a relatively simple one in which 1 to 3 mL of anticoagulated blood is added to a vial containing stannous chloride. After a few minutes, there is addition of sodium hypochlorite to oxidize the extracellular tin, followed by a mixture of citric acid, sodium citrate, and dextrose. Finally, ^{99m}Tc-pertechnetate is introduced, and after about 20 minutes the cells are reinjected into the patient. Labeling efficiency is greater than 95% with this method.

Imaging to detect GI bleeding by using labeled RBCs may commence with an initial rapid perfusion sequence of 2- to 3-second abdominal and pelvic images obtained over 30 to 60 seconds. Static images (500 to 1000 k) may then be performed at 5-minute intervals for 60 minutes, with images taken thereafter at intervals of 15 to 60 minutes, depending on the clinical setting. More commonly, a continuous dynamic computer acquisition with a 128 × 128 matrix is used and the results viewed in cine format, which may increase the accuracy of the study. Static images may be formatted at appropriate intervals for hard-copy results as needed. As discussed, 6-, 12-, or 24-hour delayed images may substantiate an interval bleed but usually do not accurately disclose the actual site of hemorrhage.

Interpretation

A positive scan shows a focal site of increased activity within the abdomen or pelvis, which progresses distally in the bowel (Figs. 8–13 and 8–14; Table 8–7). Once bleeding is identified, multiple sequential images aid greatly in establishing its origin by recording the pattern of progression of the radionuclide within the bowel. Optimally, the images are viewed in cine mode. Because blood is an irritant to the intestine, movement of activity is often rapid and can be bidirectional. This is often true in the small bowel where a rapid serpiginous course of the labeled red blood cells from the left

upper abdomen to the right lower quadrant is characteristic. The earlier in a study that the bleeding is seen, the more accurate is the localization. Because the main purpose of the examination is to localize the site of bleeding, the study should be continued for a sufficient length of time to follow the progress of the labeled blood and permit mapping of bowel anatomy, which may vary somewhat from patient to patient. An area of activity that remains fixed in location over time should raise the suspicion of other causes than intraluminal bleeding. Occasional confusion of bladder activity with a rectosigmoid bleed can usually be resolved on postvoid views or lateral pelvic images. Interfering genital activity is usually identified by its location on anterior oblique or lateral pelvic views. Carefully performed labeled red blood cell studies show a high degree of sensitivity (>90%), with a low false-negative results rate. In addition to providing evidence of active GI bleeding and its location, the examination may also be used as a guide for selective abdominal arteriography and to assess the results of interventional therapy.

MECKEL'S DIVERTICULUM IMAGING

Meckel's diverticulum occurs in about 2% of the population and predominantly affects male patients. Although most (96%) of the lesions remain asymptomatic throughout life, complications (obstruction, hemorrhage, intussusception, and volvulus) occur in a small percentage of patients. The most common presentation in a child is painless rectal bleeding. In virtually all cases accompanied by bleeding, ectopic gastric mucosa with or without associated ulceration can be demonstrated in the diverticulum. The traditional method of radionuclide investigation of a patient with bleeding from suspected Meckel's diverticulum is based on visualization of the ectopic mucosa with intravenously administered ^{99m}Tc-pertechnetate. Negative results are common in patients whose diverticula do not contain ectopic gastric tissue (Table 8–8).

Technique

The study consists of intravenous injection of 10 to 15 mCi (370 to 555 MBq) of ^{99m}Tc-pertechnetate in adults or about 200 to 300 µCi/kg (7.4 to 11.1 MBq/kg) in children. Sequential anterior abdominopelvic images are then obtained for 45 to 60 minutes. A typical positive scan consists of a focal area of increased activity in the right lower

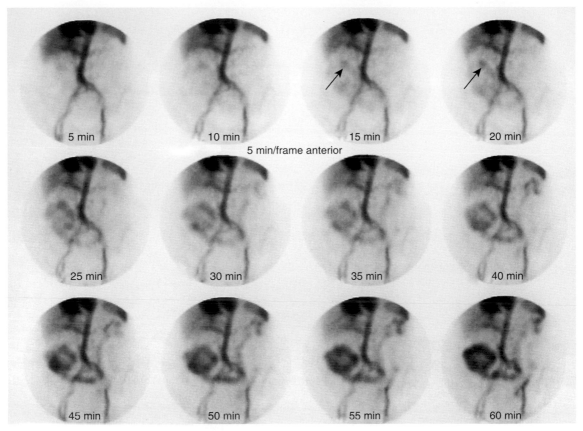

5 min/frame anterior

FIGURE 8–13. Small-bowel bleeding. This study was performed with technetium-99m labeled red blood cells and a demonstrates a focus of active bleeding in the proximal small bowel (*arrow*) and subsequent activity in the mid-abdomen and right lower quadrant.

TABLE 8–7.	Interpretation of Labeled Red Blood Cell Scans for Gastrointestinal Bleeding

CRITERIA FOR ACTIVE BLEEDING
Activity appears and conforms to bowel anatomy
Usually increase in activity with time
Must move antegrade and or retrograde in bowel

FALSE-POSITIVE
Free technetium-99m pertechnetate
Urinary tract activity
Uterine or penile blush
Accessory spleen
Hemangioma (hepatic)
Varices

FALSE-NEGATIVE
Bleeding rate too low
Intermittent bleeding

quadrant or mid-abdomen, which on lateral view is seen to be anterior and unrelated to any ureteral activity (Fig. 8–15). This finding generally appears in the first 30 minutes of the study but may take up to 1 hour to appear, depending on the amount of gastric mucosa present. False-positive results have been reported secondary to intussusception (possibly related to the associated hyperemia), urinary tract activity (often secondary to obstruction), various small-bowel lesions, inflammatory bowel disease, vascular lesions, and rarely, intestinal duplication cysts containing gastric mucosa. False-negative scans have been reported in patients with malrotation of the ileum, small amounts of ectopic mucosa, and localized bowel irritability, which causes rapid clearance of the pertechnetate from the area. The overall specificity and sensitivity of the examination, however, are about 90%.

Several pharmacologic interventions have been proposed to increase the sensitivity of Meckel's

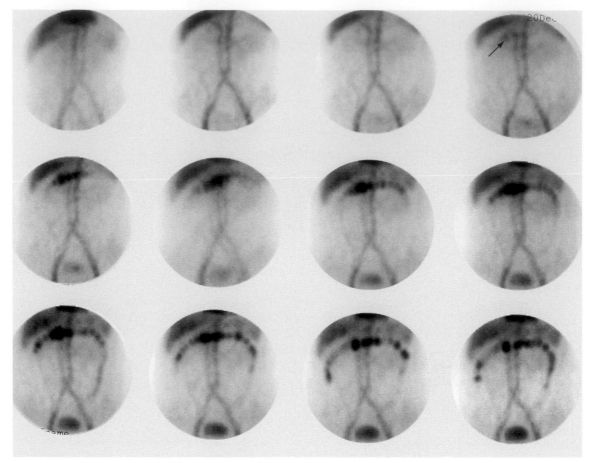

FIGURE 8–14. Lower gastrointestinal bleeding. Bleeding is seen as a focus of activity that initially appears in the right transverse colon (*arrow*) which then subsequently moves both antegrade and retrograde from the site of bleeding.

TABLE 8–8.	Interpretation of Meckel's Scans

Usually right lower quadrant and anterior
Appear and fade in same temporal pattern as stomach
  mucosa

FALSE-POSITIVE
Urinary tract activity
Other ectopic gastric mucosa
Hyperemic inflammatory lesions
Arteriovenous malformation, hemangioma, aneurysm
Neoplasms
Intussusception

FALSE-NEGATIVE
Minimal amount of gastric mucosa
Rapid washout of pertechnetate
Meckel's diverticulum with impaired blood supply
Sensitivity may be enhanced using pentagastrin,
  cimetidine, or glucagon (see text).

diverticulum imaging, with varying degrees of success. These include the use of cimetidine to block release of pertechnetate from the ectopic mucosa, pentagastrin to enhance mucosal uptake of ^{99m}Tc-pertechnetate (^{99m}TcO$_4^-$), and glucagon to decrease small-bowel (diverticular) motility. Cimetidine is administered in an oral dose of 300 mg four times daily for adults or 20 mg/kg/day for children for 2 days before the study. Some laboratories use glucagon, given intravenously 10 minutes after the start of the study.

Actively hemorrhaging patients with suspected Meckel's diverticulum may be initially investigated with radionuclide techniques intended to detect the bleeding site rather than the ectopic gastric mucosa. When technetium colloid is used for this purpose, a negative bleeding examination may be immediately followed by a technetium pertechnetate gastric mucosa imaging study.

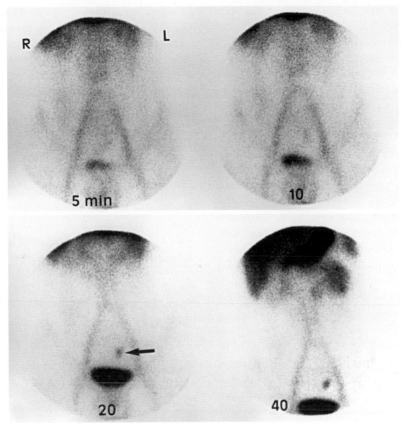

FIGURE 8–15. Meckel's diverticulum. In this 2-year-old boy with rectal bleeding, sequential technetium-99m pertechnetate scans reveal a focus of activity (*arrow*) that appears at 20 minutes in the mid-abdomen. This did not move over time and was located anteriorly in the abdomen on a lateral view (not shown).

HEPATOBILIARY IMAGING

The ^{99m}Tc-labeled hepatobiliary agents enable accurate and convenient imaging in acute and chronic biliary disease. Common indications are for acute (calculous or acalculous) cholecystitis, biliary patency, identification of biliary leaks, and, in neonates, differentiation of biliary atresia from neonatal hepatitis. Less common uses are for evaluation of biliary dyskinesia and sphincter of Oddi dysfunction.

Radiopharmaceuticals

A number of ^{99m}Tc–iminodiacetic acid (IDA) analogs are available, providing excellent quality routine imaging of the biliary system. The IDA imaging agents have strong chelating properties and therefore bind readily to ^{99m}Tc, forming a stable complex. In general, increasing the length of the alkyl chain substituted on the benzene ring of IDA increases the biliary excretion of the radiopharmaceutical and reduces renal clearance. This added biliary excretion can be of great value in imaging patients with elevated bilirubin levels.

Perhaps the most widely used IDA compound is diisopropyl IDA (DISIDA; disofenin or Hepatolite), which with its longer substituted chain allows for increased biliary excretion and visualization of the hepatobiliary system at serum bilirubin levels approaching 20 mg/dL. Mebrofenin (trimethyl-bromo IDA or Choletec) is also used and can demonstrate biliary visualization with bilirubin levels up to 30 to 40 mg/dL. Although biliary duct visualization with these agents can occur at high bilirubin levels, visualization of the gallbladder is not ensured. Persistent visualization of the cardiac blood pool after 5 to 10 minutes and renal excretion are signs of hepatic dysfunction. The radiopharmaceutical is normally rapidly removed from the circulation by active transport into the hepatocytes and secreted into the bile canaliculi and then into the biliary radicles, bile duct, gallbladder, and small intestine. In contrast to bilirubin, the IDA is excreted without being conjugated. Hepatic uptake is normally about 90% for disofenin and 98% for mebrofenin. The half-time of liver clearance for both agents is 15 to 20 minutes.

Technique

For elective studies, patients are given nothing by mouth beginning at midnight the night before the examination. In patients with acute disease, a minimum of 2 hours' fasting is suggested. Fortunately, in emergency patients with suspected acute cholecystitis, fasting has generally been self-imposed. In patients whose gallbladders are being stimulated by the presence of food in the upper GI tract, the intermittent contraction of the gallbladder interferes with biliary filling and therefore may render a false-positive study. In 65% of patients who have eaten 2 to 5 hours before the study, the gallbladder will not be visualized in the first 60 minutes of the study. In addition, prolonged fasting in some patients has been implicated as a source of false-positive examinations, because a gallbladder distended with bile may not be able to accept IDA excreted by the liver in order to visualize the gallbladder.

Subsequent to the intravenous injection of 3 to 10 mCi (111 to 370 MBq) of ^{99m}Tc-labeled IDA, sequential anterior gamma camera images of the abdomen are obtained with the patient in the supine position. Images of 500- to 1000-k counts are obtained at 5-minute intervals for the first half-hour of the study. Similar images are then obtained at 10-minute intervals. Continuous, dynamic imaging may also be used. Normally, the gallbladder is visualized within the first half-hour of the study, as are the common bile duct and duodenum (Fig. 8–16). If these structures are not identified at 1 hour, delayed images should be obtained hourly for up to 4 hours after injection, or as discussed below, intravenous morphine may be used to shorten the examination.

In jaundiced patients with increased renal excretion of the radiopharmaceutical, a right extrarenal pelvis may be confused with gallbladder activity (Fig. 8–17). This activity may be differentiated from gallbladder activity by obtaining a right lateral image, on which the characteristic anterior abdominal location of the gallbladder can be identified. At times, the gallbladder activity may be obscured by activity collecting in the adjacent duodenal loop,

or on delayed images, in the transverse colon. In the case of duodenal activity, an additional view in the left anterior oblique or right lateral position can be used to distinguish the two structures. If this fails to provide the answer, the patient may drink water to clear the duodenum of activity.

Normal Scan

In the normal patient, sufficient ^{99m}Tc-IDA is present in the liver in 5 minutes to allow good visualization of that organ. If for any reason additional views of the liver are sought, they should be obtained in the first 10 or 15 minutes of the examination. After this time, there is progressive clearance of the radiopharmaceutical from the liver, and it becomes less apparent. As the radiopharmaceutical is excreted into the biliary tree, the major hepatic ducts and common duct are visualized first. Next, the gallbladder is filled as labeled bile flows through the cystic duct. About two thirds of biliary flow bypasses the gallbladder and enters the duodenum, and about one third enters the gallbladder. The amount and timing of entry into the gallbladder depends on a number of factors, including the nutritional state of the patient, administration of various drugs, and the tone in the sphincter of Oddi. In the presence of a patent common duct, activity flows promptly into the duodenal sweep and proximal small bowel. Normally, visualization of these structures is complete by 1 hour. Occasionally, a small amount of bile reflux into the stomach can be seen as a normal variant, but it should not be a large amount or persistent.

Clinical Settings

Acute Cholecystitis

Hepatobiliary imaging has proved to be of greatest value in the diagnosis of acute cholecystitis. More than 95% of patients with acute cholecystitis have cystic duct obstruction. In this group of patients, radiopharmaceuticals excreted into the bile by the liver cannot enter an inflamed gallbladder through the obstructed cystic duct. This fact provides the theoretical basis for using ^{99m}Tc hepatobiliary agents to diagnose the disease.

In the proper clinical setting, the diagnosis of acute (calculous or acalculous) cholecystitis in a fasting patient may be reliably made in the presence of normal hepatic uptake and excretion of the radiopharmaceutical through the common duct, but without visualization of the gallbladder over a period of 4 hours after injection (Fig. 8–18). In

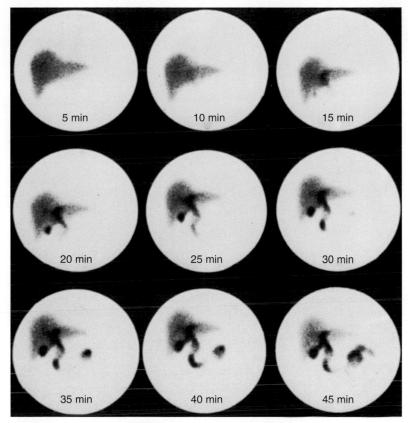

FIGURE 8–16. Normal technetium-99m diisopropyl iminodiacetic acid hepatobiliary scan. Activity is seen within the gallbladder and common bile duct by 20 minutes. The small-bowel activity is clearly identified at 35 minutes.

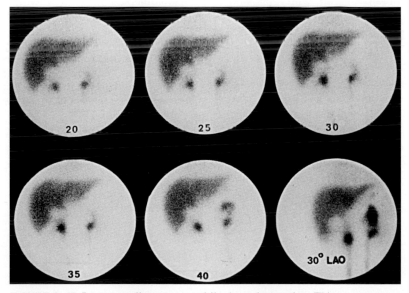

FIGURE 8–17. Long-standing common bile duct obstruction. This scan was performed with technetium-99m diisopropyl iminodiacetic acid. A significant amount of renal excretion but no hepatic excretion is noted.

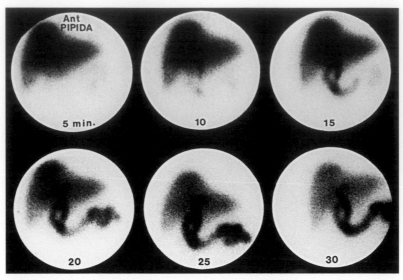

FIGURE 8–18. Acute cholecystitis. There is activity in the small bowel and common duct at 15 minutes on this technetium-99m hepatobiliary scan as well as some reflux into the proximal duodenum. This study was continued for 4 hours, with no visualization of the gallbladder.

several large series, accuracy of cholescintigraphy for diagnosis of acute calculous cholecystitis has been greater than 95% and the accuracy for acute acalculous cholecystitis is only slightly less. In addition, this imaging modality is usually unaffected by modest levels of jaundice. The accuracy of ultrasound for detection of acute cholecystitis is only about 80% to 85%, even if liberal criteria are used. A normal hepatobiliary scan with gallbladder visualization almost always excludes a diagnosis of acute cholecystitis.

Occasionally, the gallbladder may not be seen in a patient with chronic cholecystitis, but this is uncommon. Usually, the gallbladder is visualized within 4 hours after injection. Visualization of the gallbladder during this period effectively excludes the diagnosis of acute gallbladder disease. Thus, it is essential that this delayed sequence of images be a routine part of IDA imaging for acute cholecystitis. As discussed later, use of morphine may be used to shorten the study. Table 8–9 lists some sources of error in IDA scan interpretation when a diagnosis of acute cholecystitis is being considered.

The *rim sign* has been described in patients with acute cholecystitis. This has also been called the *pericholecystic hepatic activity sign*, and it refers to a curvilinear band of increased activity along the right inferior hepatic edge above the gallbladder fossa (Fig. 8–19). This sign is seen in about 20% of patients whose gallbladders are not visualized on hepatobiliary scans. The rim sign is important because about 40% of such patients have either a perforated or a gangrenous gallbladder, and 70% to 85% have acute cholecystitis. The mechanism involved in production of the rim sign is uncertain. It may be the result of inflammation causing regional hepatic hyperemia, with more radiophar-

TABLE 8–9.	Interpretative Difficulties in Diagnosis of Acute Cholecystitis by Hepatobiliary Scan

FALSE-POSITIVE
Recent meal within 4 h of imaging
Total parenteral nutrition
Alcoholism
Pancreatitis (some cases)
Chronic cholecystitis
Hepatocellular dysfunction
Cholangiocarcinoma of cystic duct
Prolonged fasting for 24 h or hyperalimentation
Severe intercurrent illness

FALSE-NEGATIVE
Acalculous cholecystitis
Duodenal diverticulum simulating gallbladder
Accessory cystic duct
Biliary duplication cyst

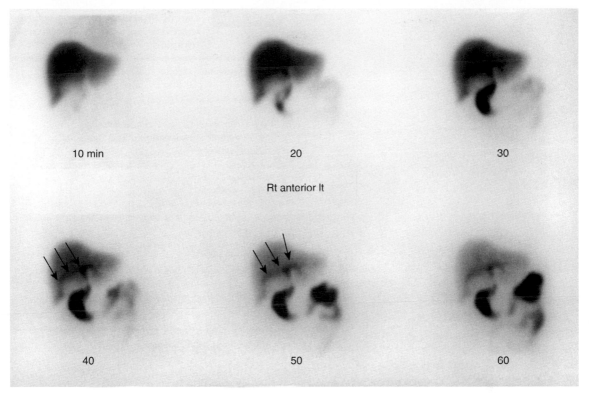

FIGURE 8–19. Rim sign of acute cholecystitis. A rim of increased activity outlining the gallbladder fossa is seen at the inferior edge of the right lobe of the liver (*arrows*).

maceutical being delivered to this area of hepatic parenchyma; or it may be caused by edema causing localized delayed biliary excretion; or both.

The *cystic duct sign* has also been described in acute cholecystitis (Fig. 8–20). This is seen as a small nubbin of activity in the cystic duct proximal to the site of obstruction. It is usually seen between the common hepatic duct and the gallbladder fossa.

Various pharmacologic adjuncts have been suggested to increase the sensitivity of hepatobiliary imaging in the evaluation of patients for acute cholecystitis (Table 8–10). The sensitivity of the hepatobiliary scan may be increased by emptying the gallbladder before the administration of the radiopharmaceutical; this, theoretically, reduces the false-positive rate of the test in patients with chronic cholecystitis, viscous bile, parenteral nutrition, or prolonged fasting. Initially, fatty meals were used, but these proved variable in their ability to produce gallbladder contraction. Consequently, a synthetic octapeptide of cholecystokinin (CCK-8, or sincalide, Kinevac) can be used. This causes gallbladder contraction, relaxation of the sphincter of

Oddi, and increased bile secretion and bowel motility. In normal patients, there is prompt gallbladder contraction, reaching a maximum effect at 5 to 15 minutes after slow (over 5 to 10 minutes) intravenous administration of sincalide. The standard dose is 0.02 to 0.04 μg/kg in 10 mL of saline. Intravenous bolus administration should be avoided because it produces abdominal discomfort and less complete gallbladder emptying, due to inducement of gallbladder neck spasm.

Although these maneuvers may reduce the false-positive rate, such premedication may potentially obscure the diagnosis of chronic cholecystitis by speeding up the visualization of the gallbladder in patients who would otherwise present with delayed visualization. Further, delayed biliary to bowel transit occurs in half the patients given sincalide before cholescintigraphy, which raises a question of partial common duct obstruction. These problems may be obviated by reserving the administration of CCK or sincalide until failure to visualize the gallbladder at 30 to 60 minutes is demonstrated. At this time, intravenous CCK can be administered, fol-

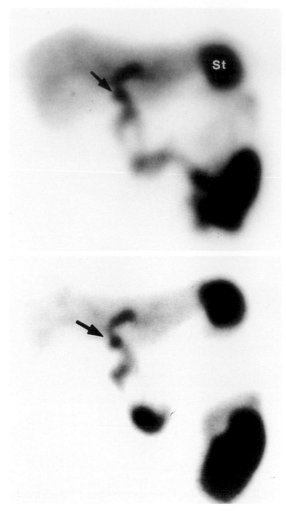

FIGURE 8–20. Cystic duct sign. In this patient with right upper quadrant pain, 30- and 60-minute images (*top* and *bottom*) from a technetium-99m hepatobiliary scan show activity in the liver, hepatic ducts, and common bile duct. The gallbladder is not seen, but there is a small focus of activity adjacent to the common duct (*arrow*), which represents activity in the portion of the cystic duct proximal to the obstruction. Incidental note is made of a large amount of bile reflux into the stomach (St).

TABLE 8–10.	Use of Pharmacologic Intervention with Hepatobiliary Imaging

Cholecystokinin (sincalide)
    0.02–0.04 μg/kg slow IV infusion
    Empty the gallbladder in a patient fasting >24 h
      before DISIDA scan
    Evaluate sphincter of Oddi dyskinesia
    Differentiate functional from anatomic duct
      obstruction
    Calculate gallbladder ejection fraction
Morphine
    0.04 mg/kg IV
    Use to shorten the imaging time when gallbladder is
      not visualized at 1 h and sufficient activity is still in
      hepatobiliary tree
    Use advisedly in patients with cystic duct sign
Phenobarbital
    5 mg/kg/day orally for 5–7 days before examination
    Use to prime hepatic enzymes to increase IDA
      excretion in distinguishing between biliary atresia
      and neonatal hepatitis

DISIDA, diisopropyl iminodiacetic acid; IDA, iminodiacetic acid.

lowed 15 to 30 minutes later by reinjection of the IDA radiopharmaceutical.

Intravenous morphine is commonly used to improve the diagnostic accuracy of hepatobiliary scanning. Morphine causes increased tone in smooth muscle and decreases peristalsis. Because morphine causes constriction of the sphincter of Oddi, there is a rise in intraductal pressure in the common duct by 60%, producing increased flow of the radiopharmaceutical into the gallbladder. Thus, if after passage of the radiopharmaceutical into the common duct and small bowel there is no gallbladder visualization, intravenous morphine can be administered. The typical dose is 0.04 mg/kg diluted in 10 mL of saline and administered over 2 to 5 minutes. This is usually well tolerated by patients, without significant aggravation of symptoms. If there is enough residual radiopharmaceutical in the liver and if the cystic duct is patent, the gallbladder usually fills in 5 to 10 minutes (Fig. 8–21). Peak effect is in about 5 minutes. If there is not enough activity remaining in the liver and common duct, it is best to first reinject the patient with more hepatobiliary agent and then to administer morphine 15 to 20 minutes later. Nonvisualization of the gallbladder 30 minutes after morphine administration has the same implication as lack of visualization on 4-hour images and indicates acute cholecystitis. Morphine should be used advisedly if a cystic duct sign is present because the back pressure may force activity past the cystic duct obstruction into the gallbladder. This nonphysiologic maneuver may convert a true-positive result into a false-negative result. Further, after morphine administration, CCK should not be used because it induces gallbladder contraction against a contracted sphincter of Oddi, increasing patient discomfort.

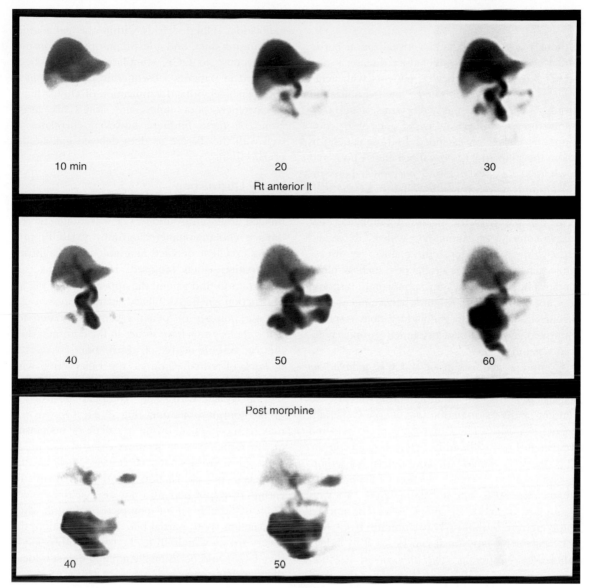

FIGURE 8–21. Morphine augmentation. In this technetium-99m hepatobiliary scan, the gallbladder is not visualized by 60 minutes, indicating either acute or chronic cholecystitis. Rather than wait 4 hours for a delayed image, morphine was given. Even 50 minutes after morphine administration, the gallbladder was not seen, indicating acute cholecystitis.

Chronic Cholecystitis

Although delayed gallbladder visualization corre-lates well with chronic gallbladder disease, it also occurs in a small number of patients with acute cholecystitis. Thus, although late visualization strongly suggests chronic cholecystitis, acute acal-culous disease with partial cystic duct obstruction cannot be completely excluded. In those patients in whom the gallbladder is visualized after 1 hour and in whom acute disease is strongly suspected on clin-ical grounds, the contractile response of the gall-bladder to administered CCK may provide a clue to the true nature of the disease. A gallbladder that fails to contract on stimulation with CCK should be held in suspicion for acute gallbladder disease until excluded by other modalities, such as ultra-sonography. However, an abnormal response does not definitively distinguish between acute and chronic disease. If the gallbladder does respond, continued investigation of presumed chronic chole-cystitis is indicated.

Computer acquisition of a CCK gallbladder stimulation study allows calculation of a gallblad-der ejection fraction obtained over the first 30 minutes of the examination (Fig. 8–22). Generally, ejection fractions of less than 35% are considered abnormal (Fig. 8–23), and ejection fractions in the 35% to 50% range are considered borderline. Unequivocally normal ejection fractions are greater than 50%. The normal mean is 75% with a standard deviation of about 20%. The normal emptying rate is about 6% per minute. If CCK is not available, a fatty meal can be used to induce gallbladder emptying, but the mean ejection fraction is lower (≈ 50% with a standard deviation of 20%) and the emptying rate is slower (≈2% per minute). An abnormal ejection fraction can be used, along with clinical information, to suggest the presence of gallbladder dysfunction. A reduced ejection fraction is suggestive, but not specific for either acute or chronic cholecystitis.

Aside from delayed gallbladder visualization, several other scintigraphic patterns demonstrate correlation with the diagnosis of chronic chole-cystitis. Delayed biliary-to-bowel transit time in the presence of normal gallbladder and common duct visualization has been reported in chronic gallbladder disease. In addition, the longer that intestinal visualization is delayed, the more likely is a diagnosis of chronic cholecystitis; however, this finding alone is by no means diagnostic.

Finally, poor but definite visualization of the gallbladder, filling defects within the gallbladder or common duct, and a less-than-optimal contrac-tile response to CCK stimulation have all been reported in patients subsequently proved to have chronic cholecystitis. Identification of cholelithiasis is extremely poor unless the stones are large. None of these findings, however, correlates as well with the disease as does delayed gallbladder visualization.

Biliary Obstruction

Suspected biliary obstruction is usually first imaged using ultrasound or CT with magnetic res-onance cholangiopancreatography (MRCP) pro-viding excellent detailed anatomic and diagnostic information when required. However, it is still important to understand the appearance of biliary obstruction on hepatobiliary scans because a sig-nificant number of patients being evaluated for acute cholecystitis have stones in the common duct that cause some degree of obstruction.

Lack of visualization of the biliary tree with good visualization of the liver (the so-called *liver scan sign*) is typical with acute complete obstruction of the common bile duct (Fig. 8–24). Obstruction may be mechanical, owing to calculi or neoplasm, or functional, as seen in some cases of ascending cholangitis. Intrahepatic cholestasis, such as that produced by obstruction of the canaliculi by certain drugs, or hepatitis may also yield a pattern indistinguishable from complete common duct obstruction. With partial bile duct obstruction, the biliary tree is visualized to the level of obstruction (Fig. 8–25), and occasionally a filling defect is iden-tified at that point.

All of these patterns depend on good hepatocyte function. In the past, severe hepatocellular dis-ease or dysfunction precluded a diagnostic study because insufficient excretion of the radiopharma-ceutical into the major biliary ducts rendered it impossible to distinguish between nonvisualization of the ducts secondary to primary liver disease and high-grade obstruction of the common duct. The use of longer-chain IDA analogs that allow good hepatic concentration and excretion, even in the presence of marked jaundice, has made this diag-nostic problem considerably less frequent.

The sequence of events occurring after acute complete distal biliary obstruction is as follows: 0 to 24 hours, hepatocyte function is normal and there is good hepatic and bile duct visualization (ultra-

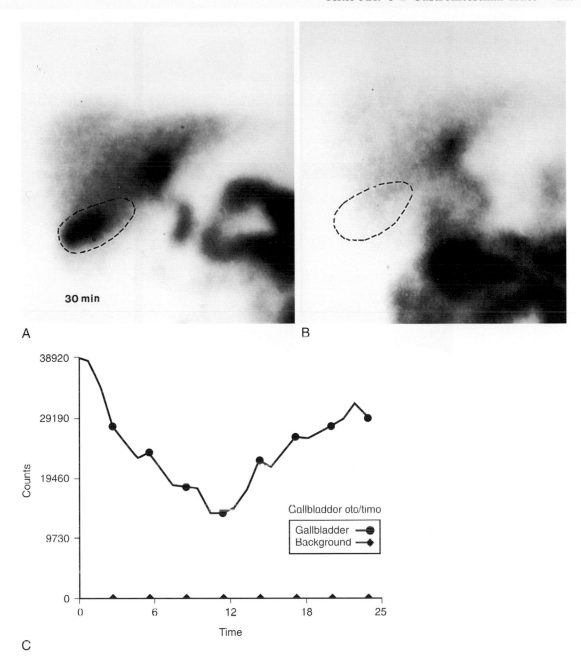

FIGURE 8–22. Normal gallbladder response to cholecystokinin (CCK). *A,* An anterior hepatobiliary image at 30 minutes after injection of technetium-99m diisopropyl iminodiacetic acid shows the gallbladder and a selected region of interest around the gallbladder. *B,* Another image taken 12 minutes after intravenous CCK administration shows almost complete emptying of the gallbladder. *C,* The time-activity curve is derived from the region of interest. The gallbladder ejection fraction is about 70%, which is clearly normal.

sound at this time is normal); 24 to 96 hours, mild to moderate reduction in hepatic and bile duct visualization (ultrasound shows enlargement of the common bile and hepatic ducts); and after 96 hours, prolonged cardiac blood pool activity and poor hepatic uptake, with no activity in bile ducts or gallbladder (ultrasound shows beginning dilatation of intrahepatic ducts). In all of these events, there is no visualization of intestinal activity unless there is only partial obstruction. In the late stage

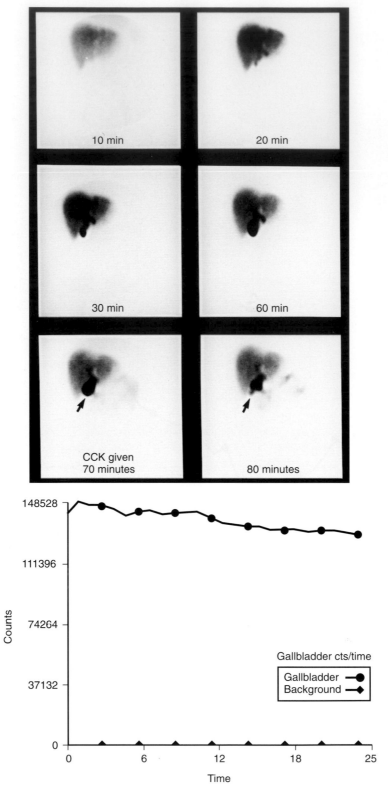

FIGURE 8–23. Abnormal gallbladder response to cholecystokinin (CCK). *Top,* Multiple images from a technetium-99m hepatobiliary scan show activity in the gallbladder by 30 minutes but no activity in bowel at 60 minutes (delayed biliary to bowel transit). After administration of CCK, the gallbladder (*arrow*) contracts minimally, and some activity is seen in the bowel at 80 minutes. *Bottom,* The gallbladder time-activity curve shows poor response to the CCK. This suggests a functional abnormality, which may be due to a number of causes, including gallbladder dyskinesia, chronic acalculous cholecystitis, cystic duct syndrome, common duct stones, stricture, or dyskinesia of the sphincter of Oddi.

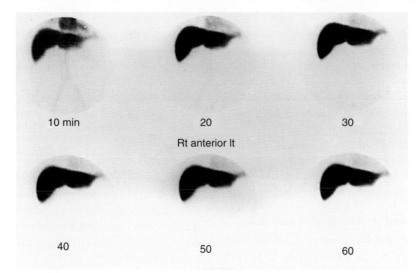

FIGURE 8–24. Liver scan sign. Anterior sequential technetium-99m (^{99m}Tc) hepatobiliary images show the liver but no biliary system or bowel activity. There is constantly increasing activity in the liver throughout the study. Also note that there is activity seen above the liver in the heart for at least 30 minutes. This blood pool activity normally should be cleared by 5 to 10 minutes. This is called the *liver scan sign* because it looks like a ^{99m}Tc colloid liver–spleen scan without the spleen. Acute high-grade common duct obstruction is the prime consideration in such cases.

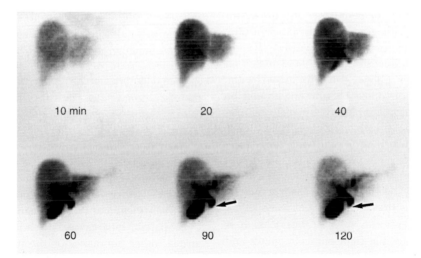

FIGURE 8–25. Partial distal common duct obstruction. The sequential images from this technetium-99m hepatobiliary scan show that the liver accumulates activity slower than normal but that there is some hepatic clearance by 120 minutes. The gallbladder and common duct are clearly seen up to the point of obstruction (*arrow*). The obstruction could have been caused by a common duct stone, tumor, or sphincter of Oddi dyskinesia, but in this case it was purely functional and iatrogenic. The referring physician had given the patient morphine for pain relief before performing the study, constricting the sphincter of Oddi and producing a false-positive scan.

(after 96 hours), differentiation of obstruction from hepatitis can be difficult or impossible without the use of ultrasound.

Partial duct obstruction is suggested by persistent visualization of the common duct or delayed clearance of activity from the duct. Delayed appearance (>60 minutes) of activity in the duodenum and small bowel is nonspecific and can occur in 20% to 25% of normal people. Partial obstruction can be caused by a common duct stone, benign or malignant stricture, or sphincter of Oddi dysfunction with elevated sphincter pressure.

Post-traumatic and Postsurgical Biliary Scans

The confirmation and localization of biliary leaks after abdominal surgery or trauma using ^{99m}Tc-IDA agents may lead to early detection and correction of the problem. This technique presents several advantages and overcomes several of the disadvantages of using conventional radiographic methods for the evaluation of suspected biliary fistula.

Hepatobiliary scintigraphy has also proved useful in the postcholecystectomy patient by allowing the identification of persistent cystic duct remnants and biliary leaks (Fig. 8–26) and the assessment of biliary patency. In attempting to detect a remnant of the cystic duct, it is important to obtain delayed images to permit sufficient time for such a structure to be visualized. Rarely, retained common duct stones may be identified on the IDA scan as photon-deficient areas in the visualized common duct. This finding should be followed by ultrasonography, although stones may be missed in the presence of a normal-caliber common bile duct. Finally, the functional significance of a dilated common duct on ultrasound after gallbladder surgery may be clarified with cholescintigraphy by determining the patency or obstruction of the duct.

When imaging for a possible bile leak, it is important to image the right paracolic gutter and to obtain pelvic images to look for subtle leaks which may accumulate in the pelvis. Often, postsurgical bile leaks may cause accumulation of labeled bile in the gallbladder fossa, producing a biloma that may mimic gallbladder visualization. Labeled bile may also track superiorly in the perihepatic spaces, coating the liver surface. When this occurs, it may give the appearance of paradoxically increasing activity in the liver after the liver has largely emptied of activity, producing the *reappearing liver sign*. It may also give the appearance of an alteration of liver shape compared to initial images.

On occasion, cholescintigraphy may be used to investigate surgically altered biliary and GI anatomy or stent patency evaluation by providing appropriate functional information. As with all postsurgical studies, it is important to obtain a precise understanding of the type of surgical procedure performed and the postsurgical anatomy before proceeding with the examination.

Biliary Atresia and Neonatal Hepatitis

Radionuclide techniques have traditionally been used to differentiate between biliary atresia and neonatal hepatitis in the jaundiced infant. Because the successful surgical treatment of biliary atresia depends greatly on early intervention, prompt diagnosis is essential. Frequently, the diagnosis cannot be made on clinical, laboratory, or even needle biopsy grounds, and cholescintigraphy may provide the only clue to the proper diagnosis.

Imaging with ^{99m}Tc-IDA analogs has been used to exclude a diagnosis of biliary atresia by demonstrating patent extrahepatic biliary systems in jaundiced neonates (Fig. 8–27). In the absence of visualization of the biliary tree, however, atresia may not be successfully differentiated from severe hepatocellular disease produced by neonatal hepatitis (Fig. 8–28). Thus, every effort should be made to permit visualization of the biliary tree, including delayed imaging at 24 hours. The relatively short physical half-life of ^{99m}Tc is disadvantageous in that imaging beyond 24 hours is not practical, and therefore, biliary flow into the small bowel more than 24 hours after injection may not be detected. There is some evidence that the examination using ^{99m}Tc-IDA analogs is more diagnostic when the liver is primed first with 5 to 7 days of phenobarbital therapy, 2.5 mg/kg orally twice a day, which stimulates better hepatic excretion of the radiopharmaceutical and therefore earlier identification of a patent biliary tree. In addition to biliary atresia, other anomalies of the biliary tract, such as choledochal cysts and Caroli's disease, have been identified successfully by using ^{99m}Tc-IDA imaging.

GASTROESOPHAGEAL FUNCTION STUDIES

Radionuclide techniques provide a convenient, noninvasive, and direct method to assess GI motility. By using imaging and computer-assisted quantitation, numerous physiologic parameters of upper GI function may be evaluated. These include (1)

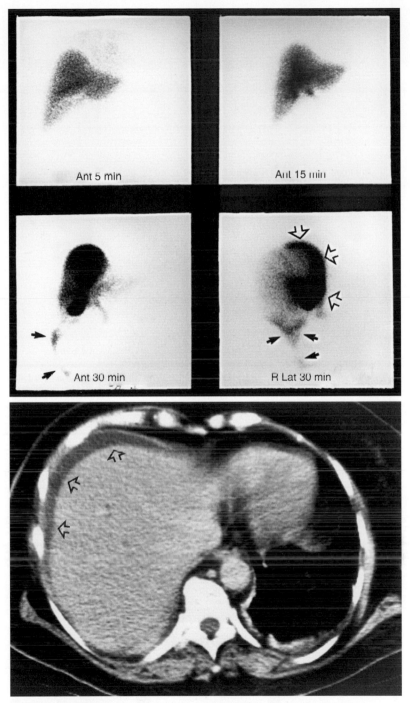

FIGURE 8–26. Bile leak. *Top,* Sequential images from a hepatobiliary scan show increasing perihepatic activity by 30 minutes that no longer conforms to the shape of the liver that was seen at 5 or 15 minutes. Also, activity has tracked inferiorly in the right pericolic gutter (*small arrows*). Most of the activity on the 30-minute images is along the anterior surface of the liver (*open arrows*). *Bottom,* Fluid (*arrows*) is also seen anterior and lateral to the liver on the computed tomography scan.

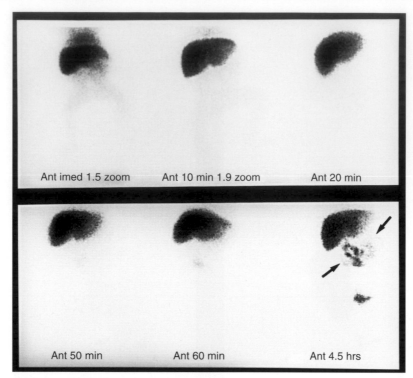

FIGURE 8–27. Neonatal hepatitis. Sequential images from a technetium-99m hepatobiliary scan in this 2-week-old, jaundiced infant show only liver activity on the initial images; however, on the 4.5-hour image, activity is seen in the bowel of the central abdomen (*arrows*), indicating a patent biliary system. This finding excludes a diagnosis of biliary atresia.

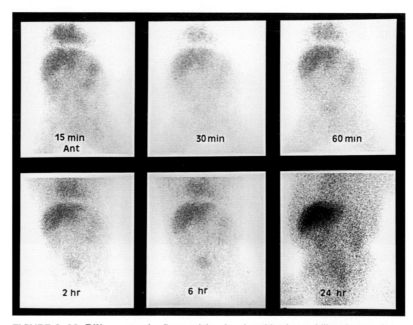

FIGURE 8–28. Biliary atresia. Sequential technetium-99m hepatobiliary images show markedly delayed clearance of radiopharmaceutical from the blood pool (heart) and poor concentration by the liver, even at 6 hours. The 24-hour image shows a great deal of residual liver and soft-tissue activity, with some excretion by the kidneys but no evidence of biliary or bowel activity. The resultant bladder activity must be distinguished from bowel activity and catheterization may be helpful.

esophageal transit, (2) the detection and quantitation of gastroesophageal and enterogastric reflux, and (3) gastric emptying rates.

Esophageal Transit

Scintigraphic methods are useful to quantitate esophageal transit. Several methods are used, and most of these use an orally administered liquid bolus and measure the time to esophageal clearance. Although the scintigraphic study is useful as a quantitative measure, it has limited anatomic resolution and therefore is not a replacement for a barium esophagram. The initial evaluation of a patient with esophageal symptoms should include a barium study.

Radiopharmaceuticals

A number of radiopharmaceuticals can be used with success; however, ^{99m}Tc-sulfur colloid is used most often. It has the advantages of being readily available, nonabsorbable, and inexpensive. The radiation absorbed dose from this procedure is about 20 mrad (0.2 mGy), compared with several rads for a barium esophagram.

Technique

The patient should fast for at least 6 hours before the procedure. The patient is placed supine under a gamma camera, with the field of view including the entire esophagus and proximal stomach. The supine view negates the effects of gravity. An upright view may be better to assess results of therapy in abnormalities such as achalasia and scleroderma. The patient is instructed to swallow 300 μCi (11.1 MBq) of ^{99m}Tc-sulfur or albumin colloid in 10 mL of water at the same time that acquisition by the camera and computer is begun. The patient then "dry" swallows every 15 seconds for 5 minutes. Because there may be variability between swallows, many laboratories repeat the procedure up to five times. After the acquisition is complete, regions of interest are outlined on the computer image to generate time-activity curves. A global esophageal region is used with optional divisions of the esophagus into thirds, with each as an additional region of interest. The global esophageal emptying time measures the time from the appearance of the radionuclide bolus in the proximal esophagus to the clearance of more than 90% from the entire esophagus. The esophageal transit time consists of the time interval between peak activity in the time activity curve from the proximal third of the esophagus and the peak in the distal third of the esophagus.

Normal and Abnormal Studies

In normal persons, esophageal transit time for water is 5 to 11 seconds, and at least 90% of the activity should have traversed the esophagus globally by the end of 15 seconds. In patients with scleroderma and achalasia, transit may be reduced to levels as low as 20% to 40%. Patients with various other motor disorders of the esophagus usually have intermediate values.

Gastroesophageal Reflux

In patients with symptoms of heartburn, regurgitation, or bilious vomiting, computer-assisted scintigraphic studies provide a sensitive and useful method for reflux determination and quantitation. Alternative methods are limited in usefulness. Fluoroscopic barium studies are not sensitive and depend on the expertise and persistence of the fluoroscopist. Acid-reflux testing is the standard that is used for comparison but requires intubation. Esophageal manometry is sometimes used, but it also requires intubation to measure the decreased resistance of the lower esophageal sphincter in cases of reflux.

Radiopharmaceuticals and Technique

Technetium-99m colloids are the radiopharmaceuticals of choice. The procedure calls for the oral administration of 300 μCi (11.1 MBq) of ^{99m}Tc sulfur colloid in 150 mL of orange juice combined with 150 mL of 0.1 normal hydrochloric acid. The patient should fast overnight or for at least 2 hours after a liquid meal. An abdominal binder is placed around the upper abdomen. While in a sitting position, the patient drinks the 300 mL of solution, and after 30 seconds, a single image is obtained to see that all the liquid is in the stomach. An additional 30 mL of water is then given to rinse residual activity from the esophagus. The patient is placed under the gamma camera in the supine position with a field of view that includes the esophagus and stomach. Serial 30-second images are then obtained with the abdominal binder at 0, 20, 40, 60, 80, and 100 mmHg. In this method, position, pressure, and the presence of acid are all used to aggravate reflux. In addition to visual interpretation, regions of interest drawn over the stomach and the esophagus are used to calculate the percentage of gastric radiopharmaceutical refluxing into the esophagus.

A variation of this scintigraphic method using ^{99m}Tc colloid mixed with milk or infant formula may be used to study gastroesophageal reflux and pulmonary aspiration of gastric contents in infants; it is often referred to as a "milk scan." In this case, an abdominal binder is not used, and imaging for reflux is performed in the left anterior oblique position rather than supine. If aspiration is suspected, anterior delayed images are obtained 2 to 4 hours later to look for activity in the lungs. In older children, ^{99m}Tc sulfur colloid, or preferably, indium-111 (^{111}In)–diethylene triamine pentaacetic acid (DTPA), can be administered as a liquid meal at bedtime with imaging performed over the lungs the following morning. The detection of aspiration occurring during esophageal reflux studies is reported to be 0% to 25%.

Normal and Abnormal Studies

By this technique, esophageal reflux is expressed as the percentage of the gastric counts obtained at the beginning of the study (before reflux) that subsequently reflux into the esophagus. The upper limit for gastroesophageal reflux in normal people is 3%. Between 3% and 4% is considered indeterminate, and more than 4% reflux is abnormal (Fig. 8–29). The sensitivity of this study is about 90%; however, if acidified liquid, abdominal binder, and supine position are not used, the sensitivity of the study decreases. The study can be used in the initial diagnosis of reflux as well as in the evaluation of various therapeutic modalities.

Gastric Emptying

Scintigraphic studies of gastric emptying are complicated by the facts that liquid and solid contents empty from the stomach at different rates and a host of factors regulate this process. Liquids empty from the stomach in an exponential fashion, whereas solid foods empty in a more linear manner. Osmolality, pH, volume, caloric content, amount of protein, carbohydrate, fat, weight, time of day, position, drugs, and sex of the patient all affect emptying rate. For example, distention of the stomach accelerates gastric emptying, whereas lipids are potent inhibitors.

Radiopharmaceuticals and Technique

A wide variety of radiopharmaceuticals have been used for evaluation of gastric emptying. Two main classes are used: those for the solid phase and those for the liquid phase. The solid phase may use ^{99m}Tc colloid to label chicken liver, whole eggs, or egg whites. Perhaps the most widely used method is to mix 0.5 to 1 mCi (18.5 to 37 MBq) of ^{99m}Tc sulfur colloid with beaten eggs, which are then cooked as scrambled eggs. If a liquid phase alone is desired for infants, ^{99m}Tc colloid can be given in milk or formula. Under these circumstances, 2.5 to 5.0 μCi (0.09 to 0.18 MBq) is added per milliliter of liquid.

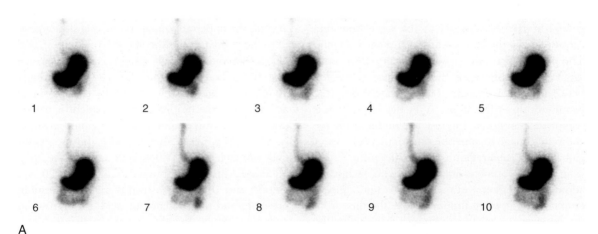

A

FIGURE 8–29. Gastroesophageal reflux. *A,* Anterior view of the chest and upper abdomen shows activity within the stomach; however, sequential views show intermittent activity in the esophagus. *B,* Three regions of interest over the proximal, mid, and distal esophagus allow time activity curves (*C*) to be generated. These show the spikes of refluxed activity in the esophagus.

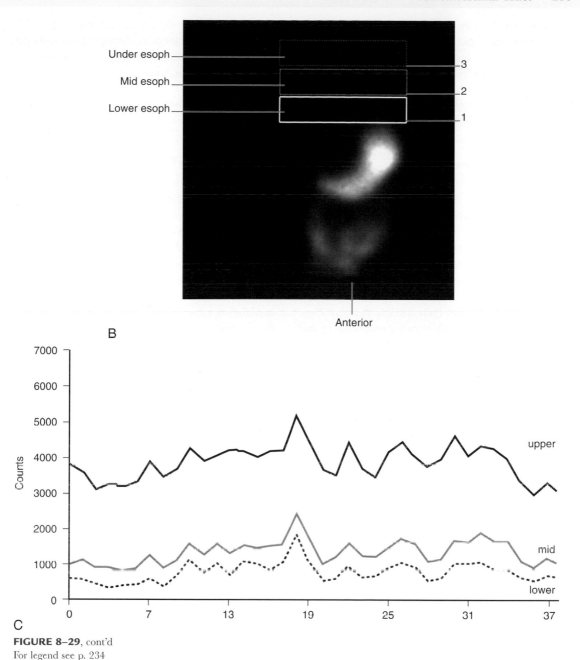

FIGURE 8–29, cont'd
For legend see p. 234

Rarely, a simultaneous liquid-phase study is desired while performing a solid-phase gastric emptying study. This can be accomplished by using another radionuclide, such as ^{111}In-DTPA (125 μCi [4.6 MBq] in 300 mL of water) and performing computer analysis of different photopeaks. Because dual-phase studies add cost and radiation dose, and because the solid phase is more sensitive than is the liquid phase for detection of delayed gastric emptying, usually a solid-phase study is all that is needed.

The patient should consume the radiolabeled solid meal within 10 minutes along with about 150 mL of water. The patient may be imaged in the upright or supine position with images obtained every 5 to 15 minutes or during continuous dynamic acquisition until half of the activity is gone, or for up to 90 minutes. The patient should sit up between the images. Computer acquisition is mandatory, and regions of interest are selected over the stomach and appropriate background areas. Anterior and posterior images can be obtained if one wishes to use the geometric mean value for calculations, although left anterior oblique view acquisition with a single-headed camera is generally satisfactory.

Normal and Abnormal Studies

In most facilities, only a solid-phase study is performed. In normal people, the approximate time for half of the activity (using scrambled eggs) to leave the stomach is 90 (45 to 110) minutes using the technique described in Appendix E–1. A computer time-activity curve is obtained from a region of interest drawn over the stomach. Emptying curves for solid meals typically display a flat initial portion (lag phase) and then a linear portion (Figs. 8–30 and 8–31). The half-time for emptying of the liquid phase is 40 (12 to 65) minutes. The normal half-time reported for infants given milk or formula varies widely in the literature from 25 to 48 minutes with breast milk, to 60 to 90 minutes with formula and bovine milk. Major uses of gastric emptying studies are to confirm gastroparesis as a cause for persistent nausea and vomiting and to monitor the effects of therapy in patients with abnormal gastric motility (Table 8–11), such as diabetic patients. As is the case with esophageal transit studies, the initial workup of a patient with symptoms of gastric outlet obstruction should include a radiographic barium examination rather than a scintigraphic study.

ABDOMINAL SHUNT EVALUATION

Various shunt procedures have been developed that involve the peritoneal cavity. Evaluation of ventriculoperitoneal shunts for relief of hydrocephalus is discussed in Chapter 4. LeVeen shunts are some-times placed for relief of intractable ascites. They drain the peritoneal cavity through a one-way pressure valve into the superior vena cava. In the event of suspected shunt failure, a pulmonary perfusion agent, such as ^{99m}Tc-MAA, can be introduced into the ascites by paracenteses. Subsequent activity in the lung indicates a patent shunt (Fig. 8–32).

SCHILLING TEST

The Schilling test is used to study GI absorption of vitamin B_{12} in the small bowel, which requires the presence of intrinsic factor from the stomach.

The patient usually fasts the night before the examination, and 0.5 mg of cobalt-57 (^{57}Co) vitamin B_{12} containing 0.5 μCi (18.5 kBq) is then given orally. This is immediately followed by an intramuscular injection of about 1000 mg of nonlabeled vitamin B_{12}. This intramuscular injection is given to saturate the liver and blood B_{12}-binding sites and thus to promote urinary excretion of the radiolabeled vitamin B_{12}. A 24-hour urine sample of at least 1 L is then collected and measured for excreted activity, which indicates whether there is significant intestinal absorption of radiolabeled B_{12}. Normal 24-hour values for urinary excretion are in the range of 10% to 40% of the administered dose. Values lower than 7% indicate a significant abnormality compatible with either pernicious anemia (intrinsic factor deficiency) or significant malabsorption problems. To differentiate between the two, a stage 2 Schilling test is needed.

A stage 2 Schilling test may be performed by repeating the test with labeled vitamin B_{12}, but with intrinsic factor also given to see if absorption of B_{12} is improved. If this still reveals low urinary excretion, a malabsorption problem, such as sprue, regional enteritis, or blind loop syndrome, may exist.

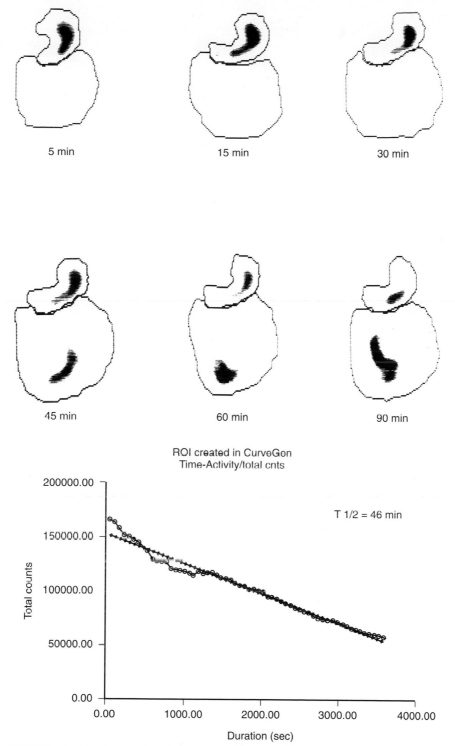

FIGURE 8–30. *Top,* **Normal gastric emptying.** Sequential images are shown with computer regions of interest around the stomach and small bowel. By 45 minutes, about half of the activity is in the stomach and half in the small bowel. By 90 minutes, most of the activity is in the small bowel. *Bottom,* The region of interest around the stomach has been used to generate a time-activity curve and thus calculate the half-time for the radiotracer to leave the stomach.

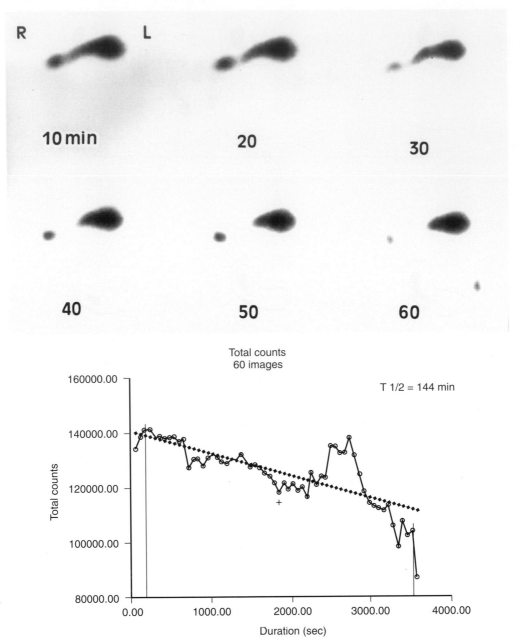

FIGURE 8–31. Delayed gastric emptying. *Top,* Sequential images taken after the patient ingested technetium-99m colloid–labeled scrambled eggs show that almost all of the activity has remained in the stomach at 60 minutes. *Bottom,* A time-activity curve shows a prolonged half-time for gastric emptying of 144 minutes.

TABLE 8–11.	Causes of Abnormal Gastric Emptying

DELAYED
Hyperglycemia
Acidosis
Connective tissue diseases
Ileus
Diabetes mellitus
Gastroesophageal reflux
Vagotomy
Proximal partial gastrectomy
Chronic gastritis
Gastric ulcer disease
Malignancies
Psychiatric disorders
Drugs
Opiates
Antacids
Anticholinergic agents
Tricyclic antidepressants
Cholecystokinin
Gastrin
Progesterone
Calcium-channel blockers
Levodopa

RAPID
Zollinger-Ellison syndrome
Duodenal ulcer disease
Sprue
Pancreatic insufficiency
Distal partial gastrectomy with vagotomy
Drugs
Metoclopramide
Domperidone
Cisapride
Erythromycin
Motilin

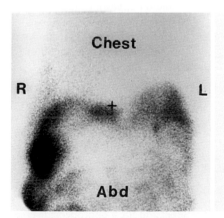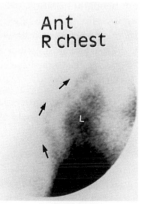

FIGURE 8–32. Patent LeVeen shunt. In this patient with intractable ascites, intraperitoneal injection of technetium-99m macroaggregated albumin allows evaluation of the shunt. *Left,* An initial anterior image of the abdomen shows the activity throughout the peritoneal cavity outlining viscera and bowel. *Right,* An anterior image of the right chest shows the tracer progressing through the shunt (*arrows*) and localizing in the lungs (L).

PEARLS & PITFALLS

Hepatobiliary

The most common indications for a hepatobiliary study are to differentiate between acute or chronic cholecystitis, to look for suspected bile leaks or biliary obstruction, and, in the setting of neonatal jaundice, to differentiate neonatal hepatitis from biliary atresia.

Technetium-99m hepatobiliary (IDA) agents are cleared and excreted by the hepatocytes, but not conjugated.

Cardiac blood pool activity should clear by 5 to 10 minutes. Lack of clearance indicates poorly functioning hepatocytes.

If there is persistent cardiac blood pool activity, poor liver activity, and no biliary excretion, the differential diagnosis includes hepatocellular diseases (hepatitis) and severe biliary obstruction.

If there appears to be only liver activity on sequential images and no cardiac, biliary, or bowel activity, this may be the liver scan sign of complete biliary obstruction, although this sign is not specific.

Renal and bladder activity may be seen if the liver cannot efficiently excrete the radiopharmaceutical.

Bowel activity should be seen by 1 hour. Delayed biliary-to-bowel transit can be the result of a number of entities, including common duct calculus, tumor, stricture, morphine, sphincter dyskinesia, or chronic cholecystitis.

For hepatobiliary scans performed to differentiate biliary atresia from neonatal hepatitis, delayed 24-hour images to look for evidence of excretion into the bowel are often necessary. If bowel activity is present, biliary atresia is excluded. If no bowel activity is seen, the child may have either severe hepatitis or biliary atresia.

The normal gallbladder with a patent cystic duct is usually seen by 30 minutes and should almost always be seen by 1 hour.

Gallbladder activity can be confused with duodenal activity. To differentiate between these, either have the patient drink water and repeat the image or use a right lateral view and a left anterior oblique view (the gallbladder is anterior).

Nonvisualization of the gallbladder is most likely the result of acute or, less often, chronic cholecystitis. Always determine whether the patient has had a cholecystectomy before interpreting the study.

Nonvisualization of the gallbladder at 4 hours or after administration of morphine at 1 hour is most likely due to acute cholecystitis.

Nonvisualization of the gallbladder at 1 hour but visualization at 4 hours or after morphine administration is most likely due to chronic cholecystitis.

Look for either the rim sign or cystic duct sign of acute cholecystitis if the gallbladder is not seen by 1 hour. A rim sign increases the likelihood of complicated cholecystitis (gangrene, abscess, or rupture).

Bile leaks often pool in the region of the porta hepatitis, along the right lateral aspect of the liver, in the right pericolic gutter, and in the lower pelvis. If the gallbladder was recently removed, the bile may pool in the gallbladder fossa and mimic a gallbladder.

Subtle bile leaks are often identified by comparing the shape and intensity of the liver on the first image to its apparent shape on the delayed views. When the liver appears to change shape or grow more intense owing to perihepatic accumulation of radiolabeled bile, a bile leak is likely.

An unequivocally normal gallbladder ejection fraction after CCK is more than 50%. Values of 35–50% are borderline. Values below 35% are abnormal.

Colloid Liver–Spleen Imaging

Common indications are for evaluation of hepatocellular disease (cirrhosis), hepatomegaly, splenomegaly, and focal abnormalities in the liver or spleen seen on ultrasound or CT.

These studies are performed with ^{99m}Tc sulfur colloid. On the posterior view, the spleen should be equal to or less intense than the liver. With colloid shift, usually indicative of hepatocellular disease, the bone marrow is easily visualized, and increased splenic activity relative to the liver is seen.

If there is colloid shift, look for ascites (a space between the ribs and the lateral right lobe of the liver) and for a photopenic liver lesion that may represent a hepatoma.

Photopenic lesions in the liver can be due to anything that does not have reticuloendothelial activity (cyst, hematoma, abscess, fatty

PEARLS & PITFALLS—cont'd

infiltration, hepatic adenoma, hepatoma, metastasis). Cold splenic lesions are usually infarct, tumor, or cyst.

If there is a photopenic lesion, make sure that it triangulates in the same place in the organ on all images; otherwise, it may be due to an artifact (such as barium in the colon or a bad photomultiplier tube).

Focal nodular hyperplasia can accumulate ^{99m}Tc sulfur colloid, but hepatic adenomas and other tumors do not.

Focal hot lesions in the liver are often the result of focal nodular hyperplasia, regenerating nodule in cirrhosis, or flow abnormalities. Collateral flow can deliver radiopharmaceutical to a specific portion of the liver. A hot area in porta hepatis region (quadrate lobe) suggests superior vena caval obstruction, and a hot caudate lobe suggests Budd-Chiari syndrome.

Meckel's Diverticulum Imaging

These scans are performed with ^{99m}Tc-pertechnetate, which concentrates in normal and ectopic gastric mucosa.

Most Meckel's diverticula do not contain ectopic gastric mucosa, but the ones that bleed almost always do.

Look for a focus of activity in the mid-abdomen or right lower quadrant. It should increase in activity similar to the stomach mucosa and should remain in a fixed spot.

A Meckel's diverticulum should be seen anteriorly on lateral or oblique views.

Cimetidine can be used to fix the radiopharmaceutical, and pentagastrin can increase the uptake in the gastric mucosa, thus increasing the sensitivity of the study.

Bladder activity from the ^{99m}Tc-pertechnetate is normal. The patient may need to void or be catheterized if there is a suspicious lesion nearby.

Gastrointestinal Bleeding Studies

Usually these are performed with ^{99m}Tc-labeled red blood cells, but ^{99m}Tc sulfur colloid can also be used.

A focus of bleeding should change shape and location on sequential images. If the activity does not move, it may represent a vascular abnormality, such as an aneurysm, or an intussusception.

The best way to pinpoint the bleeding site is to find an image in which there is a definite abnormality and then to look at the earlier images and find the first image in which the activity can be seen. This is necessary because activity seen as a result of bleeding can go both antegrade and retrograde in the bowel.

Bladder activity from free ^{99m}Tc-pertechnetate can be confusing, and sometimes it is necessary for the patient to void or be catheterized.

If bleeding is intermittent, use ^{99m}Tc-labeled red blood cells. If bleeding is active, either ^{99m}Tc-labeled red blood cells or ^{99m}Tc sulfur colloid can be used.

Gastric Emptying Studies

These studies usually are performed to assess the rate of emptying of solids from the stomach; they are most commonly performed with ^{99m}Tc colloid mixed into scrambled eggs before they are cooked.

Half of the activity of a solid meal should be out of the stomach in about 90 minutes.

Solids leave the stomach in a linear fashion, liquids exponentially.

Blood Pool Imaging of the Liver

This study is commonly performed to differentiate cavernous hemangioma from other focal liver lesions seen on ultrasound or CT.

Hemangiomas are not seen to be hypervascular on early arterial images. On late blood pool images, a hemangioma usually shows activity that is more intense than the normal liver.

Hypovascular tumors are photopenic on early and late images, and hypervascular tumors are usually increased in activity on early images but may be hot or cold on delayed images.

SUGGESTED READING

Urbain, JC, Vekemans MM, Malmud LS: Esophageal transit, gastroesophageal reflux and gastic emptying. In Sandler MP, Coleman RE, Patton JA et al. (eds): Diagnostic Nuclear Medicine, 4th ed. New York, Lippincott, Williams and Wilkins, 2003, pp 487–502.

Ziessman HA: Acute cholecystitis, biliary obstruction and biliary leakage, Semin Nucl Med 33:279–296, 2003.

Zuckier LS: Acute gastrointestinal bleeding, Semin Nucl Med 33:297–311, 2003.

Skeletal System

9

INTRODUCTION

The availability of stable technetium-labeled bone-seeking pharmaceuticals with improved soft-tissue clearance has led to sensitive, high-resolution images, which accounts for the widespread use of these agents in bone scanning. Bone imaging with these technetium agents will probably remain clinically useful for a long time, despite the rapid advances in other technologies, such as computed tomography (CT) and magnetic resonance imaging (MRI). The bone scan often provides an earlier diagnosis and demonstrates more lesions than are found by radiographic procedures. Although the presence of a lesion on a bone scan is nonspecific, its monostotic or polyostotic status and anatomic distribution can usually be determined, and these findings often provide important clues to the differential diagnosis. For optimal performance of bone scans, both the physician and the technologist need to understand the limitations and uses of skeletal imaging procedures.

ANATOMY AND PHYSIOLOGY

The basic structure of bone is a crystalline lattice composed of calcium, phosphate, and hydroxyl ions, which form the inorganic mineral hydroxya-patite. The other major constituents of bone include collagen, ground substance, and other minerals. Anatomically, the skeleton is composed of two parts: the axial and the appendicular portions. The axial skeleton includes the skull, spine, and thoracic girdle. The appendicular skeleton includes the upper extremities, pelvis, and lower extremities. This is a relatively important distinction because some diseases favor either the appendicular or the axial skeleton.

RADIOPHARMACEUTICALS

Bone-seeking radiopharmaceuticals are analogs of calcium, hydroxyl groups, or phosphates. By far the most widely used radiopharmaceuticals for skeletal imaging are technetium-labeled diphos-phonates, most often methylene diphosphonate. Bone imaging also can be performed with fluorine-18 (^{18}F) and positron emission tomography (PET) scanning, although this has not achieved wide clinical usage. The fluoride ion exchanges with the hydroxyl ion in the hydroxyapatite crystal for localization with high initial extraction efficiency.

Diphosphonates contain organic P–C–P bonds, which are more stable in vivo than are inorganic P–O–P bonds (pyrophosphates), primarily because

243

TABLE 9–1.	Possible Mechanisms of Increased Activity on Bone Scans

Increased osteoid formation
Increased blood flow
Increased mineralization of osteoid
Interrupted sympathetic nerve supply

TABLE 9–2.	Causes of Increased Activity on Bone Scan

LOCALIZED
Primary bone tumor
Metastatic disease
Osteomyelitis
Trauma
   Stress or frank fractures
   Battering
   Postsurgical osseous changes
   Loose prosthesis
Degenerative changes
Osteoid osteoma
Paget's disease, melorrheostosis, fibrous dysplasia
Arthritis
Locally increased blood flow
   Hyperemia
   Decreased sympathetic control
Decreased overlying soft tissue (e.g., postmastectomy)
Soft-tissue activity (see Table 9–5)

GENERALIZED (SUPERSCAN)
Primary hyperparathyroidism
Secondary hyperparathyroidism
Renal osteodystrophy
Diffuse metastases
   Prostate
   Lung
   Breast
Hematologic disorders

of their resistance to enzymatic hydrolysis. Because the diphosphonates have rapid renal excretion, they provide a high target-to-nontarget ratio in 2 to 3 hours after injection, with 50% to 60% of the activity localizing in bone and the remainder being cleared by the kidneys. Factors that impair renal function result in increased soft-tissue activity, which reduces the quality of the bone scan. With most diphosphonates, maximal skeletal uptake occurs at about 5 hours. The biologic half-life is about 24 hours.

Care should be taken to avoid the injection of air into the mixing vial during preparation of phosphate radiopharmaceuticals because the resultant oxidation of technetium causes poor tagging of the phosphates. Bone radiopharmaceuticals should be routinely checked with chromatography before injection; a 95% tag is acceptable. If the radiopharmaceutical is administered more than 4 hours after preparation, gastric and thyroid visualization on bone scans may be seen as the result of free pertechnetate.

The initial accumulation of technetium-labeled radiopharmaceuticals in bone is primarily related to blood supply; however, roles are also played by capillary permeability, the local acid–base relation, fluid pressure within bone, hormones, vitamins, the quantity of mineralized bone, and bone turnover. Increased radionuclide activity in bone may result from accentuation of any one of these factors. Factors that may be responsible for greater than usual activity are listed in Tables 9–1 and 9–2. For example, regionally increased blood flow causes increased delivery of the radiopharmaceutical to the bone, with resultant increased regional deposition of the agent. The converse is also true: interference with any of these factors may cause decreased skeletal activity. For instance, in cases of decreased cardiac output, bone scans may be of poor quality, owing to inadequate delivery of radiopharmaceutical to the bone. The relation between blood flow and radionuclide bone activity,

however, is not linear; a fourfold increase in blood flow increases bone uptake by only 30% to 40%.

Initial deposition is thought to be due to *chemisorption* on the bone surface. In some patients, this accumulation can be affected by administered drugs. Technetium-99m (^{99m}Tc) diphosphonates concentrate not in osteoclasts or osteoid but rather in the mineral phase of bone, which is two thirds crystalline hydroxyapatite and one third amorphous, noncrystalline calcium phosphate.

TECHNIQUE

Technical aspects, sample protocols, and dosimetry for planar and single-photon emission computed tomography (SPECT) skeletal imaging are presented in Appendix E–1.

For routine planar scans, the patient is normally injected intravenously with 10 to 20 mCi (370 to 740 MBq) of the technetium diphosphonate radiopharmaceutical and imaged 2 to 4 hours later. The site of injection should be distant from any suspected osseous pathology and should be recorded.

Often, even a slight extravasation of isotope at the injection site causes a focus of markedly increased soft-tissue activity. In patients suspected of having either osteomyelitis or cellulitis, a radionuclide angiogram and initial blood pool image are performed after injection, and routine images are obtained at about 2 to 3 hours. This is termed a *three-phase study*. Sometimes, additional images are performed 18 to 24 hours after injection (*four-phase study*). A four-phase study is rarely needed but can be useful in patients in renal failure who have poor soft-tissue clearance.

Gamma camera imaging consists of either multiple spot views or whole-body imaging, the latter of which results in a single skeletal image. If multiple spot films are obtained, the entire skeleton should be imaged. The patient is normally scanned in both the anterior and posterior projections. Detailed spot views of particular regions may be obtained as dictated by patient history or symptoms. In addition, selective pinhole or high-resolution collimator views allow for enhanced resolution in any areas of interest. These are especially useful when imaging small bones and pediatric patients.

The rapid urinary excretion of phosphate radiopharmaceuticals causes large amounts of activity to accumulate within the bladder, which may obscure pelvic lesions; therefore, voiding before imaging should be routine. Voiding, however, particularly in incontinent patients, may result in radioactive contamination of skin or clothing; this may obscure underlying pathology or mimic a lesion. Removal of contaminated clothing and cleansing of skin may be necessary to obtain accurate results. After injection and before scanning, patients should be hydrated. The resultant more-frequent voiding decreases the bladder radiation dose.

SPECT imaging may significantly improve skeletal lesion detection in patients with specific regional complaints and may establish or better localize an abnormality suspected on routine planar images. SPECT is most valuable in complex bony structures, such as large joints, the spine, and the pelvis.

NORMAL SCAN

The normal scan (Fig. 9–1) varies significantly in appearance between children and adults. In children, areas of growth in the region of the epiphyses show intense radionuclide accumulation (Fig. 9–2). In adults, the quality of the bone scan can be related to age; in general, the older the patient, the higher the proportion of poor-quality scans. There usually is good visualization of the skull, with relatively increased accumulation of activity in the region of the nasopharynx, which may be secondary to the high proportional blood flow in this region. Activity in the skull is often patchy, even in normal patients, so care must be taken in assessing skull lesions without an accompanying radiograph. Often, there is focal maxillary or mandibular alveolar ridge activity in adults, owing to dental disease. There is activity throughout the spine, and it is common to see focal areas of increased activity in the lower cervical spine even on anterior images, usually representing degenerative changes or simply due to the lordosis of the cervical spine rather than activity in the thyroid cartilage or the thyroid itself. Areas of tendon insertion, chronic stress, and osseous remodeling due to any reason also demonstrate increased activity. On the anterior view, there is prominent visualization of the sternum, sternoclavicular joints, acromioclavicular joints, shoulders, iliac crests, and hips. Increased activity in the knees in older patients is relatively common because of the propensity for arthritic changes. On the posterior view, the thoracic spine is well seen, as are the tips of the scapulae. The spine often demonstrates increased activity in areas of hypertrophic degenerative change, and the sacroiliac joints are usually pronounced.

Because the human skeleton is symmetric, any asymmetric osseous activity should be viewed with suspicion. In addition, it is important on the posterior view to examine the scan for the presence and location of renal activity; on the anterior view, for bladder activity. The kidneys and bladder should be routinely scrutinized for focal space-occupying lesions producing photopenic defects in the renal cortex or displacement of the kidneys or bladder. Asymmetric renal activity is not uncommon. Because the scans are usually obtained in the supine position, activity may accumulate in extrarenal pelves. If urinary tract obstruction is suspected, kidney views should be repeated after the patient has ambulated to distinguish obstruction from position-related collecting system activity (Fig. 9–3).

If there is extravasation of the radiopharmaceutical at the site of injection, the radiopharmaceutical will be slowly resorbed. In such cases, lymphatic drainage may also occur, resulting in the visualization of one or more lymph nodes, not infrequently seen in the axilla or supraclavicular region on the side of an upper extremity injection. (Fig. 9–4).

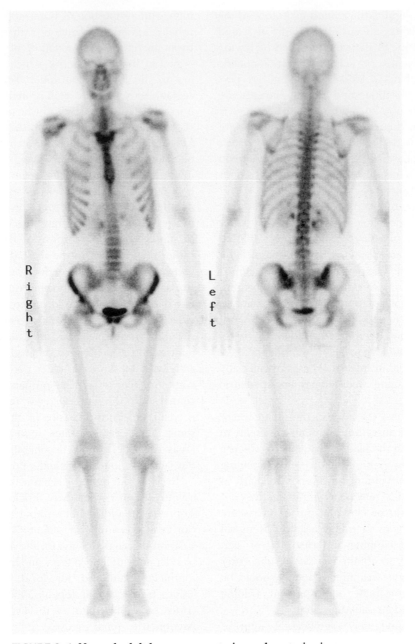

FIGURE 9–1. Normal adult bone scan, anterior and posterior images.

Localized areas of increased soft-tissue or skeletal activity in an extremity distal to the site of injection (the *glove phenomenon*) may be due to inadvertent arterial injection of the radionuclide. Regional blood flow changes may also be reflected in the scan (either relative ischemia if the activity is decreased, such as with atherosclerotic disease or gangrene, or hyperemia if the activity is locally increased, such as with cellulitis or other inflam-

mation). When pathology is suspected in the hands, wrists, or forearms, and a three-phase study is being performed, it is important to release the venous tourniquet and wait for about 1 minute before injecting the radiopharmaceutical. If this is not done, there can be confusion of actual pathology, with transient hyperemia resulting from vasodilatation caused by the tourniquet (Fig. 9–5). Differential blood flow also may be secondary to

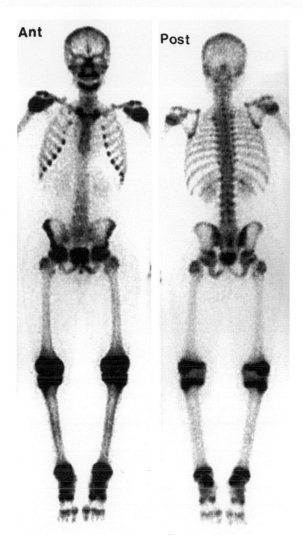

Ant   Post

FIGURE 9–2. Normal bone scan. This scan was performed on a 15-year-old boy. Anterior (*left*) and posterior (*right*) images demonstrate markedly increased activity around the epiphyseal plates. This is usually best seen around the knees, ankles, shoulders, and wrists.

rior elements. Transverse images of the spine resemble those of CT sections, whereas coronal and sagittal SPECT images are analogous to anteroposterior and lateral radiographic tomograms, respectively. The curvature of the thoracolumbar spine results in sequential rather than simultaneous visualization of the anatomic parts of adjacent vertebrae. With careful view of the sequential images on a computer monitor display, proper orientation generally is not difficult.

CLINICAL APPLICATIONS

The following are some common indications for bone scanning:

- Detection and follow-up of metastatic disease
- Differentiation between osteomyelitis and cellulitis
- Determination of bone viability: infarction or avascular necrosis
- Evaluation of fractures difficult to assess on radiographs (stress fractures, fractures of complex structures, and possible fractures in battered children)
- Evaluation of prosthetic joints for infection or loosening
- Determination of biopsy site
- Evaluation of bone pain in patients with normal or equivocal radiographs
- Evaluation of the significance of an incidental skeletal finding on radiographs

Metastatic Disease

The high sensitivity of radionuclide bone imaging in determining the presence and the extent of metastatic disease makes it an extremely important tool in decision making, particularly because survival rates in patients with multiple distant osseous metastases from many tumors are worse than for those patients with localized disease. Although the prognostic value of bone scanning for some tumors is disputed, the answer probably depends on the natural history of each tumor type and adequate actuarial analysis. Finding metastases is frequently important to clinical decisions affecting quality of life. Serial bone scanning in patients with known metastases is thought to be valuable in therapeutic decision making (Fig. 9–6), particularly if it is used in combination with other clinical information. This may prove of particular value in the detection of lesions in critical weight-bearing areas, such as the femur.

neurologically or autonomically mediated abnormalities (sympathectomy or neuropathy), or even to altered stress.

Recognition of the details of normal imaging anatomy becomes even more important when SPECT images of specific skeletal regions are obtained. Reviewing the images in three orthogonal planes generally aids interpreter orientation and thus allows more accurate localization of pathology. The specific reconstructions of greatest value depend on the area being evaluated. The complexity of the spine makes it particularly amenable to SPECT imaging to localize an abnormality in the vertebral body, disk space, or poste-

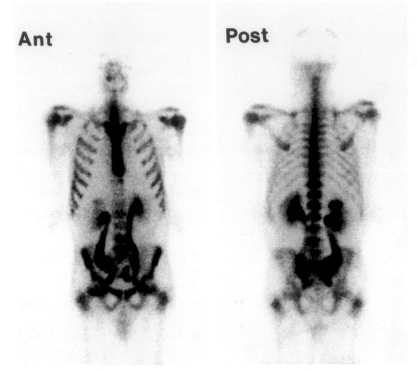

FIGURE 9–3. Hydronephrosis. This 50-year-old woman with cervical cancer had a bone scan because of back pain and suspected metastatic disease. Anterior (*left*) and posterior (*right*) images show markedly increased activity in both kidneys and ureters 3 hours after injection.

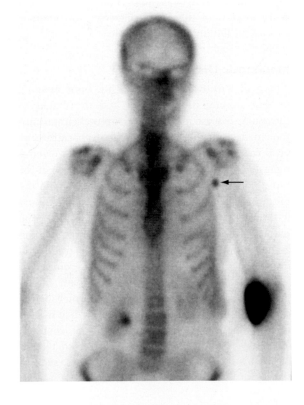

FIGURE 9–4. Activity in axillary lymph node (*arrow*) after extravasation of injection into left antecubital fossa.

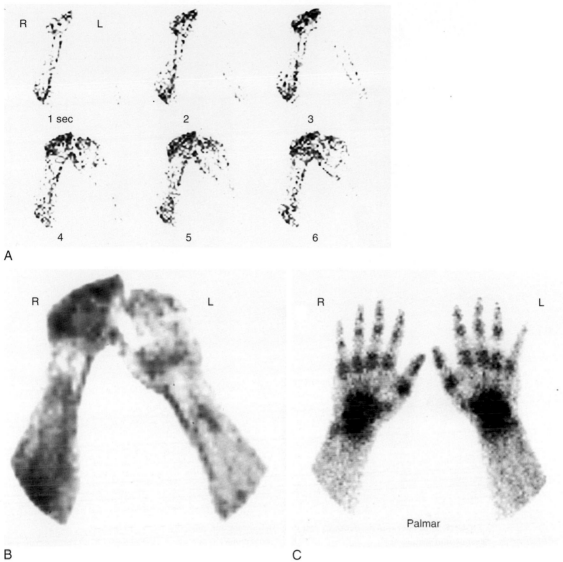

FIGURE 9-5. Tourniquet phenomenon in a normal patient. A tourniquet applied to the arm before intravenous administration of radiopharmaceutical causes distal ischemia and physiologic vasodilatation. When the tourniquet is released and the injection made within 30 to 60 seconds, there is increased blood flow (*A*) and blood pooling in the forearm and hand (*B*). In this patient, the tourniquet was applied to the right arm, and the injection was made quickly because the patient was uncooperative and moving. Note that the delayed 3-hour images (*C*) of the hands are normal.

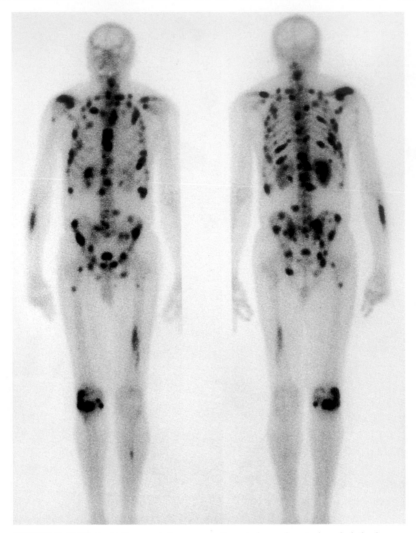

FIGURE 9–6. Metastatic prostate cancer. An anterior and posterior whole-body technetium-99m methylene diphosphonate bone scan shows the metastatic deposits as areas of increased activity.

For a lytic lesion to be visualized by radiography, localized demineralization of about 30% to 50% must occur, and there is little question that bone scans usually demonstrate metastatic lesions much earlier than radiography does. The false-negative rate of radiographic skeletal surveys may be as high as 50% with certain tumors, whereas the overall false-negative rate of bone scanning for the most common neoplasms may be as low as 2%. Some tumors are more likely than are others to produce a false-negative bone scan. These include highly aggressive anaplastic tumors, reticulum cell sarcoma, renal cell carcinoma (Fig. 9–7), thyroid carcinoma, histiocytosis, neuroblastoma, and especially multiple myeloma. When multiple myeloma is seen on a bone scan, it is often secondary to a pathologic fracture or impending fracture. For patients in whom some lesions cannot be identified easily by bone scanning, the radiographic skeletal survey remains the procedure of choice.

About 80% of patients with known neoplasms and bone pain have metastases documented by the bone scan. Because 30% to 50% of patients with metastases do not have bone pain, a good case may be made for scanning patients with asymptomatic tumors that have a propensity to metastasize to bone (e.g., breast, lung, and prostate); but for tumors with low rates of osseous metastases (e.g., colon, cervix, uterus, head, and neck), the procedure may not be cost-effective.

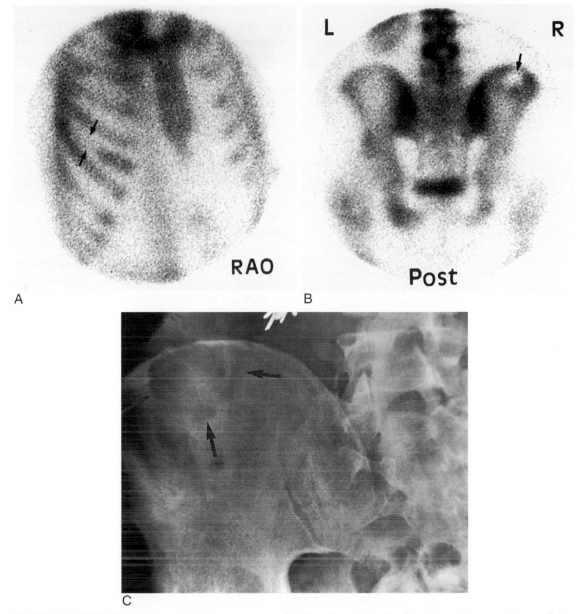

FIGURE 9–7. Cold defects caused by lytic metastases. In this patient with renal cell carcinoma, bone scan images of the anterior right chest (*A*) and the pelvis (*B*) show areas that have no bony activity (*arrows*). *C*, A radiograph of the right iliac crest shows a dark area that was originally thought to be overlying bowel gas but proved to be a lytic bone lesion.

Even though most metastases are multiple and relatively obvious, there are times when the interpretation may be difficult. If a single lesion is identified, the false-positive rate for attributing the finding to a metastasis is high. Only about 15% to 20% of patients with proven metastases have a single lesion (most commonly in the spine). A single focus of increased activity elsewhere is often secondary to benign disease, especially in a rib

where this is due to metastasis in only about 10% of cases. A notable exception to this is a single sternal lesion in a patient with breast cancer (Fig. 9–8), which can be due to metastasis in almost 80% of cases. If two consecutive ribs are involved by adjacent discrete foci of increased activity, the lesions are almost always secondary to trauma. In a patient with a known malignancy and a solitary abnormality on bone scan without an obvious

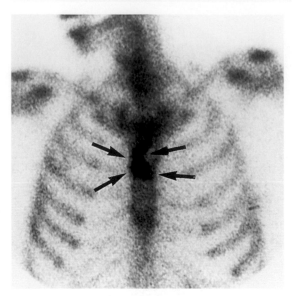

FIGURE 9–8. Sternal metastasis. This young woman was treated for breast cancer 1 year earlier. The follow-up bone scan reveals only one focus of increased activity, which is in the sternum. Round or eccentric sternal lesions in breast cancer patients have about an 80% chance of being a metastasis.

benign explanation on radiographs, additional imaging is often warranted to exclude the possibility of metastases.

When multifocal areas of increased activity are seen in noncontiguous ribs, especially if in a linear configuration along the rib, however, the likelihood of metastatic disease is high. In multifocal metastatic disease, the regional distribution of lesions for common bone-seeking primary tumors is as follows: thorax and ribs, 37%; spine, 26%; pelvis, 16%; limbs, 15%; and skull, 6%. The reason for this distribution is that most bone metastases are caused by hematogenous spread to the red marrow, which subsequently erodes the surrounding bone.

Follow-up bone scans in patients undergoing treatment for advanced breast and prostate cancer should be interpreted with caution. Within the first 3 months of chemotherapy, a favorable clinical response by focal bone metastases may result in healing that causes increased uptake at involved sites, which is usually a good prognostic sign. If not clinically correlated, this *flare phenomenon* can give the false impression of new lesions or extension of existing metastatic sites. Bone lesions that appear 6 months or later after treatment almost always indicate disease progression.

Diffuse involvement of the skeleton by metastases can be deceptive; it may initially appear as though there has been remarkably good, relatively uniform uptake in all the bones. This has been referred to as a *superscan* (Fig. 9–9). A hallmark of the superscan due to metastases is significantly decreased renal activity with diffusely increased activity noted throughout the axial skeleton. A superscan is most commonly due to prostatic carcinoma, although diffuse metastases from other tumors, such as breast cancer and lymphoma, may also cause this appearance. In the absence of neoplasm, a superscan involving bones throughout the entire skeleton (both axial and peripheral) should raise suspicion of metabolic conditions, such as primary or secondary hyperparathyroidism. Increased activity primarily in the peripheral skeleton may be seen in hematologic disorders. For example, a patient with chronic anemia, such as occurs in sickle cell disease or thalassemia, may show increased activity in the skull and around the knees and ankles as a result of expanded marrow and an accompanying increase in blood flow to these regions.

In some patients who have metastatic disease, chemotherapy results in immunosuppression, and treatment may involve use of granulocyte-macrophage colony-stimulating factor. This treatment causes marrow hyperplasia and increased marrow blood flow, resulting in bone scans with symmetrically increased activity around the major joints (particularly the knees).

Detection of bone metastases from prostate cancer is best assessed using a bone scan. Prostate-specific antigen (PSA) has been shown to be a marker for both primary and metastatic prostatic cancer. In asymptomatic patients presenting with well or moderately differentiated prostate cancer and PSA levels of less than 10 to 15 ng/mL, the likelihood of bone metastases is low. Unless these patients have focal bone pain, a bone scan is likely not indicated. In patients, who are not receiving adjuvant hormonal therapy, it is rare to see a positive bone scan if the serum PSA does not exceed 40 ng/mL. Contrarily, PSA levels can be normal in patients with osseous metastases receiving hormonal therapy.

In searching for metastatic disease, it is important not only to delineate the areas of increased activity (see Table 9–2) but also to look for cold lesions (Table 9–3), which are usually much more difficult to identify. In cancer patients, focal photon-deficient lesions are due to metastatic disease in

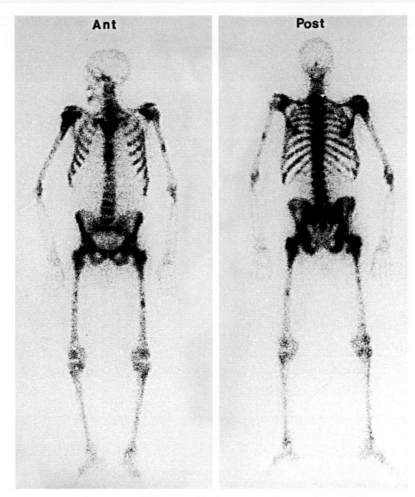

FIGURE 9–9. Superscan. Diffuse osteoblastic metastases from carcinoma of the prostate. There is involvement of the entire axial and proximal appendicular skeleton. Essentially no renal or bladder activity is identified because the metastases have accumulated most of the radionuclide. Several smaller lesions are identified in the long bones as well. *Left,* Anterior. *Right,* Posterior.

more than 80% of cases. They may occur if the tumor is extremely aggressive, if there is disruption of the blood supply to the bone, or if there is significant marrow involvement, particularly in a vertebral body. When multiple adjacent bones have a decreased radionuclide accumulation, other causes, such as radiation therapy, should be considered (Fig. 9–10). Other causes of cold lesions include infarction (particularly in patients with sickle cell anemia) and avascular necrosis. Both infarction and aseptic necrosis in the healing phase can show increased activity.

Malignant Bone Tumors

The bone scan appearance of *osteogenic sarcoma* varies widely, depending on the vascularity and

aggressiveness of the tumor and on the amount of neoplastic and reactive bone production (Fig. 9–11). Increased activity in these lesions is usually intense and often patchy with photopenic areas. Only about 2% of these patients present with osseous metastases from the primary site. Exact assessment of tumor extent by bone scanning is often complicated by reactive hyperemia in the affected limb, which may produce increased activity in the entire extremity. In this setting, MRI may provide more exact information regarding tumor extent, particularly in soft tissues.

In the past, follow-up bone scans were not thought to be worthwhile in patients with osteosarcoma because pulmonary metastases almost always developed before osseous metastases. Aggressive

TABLE 9–3.	Causes of Cold Lesions on Bone Scan

LOCALIZED
Overlying attenuation artifact caused by pacemaker, barium, etc.
Instrumentation artifact
Radiation therapy
Local vascular compromise
   Infarction
   Intrinsic vascular lesion
   Early aseptic necrosis
   Marrow involvement by tumor
Early osteomyelitis
Osseous metastases from:
   Neuroblastoma
   Renal cell carcinoma
   Thyroid carcinoma
   Anaplastic tumors (e.g., reticulum cell sarcoma)
Cyst

GENERALIZED
Age (old)
Inadequate amount of radiopharmaceutical
Chemotherapy

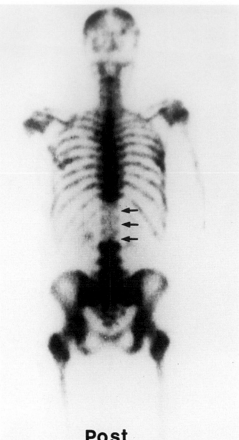

Post

FIGURE 9–10. Radiation therapy defect. This patient with diffuse osseus metastases as well as multiple bony lytic (cold) metastases in the ribs has had radiation therapy to the spine. Multiple contiguous vertebral bodies (T12 to L2) with decreased activity (*arrows*) are the result of radiotherapy, not metastases.

chemotherapy, however, has altered the natural history of osteosarcoma, and now about 20% of patients develop osseous metastases before pulmonary disease. Thus, follow-up bone scans are now recommended. In interpreting follow-up scans, care must be taken not to mistake postamputation reactive changes at the amputation site for tumor recurrence. Because osteosarcomas are bone-forming lesions, soft-tissue metastases may be seen as foci of extraskeletal increased activity, especially in the liver and lung.

Ewing's sarcoma is a relatively common primary bone tumor, frequently occurring in the pelvis or femur. Activity is often intense and homogeneous. The tumor is very vascular and may mimic osteomyelitis on three-phase bone imaging. Up to 11% of patients present with osseous metastases (Fig. 9–12). About 40% to 50% of patients with either Ewing's sarcoma or osteosarcoma develop osseous metastases within 2 years of presentation, and follow-up bone scans are recommended. Reactive hyperemia producing increased activity in the adjacent uninvolved bone is not usually seen with Ewing's sarcoma.

Benign Osseous Neoplasms

Benign osseous neoplasms have variable appearances on bone scan (Table 9–4). Angiographic and blood pool images obtained shortly after injection of bone scanning agents indicate that most malignant lesions are hyperemic and that most benign lesions initially accumulate little radiopharmaceutical. An early blood pool image may therefore be helpful in identifying benign lesions because it may show little or no increased uptake. The major exception to this is osteoid osteoma (Fig. 9–13), which demonstrates intense activity at the site of the vascular nidus. Bone scans are often of value in detecting these lesions when they occur in sites that are difficult to evaluate on a radiograph, such as the spine. On delayed images, benign lesions may show a wide range of activity. Osteoblastomas, osteoid osteomas, chondroblastomas, and giant-cell tumors usually have intense activity on delayed

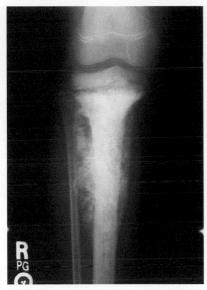
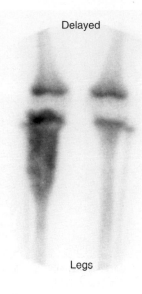

Delayed

Legs

FIGURE 9–11. Osteogenic sarcoma. An x-ray (*left*) reveals mottled sclerosis and periosteal reaction in the proximal tibia of a teenager. *Right,* Increased activity is seen on the bone scan as well. There is normal physiologic activity seen at the epiphyseal plates.

images. Enchondromas can be warm or hot (Fig. 9-14), chondroblastomas are usually of intermediate activity (Fig. 9–15), and fibrous cortical defects and nonossifying fibromas are of normal intensity or warm. Bone islands, hemangiomas, and cortical desmoid tumors rarely show increased activity and usually cannot be distinguished from normal bone. Bone cysts are usually cold centrally but may have a warm rim due to increased bone remodeling (Fig. 9–16), or even a hot area due to a pathologic fracture. *Fibrous dysplasia* is another benign disease of bone that may present as single (Fig. 9-17) or multiple areas of increased activity. Both polyostotic fibrous dysplasia and Paget's disease are sometimes confused with multifocal metastatic disease, although the distribution and radiographic presentation of lesions are frequently characteristic. Both osteochondromas and enchondromas are frequently seen as areas of increased activity.

Soft-Tissue Uptake

Activity may be seen in soft-tissue structures on the bone scan, and many possibilities can be considered when this occurs (Table 9–5). Soft-tissue activity may be secondary to any process that evokes soft-tissue calcification or infarction. The first and most obvious items to be excluded are surface contaminations by urine or by the radionuclide during injection.

TABLE 9–4.	Typical Activity of Benign Bone Tumors on Bone Scans

INTENSE
Fibrous dysplasia
Giant cell tumor
Aneurysmal bone cyst
Osteoblastoma
Osteoid osteoma

MODERATE
Adamantinoma
Chondroblastoma
Enchondroma

MILD OR ISOINTENSE
Fibrous cortical defect
Bone island
Cortical desmoid
Non-ossifying fibroma
Osteoma

"COLD"
Bone cyst without fracture

VARIABLE
Hemangioma
Multiple hereditary exostosis

Text continued on p. 260

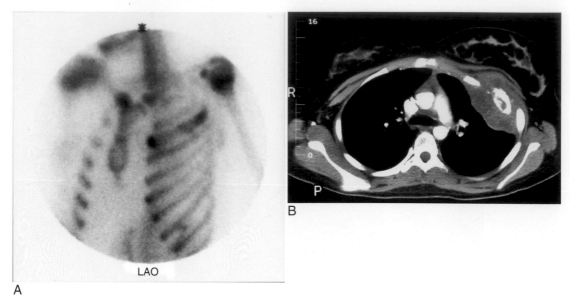

FIGURE 9–12. Ewing's sarcoma of the left third rib. *A*, On the bone scan, an oblique view of the ribs shows abnormal uptake in the anterior-lateral left third rib. *B*, A computed tomography scan shows the soft-tissue mass associated with rib destruction.

TABLE 9–5.	Causes of Extraosseous Activity on Bone Scans

GENERALIZED
Poor radiopharmaceutical preparation
Renal failure

LOCALIZED
Injection sites
Kidney (normal)
Obstructed kidney or ureter
Urine contamination
Hepatic necrosis
Tissue infarction (brain, muscle, heart, spleen)
Myositis ossificans
Polymyositis
Pulmonary or stomach calcification
  (hyperparathyroidism)
Vascular calcification
Hematoma
Steroids (breast uptake)
Sites of intramuscular iron injection or calcium
  injection extravasation

Chemotherapy (kidneys)
Radiotherapy treatment portals
Tumoral calcinosis, dystrophic and metastatic
  calcification
Calcific tendinitis
Free pertechnetate (stomach, thyroid)
Amyloidosis
Soft tissue (tumors)
  Breast
  Ovary (especially mucinous)
  Gastrointestinal (especially colon)
  Neuroblastoma
  Endometrial carcinoma
  Uterine fibroids (leiomyoma)
  Gastrointestinal lymphoma
  Hepatic metastases
  Meningioma
  Lung carcinoma
Malignant ascites or effusions

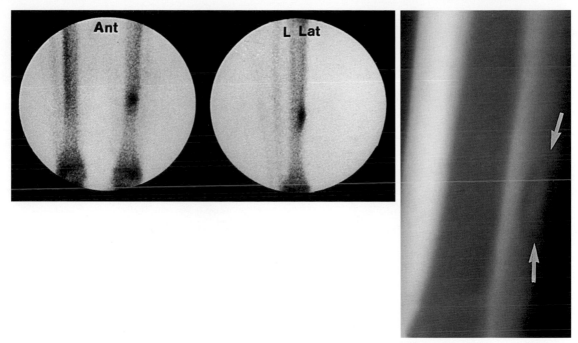

FIGURE 9–13. *Left,* **Osteoid osteoma of the left mid-tibia.** The intense uptake is characteristic of these lesions. *Right,* Lateral radiographic tomogram demonstrates the lesion (*arrows*) with a central nidus.

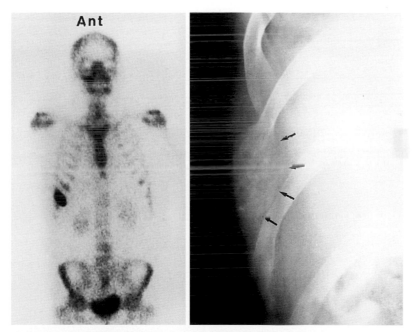

FIGURE 9–14. Multiple enchondromas. *Left,* On the anterior bone scan, areas of increased activity are noted, including in the ribs. *Right,* A rib radiograph shows a characteristic expansile lesion with central matrix.

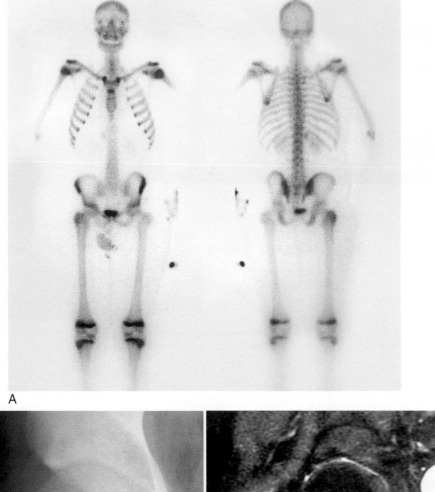

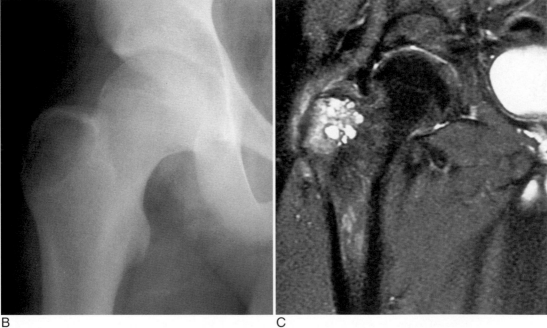

FIGURE 9–15. Chondroblastoma. *A,* The whole-body bone scan shows increased activity in the greater trochanter of the right hip. *B,* The x-ray shows a lytic lesion in the same region. *C,* A magnetic resonance imaging scan demonstrates the chondroid matrix.

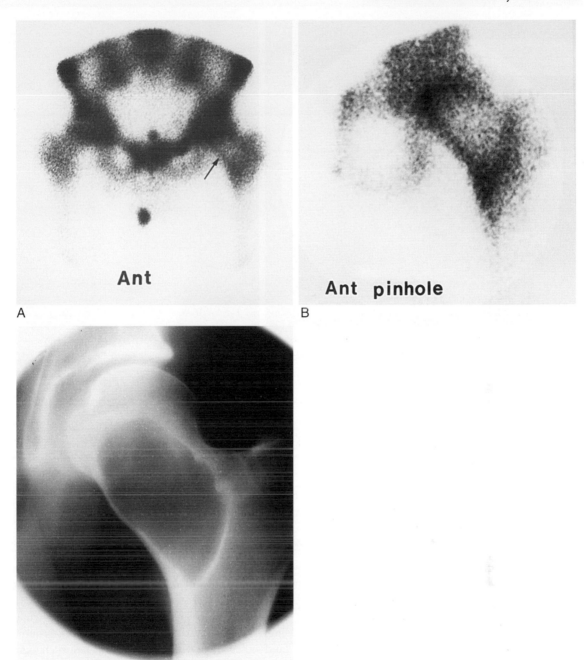

A

B

C

FIGURE 9–16. Bone cyst. *A,* A 3-hour anterior image of the pelvis from a bone scan shows a photopenic focus in the left hip with moderate peripheral activity. *B,* This is better appreciated on a pinhole image. *C,* A radiograph of the area shows a well-defined lytic lesion with a narrow zone of transition, suggesting a benign cause. In the presence of an associated pathologic fracture secondary to weakened cortex, the bone scan frequently shows much more intense activity.

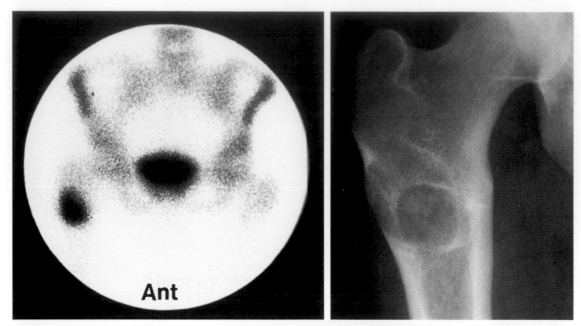

FIGURE 9–17. Fibrous dysplasia of the proximal right femur. *Left*, The anterior view of the pelvis shows markedly increased activity in the metaphysis of the promixal right femur. *Right*, The radiograph shows a well-demarcated, expansile, lucent lesion.

Soft-tissue neoplasms or their metastases (especially in the liver) may calcify, resulting in soft-tissue activity. These tumors are often mucin-producing tumors from breast (Fig. 9–18), gastrointestinal, (Fig. 9–19), and ovarian primaries (Fig. 9–20); lung cancer, lymphoma, osteogenic sarcoma (Fig. 9–21); and neuroblastoma (Fig. 9–22). Malignant pleural effusions or malignant ascites may also be demonstrated on bone scans as diffusely increased activity in the chest or abdomen (Figs. 9–23 and 9–24). Other causes of soft-tissue activity include dystrophic calcification such as occurs around joints in paraplegics; dermatomyositis (Fig. 9–25), calcific tendonitis, and other enthesiopathies; postoperative scars; inflammation; amyloidosis; and uterine fibroids.

Areas of recent infarction in skeletal muscle (rhabdomyolysis) (Fig. 9–26), brain, heart, and spleen (Fig. 9–27) may often be demonstrated on the bone scan. Renal failure evoking secondary hyperparathyroidism (renal osteodystrophy) may cause localized activity within the walls of the gastrointestinal tract (particularly in the stomach), lungs, and kidneys, owing to excessive parathyroid hormone production and subsequent calcium deposition (Fig. 9–28). Infiltration of skeletal and cardiac muscle, liver, stomach, and skin by amyloid can likewise cause soft-tissue activity. Calcification

in regions of trauma, secondary to calcifying hematomas or myositis ossificans (Fig. 9–30), has also been reported as a cause of soft-tissue accumulation of bone-imaging radiopharmaceuticals. Some surgeons use bone scans as a measure of inflammatory activity in myositis ossificans and delay possible surgery until the activity in the soft tissue is similar to activity in normal bone (Fig. 9–29), so that recurrence is minimized. Dystrophic calcification around joints as a result of trauma (Fig. 9–30) or tumoral calcinosis also shows increased activity.

Breast activity may be increased in menstruating women, breast carcinoma, mastitis, trauma and other benign conditions. Soft-tissue changes can be noted on bone scans after mastectomy. The ribs are usually more clearly seen on the mastectomy side, probably because there is less overlying soft tissue. Radiation therapy may produce increased chest wall activity in the early weeks after treatment and several months later may produce relatively decreased activity at the treatment site.

A generalized increase in soft-tissue or blood pool activity is seen in some patients receiving chemotherapy or who have chronic iron overload.

Text continued on p. 269

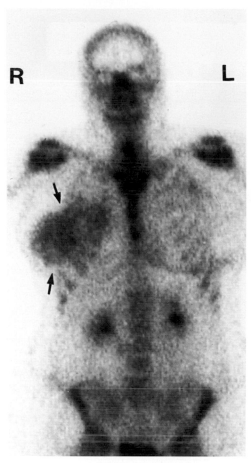

FIGURE 9–18. Activity in breast cancer. A bone scan in this patient with a right breast tumor shows marked asymmetric increased activity in the tumor (*arrows*).

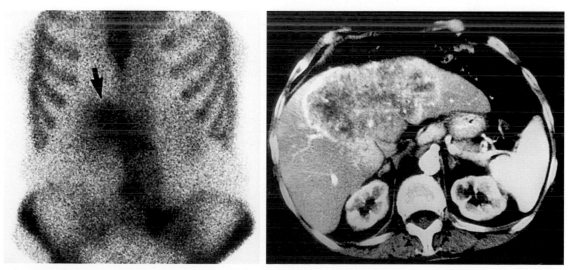

FIGURE 9–19. Liver metastases. This patient with a known mucinous colon carcinoma was thought to have hepatomegaly. *Left,* A bone scan done as part of the workup shows soft-tissue activity in the right upper quadrant (*arrow*). *Right,* A subsequent computed tomography scan clearly demonstrates a large hypervascular metastasis in the left lobe of the liver.

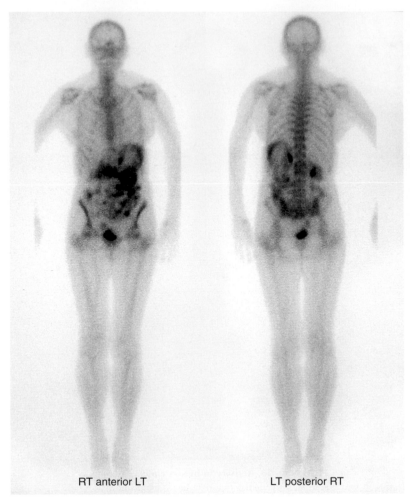

RT anterior LT   LT posterior RT

FIGURE 9–20. Omental metstases from mucinous ovarian carcinoma. The whole-body bone scan shows activity throughout the peritoneal cavity due to microscopic calcium in the metastases.

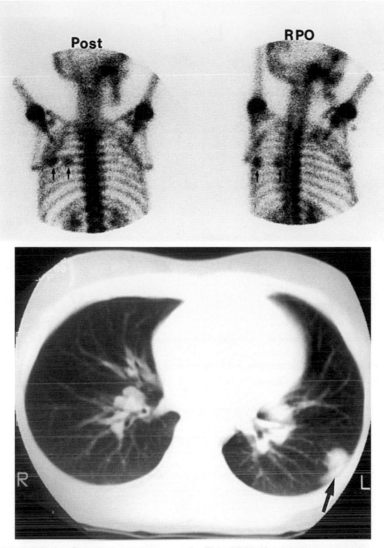

FIGURE 9–21. Osteosarcoma metastasis. This child had a right knee tumor that was resected 1 year earlier. *Top,* A follow-up bone scan showed foci of increased activity (*arrows*) projecting between posterior left ribs (and therefore probably in the lung). *Bottom,* A computed tomography scan confirmed the presence of lung metastases (*arrow*).

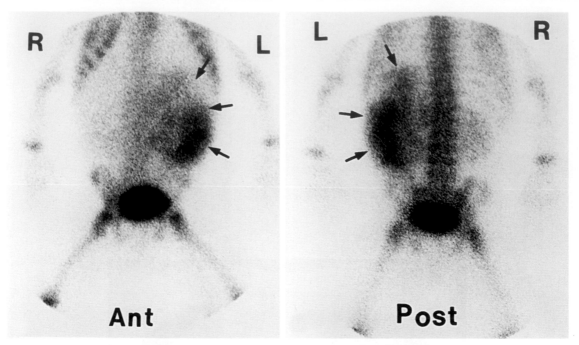

FIGURE 9–22. Neuroblastoma. A 2-year-old child with a left retroperitoneal mass was referred for a bone scan. There is increased activity (*arrows*) in the region of the mass seen on anterior (*left*) and posterior (*right*) images. The activity is too large, too lateral, and too intense to be normal renal excretion and is the result of microscopic calcification in the tumor.

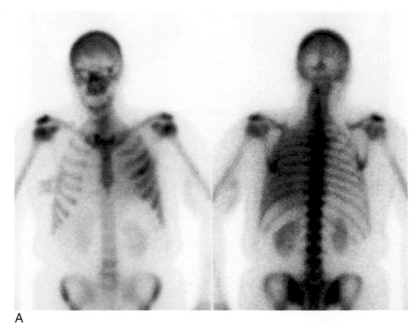

A

FIGURE 9–23. Malignant pleural effusion. *A*, Anterior and posterior bone scans show diffusely increased activity over the left hemithorax. Nonmalignant effusions uncommonly accumulate activity. The chest radiograph (*B*) and CT (*C*) demonstrate the effusion.

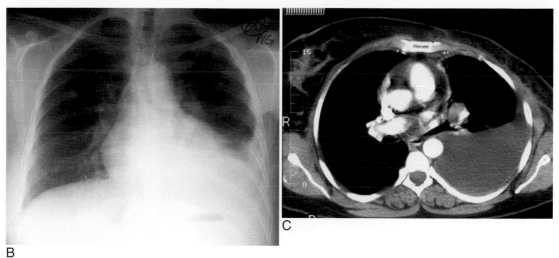

B

FIGURE 9–23, cont'd

For legend see p. 264

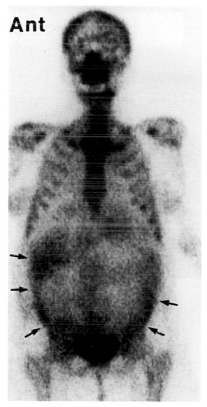

FIGURE 9–24. Malignant ascites. This 45-year-old woman has known ovarian carcinoma. Three-hour images from the bone scan show diffusely increased activity (*arrows*) over the entire peritoneal cavity.

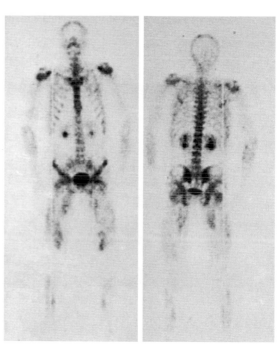

FIGURE 9–25. Dermatomyositis. Soft-tissue activity is seen on the bone scan in the large muscle groups of both lower extremities of a patient with dermatomyositis. *Left,* Anterior. *Right,* Posterior.

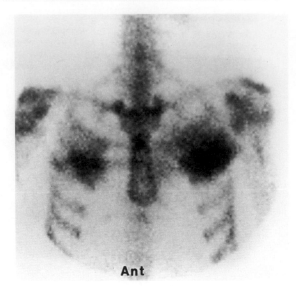

FIGURE 9–26. Muscle trauma. This young air force recruit experienced anterior chest wall pain after weight-lifting. The bone scan demonstrates increased activity in both pectoral muscles as a result of the trauma (rhabdomyolysis). Increased activity is also commonly seen for several weeks in various muscle groups after marathons or ironman competitions.

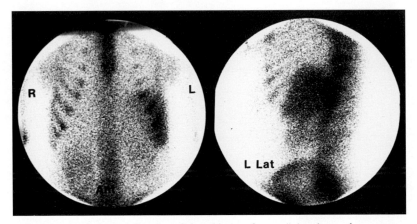

FIGURE 9–27. Splenic infarction. Selected images from a diphosphonate bone scan demonstrate increased activity in the spleen in a patient with sickle cell disease. This activity has been attributed to ongoing splenic infarction.

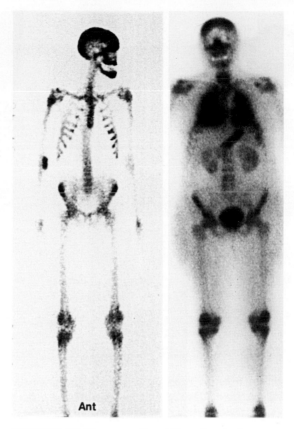

FIGURE 9–28. Hyperparathyroidism. Anterior bone scans in two different patients with hyperparathyroidism. *Left,* The first case demonstrates a typical superscan with lack of significant renal or bladder activity and with increased activity diffusely throughout the skeleton. Of note is the particularly increased activity in the calvarium, facial bones, mandible, and large joints that has been described in patients with hyperparathyroidism. *Right,* Bone scan of a second patient with hyperparathyroidism demonstrates increased activity around the major joints and significantly increased activity in the lungs, stomach, renal parenchyma, and thyroid, compatible with so-called metastatic calcification, which may be found in certain soft-tissue organs in severe cases of this disease.

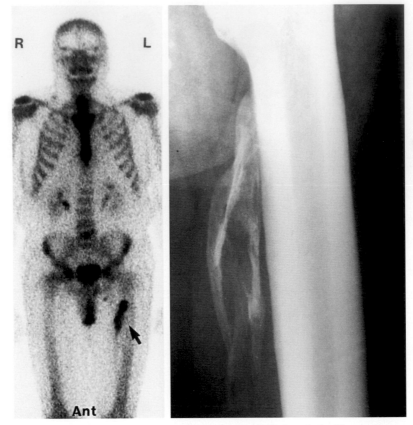

FIGURE 9–29. Myositis ossificans. This college football player had a history of trauma to the inner left thigh with residual firm swelling and limitation of motion. *Left,* The bone scan shows soft-tissue activity that is greater than the nearby bone, indicating that the process is not mature and should not yet be removed. *Right,* A radiograph shows the well-defined soft-tissue calcification.

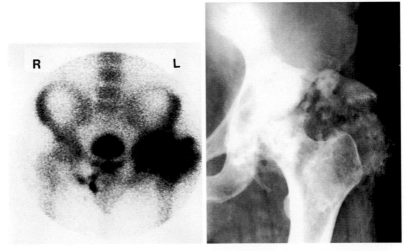

FIGURE 9–30. Heterotopic calcification. This patient was involved in a motor vehicle accident 6 months earlier and had a posterior dislocation of the left hip without fracture. *Left,* An anterior image of the pelvis from a bone scan now reveals increased activity in a periarticular soft-tissue pattern. *Right,* The radiograph shows extensive soft-tissue dystrophic calcification.

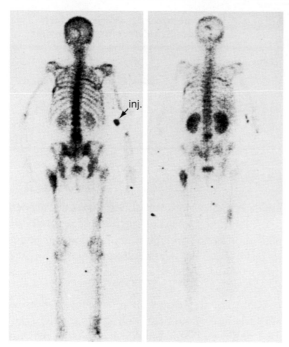

FIGURE 9–31. Diffusely increased renal activity.
Posterior bone scans in the same patient obtained for osseous metastases. *Left,* The initial scan demonstrates the osseous metastases. *Right,* The follow-up scan 2 months later after vincristine chemotherapy shows markedly decreased bone activity and relatively increased activity in the parenchyma of both kidneys.

TABLE 9–6.	Hepatic Uptake of Technetium-99m Phosphate Compounds

COMMON
Artifactual—after technetium-99m sulfur colloid study (diffuse activity)
Apparent—due to abdominal wall or rib uptake (focal activity)
Metastatic carcinoma (focal)
   Colon
   Breast
   Ovary
   Squamous cell carcinoma of esophagus
   Oat cell carcinoma of lung
   Malignant melanoma

UNCOMMON
Diffuse hepatic necrosis (diffuse activity)
Elevated serum Al^{3+} (diffuse activity)

RARE
Cholangiocarcinoma (focal activity)
Improper preparation of radiopharmaceutical causing microcolloid formation (diffuse activity)
Amyloidosis (diffuse activity)
Hepatoma

Soft-tissue injection of iron dextran may produce focal areas of increased activity. Renal failure commonly produces delayed clearance of the radiopharmaceutical and increased activity throughout the soft tissues due to diminished excretion of the radiopharmaceutical. Unilaterally increased activity in one kidney may be due to a number of causes, most commonly an extrarenal pelvis or obstruction. Persistently increased diffuse activity in the kidney parenchyma can be due to radiation treatments, chemotherapy (Fig. 9–31), hyperparathyroidism, amyloidosis, or sarcoidosis. Some reported causes of increased hepatic and renal activity on bone scans are given in Tables 9–6 and 9–7.

Trauma

Fractures not apparent on routine radiographs may be readily detected with CT, MRI, or radionuclide bone scanning (Fig. 9–32). MRI can detect the disruption of the cortex as well as the medullary fat. MRI is most useful for occult hip and knee fractures or in cases in which the site of pain is well localized. When multifocal trauma (such as child abuse) is suspected, bone scanning may be more effective.

Bone scan appearance after fracture may be divided into acute, subacute, and healing phases. The acute phase usually lasts from 3 to 4 weeks and demonstrates a generalized diffuse increase in radionuclide activity around the fracture site. The subacute phase follows and lasts 2 to 3 months, with the activity more localized and intense. The healing phase may occur over a much longer period and is accompanied by a gradual decline in intensity of radiotracer activity. The time after fracture at which the bone scan becomes abnormal is shown in Table 9–8. The percentage of fractures returning to normal at various times is shown in Table 9–9.

Most fractures show early increase in activity as a result of hyperemia and inflammation. Repair begins within a few hours and reaches a maximum in 2 to 3 weeks. The location of the fracture determines the time of appearance of increased activity on the bone scan. In the first 3 days, only 30% of pelvic and spine fractures show increased activity. Virtually all recent fractures in the axial skeleton and long bones can be seen by 14 days. Skull fractures constitute a major exception and may not show any increase in activity on bone scan. Rib fractures almost always show intense activity and

| TABLE 9–7. | Increased Uptake of Technetium-99–Labeled Bone Imaging Agents in the Kidneys |

FOCAL
Common
Urinary tract obstruction
Uncommon
Calcifying metastases (breast cancer, poorly
  differentiated lymphocytic lymphoma)
Radiation therapy to the kidney
Rare
Renal carcinoma
Renal metastasis from carcinoma of the lung

DIFFUSE
Common
Urinary tract obstruction
Idiopathic
Uncommon
Metastatic calcification
Malignant (transitional cell carcinoma of bladder,
malignant melanoma)
Hyperparathyroidism
Chemotherapy with cyclophosphamide, vincristine, and
  doxorubicin
Thalassemia major
Rare
Multiple myeloma
Crossed renal ectopia
Renal vein thrombosis
Iron overload
Administration of sodium diatrizoate after the injection
  of technetium-99m phosphate compound
Paroxysmal nocturnal hemoglobinuria
Acute pyelonephritis

TABLE 9–8. Time after Fracture at which Bone Scan Becomes Abnormal

Time after Fracture	Percentage Abnormal	
	Patients <65 yr	**All Patients**
1 day	95	80
3 day	100	95
1 wk	100	98

scan, but subsequent work has shown this to be a minor variable. However, about 3 days are needed to reliably detect an occult hip fracture in an elderly patient on bone scan. Thus, many clinicians prefer to order an MRI scan and do prompt surgery, rather than leave an elderly person in bed and wait to do a bone scan.

Return of the bone scan appearance to normal after fracture or surgical trauma is variable. Fractures and even craniotomy defects in older patients may be visible on bone scans for several years. Few fractures of weight-bearing bones return to a normal scan appearance within 5 months, whereas about 90% are normal within 2 years. More intense and prolonged uptake has been demonstrated in fractures in which open reduction was performed or a fixation device applied.

Subtle trauma, such as that from *stress fractures*, is often difficult to visualize on a plain radiograph. Often, these fractures are not visualized for 7 to 10 days, by which time interval decalcification becomes apparent radiographically around the fracture site. On the other hand, radionuclide bone scans are frequently positive at the time of clinical presentation and offer a means of early diagnosis and treatment. Bone scans are an excellent way to diagnose either fatigue or insufficiency stress injuries.

In patients with *shin splints* (*medial tibial stress syndrome*), normal blood flow and normal blood pool are seen on a three-phase bone scan (Fig. 9–34). On

can often be recognized by their location in consecutive ribs (Fig. 9–33). Single rib fractures are often difficult to distinguish from a metastasis, but eliciting a trauma history from the patient is often helpful. In addition, rib fractures present as punctate foci of increased activity, whereas neoplastic lesions frequently have a more linear distribution following the long axis of the ribs.

Age of the patient was initially thought to be relevant to time of appearance of fractures on a bone

TABLE 9–9. Time after Fracture at which Bone Scan Returns to Normal

Fracture Site	Percentage Normal			Minimum Time to Return to Normal (mo)
	1 yr	**2 yr**	**3 yr**	
Vertebrae	59	90	97	7
Long bones	64	91	97	6
Ribs	79	93	100	5

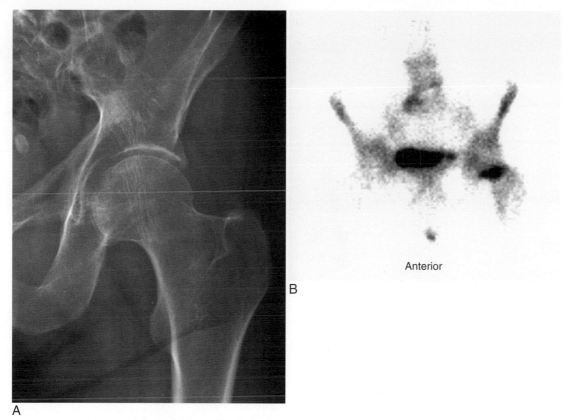

A

B

Anterior

FIGURE 9–32. Occult fracture of the left hip. An x-ray (*A*) of the hip does not show an obvious fracture; however, the anterior bone scan of the pelvis (*B*) shows increased activity in the femoral neck fracture.

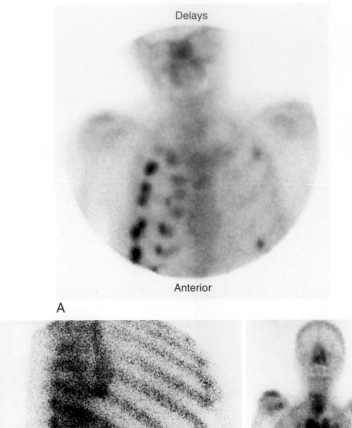

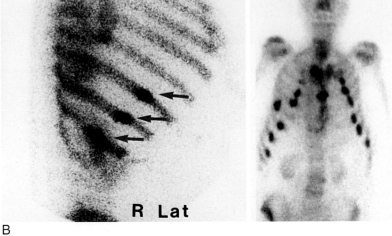

FIGURE 9–33. Rib fractures. (*A*) Rib fractures in this patient who was in an auto accident can be confidently diagnosed because consecutive ribs have distinct foci of increased activity (*arrows*). (*B*) A bone scan in another patient who was resuscitated reveals multiple anterior rib fractures as well as a mid-sternal fracture.

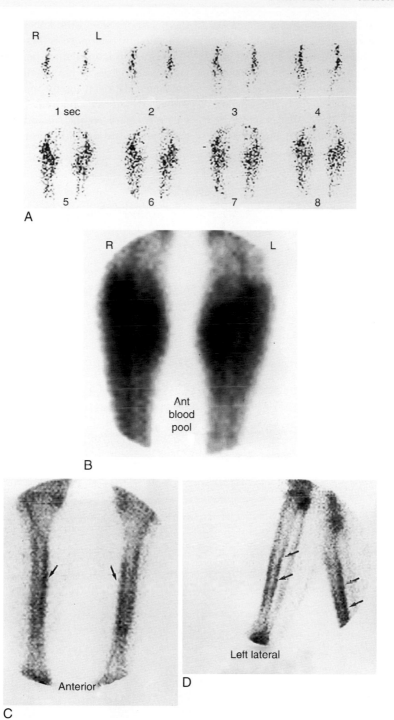

FIGURE 9–34. Shin splints. This athlete had bilateral lower leg pain. The three-phase bone scan shows normal and symmetric blood flow on the angiographic images (*A*). The blood pool image (*B*) is also normal. (There is normally a lot of blood flow to the calf muscles.) On the delayed 3-hour images (*C* and *D*), there is increased activity (*arrows*) in a long linear distribution of the posteromedial tibial shafts.

delayed images, there is typically linear increased activity along at least one third the length of the posteromedial tibial cortex at the insertion of the soleus muscle. Stress fractures tend to be more focal or fusiform on delayed images (Figs. 9–35 and 9–36) and show increased activity on blood flow and blood pool phases of a three-phase bone scan. Insufficiency-type stress fractures usually occur in the pelvis or around the knees as a result of bone weakened by osteoporosis (Fig. 9–37).

Because fractures may be identified by bone scans as early as 24 hours after occurrence, bone imaging has been useful in the assessment of suspected battered children. In infants and small children, characteristic rib and thoracic spine fractures are a strong indication of physical abuse.

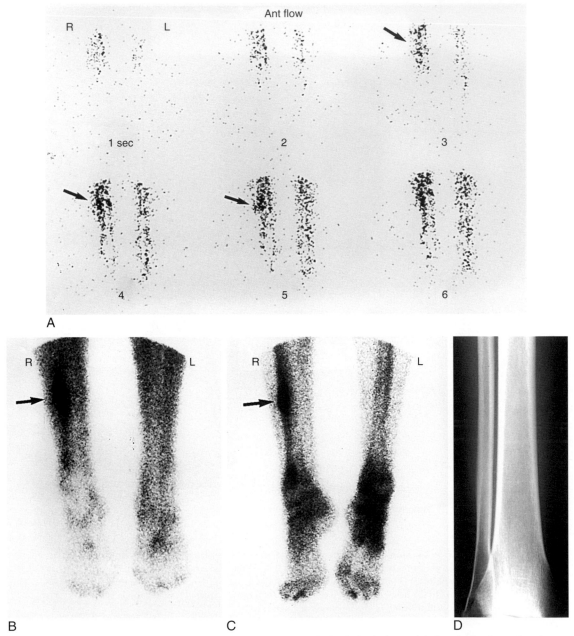

FIGURE 9–35. Fatigue stress fracture of the fibula. This jogger had pain in the lower right leg. *A,* The three-phase bone scan shows asymmetric increased activity on the angiographic phase. Note that between the blood pool image (*B*) and the 3-hour delayed image (*C*), the activity (*arrows*) becomes more intense and focal. *D,* The radiograph of the area is normal. Most tibial stress fractures occur in the proximal or middle tibia, and most fibular stress fractures occur distally.

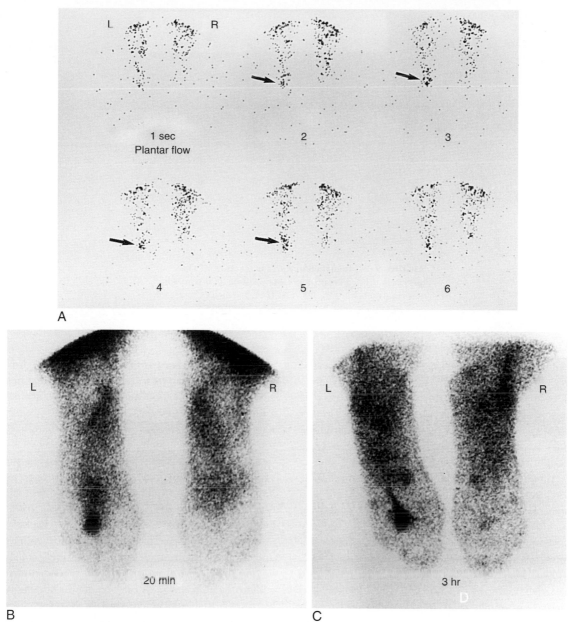

FIGURE 9–36. Fatigue stress fracture of the foot. This college soccer player had persistent foot pain. The plantar views on this three-phase bone scan reveal an abnormality of the left third distal metatarsal with increased blood flow (*A, arrows*), increased blood pooling (*B*), and a more intense and focal increase in activity on the 3-hour delayed views (*C*).

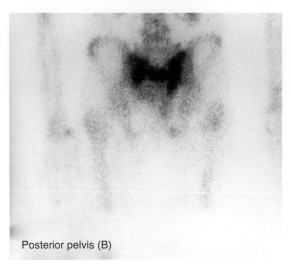

Posterior pelvis (B)

FIGURE 9–37. Insufficiency stress fracture of the pelvis. A delayed image from a bone scan in a 70-year-old woman with pelvic pain shows an H-shaped area of increased activity in the sacrum (the Honda sign).

Failure to find areas of increased activity is useful in excluding the diagnosis of child battering. Detection of trauma at the ends of long bones may be complicated by the often intense activity in the physes of children. In most cases, a combination of bone scan and radiographs is the best approach to evaluation.

In elderly patients, the bone scan may not show the fracture for several days. A negative bone scan obtained a week after trauma, however, effectively excludes an occult fracture. SPECT scans may occasionally be useful for demonstration of occult fractures, particularly in the spine (Fig. 9–38). SPECT imaging of the spine may also be helpful for detection of pseudoarthrosis. Pronounced increase in uptake more than 1 year after fusion is highly indicative of motion in a failed spinal fusion.

Another use of bone scans in trauma is in the *assessment of hip prostheses.* In the initial postsurgical period, activity is noted around cemented prostheses, although this usually rapidly decreases and returns to normal within 12 months. With a porous coated prosthesis, generalized increased activity may be seen even at 2 years because fixation depends on bony ingrowth. Persistent activity at the trochanter and at the tip of the prosthesis may be taken as an indication of loosening (77% specific and 100% sensitive) (Fig. 9–39). For both hip as well as knee prostheses, loosening may also be assessed by injecting the joint with ^{99m}Tc sulfur colloid (nuclear medicine arthrogram) to determine

if activity accumulates around the stem of the prosthesis, an indication of loosening. Postsurgical heterotopic bone formation may be visualized around a hip joint on bone scans, but this usually is easily recognized by its position predominantly lateral to the acetabulum.

Generalized increase in activity around a hip prosthesis, especially the shank (stem), may be indicative of osteomyelitis (Fig. 9–40). If there is a question of infection, a gallium scan may be useful because a normal scan effectively excludes osteomyelitis as the cause of symptoms. If gallium and ^{99m}Tc diphosphonate distributions are spatially incongruent, or if they are spatially congruent but gallium activity exceeds the technetium activity, osteomyelitis should be considered. If the gallium and technetium images are partially congruent and equal in intensity, the study is considered equivocal. An infected joint replacement is more specifically diagnosed by comparing an ^{111}In- or ^{99m}Tc-labeled leukocyte image with a technetium colloid marrow scan. When there is periprosthetic leukocyte accumulation without corresponding marrow activity on the colloid images, the study is positive for infection.

Osteomyelitis, Cellulitis, and Septic Arthritis

Early involvement of bone by an inflammatory disease process is often difficult to detect on radiographs. A number of imaging modalities can be

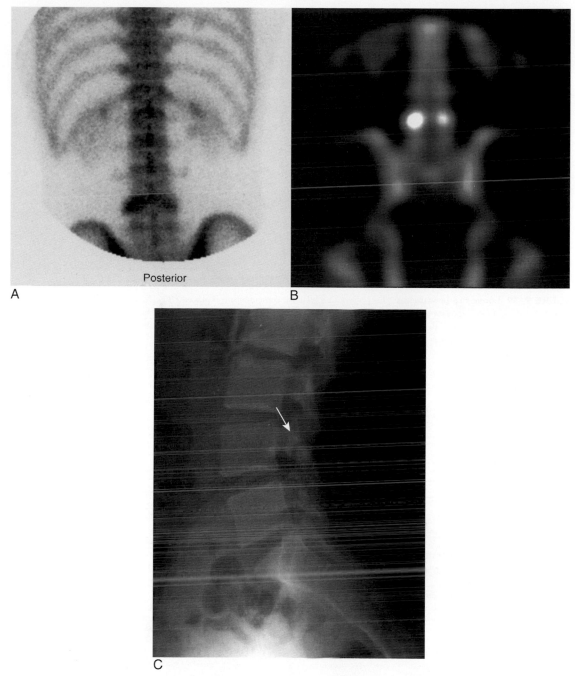

Posterior

A

B

C

FIGURE 9–38. Pars defect. A teenager with back pain was referred for a bone scan. Planar (*A*) and single-photon emission computed tomography (*B*) images show increased activity at the pedicles of L4. *C*, The lateral lumbar spine shows the pars defect as well.

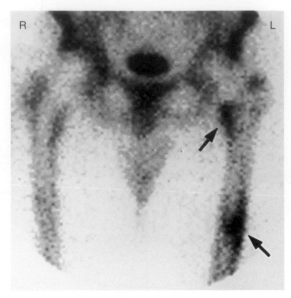

FIGURE 9–39. Loose hip prosthesis. This patient had bilateral cemented hip replacements 3 years ago. The prostheses account for the cold defects seen in the proximal femurs. The left prosthesis is loose, causing increased activity near the lesser trochanter and the distal tip of the prosthesis (*arrows*). The activity at the lesser trochanter is the fulcrum site, and the tip is the portion of the prosthesis with the greatest movement.

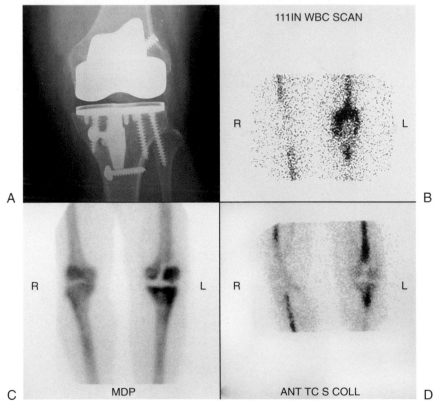

FIGURE 9–40. Infected prosthesis. *A,* An x-ray of the left knee shows a total knee arthroplasty which was painful. *B,* An indium 111 white cell scan shows activity about the proximal portion of the prosthesis and spatial nonconformity with the bone scan (*C*) activity. A bone marrow scan (*D*) done with technetium-99m sulfur colloid shows that the indium activity in not related to localized marrow hyperplasia.

used to evaluate osteomyelitis. MRI is highly effective and has excellent spatial resolution, but it is expensive and its use is limited in patients who have an infected metallic prosthesis. The earliest radiographic signs of osteomyelitis are nonspecific and include demineralization and loss of the soft-tissue fascial margins. At this stage, scanning with radionuclides often demonstrates strikingly increased activity, both in the soft tissues and in the underlying bony structures. However, if soft-tissue inflammation is a prominent feature, it occasionally may be difficult to distinguish primary bone involvement from bone activity secondary to the hyperemia that accompanies simple cellulitis.

A number of radiopharmaceuticals are available to evaluate osteomyelitis. These include ^{99m}Tc-diphosphonate, gallium-67 (^{67}Ga) citrate, and ^{111}In- or ^{99m}Tc-labeled leukocytes. In general, a three-phase ^{99m}Tc diphosphonate bone scan is performed first and if abnormal may establish the diagnosis. If the bone scan results are equivocal, further imaging with one of the other radiopharmaceuticals may be indicated.

To differentiate osteomyelitis from cellulitis on a ^{99m}Tc diphosphonate bone scan, a radionuclide angiogram and an immediate blood pool image should be obtained after injection, and routine images should be taken at 2 to 3 hours. Such three-phase scintigraphy has been widely advocated to improve bone scan specificity in this setting. Cellulitis presents as increased blood flow (perfusion) and diffusely increased soft tissue on early images, with decreasing activity on later scans (Fig. 9–41). No significant foci of increased bony activity should be seen on the delayed images in the area of concern. Osteomyelitis, on the other hand, demonstrates increased blood flow and blood pool activity with accumulation of bone activity that becomes more focal and intense on delayed scans (Fig. 9–42). The absence of increased perfusion and blood pool activity casts serious doubt on a diagnosis of osteomyelitis as a cause for a focus of increased activity in bone on delayed images. Although scintigraphy is extremely sensitive, some false-negative scans have been reported early in the disease, perhaps secondary to disruption of the blood supply to the bone. Subperiosteal collections of pus may even produce focal photopenic defects (especially in young children). If osteomyelitis is strongly suspected on a clinical basis, and if the radionuclide bone scan is negative or nondiagnostic, a gallium scan may prove useful. If the ^{67}Ga citrate study is normal, osteomyelitis is unlikely, but if the uptake of gallium exceeds the uptake of bone agent in the same location, osteomyelitis is probable. The use of labeled leukocytes in the evaluation of complicated osteomyelitis is discussed in Chapter 12.

Septic arthritis is almost always seen as increased activity in all phases of a three-phase bone scan. Usually, it can be differentiated from osteomyelitis by the presence of diffusely increased bone activity on both sides of the joint (Fig. 9–43), as opposed to osteomyelitis in which the bony activity is typically focal and increased on only one side of the joint.

Diskitis is a condition of uncertain etiology that usually occurs in children. On bone scan, there is usually increased activity of two contiguous lumbar vertebral bodies, often just the adjacent end-plates, and radiographs may show a narrowed disk space (Fig. 9–44).

Benign Non-Neoplastic Disease
Paget's disease

Paget's disease characteristically displays a marked increase in activity in large part due to the greatly increased regional blood flow. The increased activity usually conforms to the shape of all or part of the involved bone. There is often notable expansion or enlargement of the bone, and the increased activity characteristically extends to one end of the bone when a long bone is involved (Figs. 9–45 and 9–46). The disease is polyostotic in about 70% to 80% of cases. Although the osteolytic phase of the disease is often difficult to appreciate on radiographs, it is almost always represented by increased activity on bone scans. The dense sclerotic lesions seen late in the osteoblastic stage of the disease may demonstrate varying degrees of increased activity, and some "burned out" lesions may show only minimally increased or normal activity. At some institutions, serial quantitative bone scans using computer assessment of bone activity are performed to evaluate response of Paget's disease to therapy. Sarcomatous degeneration occurs in approximately 1% of Paget's disease patients. This initially results in increasing activity in the area of involvement over time. Later, the malignant area may appear photopenic, likely resulting from necrotic areas within the lesion.

Hypertrophic pulmonary osteoarthropathy

Hypertrophic pulmonary osteoarthropathy causes periosteal reaction, particularly in the long bones. It is most commonly seen in patients with lung

Text continued on p. 284

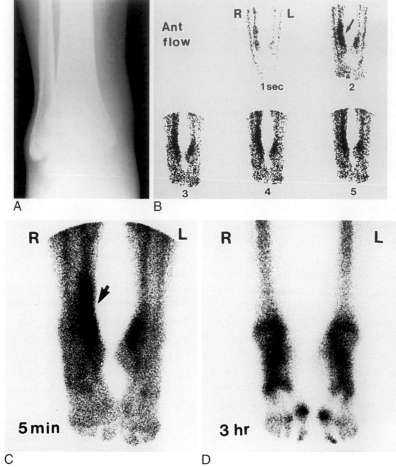

FIGURE 9–41. Cellulitis. This drug abuser had pain, redness, and swelling over the medial aspect of the right ankle. *A,* The soft-tissue swelling was evident on the anteroposterior radiograph of the ankle. On the bone scan, there is increased activity on the angiographic images (*B*) and blood pool image (*C*) at 5 minutes (*arrows*). By the 3-hour image (*D*), the activity had faded, indicating no evidence of osteomyelitis.

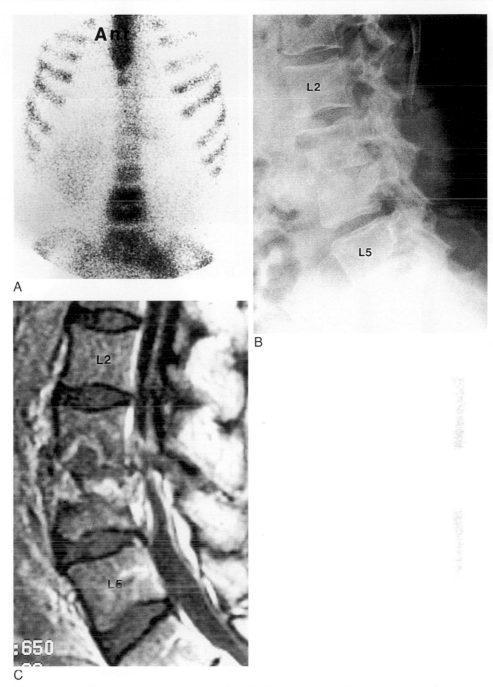

FIGURE 9–44. Diskitis. In this child with persistent back pain, the delayed bone scan image (*A*) shows increased activity in two contiguous vertebral bodies. The lateral radiograph (*B*) shows accompanying loss of L3–4 disk space. A magnetic resonance image (*C*) shows involvement of the vertebral bodies. The cause of this entity remains obscure.

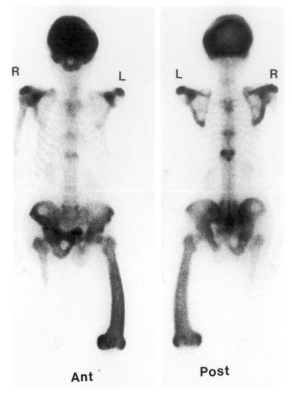

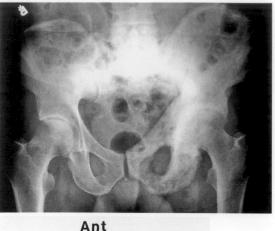

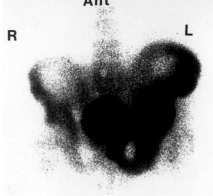

FIGURE 9–45. Extensive Paget's disease. In this deaf patient with the sclerotic form of Paget's disease, there is markedly increased activity in the skull and left femur. The femur is bowed, owing to associated bone softening. The marked increase in activity seen on the bone scan is predominantly the result of increased blood flow.

FIGURE 9–46. Paget's disease of the pelvis. In this patient, there was an unexpected finding of expansion and sclerosis in the left hemipelvis on an intravenous pyelogram scout film (*top*). The delayed images from a bone scan (*bottom*) show intensely increased activity confined to the left side of the pelvis. This is characteristic and is probably the most common presentation of Paget's disease.

cancer. The appearance on bone scan is that of distinctive parallel lines of activity along the cortex of the shafts and ends of the tibias, femurs, and radii (Fig. 9–47), especially around the knees, ankles, and wrists. This activity may decrease after treatment of the underlying disease.

Aseptic Arthritis

Bone scanning may be used as a method for documenting the early presence of various forms of arthritis as well as for assessing serial changes in the disease. Unfortunately, juxta-articular increased activity on a ^{99m}Tc diphosphonate bone scan is nonspecific and cannot reliably distinguish among synovitis, active arthritis, and old inactive disease. Both intravenously administered ^{99m}Tc pertechnetate and the diphosphonate bone imaging agents have been used for arthritis imaging. Technetium-99m pertechnetate is probably more specific for regions of synovial inflammation because it is able to diffuse across the synovial surface and into joint

effusions, whereas phosphate compounds localize primarily in adjacent bone. Because bone scanning for arthritis is limited by lack of specificity, radiologic correlation of results is mandatory.

Metabolic Bone Disease

As discussed earlier, primary hyperparathyroidism and renal osteodystrophy resulting from secondary hyperparathyroidism may produce a *superscan* with diffusely increased activity throughout the skeleton, including the skull, mandible, and long bones, and relatively diminished or absent renal activity. This may be accompanied by increased activity in the thyroid, lungs, stomach, and kidneys caused my so-called *metastatic calcification* in these organs. When brown tumors are present, focal areas of increased activity in the skeleton may be seen.

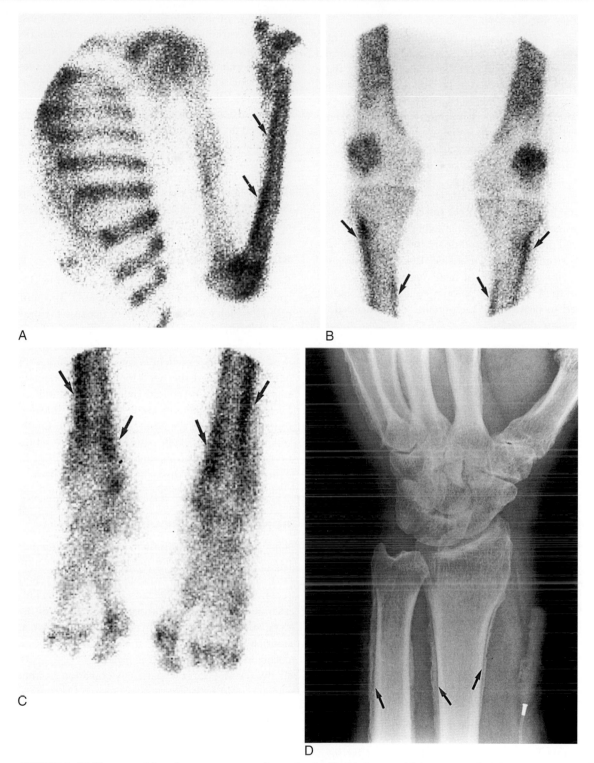

FIGURE 9–47. Hypertrophic pulmonary osteoarthropathy. In this elderly man with lung cancer, the 3-hour bone scan images show increased activity (*arrows*) in the cortical regions of the shafts of the radius (*A*) and both tibias (*B* and *C*). *D*, Radiograph of the wrist shows marked periosteal reaction (*arrows*).

Avascular Necrosis

Avascular necrosis is often due to trauma, but it may have a variety of other causes, including steroid administration and vascular disease. Initially, there is generally decreased tracer activity in the affected area. This is followed by a hyperemic or repair phase, which is characterized by increased activity. Correlation with the radiographs is mandatory to diagnose avascular necrosis accurately. MRI is probably more accurate and thus more widely used for this diagnosis. Some laboratories have used bone scans to demonstrate femoral head viability in patients with femoral neck fractures. Either diphosphonate or sulfur colloid imaging may be used. The usual procedure is to compare the normal side with the suspected abnormal side. Relatively decreased activity in the femoral head suggests avascularity. For these studies, a pinhole collimator should be used to provide the high-quality detail needed for accurate diagnosis.

Spontaneous Osteonecrosis of the Knee

Spontaneous osteonecrosis of the knee usually presents as acute knee pain, especially medially, in elderly, often osteoporotic females. Intensely increased activity in the medial femoral condyle essentially establishes or confirms the diagnosis in this setting. The disease may also occur in the medial tibial plateau or lateral femoral condyle.

Radiation Therapy

Radiation therapy constitutes a form of calculated iatrogenic trauma. Multiple factors determine the bone scan findings after radiation treatment, including the cumulative amount of radiation, fractionation of doses, and length of time after therapy that the bone scan is performed. After fractionated radiation doses of 4000 to 5000 rad (40 to 50 Gy) to bone, there is a decrease in localized vascular patency in the area of treatment within the first month. The vascularity may return to near normal in about 6 months and then is reduced again, owing to endothelial proliferation and arteriolar narrowing. An abrupt geometric area of decreased osseous activity should raise the suspicion of skeletal trauma due to radiation therapy (see Fig. 9–10).

Reflex Sympathetic Dystrophy

Reflex sympathetic dystrophy (RSD) syndrome consists of pain, tenderness, swelling, and vasomotor instability in the affected limb. Its cause is obscure, but RSD is usually precipitated by trauma, myocardial infarction, or neurologic abnormality. The most common variants are *Sudeck's atrophy* and *shoulder-hand syndrome*. Radiographically, there is usually patchy periarticular osteoporosis. Classically, three-phase bone scanning demonstrates increased blood flow to the affected limb with increased asymmetric periarticular radionuclide activity. Diffusely increased juxta-articular activity around all joints of the hand or foot on delayed images may be the most sensitive indicator of RSD (Fig. 9–48). About one third of adult patients with documented RSD do not show increased perfusion and uptake. In children, decreased perfusion and uptake is a common manifestation.

BONE MARROW IMAGING

Bone marrow scans can be used define marrow distribution. The most common agent is ^{99m}Tc sulfur colloid, which localizes in marrow because the particles are phagocytized by the resident reticuloendothelial cells in the marrow. The widespread availability and excellent anatomic resolution of MRI has reduced the need for most radionuclide marrow scans. On colloid marrow scans, intense liver and spleen activity may need to be shielded during imaging. In the adult, the marrow is usually restricted to the skull, ribs, sternum, vertebral bodies, pelvis, and proximal humerii and femurs. In children, the normal marrow extends more peripherally into the extremities.

BONE MINERAL MEASUREMENTS

The accurate measurement of bone mineral density using noninvasive methods can be of value in the detection and evaluation of primary and secondary causes of decreased bone mass. This includes primary osteoporosis and secondary disorders, such as hyperparathyroidism, osteomalacia, multiple myeloma, diffuse metastases, and glucocorticoid therapy or intrinsic excess.

By far the largest patient population is that encompassed by primary osteoporosis. Osteoporosis is an age-related disorder characterized by decreased bone mass and increased susceptibility to fractures in the absence of other recognizable causes of bone loss. Primary osteoporosis is generally subdivided into type 1 (postmenopausal osteoporosis), which is related to estrogen deprivation, and type 2 (senile osteoporosis), which occurs secondary to aging.

Primary osteoporosis is a common clinical disorder and a major public health problem because

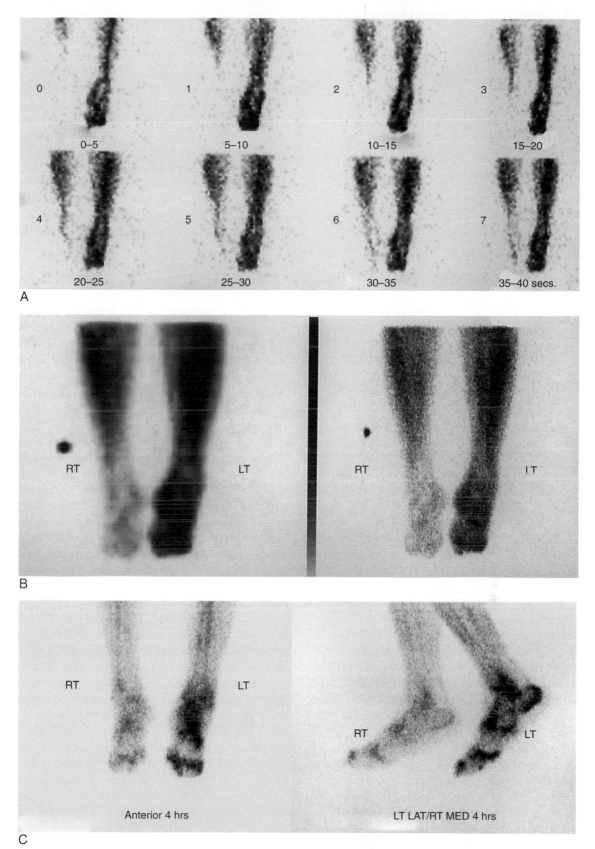

FIGURE 9–48. Reflex sympathetic dystrophy. A young female with minor ankle trauma had continuing pain. The angiographic (*A*) and blood pool (*B*) images show diffusely increased activity to the entire lower extremity. The delayed (*C*) and whole-body (*D*) images show increased activity in a periarticular distribution.

mineral. Both dual-photon absorptiometry (DPA) and DEXA use a highly collimated beam of photons or x-rays that passes through the soft tissue and bony components of the body to be detected on the opposite side by a scintillation detector. Because absorption by the body part examined (primarily by bone mineral) attenuates the photon x-ray beam, the intensity of the beam exiting the body part is indirectly proportional to the density of the bony structure being evaluated. The intensity of the exit beam is then compared with exit beam intensity from standard phantoms of known density, so that a bone mineral density can be determined. The results are expressed in grams per square centimeter.

The DPA and DEXA beams consist of photons or x-rays of two discrete energies, which obviates the need for assumptions about soft-tissue shape and attenuation. It also allows for evaluation of thicker body parts and bones involving complex geometry, such as the femoral neck and the spine. When the spine is examined, the hips are flexed to flatten the normal lumbar lordosis. When scans of the femoral neck are performed, the femur should be in slight internal rotation.

By using an x-ray tube rather than a radionuclide source, purchase of replacement radionuclide sources and recalibration are unnecessary. In addition, scan time is only 2 to 5 minutes for DEXA, compared with 20 to 40 minutes for DPA. Precision and image quality are also much better for DEXA than for DPA.

Falsely elevated bone mineral content when evaluating the spine may result from marked aortic calcification, scoliosis, hypertrophic degenerative disease, compression fractures, calcium or barium within the gastrointestinal tract, renal lithiasis, bone grafts, focal sclerotic bone lesions, or recent intake of aluminum-containing antacids. Falsely low bone mineral results may be obtained in patients who have had a laminectomy or lytic bone lesions. Most of the time, these problems can be identified from the plain radiograph, if available before the test.

The use of bone mineral measurement has been controversial. Some of this controversy is because of the wide variation of measurements in the normal population. Also, the criteria for selecting the optimal skeletal site for evaluation have not been well defined because bone mineral loss does not progress at the same rate at different body sites. Measurement of the hip bone mineral density is done to evaluate the risk for hip fracture, whereas

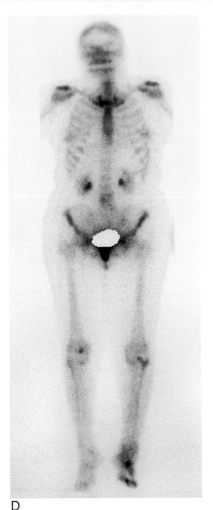

D

FIGURE 9–48, cont'd
For legend see p. 287

of the significant number of related bone fractures occurring annually. Because the risk of vertebral and femoral neck fractures rises dramatically as bone mineral density falls below 1 g/cm^2, fracture risk in individual patients may be estimated. Furthermore, in estrogen-deficient women, bone mineral density values may be used to make rational decisions about hormone replacement therapy, or other bone mineral therapies, and as follow-up in assessing the success of such treatment.

A number of methods have been devised to permit the accurate and reproducible determination of bone mineral content. The advent of radionuclide absorptiometry using dual-photon technique evoked a sustained interest in the screening of patients for osteoporosis. However, dual x-ray absorptiometry (DEXA) has replaced the radionuclide method for determination of bone

vertebral bodies are regarded as the optimal site for monitoring response to treatment. Care must be taken to look at the images to ensure that extensive degenerative changes or surgical defects are not causing erroneous values (Fig. 9–49).

Most manufacturers express results that compare the patient's bone mineral density either to age-matched controls (Z score) or to a young normal population (T score) felt to be representative of peak bone mass. These comparisons may be expressed as percentiles or as standard deviations from the normal range. As determined by the World Health Organization (WHO), a T score of greater (less negative) than −1.0 (<1 standard deviation below young normal controls) is considered normal. Between −1.0 and −2.5 is considered to be evidence of osteopenia. Less (more negative) than −2.5 is consistent with osteoporosis. Thus, the method can be used to determine the presence of osteopenia or osteoporosis and to evaluate effectiveness of a therapeutic maneuver by using serial scans in which the patient acts as his or her own control. A normal result, or a bone mineral content in the upper end of the normal range, identifies a patient in whom therapy may not be needed.

THERAPY OF PAINFUL OSSEOUS METASTASES

A large number of patients have extensive and diffuse painful blastic osseous metastases from various primary lesions that are not amenable to

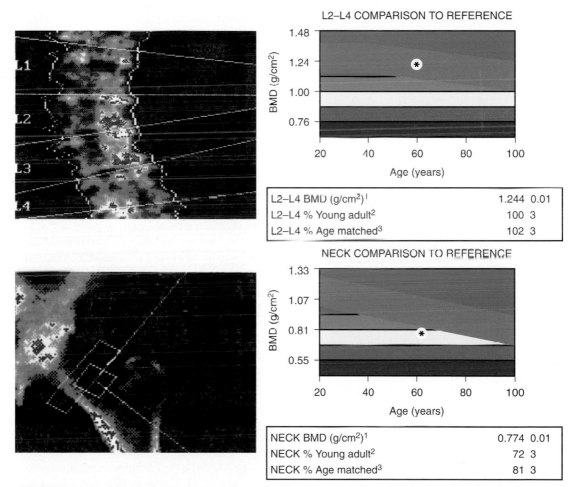

FIGURE 9–49. Dual X-ray absorptiometry. Bone mineral measurements done on the lumbar spine of a 61-year-old female with lumbar scoliosis (*upper row*) suggest that the bone mineral measurements are normal. This is actually artifact due to the extensive osteophytes. When the region of interest is taken over the femoral neck (*lower row*), it can be seen that the patient has low bone mineral density.

external beam radiotherapy or that are unresponsive to chemotherapy. Many of these patients are men with prostate cancer. Therapies with intravenously administered radionuclides are directed at palliation of pain (not at cure), decreased need for opiates, and improved quality of life. With most of the methods, the patient may have a transient increase in pain beginning 2 to 3 days after treatment and lasting for several days due to transient swelling of the treated lesions. Palliative symptomatic improvement usually begins 7 to 20 days after treatment and often lasts 3 to 6 months. Pain will not be relieved if it is caused by a pathological fracture or is of nonosseous origin (such as epidural metastases with pressure on the spinal cord or soft-tissue masses pressing on nerves). A routine bone scan should be performed before this type of therapy to ensure that there will be uptake of the therapeutic radiopharmaceutical. A normal bone scan would suggest another source of pain. External beam teletherapy is recommended if there are only one or two lesions causing the patient's pain or if there is impending spinal cord compression.

The most commonly used radionuclide is strontium-89 (^{89}Sr) chloride (Metastron). The radionuclide decays by beta emission with a physical half-life of 50.5 days. The maximum range of the beta emission in tissue is 8 mm. After intravenous administration, localization in bone occurs in areas of active osteogenesis. Metastases with a blastic response have significantly more concentration and longer retention than does normal bone. Excretion is primarily urinary and to a lesser extent fecal. For the first week, medical staff handling these items should wear gloves and follow local disposal regulations.

Strontium-89 therapy depresses the bone marrow and should not be used if the leukocyte count is below $2400/\mu L$ or if the platelets are below $60,000/\mu L$. The typical dose is 40 to 60 $\mu Ci/kg$ (1.5 to 2.2 MBq/kg) up to 4 mCi (148 MBq) given by slow (1 to 2 minutes) intravenous injection using syringe shielding (especially plastic) appropriate for a beta-emitting radionuclide. After administration, peripheral leukocyte counts are usually obtained every 2 weeks until marrow recovery occurs. Repeated doses are usually not given at intervals of less than 3 to 4 months, and it is unusual to give more than three doses without being cautious about bone marrow reserve. Because excretion is primarily urinary, ^{89}Sr therapy should be used advisedly in patients with decreased renal function.

Pain relief typically takes 1 to 3 weeks to become apparent, and generally this therapy should not be used in patients with a life expectancy of less than 3 months. In addition, issues relative to handling of a deceased patient recently treated with ^{89}Sr need to be addressed. Many states have regulations prohibiting cremation in this setting, and some have allowed only certain funeral homes to service these patients.

Other radiopharmaceuticals have been developed and used with some success. These are rhenium-186 (^{186}Re) hydroxyethylenediphosphonate (HEDP or etidronate) and samarium-153 (^{153}Sm) ethylenediaminetetramethylene phosphonic acid (EDPMT), also known as ^{153}Sm lexidronam (Quadramet). These agents have been used in patients with more metabolically active metastases from prostate and breast cancer, as well as in those from osteogenic sarcoma. Rhenium is in the same chemical family as technetium, and much of the same chemistry can be used. The physical half-life is 90 hours, which allows a large radiation dose to be delivered in a relatively short time. In addition to beta emissions, there is gamma emission (187 keV), which allows imaging. Unfortunately, the dose to normal bone is high. This has not been approved for use in the United States but is widely used in Europe.

Samarium-153 (lexidronam or Quadramet) EDPMT has many of the advantages of rhenium, including a short half-life (46 hours) and, in addition to beta rays, a gamma photon (103 keV, 30% abundance) that can be imaged. Imaging is usually done at 6 hours after administration. There may be an initial increase in bone pain within 72 hours, which usually responds to analgesics. Pain relief may begin at about 1 week and reaches a maximum in about 3 weeks. About 70% of patients report pain relief, and about 35% report to be "much better" or "completely improved." No additional advantage is obtained by dose escalation. There can be bone marrow suppression, and about 95% of patients will have a nadir of white blood cell counts and platelets to about 40% to 50% of baseline at 3 to 5 weeks. As a result, it should not be given concurrently with radiation therapy or chemotherapy unless marrow status has been adequately evaluated. The recommended dose is 1.0 mCi/kg (37 MBq/kg) administered intravenously over a period of 1 minute followed with a saline flush. Hydration following injection is recommended to reduce bladder dose because about one third of the administered activity is eliminated in the urine in the first 6 hours. Precautions should be in place for 12 hours by using a toilet instead of urinal and flushing several times. Blood counts should be monitored weekly for at least 8 weeks. No other radiation protection precautions are necessary relative to family members and the public.

PEARLS & PITFALLS

Musculoskeletal

Common indications for bone scans include evaluation of primary osseous or metastatic neoplasms, avascular necrosis of the hips or shoulders, trauma, infection, and, less commonly, arthritis or RSD in the peripheral skeleton.

When bone scans are performed with ^{99m}Tc diphosphonate agents, normal skeletal activity should be reasonably symmetric on the left and right sides.

Look at kidney activity for potential abnormalities. A large amount of diffuse soft-tissue activity remaining at 4 hours is frequently due to renal insufficiency.

Activity in the lower cervical region is frequently due to benign causes such as degenerative arthritis.

A lesion that is hot on all three phases of a bone scan can be osteomyelitis but also may be an acute fracture, hypervascular tumor, neuropathic joint, or RSD.

Most osseous metastases begin in the red marrow and therefore are predominantly located in the skull, ribs, spine, pelvis, and proximal extremities.

In a patient with known metastases, an increasing apparent number and intensity of lesions compared with prior bone scans can indicate more disease or may indicate the flare phenomenon from recent treatment. A flare phenomenon is most likely seen within 1 to 3 months of therapy completion.

Not all multifocal hot lesions are metastases; also consider fractures, multifocal osteomyelitis, multiple enchondromas, polyostotic fibrous dysplasia, or Paget's disease.

Paget's disease is commonly seen as intense activity in the skull, femur, vertebral body, or half of the pelvis. It is usually polyostotic (80%), but it may be monostotic and may cause bowing of a femur.

Good visualization of the bones and not of the kidneys may indicate a superscan due to diffuse metastases or hyperparathyroidism. If the skull is hot and the distal extremities are well seen, it is probably the latter.

Focal hot lesions in multiple adjacent ribs are essentially always due to fractures. Long lesions running along the length of a rib are not usually fractures.

Cold lesions can be due to poor perfusion of an area of bone, lack of bony matrix (aggressive tumor), overlying attenuating material, or gamma camera dysfunction, such as a bad photomultiplier tube.

Multiple sequential cold vertebral bodies are almost always due to radiation therapy.

Tumors that commonly cause cold (photopenic) metastatic lesions include kidney, lung, thyroid, and breast tumors.

Stress fractures usually occur in the pelvis and below the knees. They can be seen as focal or fusiform, primarily cortical activity.

Bilaterally increased activity along the cortex of the tibias may be due to shin splints, hypertrophic osteoarthropathy, or periosteal reaction of other causes.

A loose hip prosthesis is suggested by activity at the tip and near the lesser trochanter. An infected prosthesis usually has activity all along the length of the shaft. Postoperative activity around a cemented prosthesis can normally persist for 6 months to 1 year, and activity around a noncemented prosthesis can normally persist for 2 to 3 years.

Focal soft-tissue activity can be due to a process that makes bone (osteosarcoma metastases), calcifies (cancer of the colon, ovary, breast, neuroblastoma), or causes dystrophic calcification (infarction, myositis ossificans, tumoral calcinosis, dermatomyositis, polymyositis).

Diffuse liver activity on a bone scan is probably due to hepatic necrosis or to a radiopharmaceutical problem. Focal liver activity is often due to metastases from colon, breast, ovary, or lung. Diffuse splenic activity is probably

PEARLS & PITFALLS—cont'd

due to splenic infarction (e.g., sickle cell disease). Diffuse renal parenchymal activity is probably due to chemotherapy, especially if bone metastases are present.

Increased activity in two adjacent vertebral bodies in the absence of compression fractures suggests diskitis, especially in a child.

Osteomyelitis, acute fractures, vascular tumors, such as Ewing's sarcoma, and RSD are hot on angiographic, blood pool, and delayed bone scan images. Cellulitis is hot on the first two phases but fades on delayed images. Shin splints have normal angiographic and blood pool images but are hot on delayed views in the posteromedial aspects of the tibias (insertion of the soleus muscle).

Osteomyelitis usually does not cross joints. Increased activity seen on both sides of a joint is more likely the result of septic arthritis.

SUGGESTED READINGS

Charron M, Brown ML: Primary and metastatic bone disease. In Sandler MP, Coleman RE, Patton JA, et al. (eds): Diagnostic Nuclear Medicine, 4th ed. New York, Lippincott Williams and Wilkins, 2003, pp 413–428.

Chengazi VU, O'Mara RE: Benign bone disease. In Sandler MP, Coleman RE, Patton JA, et al. (eds): Diagnostic Nuclear Medicine, 4th ed. New York, Lippincott Williams and Wilkins, 2003, pp 429–462.

De Maeseneer M, Lenchik L, Everaert H, Marcelis S, Bossuyt A, Osteaux M, Beeckman P: Evaluation of Lower Back Pain with Bone Scintigraphy and SPECT. RadioGraphics 19:901–912, 1999.

Fogelman I, Blake GM: Different approaches to bone densitometry, continuing education. J Nucl Med 41:2015–2025, 2000.

Love C, Din A, Tomas M, et al: Radionuclide bone imaging: an illustrative review. Radiographics 23:341–358, 2003.

Love C, Tomas M, Marwin S., et al: Role of nuclear medicine in diagnosis of the infected joint replacement. RadioGraphics 21:1229–1238, 2001.

Pandit-Taskar N, Batraki M, Divgi CR: Radiopharmaceutical Therapy for Palliation of Bone Pain from Osseous Metastases. J Nucl Med 45:1358–1365, 2004.

Silberstein EB: Treatment of pain from bone metasases employing unsealed sources. In Sandler MP, Coleman RE, Patton JA, et al. (eds): Diagnostic Nuclear Medicine, 4th ed. New York, Lippincott, Williams and Wilkins, 2003, pp. 1027–1034.

Genitourinary System and Adrenal Glands

10

INTRODUCTION

Radionuclide evaluation of the genitourinary system includes quantitative estimates of renal perfusion and function. With the widespread use of ultrasound and computed tomography (CT), the evaluation of renal anatomy by nuclear techniques has diminished, and the role of nuclear renal imaging has become more confined to functional analysis. Indications for renal scanning include sensitivity to radiographic contrast material, assessment of renal blood flow, and differential or quantitative functional assessment of both native and transplanted kidneys. Nuclear techniques have also proved of value in evaluating ureteral or renal pelvic obstruction, vesicoureteral reflux, and suspected renovascular hypertension, with pharmacologic interventions used when indicated. Imaging of prostatic cancer with antibodies is discussed in Chapter 11; with PET scanning, in Chapter 13. Osseous metastases from prostate cancer are discussed in Chapter 9.

PHYSIOLOGY

The excretory function of the kidneys consists of two primary mechanisms: passive filtration through the glomerulus and active secretion by the tubules. These processes are tempered by varying reabsorption of certain substances by the tubules. The glomerulus acts as a semipermeable membrane, allowing only those compounds of a relatively small molecular size to pass through. Larger materials, such as proteins, do not pass through the glomerulus but may reach the urine by tubular secretion.

The rate at which a particular substance is cleared (C) from the plasma by these mechanisms is determined by the following formula:

$$C = UV/P$$

where U and P represent the urine and plasma concentrations of the substance and V is the rate of urine production in milliliters per minute. The model compound for determining glomerular filtration is inulin, which is freely filtered at the

293

glomerulus and is not secreted or reabsorbed by the tubules. Diethylenetriaminepenta-acetic acid (DTPA) and other chelates are also cleared by glomerular filtration and may be used as a measure of glomerular function. The normal glomerular filtration rate (GFR) is 125 mL/min.

Evaluation of renal tubular secretion has historically been performed with iodohippurate sodium (Hippuran). About 80% of iodohippurate sodium is eliminated by the tubular secretion pathway, although a rapid component (about 20%) reaches the urine through glomerular filtration. More recently, iodohippurate has been replaced in many clinical practices by the technetium-99m (^{99m}Tc)-labeled agent mercaptoacetyltriglycine (mertiatide or MAG3), which produces nearly identical results. In nuclear radiology practice, ^{99m}Tc-DTPA and ^{99m}Tc-MAG3 are routinely used for assessment of glomerular and tubular function, respectively.

RADIOPHARMACEUTICALS

Radiopharmaceuticals commonly used for evaluating renal function and anatomy fall into three main categories:

- Those excreted by tubular secretion
- Those excreted by glomerular filtration
- Those bound in the renal tubules for a sufficiently long time to permit cortical anatomic imaging

A thorough knowledge of the biodynamics of these classes of radiopharmaceuticals is essential for choosing the best radiopharmaceutical for a particular clinical setting. Sample imaging protocols and radiation dosimetry are presented in Appendix E–1.

Glomerular Filtration Agents

Technetium-99m DTPA is the radiopharmaceutical used for evaluation of glomerular filtration function. As the DTPA complex is cleared by the renal glomeruli, serial images may be obtained that demonstrate sequential visualization of the kidneys and collecting systems, ureters, and bladder, similar to a radiographic intravenous contrast urogram (IVP). Measurement of its excretion can also provide an accurate estimate of GFR. Because a small amount ($\approx$ 5% to 10%) of injected DTPA is bound to plasma proteins, it tends to underestimate the GFR slightly. For routine clinical applications, however, this is generally not significant. About 20% of ^{99m}Tc-DTPA is extracted from the blood

with each pass through the kidney (extraction fraction), so that about 90% of DTPA is filtered by simple exchange or diffusion into the urine within 4 hours. This makes it an excellent, inexpensive agent for routine renal imaging and as a substitute for intravenous urography in patients who are allergic to radiographic contrast. Because the nephrogram phase of the examination is brief, however, it is not an ideal agent for demonstrating intraparenchymal renal lesions. In addition, it may not be the agent of choice in patients with obstruction or impaired renal function in whom tubular agents with higher extraction efficiencies allow for increased excretion and better renal visualization. Technetium-99m DTPA is normally administered in activities of 10 to 20 mCi (370 to 740 MBq).

Tubular Secretion Agents

Iodine-131 orthoiodohippurate (^{131}I-OIH) is the classic tubular imaging agent, but has been replaced in clinical practice by ^{99m}Tc-MAG3. As ^{99m}Tc-MAG3 is cleared predominately by the proximal tubules (95%) with minimal filtration (<5%), it behaves much as radioiodinated orthoiodohippurate does. Its ^{99m}Tc label produces much better images. In addition, with an extraction fraction of 40% to 50% (more than twice that of ^{99m}Tc-DTPA), it provides more satisfactory images than does ^{99m}Tc-DTPA, especially in patients with obstruction or impaired renal function. Because ^{99m}Tc-MAG3 is highly protein bound, it has significantly higher plasma concentrations than does ^{131}I-OIH, which readily distributes from the plasma into the red blood cells. Thus, even though ^{99m}Tc-MAG3 exhibits only about half of the clearance of ^{131}I-OIH, this is almost exactly compensated for by the greater proportion of MAG3 that remains in the plasma and therefore is available for extraction. This produces essentially similar rates of excretion by the kidneys of both MAG3 and OIH, producing virtually identical renogram curves. The clearance of MAG3 by the kidneys can be used to measure effective renal plasma flow (ERPF). Activities administered are 10 to 20 mCi (370 to 740 MBq) in adults.

Renal Cortical Agents

The two radiopharmaceuticals commonly used for visualization of the renal parenchyma are ^{99m}Tc-dimercaptosuccinic acid (DMSA) and ^{99m}Tc-glucoheptonate. Both of these agents bind sufficiently to the renal tubules to permit renal cortical imaging.

Technetium-99m DMSA is an excellent cortical imaging agent, with about 40% of the injected dose concentrated in the renal cortex at 6 hours and the remainder being slowly excreted. DMSA is of particular value when high-resolution images of the renal cortex are needed and when there is no need to identify abnormalities in the ureters or bladder because these structures are not effectively imaged. DMSA localizes by binding to the sulfhydryl groups in the proximal renal tubules. Only 10% of the radiopharmaceutical is excreted in the urine during the first several hours. The radiopharmaceutical activity normally used is 1 to 5 mCi (37 to 185 MBq). The radiation dose to the kidneys with DMSA is high because there is a long effective half-life of the radiopharmaceutical in the kidneys. Another disadvantage of ^{99m}Tc-DMSA is its short shelf-life after preparation. In addition, because of its slow clearance rate, delayed images 1 to 3 hours after injection are frequently necessary in patients with poor renal function to allow for improved kidney-to-background ratios.

Technetium-99m glucoheptonate is a radiolabeled carbohydrate cleared by the kidneys both by glomerular filtration and by the renal tubules. Thus, early images permit assessment of renal perfusion as well as evaluation of the renal collecting systems and ureters. Early camera images demonstrate the renal cortex and the collecting system, although the renal cortex remains well visualized 2 to 4 hours after administration. Ten percent to 15% of the injected dose remains bound to the renal tubules, and 40% is cleared through the urine at 1 hour. Thus, 1- to 2-hour images permit excellent visualization of the renal cortex. Technetium-99m glucoheptonate is stable and may be used for up to 5 hours after preparation. The usual administered activity is 10 to 20 mCi (370 to 740 MBq).

RADIONUCLIDE RENAL EVALUATION

Evaluation of the kidneys with radiopharmaceuticals may be performed by using a variety of methods, each providing a slightly different approach to assessment of renal function or anatomy. These methods include the following:

- Functional imaging (visual assessment of perfusion and function)
- Renography (time-activity curves representative of function)
- Quantification of renal function (GFR and ERPF determinations)

- Anatomic imaging (visual assessment of renal cortex)

Functional Renal Imaging

Radionuclide imaging with ^{99m}Tc-labeled agents is an excellent alternative to intravenous urography that provides anatomic, functional, and collecting system patency information. Imaging may be adequately performed in most patients by using either ^{99m}Tc-MAG3 or ^{99m}Tc-DPTA.

Functional imaging of the kidneys may be divided into assessment of blood flow, parenchyma, and excretion. Normally, both kidneys can easily be imaged on a standard- or large-field-of-view gamma camera with a parallel-hole collimator. Image information is usually collected in digital dynamic mode or on an interfaced computer and reformatted in temporal sequences that reflect both initial renal perfusion and subsequent function.

Renal Perfusion Imaging

Evaluation of renal blood flow and function of native kidneys is performed from the posterior projection, whereas evaluation of transplant blood flow and function is performed from the anterior projection. Normally, a small bolus of high-activity (10 to 20 mCi [370 to 740 MBq]), ^{99m}Tc-labeled radiopharmaceutical (^{99m}Tc-DTPA or ^{99m}Tc-MAG3) is injected intravenously, preferably into a large antecubital vein. Imaging renal perfusion is usually begun as the bolus is visualized in the proximal abdominal aorta, with subsequent serial images made every 1 to 5 seconds, depending on the instrumentation available and the preferences of the interpreter. A typical renal blood flow study is seen in Figure 10–1. The activity reaches the kidneys about 1 second after the bolus in the abdominal aorta passes the renal arteries. Time-activity curves reflecting renal perfusion during the first minute may be generated by drawing regions of interest over the aorta and each kidney. Each of the renal curves may then be compared with the time-activity curve of the abdominal aorta to assess relative renal perfusion. Occasionally, the spleen overlies the left kidney, giving a false impression of asymmetrically increased left renal perfusion or of a "phantom kidney" in patients with prior left nephrectomy.

Renal Function Imaging

At the end of the renal perfusion sequence, imaging for renal function begins. Dynamic or sequential static, 3- to 5-minute ^{99m}Tc-DTPA or ^{99m}Tc-MAG3

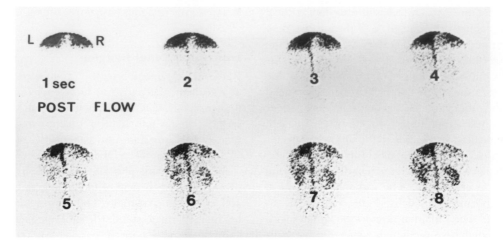

FIGURE 10–1. Normal renal blood flow. A bolus of technetium-99m DTPA in the lungs is visualized at the top of the serial images at 1 second. By 3 seconds, the aorta is fully visualized. By 5 to 6 seconds, both kidneys are clearly seen. The flow is symmetric to both kidneys. Note that in normal perfusion, the activity seen in the kidneys is about equal to that seen in the aorta just above the bifurcation. Maximal activity in the kidneys usually is reached later between 30 and 60 seconds.

(Fig. 10–2) images are then obtained over 20 to 30 minutes. Evaluation of the images is similar to that of an intravenous pyelogram, with attention to renal anatomy and position, symmetry and adequacy of function, and collecting system patency. With ^{99m}Tc-MAG3, the maximal parenchymal activity is seen at 3 to 5 minutes, with activity usually appearing in the collecting system and bladder by about 4 to 8 minutes. Some laboratories routinely use furosemide to clear activity from the renal collecting systems. However, postvoid or post-ambulation images to enhance collecting system drainage may be obtained as needed. Time-activity (renogram) curves for each kidney, reflective of relative renal function, are also usually created from regions of interest over the renal parenchyma, as discussed below.

Renography

A renogram is simply a time-activity curve that provides a graphic representation of the uptake and excretion of a radiopharmaceutical by the kidneys. Information is displayed from the time of injection to about 20 to 30 minutes after injection. The classic renogram curve is obtained by using agents that are eliminated by tubular secretion (e.g., ^{99m}Tc-MAG3). Renogram curves are generated by placing a region of interest around each kidney, usually the entire kidney, but occasionally just around the renal cortex if a considerable amount of collecting system activity is present. Background subtraction regions of interest are selected just inferior to each

kidney (Fig. 10–3). An aortic region of interest may be used to assess the discreteness and adequacy of the injected bolus as well as relative renal perfusion.

The normal computer-generated renogram curve using a tubular radiopharmaceutical consists of three phases (Fig. 10–4). Initial renal perfusion, or the *vascular transit phase*, lasts about 30 to 60 seconds and represents the initial arrival of the radiopharmaceutical in each kidney. Reconstruction of the first 30 to 60 seconds of the curve by using different axes may be performed to assess more carefully the renal perfusion phase. Generally, renal peak activity during the perfusion phase equals or exceeds that of the aorta and should be reasonably symmetric between the two kidneys. The second phase is the *cortical* or *tubular concentration phase* of initial parenchymal transit. This phase occurs during minutes 1 through 5 and contains the peak of the curve. The initial uptake slope closely correlates with ERPF values. The third phase is the *clearance* or *excretion phase*, which represents the down slope of the curve and is produced by excretion of the radiopharmaceutical from the kidney and clearance from the collecting system.

Patients should be well hydrated when renography is performed because in the presence of dehydration, an abnormal renogram curve demonstrating delayed peak activity, delayed radiopharmaceutical clearance, or an elevation of the excretion slope may result.

Overall, the renogram curves for each kidney should be reasonably symmetric, although slight

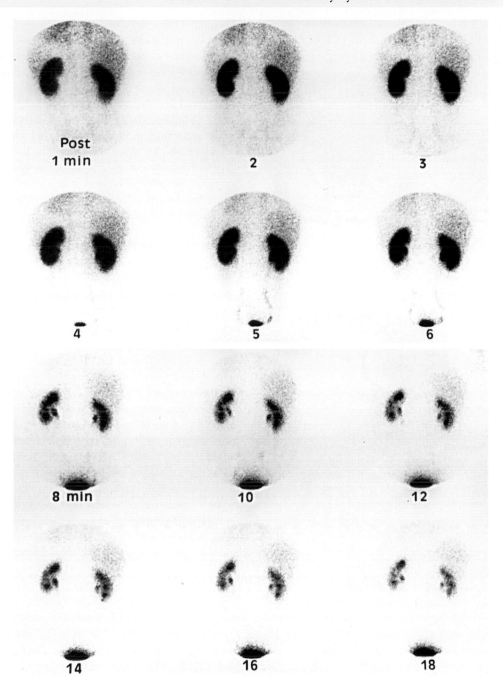

FIGURE 10–2. Normal renogram. After administration of technetium-99m mertiatide (MAG3), maximal kidney activity is seen at about 3 to 5 minutes, and by 4 to 5 minutes, the bladder can be identified at the bottom of the images. By about 8 to 12 minutes, most of the activity has cleared the parenchyma and is seen in the collecting systems, making the kidneys appear slightly smaller than on the early images. The temporal sequence here is similar to that identified on intravenous pyelogram.

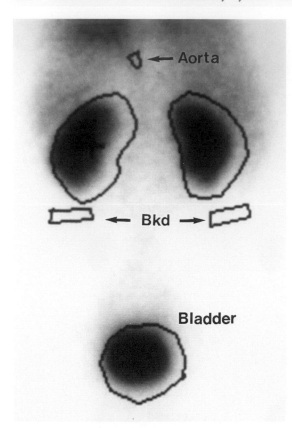

FIGURE 10–3. Typical regions of interest for computer analysis. Outlined regions of interest are drawn over the aorta, the kidneys, and the bladder. Areas of background activity (Bkd) are also drawn. Time-activity curves are then generated for each of these after appropriate background subtraction has been made.

asymmetries are not unusual. The shapes of curves should also be inspected individually for alterations in the normal configuration. Semiquantitative indices derived from the curves may be helpful in this respect. Data commonly derived from ^{99m}Tc-MAG3 renograms include the following:

Time to peak activity. Normal is about 3 to 5 minutes.
Relative renal uptake ratios at 2 to 3 minutes. This is an index of relative renal function between the two kidneys. Activity in each kidney should be equal, ideally 50%. A value of 40% or less in one kidney should be considered abnormal.
Half-time excretion is the time for half of the peak activity to be cleared from the kidney. Normal is about 8 to 12 minutes.
Differential cortical retention at 15 minutes. The percentage of retained activity about 15 minutes after injection in each kidney should be relatively

equal. Differences of 20% or more should be considered abnormal.
The 20-minute–to–peak count ratio. This is the activity measured in each kidney at 20 minutes and expressed as a percentage of peak curve activity. As renal function deteriorates, delayed transit of the radiopharmaceutical in the kidney results in an abnormal renogram curve, which can be quantitated by using this index. In the absence of pelvic calyceal retention, or if only a cortical region of interest is used, a normal 20-minute maximal cortical ratio for ^{99m}Tc-MAG3 is less than 0.3 (or 30%).

Quantitation of Renal Function

Quantitative assessment of renal function by using radionuclide techniques is an important part of nuclear nephrology and is routinely performed in some clinical settings. Because up to half of renal function, including GFR, may be lost before serum creatinine levels become abnormal, direct measurement of GFR and ERPF by using radiopharmaceuticals plays an important role in the assessment of renal function.

The classic measures of renal function involve the ability of the kidneys to clear certain substances from the plasma. These so-called clearances are expressed as volume of plasma cleared of a particular substance per minute (mL/min) as the plasma passes through the kidneys. The significance of the clearance depends on the substance used. The clearance of inulin, which is entirely filtered, defines the GFR; and the clearance of para-aminohippurate (PAH), which is both filtered and secreted by the tubules, defines renal plasma flow. The radiopharmaceutical analogs for calculation of these clearances are the totally filtered radiopharmaceutical ^{99m}Tc-DTPA for inulin clearance and GFR estimation, and ^{99m}Tc-MAG3, which is primarily secreted by the tubules, for PAH clearance and ERPF. The latter index is termed *effective* because the radiopharmaceuticals used closely estimate but do not equal the PAH clearance.

Two dominant radionuclide methods of determining GFR and ERPF are used: (1) plasma sample-based clearances, which are more tedious but more accurate, and (2) camera-based clearances, which do not require sampling of plasma or urine.

Plasma Sample-Based Clearances

These measurements are generally obtained by determining the plasma levels of the injected radio-

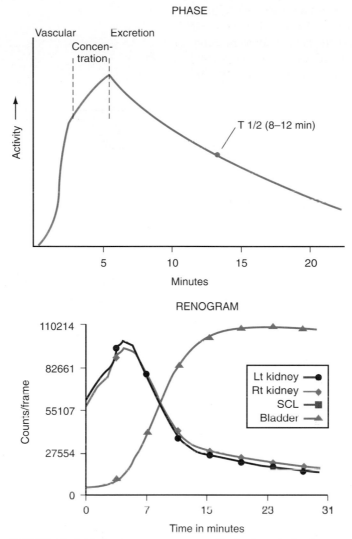

FIGURE 10–4. Typical renogram curves. *Top,* A schematic drawing demonstrates the conceptual portions of the time-activity curve within the kidney. *Bottom,* An actual renogram shows symmetric activity between right and left kidney, rapid dropoff after the peak, and a long tail extending to the right. The curve also shows increasing activity within the bladder after about 4 minutes.

pharmaceutical at a specified time, although some techniques require urine collection as well. For tubular agents such as ^{99m}Tc-MAG3, ERPF can be estimated by a single, timed blood sample obtained about 45 minutes after injection. Because the glomerular agent ^{99m}Tc-DTPA is cleared more slowly than are tubular agents, plasma samples are obtained 60 and 180 minutes after injection. The amount of activity remaining in the blood at these times is a measurement of activity not yet cleared by the renal mechanism and therefore is indirectly a measure of activity already cleared.

These techniques require meticulous attention to detail and must employ personnel expertly trained in in-vitro techniques. When performed correctly, GFR and ERPF measurements are theoretically more accurate than are those based on camera measurements.

Camera-Based Clearances

State-of-the-art gamma cameras and computers have allowed the development of methods for estimating GFR and ERPF without collecting blood or urine samples. Commonly, calculations are made by using counts acquired from the syringe containing the radiopharmaceutical before injection and subsequent counts over the kidneys after injection. Commercially available software for camera-based clearances simplifies corrections for patient and acquisition variables and provides reasonably accurate computer-derived clearance values. Although camera-based clearances are not as accurate as are those based on plasma samples, they are highly reproducible and sufficiently reliable to be used in clinical practice.

A renal functional measurement expressed simply as *MAG3 clearance*, without a need for corrections to estimate ERPF, has been developed by using both single plasma sample-based and camera-based techniques. MAG3 clearance may be used to follow the course of renal disease and has proved useful in individual laboratories in which its own range of normal values can be determined. Both MAG3 clearance and GFR determination are as useful and accurate measurements of renal function as is creatinine clearance.

Anatomic (Cortical) Imaging

Renal cortical imaging is usually performed for evaluation of space-occupying lesions, functioning pseudotumors such as cortical columns of Bertin, or edema or scarring associated with acute or chronic pyelonephritis, especially in children. These images of the renal cortex are generally taken by using ^{99m}Tc-DMSA or glucoheptonate and by using a pinhole or a high-resolution collimator, or single-photon emission computed tomography (SPECT) (Fig. 10–5).

CLINICAL APPLICATIONS
Diffuse Renal Disease

In evaluation of diffuse renal diseases producing acute or chronic impairment of renal function, such as acute pyelonephritis or chronic glomerulonephritis, radionuclide techniques are often sensitive but not disease specific. Most often, there is simply demonstration of unilaterally or bilaterally poor vascular perfusion and poor radiopharmaceutical excretion (Fig. 10–6). The renogram provides quantitative estimates of the function of each kidney, information that is not easily obtained by other methods. Generally, poor renal function results in flattening of the renogram curve as concentration and excretion of the radiopharmaceutical become increasingly impaired.

In patients with *acute tubular necrosis (ATN)*, there may be normal or only modestly reduced renal per-

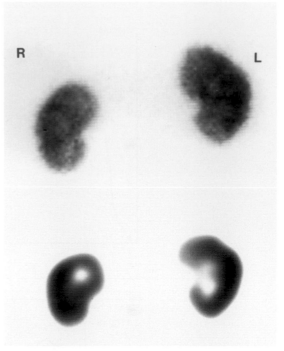

FIGURE 10–5. Cortical imaging of the kidneys. *Top,* Planar images after administration of technetium-99m dimercaptosuccinic acid. This radiopharmaceutical is essentially fixed in the renal tubules, permitting images of the renal parenchyma. *Bottom,* Better delineation of the activity seen within the cortex is identified on the coronal single-photon emission computed tomography scan.

fusion and preserved parenchymal accumulation but bilaterally poor excretion of ^{99m}Tc-MAG3 (Fig. 10–7). This frequently presents as bilateral persistent nephrograms with rising renogram curves. Reasonably good visualization of the kidneys indicates a favorable prognostic outcome, whereas poor visualization correlates with a prolonged or absent recovery.

Vascular Abnormalities

Renal perfusion abnormalities may be encountered in patients evaluated for unexplained renal failure. Renal artery occlusion, avulsion or stenosis, venous thrombosis, and renal infarction can be demonstrated by nuclear techniques, but other radiographic studies remain the procedures of choice. The image presentations of these disorders and the detection rates are not significantly different from those demonstrated by conventional radiographic techniques.

In *acute renal vein thrombosis*, there is generally decreased or absent perfusion and delayed and diminished accumulation and excretion of ^{99m}Tc-

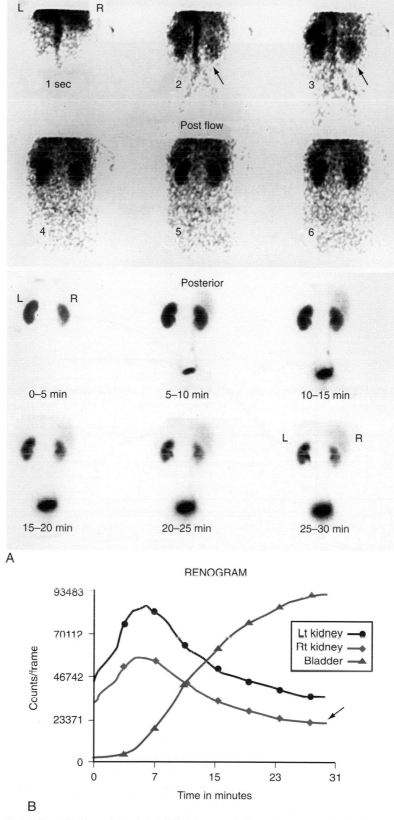

FIGURE 10–6. Acute pyelonephritis. *A,* Posterior perfusion images obtained after intravenous administration of technetium-99m mertiatide (MAG3) show decreased perfusion to the right kidney (*arrows*). The subsequent static images show decreased general activity in the right kidney throughout the study. *B,* The right renogram curve (*arrow*) demonstrates a near-normal shape but depressed function.

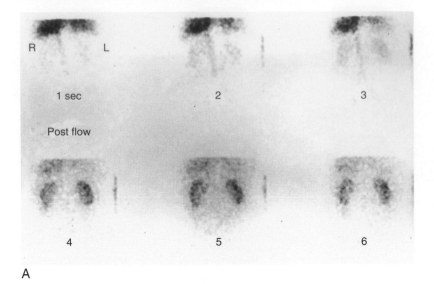

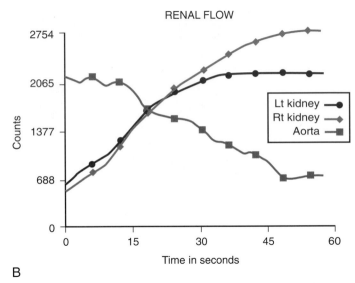

FIGURE 10–7. Acute tubular necrosis. *A*, Posterior flow images done after intravenous administration of technetium-99m mertiatide (MAG3) show symmetric and normal perfusion to both kidneys. *B*, Computer curves of blood flow during the first minute demonstrate a normal pattern, with aortic activity decreasing quickly after about 10 seconds and renal activity increasing rapidly up to about 30 seconds after injection, ultimately exceeding the peak aortic activity. *C*, Renogram images demonstrate poor function on the 0- to 5-minute image and increasing parenchymal activity throughout the remainder of the study, with no obvious excretion. *D*, This is confirmed by the continuously-rising renogram curves.

MAG3 by an enlarged, engorged, edematous kidney.

Obstructive Uropathy

The diagnosis of urinary tract obstruction and assessment of its functional significance are common indications for radionuclide imaging in both adults and children. Obstruction may be suspected on the basis of clinical findings or as an incidental finding of a dilated renal collecting system on IVP, CT, ultrasound, or radionuclide renal imaging. Standard imaging techniques, such as IVP and ultrasonography, evaluate structure but do not depict urodynamics.

Routine Functional Imaging and Renography

With acute high-grade obstruction, routine radionuclide renal function imaging frequently dis-

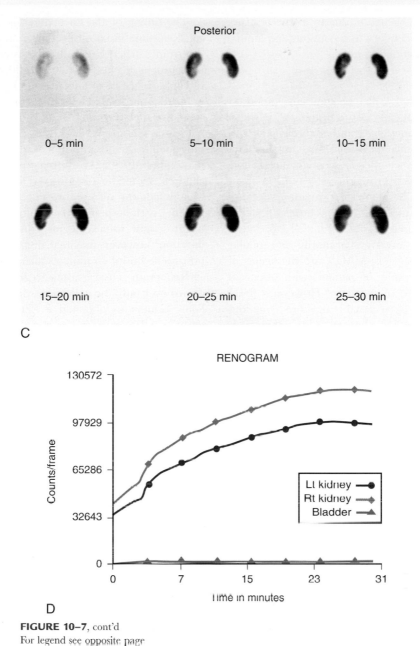

C

D

FIGURE 10–7, cont'd
For legend see opposite page

closes reduced renal perfusion. The renogram curve demonstrates a rising excretion slope determined by the severity of the hydronephrosis or the degree and duration (acute or chronic) of the underlying obstruction and by the amount of preserved renal function. To obtain an adequate image, there must be enough residual function to allow excretion of the radionuclide into the collecting system. The classic acute or subacute high-grade obstructive renogram is a steeply rising continuous arched curve with no definable excre-

tion downsloping. In long-standing high-grade obstruction, no renal perfusion or function may be seen, and the renogram curve may be uniformly flattened.

Similar to anatomic imaging, however, routine renography may not differentiate obstructive collecting system dilatation from hydronephrosis of a nonobstructive nature, so that appropriate management can be instituted before significant renal damage occurs. In this setting, diuretic renography provides a noninvasive method to distinguish collecting system dilatation due to a true obstruction from that secondary to a patulous and atonic, but patent, collecting system.

Diuretic Renography

Diuretic renography has become an important diagnostic radionuclide test to distinguish between obstructive hydronephrosis and nonobstructive collecting system dilatation due to vesicoureteral reflux, urinary tract infection, congenital malformations, previous obstruction, or a noncompliant bladder. Generally, glomerular function declines earlier and more rapidly than does tubular function in response to ureteral obstruction. Thus, radiopharmaceuticals excreted primarily by tubular secretion, such as ^{99m}Tc-MAG3, are the agents of choice for renography of patients with suspected collecting system obstruction. However, ^{99m}Tc-DTPA may also be acceptable in more acute and less severe obstructions. Diuretic renography evaluates both renal function (obstructive nephropathy) and urodynamics (hydronephrosis) in a single test.

In patients with nonobstructive hydronephrosis and/or hydroureter due to vesicoureteral reflux, previous obstruction, or functional ureteropelvic disorders, the dilated intrarenal collecting system may fill but not reach pressures sufficient to "open" the ureteropelvic junction to permit flow of urine under normal conditions of urine production. This may give the impression of a fixed anatomic abnormality rather than a functional abnormality. By increasing urine flow using a diuretic (such as furosemide), a functional obstruction may be overcome by increasing pressure in the renal pelvis and thus allowing urine to flow from the collecting system into the ureter to the bladder. A fixed, anatomic obstruction would not be expected to be overcome by the diuresis. Thus, performing this maneuver during functional renal imaging permits documentation of the diuretic urodynamics and differentiation of a fixed anatomic from functional abnormality. Patients should be well hydrated before the examination, and the bladder should be emptied before the administration of furosemide because a full bladder can slow drainage from the upper part of the urinary tract and result in the false appearance of obstruction. In adults or infants who cannot empty their bladders, a bladder catheter may be used. The study is best performed by using 10 mCi (370 MBq) of ^{99m}Tc-MAG3, although ^{99m}Tc-DTPA may also be used. Standard renal perfusion and functional imaging techniques are employed.

The timing of the furosemide injection is critical. Real-time visual inspection of renal excretion determines when the collecting systems are full. This usually occurs about 15 to 20 minutes after radiopharmaceutical injection but may occur later in hydronephrotic kidneys. Injection of the diuretic should be delayed until the dilated renal pelvis is full or the renogram curve is near its peak. At that time, an intravenous injection of furosemide, 40 mg for adults and 1 mg/kg to a maximum of 40 mg for children, should be administered. A larger dose, up to a maximum of 80 mg, may be required in patients with impaired renal function. Response to furosemide usually begins 2 to 5 minutes after injection; however, maximal diuresis is frequently not reached until 15 minutes after injection.

Renogram curves using regions of interest drawn over only the collecting systems or over the entire kidneys are obtained. Preference is generally given to collecting system regions of interest, which should also include the ureters if they appear to retain the radiopharmaceutical. Calculating the half-time excretion for diuretic renography is often performed either from the time of injection of the diuretic or at the beginning of the diuretic response. However, determination of the time of onset of the diuretic response can be subjective if the response is not discrete.

Interpretation of the data is generally performed by visual analysis of the renogram washout curve with assessment of the half-time excretion (Fig. 10–8). Dilated collecting systems secondary to either fixed or functional "obstruction" may produce continuously rising renogram curves before furosemide administration, with minimal or no evidence of excretion downsloping. After furosemide administration, the curve is inspected for any change. In dilated, nonobstructed systems, furosemide causes increased urine flow through the collecting system, which washes out the initial increase in activity and causes a decline of the excretion slope in the computer-generated time-activity curves (Fig. 10–9).

In the case of significant mechanical obstruction, there is very little decrease in renal collecting system activity after furosemide administration, owing to the narrowed fixed lumen of the ureter. The rising renogram curve is changed little or is unaffected.

Assessment of the half-time excretion may aid in the interpretation of the renogram. In general, in a normally functioning kidney, a half-time of less than 10 to 15 minutes from the time of diuretic

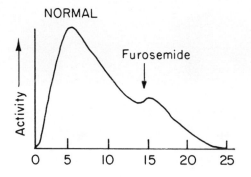

NORMAL

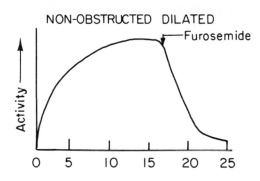

NON-OBSTRUCTED DILATED

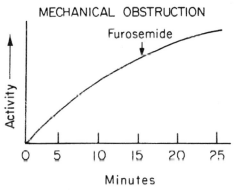

MECHANICAL OBSTRUCTION

Minutes

FIGURE 10–8. Characteristic time-activity curves in a diuretic renogram.

- Poor hydration, resulting in poor diuretic response
- Poor underlying renal function, resulting in a diminished diuretic response
- A noncompliant or rigid renal pelvis, producing increasing resistance to urine flow as diuresis increases urine volume
- High filling pressure of the bladder due to a distended or noncompliant bladder, which may impair washout from the upper urinary tract
- An overcompliant or patulous renal pelvis. During the diuretic response, increased urine flow may be sufficient to fill this large reservoir without being sufficient enough to wash out the tracer, producing a rising renogram curve.
- A large hydronephrotic volume, especially in the presence of diminished function. With a larger volume in the system, a larger diuretic response is needed to clear that system of accumulated activity. This is the so-called *reservoir effect.*

Pediatric Hydronephrosis

Perinatal ultrasonography has resulted in increased diagnosis of hydronephrosis and hydroureteronephrosis in newborns. Differentiation of obstructive from nonobstructive causes is therapeutically important. Obstruction commonly occurs in the regions of the ureteropelvic or ureterovesical junctions. Technetium-99m MAG3 diuresis renography appears to be reliable in the diagnosis of unilateral and bilateral ureteropelvic junction and ureterovesical junction obstruction (Fig. 10–11). In infants and children older than 1 month, glomerular filtration has usually matured to the level at which its measurement becomes reliable by using either glomerular or tubular agents. One difficulty is the diagnosis of coexisting ureteropelvic junction and ureterovesical junction obstructions—one or the other may be missed using this technique.

Angiotensin-Converting Enzyme Inhibitor (Captopril) Renography

Renovascular hypertension constitutes about 1% to 4% of all cases of hypertension, but no discriminating findings allow its diagnosis on clinical grounds. In patients with renovascular hypertension, the most common cause of renal artery stenosis is atherosclerosis, predominant in the elderly; the second most common cause is fibromuscular dysplasia, occurring primarily in women younger than 35 years. When an angiotensin-converting enzyme

effect constitutes a normal response. Half-time values and renogram curves should always be considered in conjunction with the scintigraphic images and adequacy of existing renal function (Fig. 10–10). Because a spectrum of renal function is encountered in clinical practice, a spectrum of diuretic responses is to be expected.

Factors that produce a false-positive impression of mechanical obstruction or that contribute to indeterminate results include the following:

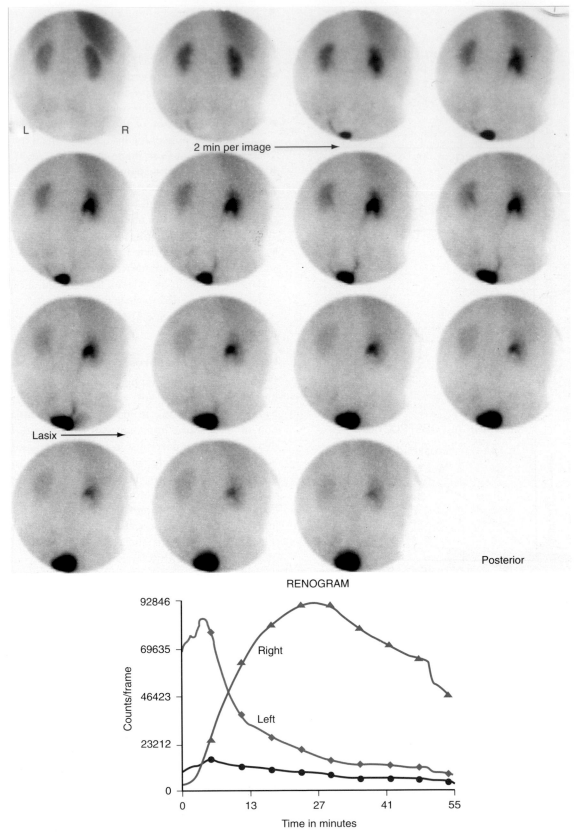

FIGURE 10–9. Non-obstructed patulous collecting system. A diuretic renogram shows that activity in the collecting system of the right kidney decreases significantly after administration of furosemide at about 20 minutes.

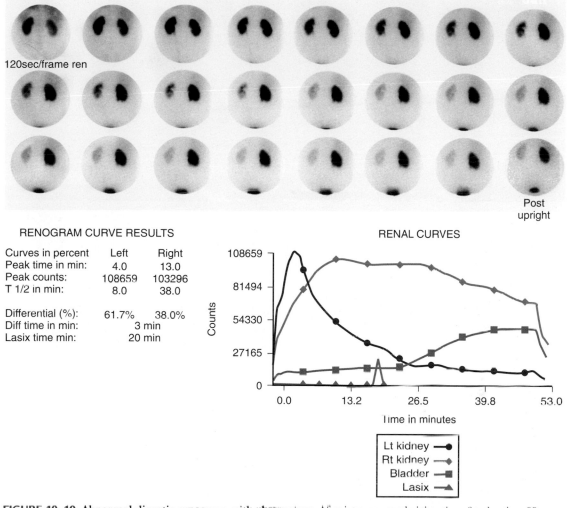

RENOGRAM CURVE RESULTS

Curves in percent	Left	Right
Peak time in min:	4.0	13.0
Peak counts:	108659	103296
T 1/2 in min:	8.0	38.0
Differential (%):	61.7%	38.0%
Diff time in min:	3 min	
Lasix time min:	20 min	

RENAL CURVES

Counts: 108659, 81494, 54330, 27165, 0

Time in minutes: 0.0, 13.2, 26.5, 39.8, 53.0

Lt kidney ●
Rt kidney ◆
Bladder ■
Lasix ▲

Post
upright

FIGURE 10–10. Abnormal diuretic renogram with obstruction. After intravenous administration of technetium-99m DTPA, the posterior 2-minute sequential images show a dilated collecting system of the right kidney. After administration of furosemide (beginning of the second row of images), the activity in the collecting system on the left decreases normally, however, the activity in the right kidney decreases only slightly.

(ACE) inhibitor is given to a patient with renal artery stenosis that has been compensated by the renal angiotensin mechanism, there is a decrease in GFR that is scintigraphically detectable. The test is highly specific for renal artery stenosis as a cause for the patient's hypertension, which may eliminate the need for diagnostic angiography.

Significant renal artery stenosis (60% to 75%) decreases *afferent* arteriolar blood pressure, which stimulates renin secretion by the juxtaglomerular apparatus. Renin elicits the production of angiotensin I, which is acted on by ACE to yield angiotensin II. Angiotensin II induces vasoconstriction of the *efferent* arterioles, which restores glomerular filtration pressure and rate. ACE inhibitors, such as captopril and enalaprilat, prevent the production of angiotensin II, so that in patients with renal artery stenosis and compensated renal function, preglomerular filtration pressures are no longer maintained. This results in a significant sudden decrease in glomerular filtration. This induced decompensation can be documented by performing ^{99m}Tc-MAG3 or ^{99m}Tc-DTPA studies before and after the administration of captopril. Sensitivity and specificity may be higher with MAG3 than with DTPA, although excellent results may be obtained with either radiopharmaceutical in most patients. A positive study indicates that a

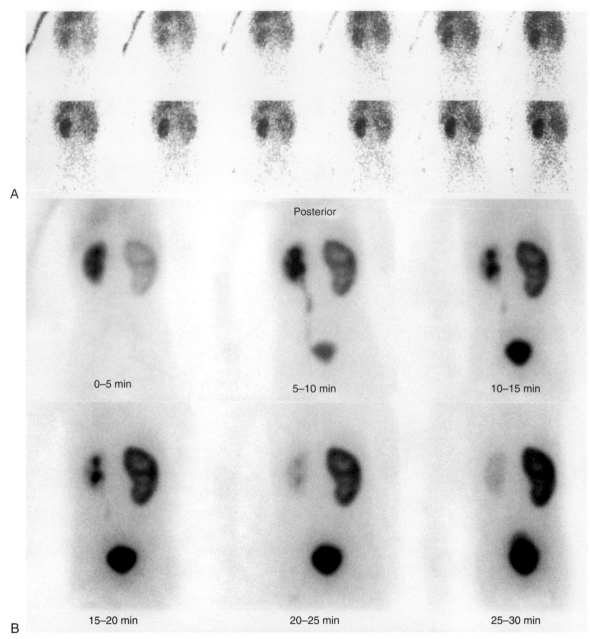

FIGURE 10–11. Hydronephrosis in a child. *A,* Posterior images obtained after intravenous administration of technetium-99m DTPA show decreased perfusion to an enlarged right kidney. *B,* The renogram shows a dilated collecting system of the right kidney. *C,* Computer-generated time-activity curves show that after administration of furosemide (at 15 minutes), there is no decrease in activity, indicating a high-grade obstruction on the right.

patient's hypertension is renin dependent (renovascular hypertension), most commonly produced by renal artery stenosis, and that it is likely to be improved by renal revascularization.

ACE inhibition (ACEI) scintigraphy should not be used as a screening procedure for all patients with hypertension because it is not cost-effective and because screening a population with low prevalence for renal artery stenosis will lead to an unacceptably high false-positive rate and incite further unnecessary invasive testing. Patients should be selected carefully and limited to those with a moderate to high probability of renovascular hypertension. Selection criteria include the following:

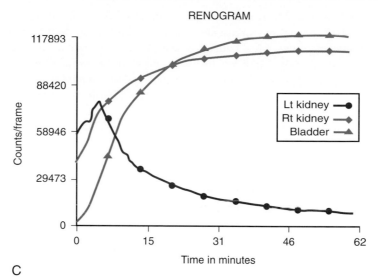

C

FIGURE 10–11, cont'd
For legend see opposite page

- Initial presentation of hypertension in patients older than 60 years or younger than 20 years
- Severe or accelerated hypertension resistant to medication therapy
- Hypertension previously well controlled but now difficult to manage medically
- Hypertension in patients with other evidence of vascular disease
- Unexplained renal dysfunction in patients with recent onset of hypertension
- Unexplained hypertension in patients with abdominal bruits

Patients taking ACE inhibitors therapeutically should have their medication halted for about 48 hours for captopril and for about 1 week for lisinopril or enalaprilat before the examination. The patient's ACEI medication may be maintained, if it is deemed medically necessary and inadvisable to halt administration for more than 24 hours. However, the patient should refrain from taking ACEI medication on the day of the study. Antihypertensive drugs of non-ACE inhibitor classes do not appear to affect the test results. The patient should be fasting to allow for maximum absorption of oral captopril and should be well hydrated.

Although ACEI scintigraphy protocols vary, the basics of the examination are well defined and include the following:

- Twenty-five to 50 mg of oral captopril is administered with sitting blood pressure recordings at 15-minute intervals for 1 hour. As an alternative, in patients with uncertain gastrointestinal absorption of oral medication, intravenous enalaprilat (Vasotec), 0.04 mg/kg up to a maximum of 2.5 mg, may be administered over 3 to 5 minutes.
- One hour after captopril administration or 15 to 20 minutes after enalaprilat infusion, 10 mCi (370 MBq) of ^{99m}Tc MAG3 (preferred in most patients, especially those with impaired renal function) or ^{99m}Tc-DTPA is administered intravenously and routine renal scintigraphy with renography is performed. Some protocols use intravenous furosemide (40 to 60 mg) shortly after the administration of the radiopharmaceutical to clear the renal collecting systems of activity, which may interfere with calculation of cortical indices. At the termination of imaging, a final blood pressure reading should be obtained before the patient leaves the imaging department.

In patients with unilateral renal artery stenosis and renal insufficiency, bilateral renal artery stenosis, or stenotic solitary or transplanted kidneys, captopril or enalaprilat should be used advisedly for diagnosis, especially if severe stenosis is known to be present. Under these circumstances, acute renal failure may be induced, which is generally self-limited, although persistent anuria may occasionally develop. Furthermore, in any patient undergoing captopril intervention studies, the possibility of severe hypotension induction exists. This complication usually responds to intravenous volume expanders (normal saline). Thus, it is prudent to maintain intravenous access throughout the study.

Two primary protocols may be used that employ one- and two-stage examinations. Choice of the examination depends primarily on patient scheduling and department preferences. Because establishing a diagnosis of renal artery stenosis as a cause for hypertension depends on the induction or worsening of renal dysfunction after ACE inhibitor administration, a baseline study is extremely useful in assessing the effects of the medication on renal function.

The *single-day, two-stage protocol* consists of an initial baseline noncaptopril study, usually performed early in the day with a low radiopharmaceutical dose (1 to 2 mCi, 74 MBq of ^{99m}Tc-MAG3). This allows a repeat examination using captopril intervention several hours later, after clearance of the tracer from the kidneys and urinary tract. By administering 40 mg of furosemide during or after the first study to ensure good washout of residual activity, the waiting time between studies may be shortened further.

The *one-stage protocol* is generally performed on patients without evidence of pre-existing renal dysfunction or failure. In this protocol, the captopril challenge study is performed first. If normal, a diagnosis of renovascular hypertension is unlikely (10% probability) and the baseline study is not needed.

The principal diagnostic criterion and the hallmark of renovascular hypertension is a postcaptopril renogram that becomes abnormal or more abnormal, usually unilaterally, than a baseline renogram in which an ACE inhibitor is not given. Using the glomerular agent ^{99m}Tc-DTPA, the principal finding is diminished uptake and excretion caused by a drop in glomerular filtration. There may also be prolonged parenchymal transit manifested by delay in time to peak activity of the renogram curve. If the fall in GFR is severe enough, there may be nonvisualization of a previously functioning kidney. Using the primarily tubular agent ^{99m}Tc-MAG3, reasonably adequate initial uptake and secretion is preserved. The reduced GFR, however, results in decreased urine production and flow and therefore in decreased washout of the secreted agent from the collecting tubules. This results in increased cortical retention, which is the principal finding (Fig. 10–12). This results in an abnormal renogram curve with an elevated cortical retention index (increased cortical activity at 20 minutes compared with the renogram peak). Occasionally, in very severe stenosis, early decreased uptake of ^{99m}Tc-MAG3 may also be identified.

A number of quantitative renogram parameters have been devised to assist in visual interpretation and to facilitate comparison of the baseline and the postcaptopril examinations. These criteria differ with respect to the radiopharmaceutical used. Several criteria frequently used to indicate an abnormality on ^{99m}Tc-MAG3 ACEI renography are as follows:

■ Percentage of renal uptake at 2 to 3 minutes by one kidney less than 40% of total uptake
■ Retained cortical activity at 20 minutes expressed as a fraction of peak activity differing from the contralateral kidney by more than 20%; or an increase from the baseline study of 0.15. Normal is less than 0.3
■ Delay in the time to peak activity in the affected kidney of more than 2 minutes when compared with the baseline study or the unaffected kidney

These parameters have met with various levels of reported success and should be used only in conjunction with visual analysis of the renogram curves and review of the scintigraphic images.

In addition to unilateral renal artery stenosis, bilateral abnormalities produced or demonstrating worsening from baseline may be noted in bilateral renal artery stenosis, although detection becomes more difficult. Bilateral renal artery stenosis often behaves in an asymmetric fashion in response to ACEI renography and is therefore distinguishable from the usually symmetric appearance seen in patients with either essential hypertension or chronic parenchymal renal disease after captopril administration. Further, bilateral worsening of the renogram curves after ACEI administration may also be caused by hypotension induced during the study, dehydration, and bladder distention resulting in poor collecting system drainage. The diagnosis of renovascular hypertension due to segmental renal artery stenosis and after renal transplantation has been reported.

Both the sensitivity and specificity of ACEI renography surpass 90%. When strict attention

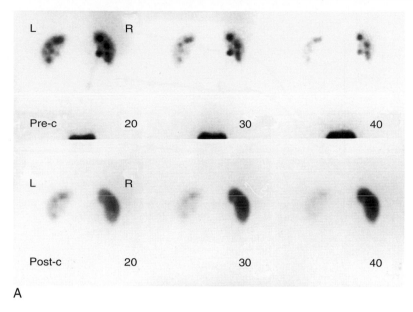

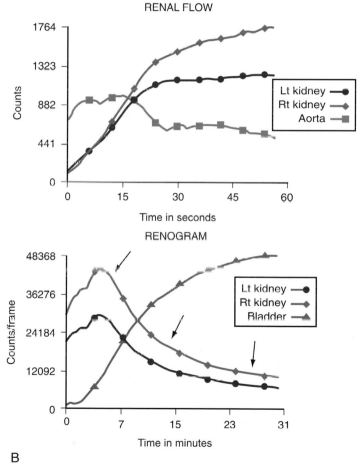

FIGURE 10–12. Right renal artery stenosis. *A,* The precaptopril ^{99m}Tc-MAG3 renogram (*upper row*) shows slightly asymmetric activity. The postcaptopril MAG3 renogram (*lower row*) shows markedly abnormal retention of activity in the right kidney as late as 40 minutes. *B,* Computer-generated curves for renal perfusion and renograms done before captopril administration actually show normal blood flow to the right kidney and a normal right renogram curve (*arrows*). *C,* Curves after captopril administration again show essentially normal renal blood flow to the right kidney, but the right renogram curve (*arrows*) shows markedly increasing activity owing to retention of technetium-99m (MAG3) mertiatide after administration of captopril.

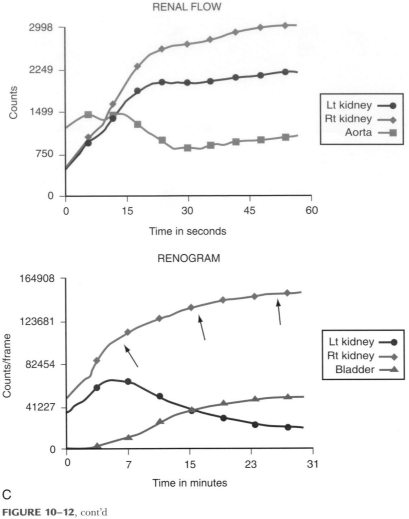

FIGURE 10–12, cont'd
For legend see 313

is paid to patient preparation and examination protocol, false-positive studies are uncommon. As with most tests, however, its limitations should be recognized.

Scintigraphic abnormalities with captopril renography are best demonstrated in patients with renal artery stenoses of 60% to 90%. Abnormalities may not be demonstrated in stenoses of less than 60% because of the lack of significant renin-angiotensin compensation. Severe renal artery stenosis of greater than 90% may not be compensated sufficiently by the renin-angiotensin system at baseline to allow for a scintigraphically-detectable change to occur after administration of ACE inhibitors. False-negative examinations may be caused by accommodation to the drug by patients receiving ACEI therapy, even with continued ther-

apeutic response. This can be avoided by withholding captopril therapy for 2 to 4 days or the long-acting enalapriat for 1 week before the study. In addition, using a patient's chronic medication regimen of ACE inhibitor to perform the ACEI renogram is not advisable.

The sensitivity and specificity of captopril renography may be diminished in patients with renal insufficiency, especially in those with small, poorly functioning kidneys. In patients with unilateral renal disease at baseline that does not demonstrate change after captopril administration, renal stenosis cannot be reliably differentiated from unilateral parenchymal disease. Also, asymmetric hydronephrosis or poor drainage from an intrarenal collecting system may cause confusion between cortical and parenchymal retention of activity, producing a false-positive examination. Visual inspection of the images or administration of furosemide may prevent this problem.

A profound drop in blood pressure after ACE inhibitor administration may induce acute oliguria and cortical retention of the radiopharmaceutical not only in patients with renovascular hypertension but also in patients with essential hypertension or even in normal control subjects, causing false-positive results. Poor hydration of patients may cause diminished urine formation and delayed transit and retention of the radiopharmaceutical in the renal cortex, mimicking a poststenotic kidney on the ACEI study.

Acute Pyelonephritis

The diagnosis of acute pyelonephritis in children based on clinical and laboratory observations is frequently difficult, even in the presence of fever, flank pain, or pyuria and a positive urine culture. Intravenous urography and renal sonography have a low sensitivity and underestimate the degree of parenchymal involvement. Radionuclide renal cortical imaging is a highly sensitive technique for diagnosis of renal parenchymal infection and should be considered for the diagnosis of acute pyelonephritis in children. Normal cortical imaging effectively excludes a diagnosis of acute pyelonephritis. Imaging studies are usually not necessary for the diagnosis of acute pyelonephritis in adults.

Technetium-99m DMSA in a dose of 50 μCi (1.85 MBq)/kg is the radiopharmaceutical of choice, with a minimum administered dose of 300 μCi (11.1 MBq). Although ^{99m}Tc glucoheptonate (150 μCi [5.55 MBq]/kg) may be used, the lesser accumulation of activity in the bladder when using ^{99m}Tc-DMSA significantly reduces gonadal radiation dose and is therefore preferable in infants and young children. SPECT imaging may be used as needed.

In normal patients, cortical uptake of DMSA appears homogeneous throughout the kidneys on routine imaging, except for relative defects in the regions of the collecting systems. High-resolution magnified images, however, especially with the use of a pinhole collimator, may show heterogeneous uptake owing to prominent cortical columns and may provide better differentiation of the cortex from the medulla. Normal variants include smooth variations in cortical contour caused by fetal lobulation, which are distinguished from scars by preservation of cortical thickness.

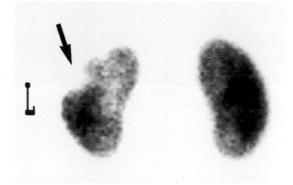

FIGURE 10–13. Pyelonephritis. The posterior planar image from a technetium-99m dimercaptosuccinic acid (DMSA) scan in a young child shows cortical defects in the upper pole of the left kidney (*arrow*).

In patients with acute pyelonephritis, there are three common patterns of presentation: (1) focal cortical defects (Fig. 10–13), (2) multifocal cortical defects, and (3) diffusely decreased activity.

In the acute phase, defects may be associated with edema presenting as a bulging renal contour. Because diminished activity of ^{99m}Tc-DMSA in areas of acute inflammation reflects early ischemia that precedes functional abnormalities, DMSA scans likely become positive before any significant tissue damage has occurred. These findings may resolve completely and return to normal within several months or may evolve into permanent damage with scar formation. If the disease progresses, scarring becomes prevalent, and the cortical defects become associated with contraction and volume loss.

Renal Masses

Renal space-occupying lesions identified by sonography, CT, or magnetic resonance imaging (MRI) may occasionally warrant further evaluation with renal cortical imaging using ^{99m}Tc-DMSA or glucoheptonate to distinguish nonfunctioning from functioning renal tissue. Masses not representing renal parenchyma, such as neoplasms, abscess, cysts, hematoma, or infarcts, present as photopenic lesions in the renal parenchyma. Pseudotumors consisting of normally functioning renal tissue but simulating neoplasm may be caused by fetal lobulation, dromedary humps, and columns of Bertin, which are generally the most worrisome. These columns represent normal cortical tissue extending into the renal medulla between the renal pyramids and are frequently found at the junction of the

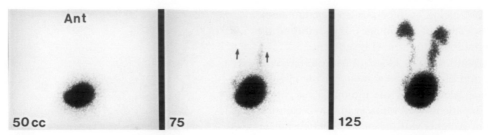

FIGURE 10–14. Ureterovesicular reflux. In this child, the bladder was filled with technetium-99m sulfur colloid. At 75 mL, activity is seen refluxing into both ureters (*arrows*). At 125 mL, the bilaterally dilated ureters and renal pelves are identified.

upper and middle thirds of the kidney. Demonstration of functioning renal tissue in the region of the suspected mass confirms its benign nature.

Radionuclide Cystography

Radionuclide cystography is the technique of choice for the evaluation and follow-up of children with suspected vesicoureteral reflux. Radionuclide cystography is more sensitive than is iodinated contrast cystography, with reflux volumes as low as 1 mL being detected. There is also significantly less radiation exposure. For direct radionuclide cystography, 0.5 to 1 mCi (185 to 37 MBq) of ^{99m}Tc pertechnetate, ^{99m}Tc DTPA, or ^{99m}Tc sulfur colloid is instilled through an indwelling bladder catheter, in a volume of normal saline sufficient to fill the bladder. A sample protocol and dosimetry are provided in Appendix E–1.

In normal patients, no radiopharmaceutical reflux from the bladder into the ureters or the kidneys is seen. When vesicoureteral reflux occurs, it may be identified during the bladder filling, voiding, or postvoid phases of the examination. For purposes of reporting, reflux is usually described as follows:

- Minimal—confined to the ureter
- Moderate—involving the pelvicalyceal system
- Severe—reflux into the pelvicalyceal system accompanied by a dilated intrarenal collecting system or a dilated tortuous ureter (Fig. 10–14)

Minimal reflux is the most difficult to discern on images, and false-negative studies are not uncommonly those in which the reflux is confined to the distal ureter.

When required, residual urine volume in the bladder can be calculated by measuring the change in bladder count rate before and after voiding and comparing it to the voided urine volume. In addition, information concerning volume of reflux into the upper tracts also can be calculated by using regions of interest over the intrarenal collecting systems on computerized images.

Renal Transplant Evaluation

The transplantation of kidneys from living or cadaveric donors is a well-established organ transplantation procedure both surgically and medically. Transplants are placed in the anterior iliac fossa with vascular anastomosis to the hypogastric artery and the external iliac vein, and with ureteral anastomosis or implantation into the bladder. Radionuclide imaging using ^{99m}Tc-DTPA or ^{99m}Tc-MAG3, is a useful tool in evaluating the medical and surgical complications of renal transplantation. Imaging of renal transplants is performed with the patient supine. Anterior images are obtained over the iliac fossa containing the transplanted kidney. Baseline functional renal imaging and renography are generally performed shortly after surgery. Subsequent serial imaging may be obtained if abnormalities are noted on the baseline study to assess improving or deteriorating renal function or as medical or surgical complications are suspected.

In the normal transplant perfusion study, the radioactive bolus reaches the renal transplant at almost the exact time it is seen in the iliac vessels. As with a renogram of a native kidney, the maximal parenchymal phase is normally seen at 3 to 5 minutes, with bladder activity present at 4 to 8 minutes (Fig. 10–15). Immediately after transplantation and for up to 2 weeks, there may be fairly prominent visualization of the ureter, owing to edema at the ureterovesical anastomotic site.

Complications of renal transplantation are generally acute tubular necrosis (ATN), rejection, antirejection medication (cyclosporin) toxicity, and surgical mishaps.

ATN commonly occurs in cadaveric transplants and results from ischemia in the renal transplant

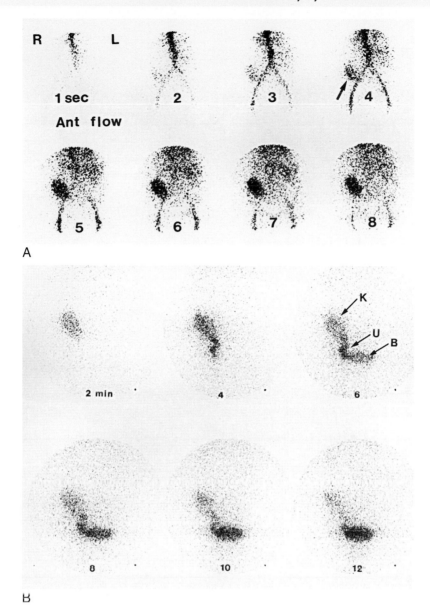

FIGURE 10–15. Normal renal transplant. *A,* Anterior perfusion images done with technetium-99m DTPA show prompt perfusion of the transplanted kidney in the right renal fossa *(arrow).* Note that in the early phases, the activity in the transplanted kidney is essentially equal to the intensity of activity in the iliac vessel directly next to the transplant. *B,* The renogram images done with ^{99m}Tc-mertiatide (MAG3) show activity in the kidney (K) and ureter (U) by 6 minutes. Activity in the kidney is greatest at 4 minutes, and this washes out almost completely by 12 minutes, with most of the activity in the bladder (B) occurring at this time.

after harvesting and before transplantation. The scintigraphic presentation of ATN consists of preserved or only mildly reduced perfusion but diminished renal function and progressive cortical retention of tubular agents, such as ^{99m}Tc- MAG3, with a consequent decrease in or absence of urine production (Fig. 10–16). ATN is generally observed

during the first 3 to 4 days after surgery and usually resolves during the next several weeks.

Renal transplant rejection is primarily a small-vessel obliterative disease, with perfusion deteriorating faster and more severely than function in the early stages. The dynamic perfusion study often reveals poor perfusion, which usually worsens on serial

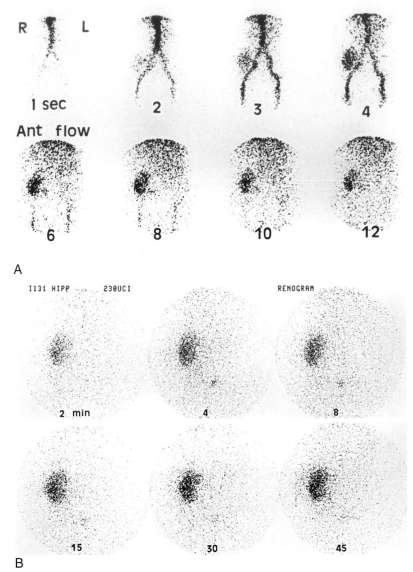

FIGURE 10–16. Acute tubular necrosis. *A*, Anterior perfusion images of the right iliac fossa transplant demonstrate normal perfusion. *B*, The renogram images done with iodine-131 hippuran (a tubular agent similar to MAG3) show increasing parenchymal activity over 45 minutes, compatible with acute tubular necrosis.

examinations. The renogram is equally poor, demonstrating a diminished nephrogram phase and delayed appearance of bladder activity (Fig. 10–17), which may be largely due to the decreased perfusion and inability of the radionuclide to reach functional renal structures. Renal transplant rejection is usually classified according to its time of onset (hyperacute, acute, or chronic), with each form having a characteristic mechanism.

Hyperacute rejection occurs immediately (0 to 24 hours) after transplantation as a result of pre-

formed antibodies in the recipient's blood. Hyperacute rejection produces rapid vascular thrombosis in the donor kidney, presenting as absent perfusion and severely reduced or absent function.

Acute rejection is a cell-mediated process characterized by lymphocytic infiltration. This generally occurs within the first 2 to 3 months after transplantation but may occur during the first several weeks. Acute rejection presents as decreased transplant perfusion with diminished radiopharmaceutical uptake and excretion. Acute rejection may also

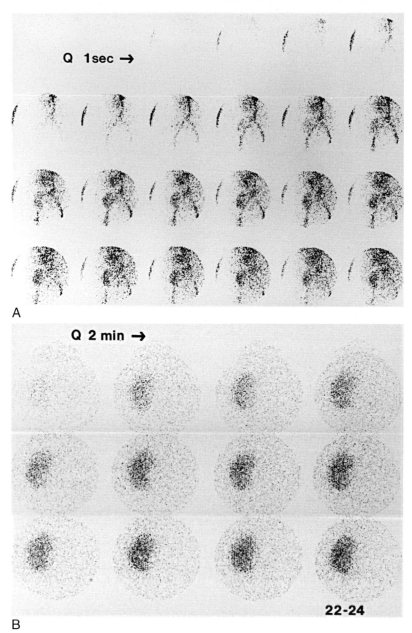

FIGURE 10–17. Renal transplant rejection. *A,* The ^{99m}Tc-diethylenetriaminepenta acetate (DTPA) flow study demonstrates poor flow to the transplant, which can be seen several seconds after the iliac vessels. *B,* The renogram demonstrates delayed parenchymal activity, with no evidence of activity in the collecting system or bladder.

be imaged by using ^{99m}Tc sulfur colloid, which localizes in the rejecting transplant by trapping of the labeled colloid particles in fibrin thrombi. It appears to be less sensitive for detection of chronic rejection.

Chronic rejection is an antibody-mediated process that occurs 6 months to years after transplantation. It is a slow process that produces a gradual obliter-

ation of the renovascular bed with concomitant deterioration of renal transplant perfusion and function.

Cyclosporin nephrotoxicity (renal transplant toxicity from the antirejection drug cyclosporin) usually presents a scintigraphic appearance similar to that of ATN, with relatively good transplant perfusion and poor tubular function, which may result in

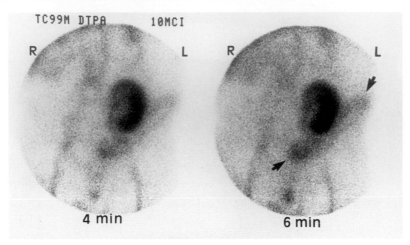

FIGURE 10–18. Urinoma. Images from a technetium-99m DTPA renogram clearly show a left iliac fossa transplant. However, the infralateral collection of activity (*arrows*) represents a urinoma.

progressive cortical retention of ^{99m}Tc-MAG3. Cyclosporin nephrotoxicity, however, characteristically occurs several weeks after transplantation when any ATN has resolved. The functional impairment associated with cyclosporin toxicity generally reverses after withdrawal of therapy.

Surgical complications include urine collections (urinomas), lymphoceles, hematomas, ureteral obstruction, and vascular complications. Urinomas are caused by leakage from the ureteral anastomosis. This complication occurs shortly after surgery. If the leak of urine is significant, the excreted radiopharmaceutical may appear within the urine collection (Fig. 10–18). If the leak is slow, the urinoma may present as a photopenic defect adjacent to the kidney or ureter. Photopenic defects in and around the renal transplant may also be due to hematomas in the immediate postoperative period or lymphoceles, which commonly occur several months after transplantation.

Because a transplanted kidney has no venous collaterals, renal vein thrombosis produces deficient or absent perfusion and function in the transplanted allograft in a pattern identical to that seen with arterial obstruction. In the setting of acute complete arterial or venous obstruction, the kidney presents as a photopenic reniform area outlined by background activity on radionuclide imaging. Postsurgical obstruction of the ureteral anastomosis may be diagnosed by radionuclide techniques in a similar fashion to native ureteral obstructions.

SCROTAL IMAGING

Ultrasound is preferred to scintigraphy in the evaluation of chronic or painless scrotal masses. However, scrotal scintigraphy may occasionally be a useful test to differentiate among the causes of a swollen or painful testicle (Table 10–1), although it is seldom performed. Essentially, this entails differ-

TABLE 10–1.	**Testicular Scintigraphy**	
DIAGNOSIS	**DYNAMIC STUDY (ACTIVITY)**	**DELAYED STATIC IMAGE (ACTIVITY)**
Acute torsion (<24 hr)	Normal or slightly decreased	Decreased
Late torsion (>24 hr)	Decreased, normal, or increased	Cold lesion with surrounding activity
Trauma (hematoma)	Variable	Variable
Epididymitis	Increased	Increased
Abscess	Increased	Cold lesion with surrounding activity
Tumor	Normal or increased	Decreased or increased
Hydrocele	Normal or increased	Decreased

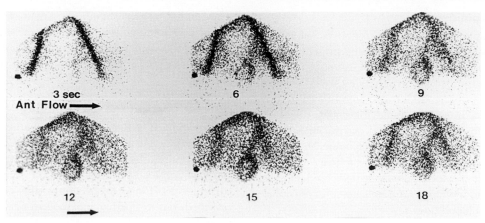

FIGURE 10–19. Testicular torsion. Serial dynamic images demonstrate hypervascularity on the left with a lucent center, consistent with a delayed diagnosis of testicular torsion.

entiating acute testicular torsion, a surgical emergency, from acute epididymo-orchitis, which may be treated conservatively with antibiotic therapy.

The purpose of the examination is to evaluate the vascularity of scrotal structures in both dynamic and static phases. Technetium-99m pertechnetate or DTPA (30 mCi) is useful because it is inexpensive and has sufficiently long residence in the blood pool and extracellular space to serve as a marker of perfusion distribution. Because blood flow to the testicles and scrotum is relatively small compared with that to surrounding anatomy, the early perfusion images reveal activity in the iliac vessels, with only a small amount of activity seen in the scrotum. Delayed images also reveal homogeneous but slight activity in the testicles, with a greater amount of activity noted at the base of the penis in the midline when it is included in the field of view.

Testicular Torsion

Clinically, testicular torsion presents as sudden onset of testicular pain with hemiscrotal swelling; it frequently is preceded by a recent history of trauma. The mechanism is that of twisting of the testicle, usually enabled by accompanying anatomic variation or anomaly, which strangulates its blood supply through the spermatic cord. The sensitivity of scrotal imaging for the diagnosis for testicular torsion in adults is greater than 90%, similar to that of Doppler ultrasound. Sensitivity of radionuclide imaging in young children is somewhat less, presumably related to small testicular size. The scintigraphic appearance of testicular torsion varies with

both the degree and the duration of ischemia and thus with the time from onset of torsion. When interpreting scrotal scans, it is important to know which side is clinically symptomatic.

Early-Phase Torsion

During the first few hours, perfusion to the affected hemiscrotum and testicle is usually perceived as normal. A *nubbin sign* may be apparent, which consists of vascular activity projecting from the ipsilateral iliac artery into the spermatic cord vessels and terminating abruptly at the site of torsion. When identified, this sign is thought to be pathognomonic of torsion. On the delayed static scrotal images, testicular activity may be decreased but without evidence of a surrounding halo of increased activity. If the study appears normal in the setting of strong clinical suspicion of torsion, then acute torsion cannot be excluded and further evaluation is needed.

Late-Phase (Missed or Delayed) Torsion

As the duration of torsion increases, perfusion to the tissues surrounding the affected testicle increases through pudendal vessels, producing a halo of increased activity around the testes. Delayed torsion presents as significantly increased perfusion and delayed activity throughout the affected hemiscrotum, with the infarcted testes presenting as a central focus of photopenia (Fig. 10–19). Although their appearances vary, testicular neoplasms, testicular trauma with hematoma, and scrotal abscesses may produce scintigraphic findings identical to delayed testicular torsion.

Acute Epididymitis

Scintigraphically, acute bacterial or viral epididymitis and epididymo-orchitis present distinctively from acute or delayed torsion. Classically, both perfusion and delayed activity are increased in the region of the epididymis, with normal testicular activity in simple epididymitis (Fig. 10–20). In epididymo-orchitis, increased activity in both the epididymis and testicle is usually seen. However, if there is sufficient edema in the testicle, activity of the testicle may occasionally be decreased. Doppler ultrasound is often helpful in these cases to confirm preserved blood flow.

ADRENAL GLAND IMAGING

Adrenal lesions can present clinically with signs and symptoms of endocrine hyperfunction or as masses or adrenal enlargement on cross-sectional imaging. Incidental adrenal masses seen on CT or MRI are common. When clinically warranted, nuclear med-

icine studies allow selection of patients for biopsy or surgical intervention. Although the sensitivity values of the studies are high, the specificity values depend strongly on the suspected pathology being evaluated.

Adrenal Cortical (NP-59) Imaging

Radioiodinated NP-59 (I-6-β-iodomethyl-19-norcholesterol) is a cholesterol analog that is bound to and transported by low-density lipoproteins to specific low-density lipoprotein receptors on adrenocortical cells. Once taken up by the cells, it is esterified, but no further metabolism occurs. This allows imaging of the adrenal cortex. NP-59 remains investigational and very difficult to obtain. As a result it is only rarely used in clinical practice.

NP-59 background clearance and accumulation in the adrenal glands occurs slowly over several days, but by 4 to 5 days, accumulation in the normal adrenal glands is greater than in any other organ. Activity is usually noted in the liver,

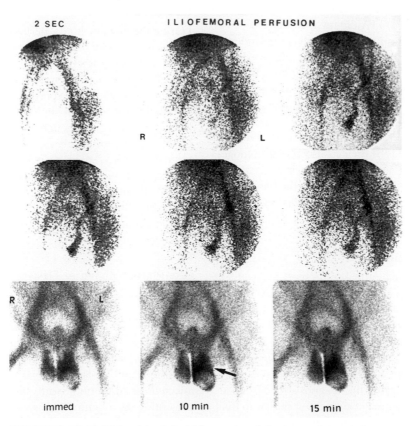

FIGURE 10–20. Epididymitis. *A*, Serial 2-second perfusion images demonstrate markedly increased flow to the region of the left testicle. *B*, On immediate blood pool and delayed static images, markedly increased activity (*arrow*) is seen in the region of the epididymis. Normal activity is seen in the testicle just below.

gallbladder, and colon. Interfering gallbladder activity at the time of imaging may be cleared by using cholecystokinin, and colon activity may be reduced with cathartics as needed. Some asymmetry of adrenal gland activity is usual. Because of liver background activity and because of less soft-tissue attenuation owing to its more posterior location, activity in the right adrenal is usually more intense than that in the left.

Clinical Applications

Cushing's syndrome (Hypercortisolism). Cushing's syndrome produces bilateral adrenal hyperplasia manifested by bilateral increased uptake of NP-59. Cushing's syndrome may also be caused by autonomous adrenal cortisol production (30% to 40% of cases). The causes include adrenal adenomas, which concentrate NP-59, and hyperfunctioning adrenal carcinomas, which do not concentrate NP-59. Thus, in this setting, increased unilateral adrenal uptake suggests hyperfunctioning adenoma, and bilateral nonvisualization is indicative of adrenal carcinoma.

Hyperaldosteronism. Hyperaldosteronism is caused by adenomas (70% of cases; aldosteronoma) or hyperplasia of the zona glomerulosa (30% of cases). In these circumstances, the sensitivity of NP-59 imaging is increased by prior suppression of the adrenocorticotrophic hormone–dependent inner cortical zona fasciculata by dexamethasone administration. This suppression delays normal adrenal cortex visualization for about 5 days. Thus, any adrenal activity seen on early imaging (3 to 4 days) indicates an abnormality. Early unilateral adrenal uptake before 5 days is seen with aldosteronoma, whereas bilateral uptake indicates hyperplasia.

Hyperandrogenism. Hyperandrogenism is a syndrome of excess secretion of weak androgens. It most commonly occurs secondary to polycystic ovarian disease but is also produced by primary adrenal cortical (zona reticularis) hyperplasia and rarely by adrenal tumors. The imaging patterns seen with dexamethasone suppression NP-59 imaging are identical to those seen in hyperaldosteronism. Early unilateral uptake is indicative of adenoma, and bilateral early uptake is compatible with hyperplasia.

Adrenal Medullary Imaging

Metaiodobenzylguanidine (MIBG) is a guanethidine analog similar to norepinephrine. It is taken up by chromaffin cells and is therefore useful for imaging normal and abnormal sympathetic adrenergic tissue, especially pheochromocytomas, whether located in the adrenal medulla or ectopically, and neuroblastomas. MIBG is localized in other neuroendocrine tumors to lesser degree, including carcinoid, medullary thyroid carcinoma, and paraganglioma. In the settings of pheochromocytoma and neuroblastoma, the sensitivity and specificity of MIBG are high, approaching 90%.

The specific radiopharmaceutical used is radioiodinated MIBG labeled with 3 to 10 mCi (81 to 370 MBq) of iodine-123 (^{123}I). Iodinated MIBG is slowly metabolized; 75% to 90% is excreted by the kidneys as unaltered MIBG. Whole-body planar images or selected spot images of the regions of interest using a low-energy parallel-hole collimator are obtained serially over 24 to 72 hours, depending on the suspected pathology.

Radioiodinated MIBG appears normally in the salivary glands and liver, with faint activity apparent in the heart and thyroid gland. Because of renal excretion, there is renal and bladder activity. Nasal, neck muscle, diffuse lung activity, and bowel activity may be noted in some patients. The normal adrenal medulla is only occasionally visualized. It is seen best on delayed images in about 30% to 40% of patients, but the intensity is usually less than that of the adjacent liver and must be distinguished from the more intense abnormal accumulation seen in pheochromocytoma or neuroblastoma.

Clinical Applications

Pheochromocytoma. Imaging with whole-body ^{123}I-MIBG is the method of choice for pheochromocytomas. Scanning for pheochromocytomas is especially helpful in diseases with a high incidence of the neoplasm, including multiple endocrine neoplasms (MEN) types 2A and 2B, neurofibromatosis, von Hippel-Lindau disease, Carney's triad, and familial pheochromocytoma. In addition to tumors of the adrenal medulla, ectopic pheochromocytomas are also imaged. The technique is sensitive in both adults and children.

Posterior adrenal images are obtained at 24, 48, or 72 hours, as needed. Whole-body planar imaging is useful if ectopic lesions are suspected. Pheochromocytomas imaged with radioiodinated MIBG present as focally increased activity whether the tumor is located in the adrenal medulla or ectopically (Fig. 10–21). Occasionally, some large

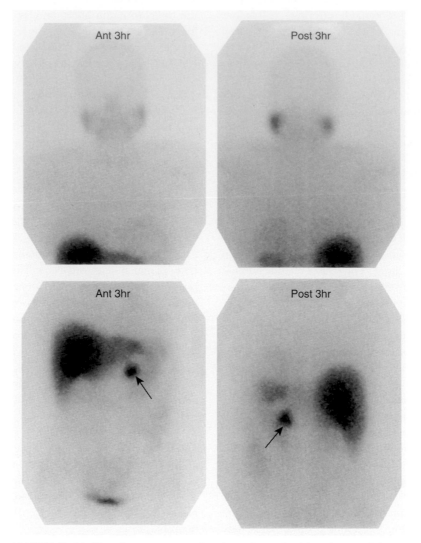

FIGURE 10–21. Pheochromocytoma. Anterior and posterior 3-hour images of the chest (*upper row*) and abdomen (*lower row*) done after administration of iodine-123 metaiodobenzylguanidine (MIBG) show a focus of abnormally increased activity (*arrow*) in the left adrenal gland.

tumors are not visualized because of extensive tumor necrosis.

Imipramine, insulin, reserpine, tricyclic antidepressants, and amphetamine-like drugs may inhibit localization of radioiodinated MIBG and thus interfere with tumor imaging. These should be withheld before imaging when practical.

Neuroblastoma. MIBG can be used to detect adrenal medullary neuroblastoma and its metastases in more than 90% of affected neonates and children. Whole-body imaging is performed 24 and 48 hours after administration. In normal subjects, the adrenal medulla may be seen on the more delayed images, and diffuse lung and gut activity can be prominent. Neuroblastomas and any metastases detected with MIBG present as foci of increased activity. Skeletal and marrow metastases are usually best seen on the 48-hour images. Aggressive chemotherapy may hinder the detection of some metastases.

Imaging of neuroblastomas and pheochromocytomas by using radiolabeled somatostatin analogues is discussed in Chapter 11.

PEARLS & PITFALLS

General

The common indications for radionuclide scanning of native kidneys include allergy to iodinated contrast material, assessment of possible renal artery stenosis, and differentiation of obstruction from a flaccid collecting system. In children, cortical scanning agents are used for evaluation of pyelonephritis.

Technetium-99m DTPA reflects glomerular filtration, whereas ^{99m}Tc-MAG3 is essentially a tubular agent. Technetium-99m-DMSA is a renal cortical agent. Technetium-99m glucoheptonate is used to evaluate both renal cortical anatomy and the collecting system.

On angiographic images, normally perfused kidneys should have the same intensity of activity as is seen at the bifurcation of the aorta. Renal transplants should have the same intensity as the adjacent iliac artery.

On serial 1- to 30-minute images of either normal native or transplanted kidneys, radiopharmaceutical excretion should follow the approximate time sequence of an IVP. Maximum parenchymal activity is seen at about 3 to 5 minutes, and bladder activity is seen by 4 to 8 minutes.

On serial 1- to 30-minute images, after the maximum renal activity peak, half of the renal activity should be cleared in about 8 to 12 minutes.

On a postcaptopril renogram using Tc-99m-MAG3 as the imaging agent, the kidney that has delayed clearance with significant renal cortical retention should be the one with the renal artery stenosis. Bilateral delayed clearance can be caused by bilateral stenosis, obstruction, medical renal disease, dehydration, or hypotension.

Technetium-99m MAG3 or DTPA in a dilated intrarenal collecting system that does not clear by 20 to 30 minutes can be either a flaccid system or an obstruction. This can often be differentiated with a furosemide renogram. Rapid washout of activity after furosemide administration indicates a flaccid system as opposed to a fixed mechanical obstruction.

In acute tubular necrosis (ATN) perfusion is usually normal with bilaterally increasing renal cortical activity and rising renogram curves when ^{99m}Tc-MAG3 is used.

Always interpret the renogram curves in light of the scintigraphic imaging findings. When faced with abnormal time-activity curves, look at the images to see if the problem is parenchymal or related to the collecting system.

Renal Transplant Imaging

Common indications are to differentiate rejection from ATN. Occasionally, surgical complications may be suspected.

ATN is usually seen within the first week after transplantation. It usually has preserved renal perfusion with progressive accumulation of tubular agents (^{99m}Tc-MAG3) in the renal parenchyma. It should improve with time.

Occasionally, severe ATN can present with enough edema immediately after surgery to have reduced perfusion and therefore look similar to acute rejection.

Cyclosporin toxicity can look like ATN but is usually not seen in the immediate postoperative period.

Rejection usually has poor perfusion and poor tubular excretion.

Look for photopenic defects around the transplant on the blood pool image that may be caused by urinomas, hematomas, and lymphoceles.

There often is a low-grade ureterovesicular obstruction during the first few days after surgery as a result of edema at the anastomotic site.

Testicular Imaging

Common indications are to differentiate between epididymitis and acute or delayed torsion.

The initial problem is to determine whether blood flow is increased or decreased. The best way to determine which side is abnormal is to obtain a patient history. If this is not available, the abnormal side is usually obvious on the blood pool and delayed images.

Epididymitis should be diffusely hot on all images and frequently focally hot in the region of the epididymis.

Acute torsion should have decreased or absent testicular flow.

Increased flow to one hemiscrotum and a rim of testicular activity with a cold center (halo sign)

PEARLS & PITFALLS—cont'd

can be a delayed torsion but also can be a testicular abscess, hematoma, or tumor.

Adrenal Imaging

NP-59 is an adrenal cortical imaging agent with imaging performed at 4–5 days. Unilateral adrenal uptake is usually an adenoma and bilateral uptake is usually due to adrenal hyperplasia.

MIBG is a medullary adrenal imaging agent which effectively localizes in pheochromocytoma and neuroblastoma. It may also localize in carcinoid, medullary thyroid carcinoma and paraganglioma.

SUGGESTED READINGS

Barron Bj, Kim EE, Lamki LM: Renal nuclear medicine. In Sandler MP, Coleman RE, Patton JA et al. (eds): Diagnostic Nuclear Medicine, 4th ed. New York, Lippincott, Williams and Wilkins, 2003, pp 865–902.

Brown ED, Chen MYM, Wolfman NT, Ott DJ, Nat E, Watson Jr NE: Complications of Renal Transplantation: Evaluation with US and Radionuclide Imaging. RadioGraphics 20:607–622, 2000.

Dubovsky EV, Russel CD: Evaluation of renal and pancreatic transplants. In Sandler MP, Coleman RE, Patton JA et al. (eds): Diagnostic Nuclear Medicine, 4th ed. New York, Lippincott, Williams and Wilkins, 2003, pp 1037–1050.

Fine EJ: Diuretic renography and angiotensin converting enzyme inhibitor renography. Radiol Clin North Am 39:979–95, 2001.

Frietas JE: Scrotal scintigraphy. In Sandler MP, Coleman RE, Patton JA et al. (eds): Diagnostic Nuclear Medicine, 4th ed. New York, Lippincott, Williams and Wilkins, 2003, pp 903–910.

Rossleigh MA: Renal Cortical Scintigraphy and Diuresis Renography in Infants and Children. J Nucl Med 42:91–95, 2001.

Conventional Neoplasm Imaging and Radioimmunotherapy

11

INTRODUCTION

It has long been recognized that many routinely used radiopharmaceuticals may incidentally accumulate in neoplasms, but it was not until the introduction of gallium-67 (^{67}Ga) citrate as the first widely used tumor imaging agent that the noninvasive localization of primary and metastatic neoplasms using nuclear medicine techniques was realized. During the past decade, new biotechnologic advances have spurred the development of increasingly sensitive and specific tumor imaging agents for use in both single-photon and positron imaging. In this chapter, tumor imaging using conventional gamma camera techniques is addressed. Positron emission tomography (PET) imaging of neoplasms is discussed in Chapter 13.

Tumor-imaging radiopharmaceuticals may be divided into two broad groups: (1) those that have a nonspecific affinity for neoplastic tissue and may be used to image a range of tumors in various organs, including ^{67}Ga, thallium-201 (^{201}Tl),

technetium-99m (^{99m}Tc) sestamibi, and fluorine-18 deoxyglucose (^{18}F-FDG); and (2) those designed to label specific tumor antigens, receptors, or metabolic processes, including monoclonal antibodies, peptides such as somatostatin, and metaiodobenzylguanidine (MIBG). Both categories of radiopharmaceuticals are used in clinical nuclear medicine practice. Typical administered activities and radiation doses for tumor-seeking radiopharmaceuticals in current use are given in Appendix E–1.

GALLIUM-67 IMAGING

Gallium-67 imaging has been used for many years as a valuable diagnostic tool in the setting of neoplastic disease. With the development of newer, more tissue-specific radiopharmaceuticals and the widespread availability of computed tomography (CT), magnetic resonance imaging (MRI), and PET, many of the original applications of ^{67}Ga

325

imaging are no longer routinely used. Nevertheless, ^{67}Ga may still be useful in some settings and in some institutions for the localization, evaluation, and follow-up of lymphoma and Hodgkin's disease. However, there appear to be few clinical indications for gallium use in other tumors.

Physical Characteristics and Biologic Behavior

Gallium-67 has a physical half-life of 78.1 hours and decays by electron capture, emitting gamma radiation over an energy range of 93 to 880 keV. The four principal energy peaks useful in diagnostic imaging are 93, 184, 296, and 388 keV. One or all of these peaks may be used in obtaining gamma camera images. In practice, several peaks are usually used to increase photon abundance. Gallium is commonly used as a trivalent citrate compound and usually arrives in the nuclear medicine laboratory in a carrier-free state ready for intravenous administration.

When injected intravenously, most ^{67}Ga is immediately bound to plasma proteins, primarily transferrin. During the first 12 to 24 hours, excretion from the body is primarily through the kidneys, with 20% to 25% of the administered dose being excreted by 24 hours. After that time, the intestinal mucosa becomes the major route of elimination. Overall, these modes of excretion account for the elimination of about one third of the administered dose. The remaining two thirds is retained in the body for a prolonged period. In addition to activity within the axial skeleton, liver, spleen, and bowel, concentration is also seen in the salivary and lacrimal glands as well as in the breasts and external genitalia. If imaging is performed in the first 24 hours, kidney and bladder activity may also be noted.

The mechanisms underlying the uptake of ^{67}Ga in neoplasms appear to be mediated by transport of ^{67}Ga to the site of localization mainly by plasma proteins and ^{67}Ga–transferrin complexes, which act as carriers for [67]Ga. Once it is taken up by neoplastic cells, ^{67}Ga is, for the most part, located in the cytoplasm and is associated predominantly with lysosomes and the endoplasmic reticulum. Although the reason for localization in certain tumors and not in others is not entirely understood, one hypothesis suggests that the mechanism is related to the presence of transferrin receptors on the tumor cells that bind ^{67}Ga–transferrin complexes.

Technique

Gallium imaging may be performed by using whole-body techniques or by using spot imaging with a large-field-of-view gamma camera and a medium-energy parallel-hole collimator. A gamma camera with a multichannel analyzer permits the several ^{67}Ga gamma peaks to be imaged simultaneously. Although imaging may be successful using a standard intravenous dose of 4 to 6 mCi (148 to 222 MBq) of ^{67}Ga citrate, doses in the range of 8 to 10 mCi (296 to 370 MBq) are often preferred for tumor imaging to provide better photon flux, especially if single-photon emission computed tomography (SPECT) imaging is anticipated. For imaging neoplasms, initial images are usually obtained at 48 hours. Images are subsequently obtained at 24-hour intervals as needed to allow for improved target-to-nontarget ratios and for improving differentiation of normal bowel activity from accumulations in pathologic entities. Use of SPECT techniques may increase sensitivity relative to planar imaging, especially in the mediastinum and abdomen. Tomographic techniques should be considered when the results of the planar study are negative and a specific site of tumor involvement is suspected, or when the planar findings are equivocal or incomplete in defining the extent of disease. Details relative to imaging protocols are presented in Appendix E–1.

Normal Scan

The interpretation of ^{67}Ga images is complicated by marginal anatomic resolution and by interfering activity in the bowel, in postoperative sites of hematoma or wound healing, and in healing fractures. Thus, careful attention to patient history and anatomic orientation and a thorough appreciation of the physiologic distribution of gallium and its excretion patterns are of utmost importance (Fig. 11–1). Normally, gallium activity is noted in the osseous structures of the skull, in the nasopharynx, and variably in the lacrimal and salivary glands. Activity in the salivary glands may be especially increased in patients who have undergone radiation therapy.

Gallium activity is prominent in the skeletal structures of the thorax, including the sternum. In early images (4 to 6 hours), blood pool activity in the heart and great vessels may be noted. Diffuse activity in the lungs is abnormal but usually due to benign causes (Table 11–1). Symmetric accumulation of gallium in the breasts occasionally interferes

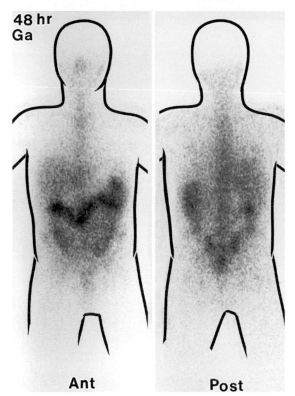

48 hr Ga

Ant   **Post**

FIGURE 11–1. Normal gallium scan. Anterior (*left*) and posterior (*right*) images are obtained at 48 hours. Some activity is seen in the bone marrow, the nasopharynx, and the liver. In addition, there is a larger amount of activity within the colon. This is normal physiologic excretion, which limits the usefulness of gallium in the abdomen. Although not present in this patient, activity is commonly seen in the lacrimal glands.

TABLE 11–2.	Persistent Gallium Activity in the Kidneys after 24 Hours
Obstruction	
Renal parenchymal pathology	
Neoplasm	
Pyelonephritis	
Vasculitis	
Acute tubular necrosis	
Infiltrative disease	
Leukemia	
Lymphoma	
Plasma transferrin saturation	
Parenteral iron injections	
Blood transfusions	
Perirenal inflammatory disease	
Faint visualization, which may be normal	

injection. After that time, renal activity should be considered abnormal, especially when it is asymmetric (Table 11–2). A common problem encountered in the interpretation of abdominal images is the physiologic presence of gallium in the bowel, which may mimic lesions or mask disease. Bowel activity is particularly notable in the colon and may be diffuse or focal. Frequently, activity is seen in the region of the cecum, hepatic and splenic flexures, and rectosigmoid. These accumulations may appear as early as a few hours after injection. Various bowel preparations have been investigated as possible means of eliminating such interfering activity in the colon, but none have proved consistently successful. The progress of excreted gallium through the colon on sequential images may provide the best evidence of physiologic activity. Persistence of gallium in a given area of the abdomen should be viewed as abnormal. Activity is seen in the osseous pelvis, particularly in the sacrum and sacroiliac joints on posterior views. On early images, bladder activity may be noted, and later, concentrations may be seen in the region of male or female genitalia. As in the abdomen, cecal or rectosigmoid accumulation may present a problem in interpretation. As a weak bone agent, gallium is noted throughout the normal skeleton and in areas of benign skeletal remodeling.

Clinical Applications

In the proper clinical setting and with meticulous attention to technique, gallium imaging can be a useful adjunctive tool in the investigation of selected neoplasms. The technique is most successful when correlated with clinical findings and

with chest imaging, especially under the stimuli of menarche, pregnancy, or hormonal agents, such as birth control pills or hormone replacement therapy.

Gallium is normally detected in the liver and, to a lesser extent, in the spleen. As the primary initial excretory route, the kidneys and bladder may be identified on images obtained up to 24 hours after

TABLE 11–1.	Diffuse Pulmonary Uptake of Gallium-67
Idiopathic pulmonary fibrosis	
Diffuse pneumonitis	
Pulmonary sarcoid	
Lymphangitic metastases	
Pneumocystis carinii pneumonia	
Miliary tuberculosis	
Bleomycin toxicity	
Radiation pneumonitis (early exudative phase)	

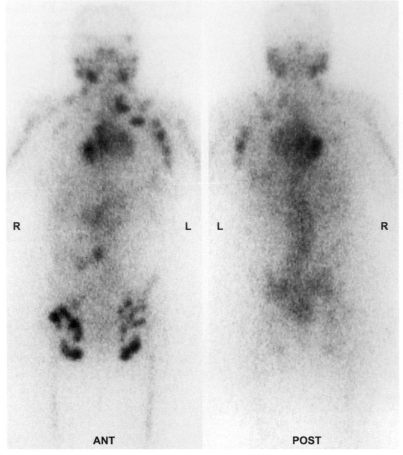

FIGURE 11–2. Lymphoma. Anterior and posterior whole-body gallium scans performed at 48 hours demonstrate multiple foci of active disease in the neck, left axillary region, mediastinum central abdomen, and both inguinal areas.

results of other imaging procedures, such as CT, MRI, or ultrasound.

Lymphoma

The malignant lymphomas constitute the neoplastic group in which gallium has been most extensively studied and was widely used before being largely replaced by ^{18}F-FDG PET imaging. The sensitivity of gallium in detecting lymphomatous disease depends greatly on the size and location of the lesions. Lesions smaller than 1.0 cm are not often detected. Sites of involvement in the abdomen and pelvis may be difficult to identify because of interfering activity within the liver and colon and their often deep-seated location.

The sensitivity value of ^{67}Ga imaging in untreated Hodgkin's disease is more than 85% to 90%, with all histologic types showing some degree of gallium concentration (Fig. 11–2). The sensitiv-

ity of ^{67}Ga imaging in non-Hodgkin's lymphoma (NHL) is less than that in Hodgkin's disease and demonstrates variability related to histologic type. Sensitivity ranges from about 90% in the histiocytic cell type to less than 60% with the lymphocytic well-differentiated type lymphoma. Significantly lower detection rates are seen in low-grade lymphomas., although success in imaging may be improved with high-dose SPECT imaging. In addition to soft-tissue disease, gallium scans can also identify osseous lymphoma (Fig. 11–3).

Gallium imaging can be used as a tool for post-treatment evaluation of lymphoma patients. Successful therapy, including radiotherapy and chemotherapy, results in decreased or absent uptake of gallium in involved sites. Thus, serial imaging may be of value in assessing the effects of therapy as well as in detecting early disease recurrence. The use of gallium in this setting requires

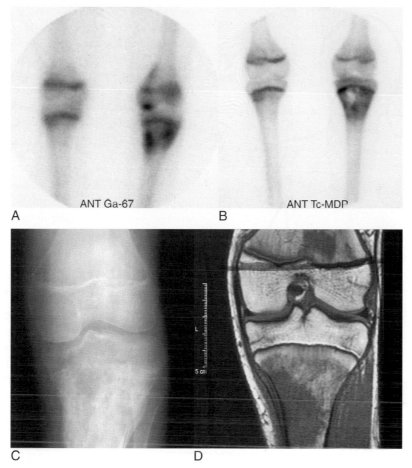

FIGURE 11–3. Lymphoma in bone. *A,* Anterior gallium scan of both knees shows an abnormal focus of activity in the left tibial metaphysis and medial tibial plateau. *B,* Similar but less intense activity is evident on the bone scan. Normal epiphseal plate activity is seen in this teenager. Abnormal mottled sclerosis is seen in the plain x-ray (*C*) and abnormal signal is seen on the magnetic resonance imaging scan (*D*).

meticulous technique. High-dose imaging with the routine use of SPECT in the neck, chest, and abdomen is essential. Imaging before therapy is mandatory to determine whether the lymphoma is gallium avid and to serve as a baseline map of existing lesions. Any gallium uptake in residual masses is an indicator of persistent viable tumor cells, and further treatment is indicated. A negative scan is considered a sign of successful treatment. Gallium-67 imaging should not be performed before about 4 to 6 weeks after completion of chemotherapy because "stunned" but still viable tumor cells may temporarily cease to take up gallium, resulting in false-negative results.

Conversion of a positive gallium scan to negative may confirm a clinical and radiologic impression of eradication of lymphomatous lesions. Because technical factors may limit the detection of small tumor deposits, however, a negative gallium study by itself cannot ensure remission. Radiation therapy can cause both the parotid glands and the thymus to accumulate gallium for several months after therapy. Thymic activity after chemotherapy or radiation can be confusing and can lead to a false-positive diagnosis of lymphoma recurrence (Fig. 11–4).

Hepatoma

Gallium-67 scanning has proved to be successful in differentiating primary hepatocellular carcinoma from regenerating nodules in patients with cirrhosis. Almost always, these studies are preceded by radionuclide or CT scans of the liver. In patients with a hepatic defect on a ^{99m}Tc colloid liver scan

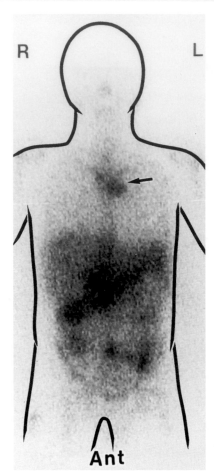

FIGURE 11–4. Reactive changes of the thymus. In this patient with known Hodgkin's disease, a gallium scan was performed after radiation therapy of the thorax. A focus of activity is seen in the mediastinum slightly to the left of midline (*arrow*). This was not present on the gallium scan performed before radiation therapy. This benign reactive change can be seen in the thymus (and occasionally in the parotid glands) after radiation therapy or chemotherapy. It is important not to mistake this for recurrent disease.

or a mass on CT that is suspected to be hepatoma, gallium uptake of greater intensity in the region of the abnormality than elsewhere in the liver is a strong indication of hepatoma (Fig. 11–5). When greatly diminished gallium uptake is identified in the suspect region, hepatoma is extremely unlikely. Gallium uptake in the anatomically abnormal region equal to that in the surrounding liver is equivocal and may be found in regenerating nodules and hepatoma as well as in tumors of other causes, such as metastatic disease.

Other Neoplasms

Although the sensitivity of gallium imaging for bronchogenic carcinoma is about 90%, there is poor specificity due to accumulation of gallium in a variety of non-neoplastic lesions, including infectious and inflammatory lesions and sarcoidosis. Therefore, gallium is not generally a useful tool in the differential diagnosis of pulmonary lesions. In general, melanoma, seminoma, and rhabdomyosarcoma are gallium-avid tumors, and gallium imaging displays excellent sensitivity for the detection of both primary and metastatic lesions within the limitations of the technique. Gallium studies exhibit low sensitivity for breast cancer, gastrointestinal tumors, and most genitourinary neoplasms and are of essentially no use in these settings. Gallium imaging is not usually recommended for the routine screening of patients with occult primary malignancies.

THALLIUM-201 CHLORIDE IMAGING

Thallium-201 chloride is a potassium analog that is avidly concentrated by some tumors. Long known for its use as a myocardial perfusion imaging agent, thallium has shown to be of value in the investigation of certain neoplastic diseases, including thyroid, lung, and breast cancer; glioblastomas; and bone and soft-tissue sarcomas. Compared with ^{67}Ga citrate, thallium generally shows less uptake in benign tumors, inflammatory processes, and remodeling bone. As with myocardial imaging, oncologic thallium imaging suffers the limitations of low administered dose, long half-life, and less than ideal, low-energy photon. After intravenous administration, ^{201}Tl localizes in the normal skeletal muscle, myocardium, liver, spleen, stomach, and colon, which may cause interference in the detection of certain lesions. Uptake is also seen in the choroid plexus, orbits, salivary glands, kidneys, and testes.

Tumor cell type, viability, and blood flow greatly influence the uptake of thallium in specific tumor masses. In tumor cells, the mechanisms of ^{201}Tl uptake are not fully defined, but penetration of the cell membrane is generally acknowledged to be related to cell membrane potential and to the Na$^+$-K$^+$ ATPase pump. Thallium rapidly localizes in active, viable neoplasms, with peak uptake in tumors such as lymphoma and breast and lung carcinomas at about 10 to 20 minutes after injection. Imaging is usually performed 2 to 4 hours after administration to permit improved target-to-background ratios. Both 15- to 20-minute and 3-hour imaging may prove of value when the object is to distinguish benign from malignant masses.

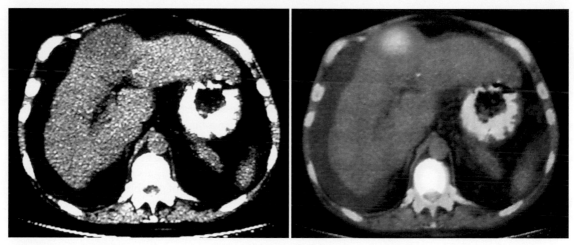

FIGURE 11–5. Hepatoma. *Left,* A narrow window computed tomography (CT) scan demonstrates a low density bulge in the anterior aspect of this cirrhotic liver. *Right,* A gallium SPECT/CT fusion image shows increased gallium activity in this hepatoma.

Early activity seen in benign lesions tends to decrease by 3 hours, whereas the activity in malignant lesions remains relatively constant. Lack of thallium uptake correlates with but is not diagnostic of a benign cause.

Clinical Applications
Brain Neoplasms

Thallium accumulates in malignant gliomas in proportion to the aggressiveness of the lesions. Low-grade lesions concentrate little or no thallium and may not be detected, whereas high-grade gliomas show markedly increased activity compared with normal brain tissue. Gliosis surrounding brain abscesses, however, may also demonstrate marked thallium accumulation, so that correlation with CT or MRI and clinical findings is important in the differential diagnosis. Thallium imaging can be useful in distinguishing postradiation necrosis from recurrent tumor in patients with recurrence of symptoms and equivocal MRI findings. This topic is discussed more fully in Chapter 4.

Acquired Immunodeficiency Syndrome-Related Neoplasms

Kaposi's sarcoma is thallium avid but does not take up gallium, whereas lymphoma concentrates both agents. Thus, use of both agents may allow differentiation. Further, gallium uptake in a thoracic lesion without corresponding thallium uptake, or with mildly increased thallium uptake that fades on delayed images, suggests tuberculosis, *Mycobacterium avium-intracellulare,* or acute infection.

Other Adult Tumors

Although most lymphomas are thallium avid, the intensity of uptake is inversely proportional to the aggressiveness of the lesions. Low histologic grades tend to show marked thallium avidity, and higher-grade lesions display less or absent uptake. Thallium may be useful in low-grade lymphomas, for which gallium imaging may demonstrate a somewhat lower sensitivity. Soft-tissue and skeletal sarcomas, including osteosarcoma, may concentrate thallium, and thallium imaging has been used to determine the success of preoperative chemotherapy and thus prognosis. Relapse rates are higher in patients exhibiting modest or no detectable change in thallium activity after treatment. Differentiated thyroid carcinoma is thallium avid, and some institutions use thallium follow-up imaging for metastatic or residual disease instead of iodine-131 (^{131}I). Thallium is also taken up by parathyroid adenomas and some breast carcinomas, but ^{99m}Tc-sestamibi appears to be a better imaging agent and is more commonly used in these settings.

TECHNETIUM-99M SESTAMIBI TUMOR IMAGING

Although ^{99m}Tc-sestamibi concentrates in a number of tumors, including breast and thyroid cancers, it is primarily used to image parathyroid adenomas (discussed in Chapter 5). Although the exact mechanism of ^{99m}Tc-sestamibi uptake by tumor cells is uncertain, primary factors include its lipophilicity, which permits passive transport through tumor cell membranes, and its active uptake by mitochondria once intracellular. Cells with higher mitochondrial content show greater ^{99m}Tc-sestamibi concentration.

After intravenous injection, ^{99m}Tc-sestamibi distributes throughout the body in proportion to blood flow, localizing in the myocardium, thyroid, and salivary glands as well as in the spleen, kidneys, bladder, lungs, skeletal muscle, liver, gallbladder, and small and large intestines.

Breast Cancer

Technetium-99m sestamibi concentrates in malignant breast tumors, with a mean contrast ratio approaching 6 : 1 when compared with normal breast tissue or surrounding fat. When used to image breast carcinomas, ^{99m}Tc-sestamibi has reported sensitivity and specificity of 85% to 90% in palpable lesions; sensitivity is somewhat less in nonpalpable and presumably smaller lesions. A negative scan in the presence of a palpable lesion is also significant, making breast cancer possible but unlikely.

Imaging of suspected breast cancer is performed 10 to 20 minutes after the injection of 20 to 30 mCi (740 to 1110 MBq) of ^{99m}Tc-sestamibi in an arm vein contralateral to the side of the suspected breast lesion. A foot injection is advised if both breasts are to be imaged. Planar imaging is best performed in a prone breast-dependent position with a breast positioning device that places the breast as close to the camera face as possible. Dedicated gamma cameras for sestamibi breast imaging have been developed that mimic conventional mammographic compression and offer greater sensitivity than do standard gamma cameras. Because there is little sestamibi washout from malignant lesions, imaging may be delayed, if needed, for up to 2 hours.

Technetium-99m sestamibi distributes homogeneously in the normal breast, regardless of the degree of breast density demonstrated on mammograms, and is usually of low intensity. A small number of patients exhibit diffusely increased activity in one or both breasts, which may be related to hormone levels at the time of imaging. This activity appears to be lowest at or about mid-cycle in premenopausal patients, especially those younger than 30 years. Although this is considered a benign finding, the increased background may obscure a lesion. A positive study presents as a discrete focus of increased activity in the breast or axilla that is greater than adjacent breast activity. The location of the abnormal focus should be carefully correlated with any palpatory and mammographic findings.

False-positive results are generally related to fibroadenomas, fibrocystic change, or inflammation but have also been reported in benign conditions that confer a higher risk for developing carcinoma, including epithelial hyperplasia and sclerosing adenosis. False-negative results may occur with small (less than 1 cm) or deep lesions, especially in the medial aspect of the breast; in lesions overlapping myocardial activity; or in tumors with less avidity for sestamibi. At this time, the use of ^{99m}Tc-sestabmibi for assessment of suspicious breast lesions has been largely replaced by other techniques (such as stereotactic needle biopsy).

LABELED MONOCLONAL ANTIBODIES

A number of monoclonal antibodies have been developed that target pancarcinoma antigens shared by various neoplastic lesions, such as carcinoembryonic antigen (CEA), or antigens specific to particular tumor types. These radiopharmaceuticals have met with mixed success in clinical application. The accuracy of the antibody depends in large part on the uniqueness of the antigen targeted and the specificity of the monoclonal antibody in recognizing the antigen. It is rare, however, to discover a monoclonal antibody that is specific to a particular normal or neoplastic tissue type. Cross-reaction with normal or other malignant tissues, with the resultant loss of specificity, is expected even under the best conditions.

The most recent generation of antineoplastic monoclonal antibodies includes indium-111 (^{111}In)- and ^{99m}Tc-labeled antibody fragments to particular tumor antigens. Imaging with these agents usually depends largely on delivering a sufficient number of labeled antibodies by the intravenous route to tumor sites to overcome background activity of various nontargeted normal tissue and organs (especially the liver, kidneys, and lungs), binding to antigens circulating in the plasma, and nonspecific leakage into the extravascular space.

Recent monoclonal imaging radiopharmaceuticals are largely focused on ovarian, prostate, and colon carcinomas. With progress in the development of monoclonal antibodies of higher specificity, an increasing number have achieved approval by the Food and Drug Administration (FDA). Unfortunately, even those with FDA approval are not widely used due to relatively low sensitivity and specificity in the range of only 50% to 70%. Perhaps the only widely used monoclonal radiopharmaceutical at this time is ibritumomab tiuxetan used for lymphoma therapy, which is discussed later in this chapter.

NEUROPEPTIDE RECEPTOR IMAGING

Neuropeptides constitute a family of highly potent substances that consist of only a few amino acids. They are synthesized and released primarily by the brain (hence the name *neuropeptides*) and the gut and also by the endocrine system and lymphatic tissue. A number of neuropeptides and tissue receptors present as potential candidates for neuropeptide receptor imaging, including somatostatin, vasoactive intestinal peptide (VIP), α-melanocyte-stimulating hormone, and substance P receptors. Of these, radiolabeled somatostatin analogs have emerged as a prime example of the clinical utility of this approach.

Somatostatin Receptor Imaging

Somatostatin is a naturally-occurring neuro-polypeptide that is synthesized and released by endocrine or nerve cells in various organs, especially the hypothalamus. It has a wide range of pharmacologic effects, including (as its name implies) the inhibition of secretion of growth hormone (somatotropin). Because a high density of somatostatin receptors is present in numerous neuroendocrine and some non-neuroendocrine tumors, radiolabeled somatostatin analogs can be used to image a variety of tumors, including primary and metastatic foci.

Neuroendocrine tumors are those derived from APUD (*a*mine *p*recursor *u*ptake and *d*ecarboxylation) system cells, including carcinoid (Fig. 11–6), pituitary adenomas, pancreatic islet cell neoplasms, medullary carcinoma of the thyroid, pheochromocytomas, neuroblastomas, paragangliomas, and small-cell lung cancers (Fig. 11–7). Most of these are successfully imaged with radiolabeled somatostatin analogs with sensitivities approaching 80% to 100%. Exceptions are insulinomas (50% to 60% sensitivity) and medullary thyroid carcinoma (65% to 70% sensitivity), in which somatostatin sensitivity values are considerably less. Some non-neuroendocrine tumors, including lymphomas, breast carcinoma, gliomas (especially low-grade tumors), and meningiomas, show variable and unpredictable uptake.

Because endogenous somatostatin has a biologic half-life of only a few minutes, radiolabeled analogs with greater in vivo stability have been developed. The eight-amino acid peptide iodine-123 (^{123}I) octreotide was the first to be used clinically. Subsequently, a cyclic structural modification of octreotide, ^{111}In-labeled pentetreotide (OctreoScan), was proven to have the additional advantages of greater stability and reduced hepatobiliary excretion, with clearance primarily through renal elimination. Less gastrointestinal activity allows for better visualization of abdominal tumor sites.

An intravenous imaging dose of 3.0 to 6.0 mCi (111 to 222 MBq) of ^{111}In-pentetreotide is used; the higher end of the dose range is preferred when SPECT is performed. Adverse effects from pentetreotide occur in less than 1% of patients. Imaging is performed at 4 and 24 hours, with 48-hour images acquired as needed to confirm a lesion suspected at 24 hours or when residual bowel or gallbladder activity is a problem. Planar images allow for survey of the whole body. SPECT images are frequently helpful and may add to the sensitivity of the examination, especially in the upper abdomen, where interfering kidney, spleen, and often gallbladder activity may hamper imaging of the pancreas and duodenum. SPECT may also be useful in better evaluating suspect liver metastases. A detailed imaging protocol in presented in Appendix E–1.

Patient preparation is important for safe, effective imaging with ^{111}In-pentetreotide. Patients should be well hydrated to enhance renal clearance. A laxative should be used to decrease interfering bowel activity. In patients with diarrheal syndromes or insulinomas, laxatives should be prescribed only after consultation with the referring physician.

Because of its ability to inhibit the secretion of hormones, stable octreotide is helpful in controlling symptoms in patients with hypersecretion syndromes associated with metastatic carcinoid tumors, gastrinomas, insulinomas, glucagonomas, and vasoactive intestinal peptide-related tumors (VIPomas). Although somatostatin receptor-positive tumors may be visualized in patients receiving stable octreotide therapy, it is preferable to discontinue the drug temporarily for 24 to 48 hours before administration of ^{111}In-pentetreotide.

In a normal patient, ^{111}In-pentetreotide activity is identified in the blood pool, normal thyroid gland, kidneys and bladder, liver, gallbladder, spleen, and, to a lesser degree, bowel on delayed images. The kidneys and spleen retain the most

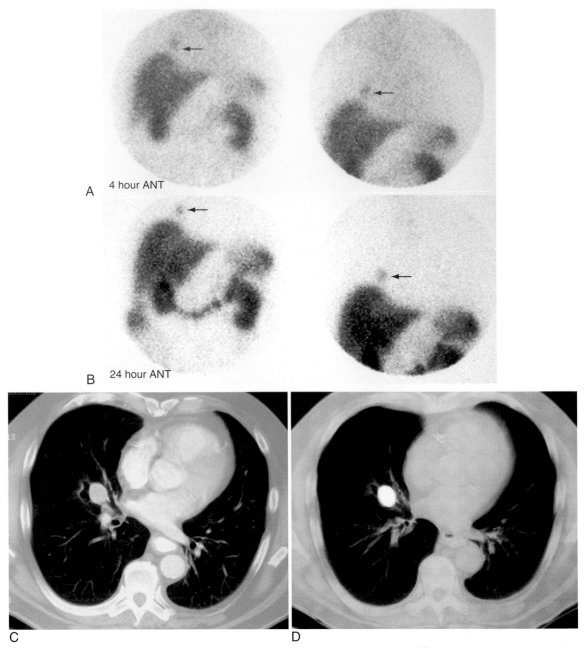

FIGURE 11–6. Pulmonary carcinoid. Four-hour (*A*) and 24-hour (*B*) anterior indium-111 (^{111}In) pentetreotide (somatostatin) images of the abdomen and chest show normal activity in the liver, kidneys, and bowel; however, an abnormal focus of activity is seen in the right lower chest (*arrow*). *C*, An abnormal enhancing lesion is seen on the computed tomography (CT) scan. *D*, The SPECT/CT fusion image clearly shows accumulation of ^{111}In pentetreotide by this carcinoid.

activity and therefore receive the highest absorbed doses. Because the radiopharmaceutical is in part retained by the renal parenchyma, the kidneys are seen even on delayed views.

In abnormal images, primary neoplasms or metastases present as foci of increased activity. Because somatostatin receptors are expressed in some non-neoplastic, chronic inflammatory processes, such as granulomatous lesions (sarcoidosis, tuberculosis), Crohn's disease, ulcerative colitis, and rheumatoid arthritis, these entities may serve as potential sources of false-positive results.

Indium-111 pentetreotide is primarily useful in evaluating neuroendocrine tumors, especially car-

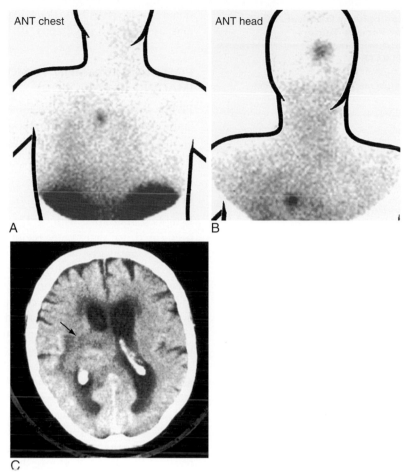

FIGURE 11–7. Small-cell lung cancer with brain metastasis. *A,* Anterior indium-111 pentetreotide (somatostatin) image of the chest shows an abnormal focus of activity in the central thorax. *B,* Another anterior image also shows a lesion in the brain. *C,* A computed tomography scan shows the metastatic brain lesion (*arrow*).

cinoids (sensitivity, 85% to 95%) and gastrinomas. A wider spectrum of tumors may be assessed with this radiopharmaceutical, however, including a number of nonendocrine solid tumors (Table 11–3). Indium-111 pentetreotide is not useful in pancreatic carcinomas of exocrine origin because they do not express somatostatin receptors. The sensitivity of pentetreotide for imaging pheochromocytomas, neuroblastomas, and paragangliomas in extra-adrenal sites is over 85%.

Whole-body gamma camera imaging provides cost-effective screening of patients with suspected or known somatostatin receptor-containing tumors. The information obtained may disclose or confirm the presence of a lesion, detect metastases from a primary tumor, or characterize neuroendocrine conditions in which multicentric lesions may exist.

In addition, because somatostatin receptor expression is seen more often in well-differentiated tumors, visualization may imply a more favorable prognosis. Patients with positive ^{111}In-pentetreotide images are also candidates for octreotide therapy because the documentation of somatostatin receptors provides a higher likelihood of controlling hormonal hypersecretion.

ADRENAL TUMOR IMAGING

Iodine-123 or 131 MIBG imaging is useful and sensitive in the detection and evaluation of primary adrenal or extra-adrenal pheochromocytomas (see Fig. 10–21), of neuroblastomas and their metastases, and of paragangliomas. Imaging adrenal neoplasms with radiolabeled MIBG and the occa-

TABLE 11–3.	Radiopharmaceutical Affinity for Various Tumors

GALLIUM-67 CITRATE
Hodgkin's disease
Non-Hodgkin's lymphoma (especially high-grade)
Hepatoma
Bronchogenic carcinoma
Melanoma
Seminoma
Rhabdomyosarcoma

THALLIUM-201 CHLORIDE
Gliomas (high-grade)
Thyroid carcinoma
Benign tumors (usually fade over 2 hr)
Osteosarcoma
Lymphoma (especially low grade)
Kaposi's sarcoma (gallium-negative)

TECHNETIUM-99m SESTAMIBI
Cancer metastases
Breast cancer
Parathyroid adenomas
Gliomas
Lymphoma
Thyroid

INDIUM-111 PENTETREOTIDE
APUD cell tumors
Pancreatic islet cell
Pituitary adenoma
Pheochromocytoma
Neuroblastoma
Paragangliomas
Carcinoid
Gastrinoma
Medullary carcinoma of thyroid
Small-cell lung cancer
Meningioma

FLUORINE-18 FLUORODEOXYGLUCOSE
Most tumors
Head and neck cancer
Esophageal cancer
Non–small-cell lung cancer
Melanoma
Lymphoma
Colorectal cancer
Breast cancer

IODINE-123 OR 131 SODIUM IODIDE
Thyroid cancer

IODINE-123 OR 131 METAIODOBENZYLGUANIDINE
Pheochromocytoma
Neuroblastoma
Paraganglioma

MONOCLONAL ANTIBODIES
Lymphoma

sional use of NP-59 for detecting adrenal adenomas are discussed in Chapter 10.

POSITRON-EMISSION TOMOGRAPHY IMAGING IN ONCOLOGY

PET is now extensively used for staging, restaging and monitoring response to therapy of many neoplasms. These applications are addressed in a dedicated PET chapter (Chapter 13).

LYMPHOSCINTIGRAPHY

Lymphoscintigraphy with ^{99m}Tc-sulfur colloid has been used to determine regional lymph node drainage pathways from malignant neoplasms, which may direct therapeutic management decisions, including radiation therapy fields and surgical approach. This technique has proved most useful in breast and skin malignancies, especially truncal and head and neck malignant melanomas.

The particles in standard colloid preparations are generally too large to be acceptable for most applications of lymphoscintigraphy. Thus, the sulfur colloid is filtered to select a more appropriate particle size (<0.22 μm). The procedure involves several injections of small volumes (0.1 mL) of filtered ^{99m}Tc-sulfur colloid into the soft tissues at, or adjacent to, the tumor site. Generally, injection of the radiocolloid directly into the tumor is not advisable as this may significantly delay or even prevent migration into the lymphatic channels. For skin lesions such as melanoma, intradermal injections are used. For other tumors, subcutaneous or interstitial injections are performed. The detailed protocol is presented in Appendix E–1.

Once injected, the radiocolloid is removed from the area through lymphatic channels to reach regional lymph nodes, which receive lymphatic drainage from the primary lesion and thus have the potential of harboring metastases. Gamma camera imaging allows mapping of lymphatics and lymph nodes, especially sentinel nodes. The sentinel node is the first node to receive regional lymphatic flow from the tumor site and is a reliable biopsy indicator of the presence or absence of metastatic tumor in a lymph node group. If the sentinel node is free of tumor cells, the patient may be spared the morbidity and cost associated with elective dissection of the remaining lymph nodes in the chain. Performing the procedure just before surgery also permits intraoperative identification of sentinel nodes for biopsy by using a hand-held gamma probe detector. Use of a gamma probe in the operating room can usually be performed 30 minutes to several hours after injection to help localize the sentinel node during surgery. The sentinel lymph node typically has 10 or more times the background count rate observed at a location remote from the injection site.

A two-phase imaging technique is preferred that includes an early-phase series of static images or dynamic imaging to map visually the lymphatic channels followed by delayed static imaging to identify lymph node retention and to visualize sentinel nodes. The early or dynamic images permit a more exact identification of the first-draining node when more than one node is identified on the delayed images. The times of imaging are determined by the rate of migration of the radiocolloid from the site of injection.

In addition to normal pathways, abnormal patterns suggestive of tumor replacement of lymph nodes and lymphatic obstruction have been described. These include lack of migration of the radiocolloid through the lymphatic channels, decreased or absent nodal accumulation, and collateral channels. These findings may indicate the advisability of inclusion of the suspect nodes in radiation treatment fields and/or their surgical removal (Fig. 11–8)

In addition to oncologic settings, lymphoscintigraphy has been used in the diagnosis of the edematous extremity. Interdigital injection of the radiopharmaceutical in the involved extremity or a single injection on the dorsum of the hand or foot generally produces satisfactory visualization of the peripheral lymphatic channels and lymph nodes. Primary (congenital) lymphedema usually presents with only a few lymphatic channels, which are frequently unobstructed. Patients with secondary (obstructive) lymphedema may show evidence of obstructed lymphatics as evidenced by lack of migration of the radiocolloid from the injection site, diffuse dermal activity, or multiple tortuous collateral channels.

TREATMENT OF LYMPHOMA WITH RADIOIMMUNOTHERAPY

Treatment of lymphomas can be accomplished by labeling a monoclonal antibody against lymphoma antigens with a beta-emitting radionuclide. Yttrium-90 (^{90}Y)-labeled anti-CD20 murine (mouse) monoclonal antibody (ibritumomab tiuxetan or Zevalin) has been developed for treatment of disseminated follicular B-cell (NHL) refractory to stable rituximab therapy, and for treatment of patients with disseminated refractory or relapsed low-grade follicular or transformed B-cell NHL, including patients with rituximab refractory NHL. The monoclonal antibody ibritumomab targets by specific binding of the IgG, kappa-monoclonal antibody to the C20+ antigen found on the surface of malignant as well as normal B lymphocytes. Radioisotopes (^{111}In for imaging or the pure beta emitter ^{90}Y for treatment) can be attached to ibritmomab by the chelating agent, tiuxetan. Yttrium-90 has a beta path length of 5 mm in soft tissue (about 100 to 200 cell diameters) and a physical half-life of 64 hours. The ^{111}In-labeled antibody is used for imaging the patient to determine that

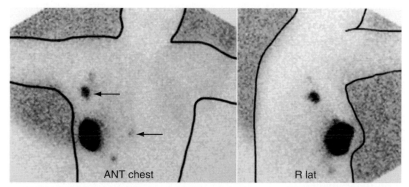

ANT chest   R lat

FIGURE 11–8. Lymphoscintigraphy. Anterior (*left*) and lateral (*right*) images after injection of radiocolloid around a cancer site in the right breast demonstrates that there are multiple routes of lymphatic drainage from this tumor, including into the right axilla (*upper arrow*), internal mammary node (*lower arrow*), and an inframammary node.

the biodistribution of the antibody is appropriate before administration of ^{90}Y-labeled therapeutic dose. The treatment has about a 75% overall response rate and works best in patients who have had fewer prior antineoplastic treatments. Plastic and acrylic materials are appropriate for shielding the syringe containing the beta-emitting ^{90}Y Zevalin, but lead shielding (appropriate for the ^{111}In Zevalin) should not generally be used as it will generate more penetrating bremsstrahlung radiation. Indium-111 is the radionuclide used for the imaging portion of the procedure.

Yttrium-90 Zevalin therapy is appropriate for diffusely disseminated disease, and the procedure occurs over a period of about 1 week as follows. On day 1, the patient receives unlabeled rituximab (Rituxan) intravenously (250 mg/m^2) followed in 4 hours by an imaging dose of 5.0 mCi (185 MBq) of ^{111}In-Zevalin injected intravenously over a period of 10 minutes. The purpose of the unlabeled ituximab is to saturate readily available C20 sites in the spleen and on normal circulating B cells. This improves the amount of ^{111}In-Zevalin available to image the tumor. The unlabeled ituximab should not be given as an intravenous bolus or push as deaths have been reported as a result of myocardial infarction, hypoxia, and acute respiratory distress syndrome.

Whole-body images of the ^{111}In-Zevalin are then obtained at 2 to 24 and again at 48 to 72 hours to assess biodistribution. These are performed with a large-field-of-view gamma camera using the 172 and 247 keV photopeaks for ^{111}In with a 15% to 20% symmetric energy window. The expected biodistribution of Zevalin is easily detectable activity in the blood pool on the first day of imaging, decreasing on the second and third days; moderately high activity in the normal liver and spleen; and low or very low activity in normal kidneys, bladder, and bowel. Biodistribution is considered unacceptable if there is diffuse uptake of ^{111}In-Zevalin in the lungs that is more intense than the cardiac blood pool on the first day or more intense than the liver on the second- and third-day images, or activity in the kidneys that is more intense than the liver on the posterior view on the second and third days, or intense uptake throughout normal bowel comparable to the liver on the second- or third-day images. As expected, areas of tumor will also be visualized on these images.

If the biodistribution is acceptable, the ^{90}Y Zevalin therapeutic administration is performed on day 7, 8, or 9. On the day of treatment, an infusion of unlabeled rituximab is followed within 4 hours by 0.4 mCi (14.8 MBq)/kg of ^{90}Y Zevalin intravenously over a period of 10 minutes. The maximum administered activity is 32 mCi (1.18 GBq). Zevalin should not be administered to patients with a platelet count of less than 100,000/mm^3. In patients with platelet counts between 100,000 to 149,000/mm^3, the administered activity is reduced to 0.3 mCi (11.1 MBq)/kg. Response rates are about 75%, but complete response is only about 15%. The most common adverse events are thrombocytopenia and neutropenia, which occur in about 90% of patients. There can be potentially fatal infusion reactions, and the treatment is contraindicated in patients with known type 1 hypersensitivity or anaphylactic reactions to murine proteins. Other infusion reactions include hypotension, angioedema, hypoxia, and bronchospasm.

The dose to caretakers and persons near a patient treated with Zevalin is less than 1 mrem (<10 μSv), and the patient can be released immediately after treatment without the need to measure dose rates or retained activity. Urinary excretion of Zevalin is about 7% during the first week. From the start of therapy and for a period of 1 week thereafter, it is recommended that a condom be used during intercourse and deep kissing should be avoided as should other transfers of bodily fluids. Patients are advised to wash their hands thoroughly after using the toilet. Despite the low radiation dose to others, patients are also advised to sleep apart for 4 to 7 days, drink plenty of liquids, wash laundry separately, avoid long trips with others, and limit time spent in public places.

Another anti-CD20 antibody radioimmunotherapeutic agent, tositumomab (Bexxar), labeled with I-131, has also proven useful in the treatment of patients with NHL, particularly those with chemotherapy-refractory disease. I-131 tositumomab has demonstrated high response rates and long durations of response in patients with relapsed low-grade and transformed low-grade NHL. In clinical trials of Bexxar, the objective response rates ranged from 54%–71% in pretreated patients. In newly diagnosed patients, the response rate has shown to be considerably higher.

TREATMENT OF HEPATOMA AND LIVER METASTASES WITH MICROSPHERES

Palliative treatment of nonresectable hepatoma and liver metastases with radioactive ^{90}Y-labeled microspheres (SIR-Spheres) has grown in use over the last several years. The microspheres are 20 to 60 microns in diameter and are delivered via angiographic catheter into the hepatic artery. The majority of administered activity will localize in the hypervascular tumor and to a lesser extent in normal parenchyma. The lower size limit of the microspheres prevents the majority from passing through the tumor into the venous system, although some do pass through to the lung. The localized microspheres remain in the liver, do not degrade, and after placement are only retrievable by surgery. The product is usually delivered in 5-mL vials with an activity of about 81 mCi (3 GBq). The typical administered activity is about 40–70 mCi (1.5 to 2.5 GBq) and is calculated based on the desired absorbed radiation dose. However, the administered activity may be modified if there has been concomitant chemotherapy.

Initial patient assessment includes issues related to tumor resectability, extent of disease in the liver, extent of extrahepatic disease, hepatic vascular anatomy, arteriovenous shunting, liver and renal function, and the general constitutional status of the patient. Radiological workup consists of a hepatic angiogram, combined angiogram CT scan, ^{99m}Tc-macroaggregated albumin scan (to assess shunting) and embolization of the gastroduodenal artery or other vessel that might result in inadvertent delivery of microspheres. If there is possible delivery of the microspheres to small arteries to the stomach, duodenum, or gallbladder, the procedure should be abandoned to avoid serious radiation damage to those organs. Treatment is questionable if there is a large amount of extrahepatic disease and the liver burden is not the life-threatening problem. If there is arteriovenous shunting of more than 10% to the lung, the dose must be reduced to prevent radiation pneumonitis, and shunting of greater than 20% is a contraindication to this form of therapy. Portal vein thrombosis is also a contraindication. After the microspheres are placed, it is possible to use SPECT imaging of the bremsstrahlung radiation from the ^{90}Y to confirm localization (Fig. 11–9).

Environmental contamination with microspheres should be taken seriously. The microspheres are very easily spread by foot traffic and hand contamination. Patients may travel home after the procedure, and at 5 hours after implantation, the dose rate at a distance of 0.5 m from a patient is about 10 μSv/hr. No special precautions are required for linens and clothing, but there is a

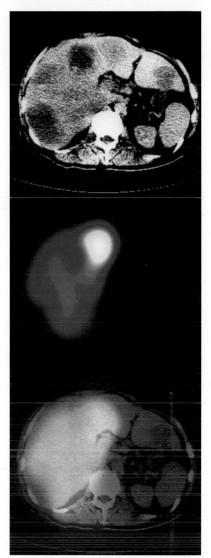

FIGURE 11–9. Yttrium-90 (^{90}Y) microsphere therapy.
Top, A CT scan in this patient with hepatoma shows multiple low density lesions. *Middle,* After hepatic artery injection of ^{90}Y microspheres, a SPECT image can be obtained by using the bremsstrahlung radiation. *Bottom,* A SPECT/CT fusion image shows where the microspheres actually localized.

small amount of activity that may appear in the urine, and as a result for the first 24 hours, a toilet (not a urinal) should be used and flushed twice. Many jurisdictions have activity restrictions in the event of patient demise. Typical limits are set for autopsy (4 mCi; 150 MBq), cremation/burial (27 mCi; 1 GBq), and embalming (4 mCi; 150 MBq).

PEARLS & PITFALLS

Gallium-67 scans for inflammatory lesions are performed 24 hours after injection; for tumors, they are usually done at 48–72 hours.

Lymphoma and hepatoma are particularly gallium-avid tumors. Other tumors (such as lung cancer) also accumulate gallium.

If a lymphoma accumulates gallium initially, but not on a post-therapy scan, there is probably a favorable therapeutic response. If, on subsequent follow-up scans, gallium again accumulates, the probability of tumor recurrence is high. ^{18}F-FDG PET/CT scans are preferred for staging and restaging lymphoma.

A gallium scan can most often be recognized by noting activity in the lacrimal glands, nasopharynx, liver, bowel, and skeleton. The images are usually count-poor (coarse).

Gallium-67 may localize in the parotid glands after radiotherapy and the thymus after chemotherapy, especially in children and young adults. Reactive thymic changes should not be mistaken for recurrent mediastinal lymphoma.

Thallium-201 and ^{18}F-FDG accumulate nonspecifically in many tumors, including recurrent brain tumors.

Many breast cancers, parathyroid adenomas and metastatic thyroid cancers accumulate the cardiac agent ^{99m}Tc-sestamibi. Some benign breast conditions accumulate this agent.

Indium-111 octreotide is accumulated by tumors with somatostatin receptors, including pheochromocytoma, carcinoid, neuroblastoma, gastrinoma, islet cell tumors, pituitary adenomas, medullary thyroid cancer, and small-cell lung cancer.

MIBG is accumulated by pheochromocytomas and neuroblastomas.

Kaposi's sarcoma is thallium-avid but does not accumulate gallium. Lymphoma concentrates both agents.

Lymphoscintigraphy is performed with intradermal or peritumoral injection of filtered ^{99m}Tc-sulfur colloid. The purpose is to identify the sentinel node which is the lymph node most likely to be involved with metastatic tumor.

SUGGESTED READINGS

Aarsvold J, Alazraki N, Grant S: Sentinel node staging of early breast cancer with lymphoscintigraphy and an intraoperative gamma detecting probe. In Sandler MP, Coleman RE, Patton JA et al. (eds): Diagnostic Nuclear Medicine, 4th ed. New York, Lippincott, Williams and Wilkins, 2003, pp 1015–1026.

Birdwell RL, Smith KL, Betts BJ, Ikeda DM, Strauss HW, Jeffrey SS: Breast Cancer: Variables Affecting Sentinel Lymph Node Visualization at Preoperative Lymphoscintigraphy. Radiology 220:47, 2001.

Borys R. Krynyckyi, Chun K. Kim, Martin R. Goyenechea, Peggy T. Chan, Zhuang-Yu Zhang, Josef Machac: Clinical Breast Lymphoscintigraphy: Optimal Techniques for Performing Studies, Image Atlas, and Analysis of Images. RadioGraphics 24:121–145, 2004.

Intenzo CM, Kim SM, Pate JI, Lin HC, Kairys JC: Lymphoscintigraphy in Cutaneous Melanoma: A Total Body Atlas of Sentinel Node Mapping. RadioGraphics 22:491, 2002.

Kwekkeboom DJ, Krenning EP: Somatostatin receptor imaging. Semin Nucl Med 32:84–91, 2002.

Machac J, Krynyckyi B, Kim C: Peptide and antibody imaging in lung cancer. Semin Nucl Med 32:276–292, 2002.

Spies SM: Imaging and dosing in radioimmunotherapy with yttrium-90 ibritumomab tiuxetan (Zevalin). Semin Nucl Med 34:10–13, 2004.

Torabi M, Aquino SL, Harisinghani MG: Current Concepts in Lymph Node Imaging. J Nucl Med 45:1509–1518, 2004.

Wahl RL: Tositumomab and [131]I Therapy in Non-Hodgkin's Lymphoma. J Nucl Med 46:128S–140S, 2005.

Warner RR, O'Dorisio TM: Radiolabeled peptides in diagnosis and tumor imaging: clinical overview. Semin Nucl Med 32:79–83, 2002.

Uren RF, Howman-Giles R, Thompson JF: Patterns of Lymphatic Drainage from the Skin in Patients with Melanoma. J Nucl Med 44:570–582, 2003.

Zhu X: Radiation safety considerations radioimmunotherapy with yttrium-90 ibritumomab tiuxetan (Zevalin). Semin Nucl Med 34:20–23, 2004.

Inflammation and Infection Imaging

12

INTRODUCTION

A variety of nuclear medicine imaging techniques provides effective methods for the detection and assessment of both clinically apparent and occult infections and inflammatory conditions. Rather than representing organ-specific techniques, these procedures use radiopharmaceuticals that localize preferentially in inflamed or infected tissue in any location in the body. The available radiopharmaceuticals exhibit varying degrees of nonspecificity and are best used with meticulous clinical correlation (Table 12–1). These agents include the following:

- Gallium-67 (^{67}Ga) citrate
- Radiolabeled white blood cells
    Indium-111 (^{111}In) leukocytes
    Technetium-99m (^{99m}Tc) leukocytes
- Radiolabeled monoclonal antibodies and antibody fragments
- Radiolabeled peptides
- Fluorine-18 Fluorodeoxyglucose (^{18}F-FDG) (discussed in Chapter 13)

The particular role of each of the readily available radiopharmaceuticals for infection imaging often depends on the clinical setting and the specific part of the body under scrutiny. Selection of the proper imaging agent is critical to the success of the procedure.

GALLIUM IMAGING

Gallium-67 imaging accumulates nonspecifically in inflammatory and infectious diseases, as well as neoplastic diseases. The nonspecificity of gallium has caused it to be supplanted for the imaging of many infectious processes by more specific imaging agents such as radiolabeled leukocytes. However, gallium has been used for over 3 decades as an infection imaging agent and continues to be a valuable radiopharmaceutical for the detection and localization of certain inflammatory lesions. The general physical and biokinetic properties of ^{67}Ga, as well as the appearance of a normal scan, are presented in Chapter 11.

Mechanisms of Localization in Inflammation/Infection

The mechanisms of gallium citrate localization in inflammatory tissues are likely different in some respects from the mechanisms associated with localization in neoplasms. The process is complex, but a few basic principles are known to be associated with such concentration: (1) gallium forms complexes with plasma transferrin that act as carriers

341

TABLE 12–1.   Infection Imaging Radiopharmaceuticals

RADIOPHARMACEUTICAL AND ADMINISTERED ACTIVITY	TIME OF IMAGING	ADVANTAGES	DISADVANTAGES	COMMON USES
[67]Ga-citrate 5–10 mCi (185–370 MBq)	24–48 hr	A variety of infections detected, including opportunistic	Interfering bowel and renal activity Delayed imaging necessary ^{67}Ga label not ideal for imaging	Immunocompromised patients Uncomplicated osteomyelitis Chronic infections Diskitis/spinal osteomyelitis FUO: chronic phase
[111]In white blood cells 300–500 μCi (10–18.5 MBq)	12–24 hr	No interfering bowel/renal activity Delayed imaging possible Simultaneous ^{99m}Tc-sulfur colloid or ^{99m}Tc-diphosphonate bone imaging possible	Less sensitivity for nonbacterial and nonpyogenic infections ^{111}In label not ideal for imaging Complex preparation	Bacterial infections Indolent inflammatory conditions: e.g., prosthetic joint infections Abdominal infections Prosthetic vascular graft infections Brain abscess Complicated osteomyelitis Extremity infections: e.g., diabetic foot Renal infections FUO: acute phase
[99m]Tc-white blood cells 5–10 mCi (185–370 MBq)	0.5–4.0 hr	Early imaging Excellent early sensitivity ^{99m}Tc label ideal for imaging	Less sensitivity for nonbacterial and nonpyogenic infections Delayed imaging not ideal Early renal activity Bowel activity after 1–2 hr Complex preparation	Bacterial infections Acute inflammatory conditions: e.g., inflammatory bowel disease Complicated osteomyelitis Extremity infections: diabetic foot Prosthetic vascular graft infections
[99m]Tc-fanolesomab (NeutroSpec) 10–20 mCi (370–740 MBq)	0.5–4.0 hr	Rapid preparation of radiopharmaceutical Early imaging ^{99m}Tc label ideal for imaging	Liver, spleen, renal activity	Equivocal appendicitis Inflammatory or ischemic bowel disease Abdominal abscess Osteomyelitis

[67]Ga, gallium-67; FUO, fever of unknown origin; ^{111}In, Indium-111; ^{99m}Tc, technetium-99m.

for ^{67}Ga to sites of inflammation; (2) gallium is also incorporated into leukocytes, bound by intracellular lactoferrin, which then migrate to inflamed areas; and (3) gallium may be taken up by pathogenic microorganisms themselves by binding to siderophores produced by the bacteria.

Technique

The technique used for gallium imaging in the setting of inflammation and infection is in many ways similar to that used when imaging neoplasms. The major difference is the temporal sequence for obtaining images. Initial images are obtained earlier in cases of suspected inflammatory disease, usually 18 to 24 hours after injection. Images are subsequently obtained at 24-hour intervals as needed to allow for improved target-to-nontarget ratios and for the possible differentiation of normal bowel activity from accumulations in pathologic entities. Suggested imaging protocol and dosimetry are presented in Appendix E–1.

Clinical Applications

The significance of an abnormal accumulation of gallium increases with the intensity of the focus as seen on appropriate images. Various grading systems for assessing intensity have been devised for particular anatomic locations. In general, however, any abnormal gallium activity equal to or greater than that seen in the liver may be considered significant.

Abdominal and Retroperitoneal Inflammation and Infection

In general, the proper interpretation of gallium images in the abdomen hinges on the differentiation of physiologic activity from abnormal accumulations of the radiopharmaceutical. A common problem in image interpretation in the abdomen is the presence of gallium in the bowel, which may mimic lesions or mask disease. Bowel activity is particularly prominent in the colon and may be diffuse or focal. Frequently, activity is seen in the regions of the cecum, hepatic and splenic flexures, and rectosigmoid. These accumulations may appear as early as a few hours after injection. Various bowel-cleansing preparations have been investigated as possible means of eliminating such interfering activity in the colon, but none have proved consistently successful. The progress of excreted gallium through the colon over time may provide the best evidence of physiologic activity, whereas persist-

ence of gallium in a given area of the abdomen should be viewed as abnormal.

The presence of liver activity in the right upper quadrant may obscure abnormal gallium concentration. In this setting, ^{99m}Tc-sulfur colloid hepatic images subtracted from the gallium images of the upper abdomen may unmask adjacent inflammation or abscess.

Abscesses in the retroperitoneum are frequently related to associated renal infection. Persistence of renal activity after 24 hours, progressively increasing activity, and unilateral discrepancy in gallium activity in the kidneys should be considered abnormal. However, abnormally increased activity in one or both kidneys can occur in nonspecific pathologic and physiologic states and may therefore present a difficult problem of differential diagnosis (see Table 11–2).

Thoracic Inflammation and Infection

Gallium accumulates nonspecifically in tumors and in a variety of inflammatory abnormalities, including pyogenic pneumonias, tuberculosis, vasculitis, idiopathic pulmonary fibrosis, and various other pulmonary, pleural, and mediastinal benign diseases (Table 12–2). The degree of gallium activity has been used to determine whether a pulmonary process is in an active or a quiescent stage. In general, increasing degrees of gallium activity correlate with increasing activity of disease. Acute inflammatory diseases of the heart and pericardium may also produce positive gallium images. In both the chest and abdomen, hematomas and healing wounds, both sterile and infected, may demonstrate gallium uptake.

Fever of Unknown Origin

An fever of unknown origin (FUO) is a fever of at least 3 weeks' duration with several episodes exceeding 38.3°C. Causes are infection in about 25% of cases and neoplasm in about 20% of cases. Miscellaneous other entities can also cause FUOs, including drugs, pulmonary emboli, and collagen vascular disease. Initial imaging for an FUO should begin with labeled leukocytes and followed with a gallium study if necessary. Although gallium is reasonably sensitive for localized pyogenic disease (80% to 90%), it is less sensitive than are radiolabeled leukocytes, especially in the abdomen, where about one third of infections responsible for FUOs are found. In addition, a gallium study should be used with caution in patients who have been treated with systemic antibiotics because false-negative

TABLE 12–2.	Nonmalignant Causes of Gallium-67 Citrate Uptake in the Lungs

INFECTIONS
Pyogenic
Viral
Pneumocystis carinii
Atypical
Granulomatous
Fungal

OCCUPATIONAL EXPOSURES
Coal workers pneumoconiosis
Silica
Talc
Beryllium

CONNECTIVE TISSUE DISEASES
Systemic lupus erythematosus
Mixed connective tissue disease
Rheumatoid arthritis

DRUG REACTIONS
Amiodarone
Bisulfan
Cytoxin
Methotrexate
Procarbazine
Vincristine

MISCELLANEOUS
Acute respiratory distress syndrome
Idiopathic pulmonary fibrosis (active)
Sarcoidosis
Radiation pneumonitis
Wegener's granulomatosis

results may occur under these circumstances. In patients with FUO and leukocytosis in whom an infectious process is suspected, radiolabeled leukocytes are often chosen as the initial radionuclide imaging study, especially if the patient has had symptoms for less than 2 weeks. A negative leukocyte examination essentially excludes an acute infection as the cause of an FUO. Because only 25% of FUOs are caused by infection, however, the source of the fever is not elucidated by a negative leukocyte study. In this setting, further evaluation with gallium imaging may disclose a chronic infectious process or neoplasm. Unlike regional anatomic imaging, such as computed tomography (CT), both gallium and radiolabeled leukocyte imaging provide rapid whole-body surveys in patients with FUOs and no localizing signs. Gallium imaging may also be useful in febrile

infants and neonates, in whom sufficient blood withdrawal for leukocyte labeling may not be possible.

Immunocompromised Patients

Because its sensitivity for detection of infection does not depend on acute pyogenic response, gallium imaging is the radionuclide procedure of choice for detecting and evaluating the varied opportunistic pulmonary infections and adenopathies common in patients with compromised immune systems due to acquired immunodeficiency syndrome (AIDS), antineoplastic chemotherapy, or immunosuppression after organ transplantation.

In immunocompromised patients, gallium scans of the thorax should always be interpreted in comparison with recent chest radiographs, which add specificity to the examination. A normal gallium scan with a normal chest radiograph essentially excludes an infectious process. A normal gallium scan in the presence of a focal mass or infiltrate on the chest radiograph, however, suggests the diagnosis of Kaposi's sarcoma, which does not accumulate gallium.

Bilateral intense diffuse homogeneous pulmonary uptake of gallium is the classic appearance of *Pneumocystis carinii* pneumonia (PCP) and occurs in 60% to 70% of cases. The gallium scan is frequently positive before chest radiographs become abnormal. Gallium imaging is 90% sensitive for the disease, and although not specific, diffuse pulmonary activity in this population should prompt investigation or treatment of the offending organism. The specificity of a diffusely positive scan is greater when the chest radiograph is negative and the pulmonary activity is intense (equal to or greater than liver activity) (Fig. 12–1). Lymph node activity can occasionally be seen as well.

Treatment of PCP or prophylaxis with aerosolized pentamidine may alter the classic appearance of diffuse uptake in active or recurrent infections. Because aerosol deposition is less efficient in the upper lobes, the resultant relative undertreatment may restrict recurrent disease to the upper lung zones. In addition, with early aggressive therapy, patients can survive long enough to develop chronic airway and parenchymal changes, which may further alter the distribution of successful treatment and thus the distribution of recurrent disease. Under these circumstances, positive gallium scans may appear as nonhomogeneous or even focal areas of increased

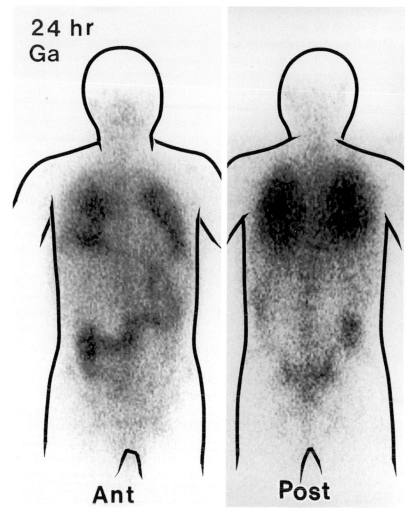

FIGURE 12–1. Pneumocystis pneumonia. Anterior (*left*) and posterior (*right*) 24-hour gallium images demonstrate normal physiologic excretion in the colon; however, there is markedly abnormal increased activity in both lungs. Note the negative cardiac defect produced by the intense lung activity.

activity. Successful treatment of PCP is generally reflected by decreasing intensity of gallium uptake or a return to a normal appearance.

The appearance of bacterial pneumonias on gallium scans in immunocompromised patients is identical to that in patients with intact immune systems. A solitary focus of gallium uptake without lymph node activity is the usual presentation. When the abnormalities are multifocal, more aggressive infections, such as actinomycosis or nocardia, should be considered. A negative gallium scan in a patient with documented progressive pneumonia has grave prognostic implications, suggesting a severe deterioration in immune inflammatory response.

In patients with AIDS, lymph node involvement by a variety of diseases is common. Gallium uptake in the generalized lymphadenopathy associated with AIDS and AIDS-related complex is variable in occurrence and degree of activity, which may be minimal. Increased gallium uptake equal to or greater than liver activity in hilar, mediastinal, periaortic, or supraclavicular nodes suggests the diagnoses of malignant lymphoma, *Mycobacterium tuberculosis*, or *M. avium-intracellulare*. However, this nodal activity is nonspecific, and other less common infectious processes cannot be excluded.

In the abdomen, abnormal gallium accumulation may be seen in bacterial abscess and gastrointestinal infections, as well as in regional lymph nodes affected by *M. avium-intracellulare* or lymphoma. The usefulness of gallium for the detection and evaluation of AIDS-related diseases of the gastrointestinal tract is limited by interfering physiologic bowel activity and the lack of correlation of abnormal uptake with specific pathogens, as is seen in thoracic disease. Intense colonic activity (greater than liver activity) that persists unchanged over 72 hours of imaging is suspicious, but not diagnostic, of infectious colitis and should be interpreted with caution.

Combined imaging with thallium-201 (^{201}Tl) and ^{67}Ga may add to the diagnostic specificity of gallium imaging in the setting of immunocompromised patients. With some exceptions, this type of combined imaging has yielded the following results:

Kaposi's sarcoma is gallium negative but thallium positive.

Lymphoma is both gallium and thallium positive.

Acute infections, tuberculosis, and *M. avium-intracellulare* are usually gallium positive and thallium negative but may show faint thallium uptake.

Osteomyelitis

The initial imaging test of choice for osteomyelitis is a routine radiograph. If this is negative, triple-phase bone imaging with ^{99m}Tc-diphosphonates is the radionuclide procedure of choice for the diagnosis of uncomplicated osteomyelitis, with a sensitivity of greater than 90%. But this test is nonspecific. In some circumstances, gallium imaging may increase the specificity of a positive bone scan and suggest the presence of osteomyelitis, especially in situations such as vertebral osteomyelitis and osteomyelitis superimposed on underlying bone disease. In these settings the following apply:

■ Osteomyelitis is likely if gallium activity exceeds bone scan activity in the same location (spatially congruent images), or when the spatial distribution of gallium exceeds that of the bone scan (spatially incongruent images).

■ Osteomyelitis is unlikely if gallium images are normal regardless of bone scan findings or when gallium distribution is less than bone scan activity on spatially incongruent images.

■ Because gallium is a weak bone agent in addition to being an inflammatory marker, a gallium scan may be considered nondiagnostic for osteomyelitis when the distribution and activity of the gallium and bone scan activity are the same.

When monitoring treated osteomyelitis, bone scans with ^{99m}Tc-diphosphonates may produce positive images during healing or in chronic but sterile disease, owing to accumulation in residual localized bony remodeling. Gallium accumulation in osteomyelitis, however, tends to decrease with successful antibiotic therapy. A negative gallium scan in such instances is generally associated with healed infections, whereas highly positive images suggest active disease indicative of unsuccessful therapy or relapse.

Triple-phase bone scans are often difficult to obtain in the spine because of overlying vascular and blood pool structures, and routine bone scans are nonspecific for infection. In addition, radiolabeled leukocyte studies have a high false-negative rate for infection in the spine. Gallium imaging in conjunction with a bone scan provides improved sensitivity for the diagnosis of both tuberculous and nontuberculous vertebral osteomyelitis, with an accuracy of more than 85% when both studies are positive.

Radionuclide bone scans are frequently nondiagnostic in the setting of suspected osteomyelitis superimposed on noninfectious conditions, such as healing fractures, that cause increased bone mineral turnover, especially when accompanied by a sterile inflammatory response producing an abnormal three-phase bone scan. This setting includes that of painful orthopedic prostheses, for which ^{99m}Tc-methylene diphosphonate (MDP) bone and gallium imaging is generally superior to bone imaging alone for the diagnosis of complicating infection. Definitive positive or negative studies, however, although highly accurate, occur in only about one third of cases. Indium-111 leukocyte imaging offers more accurate and consistently helpful results in this setting and, when available, is usually the procedure of choice for suspected infection of orthopedic appliances.

Sarcoidosis

The lesions of active sarcoidosis are quite gallium avid, especially in the chest. Both nodal and parenchymal lung involvement can be detected. In the early stages, gallium images are frequently positive before any radiographic abnormalities are noted. The finding of increased gallium activity in intrathoracic lymph nodes (right paratracheal and hilar) in a pattern resembling the Greek letter lambda (λ) is suggestive of sarcoidosis. However, a *lambda sign* in combination with a so-called *panda sign*, produced by symmetric increase in activity in the lacrimal, parotid, and salivary glands, represents a highly specific pattern for sarcoidosis (Fig. 12–2). Similarly, the panda sign by itself is not specific and may be seen in a significant percentage of patients with radiation sialoadenitis, primary Sjögren's syndrome, and in patients with AIDS.

In the presence of gallium-avid adenopathy in the mediastinal and hilar regions, the diagnoses of lymphoma or infectious disease, especially in human immunodeficiency virus (HIV)-positive patients, must also be considered. In malignant lymphomas, however, the adenopathy is frequently asymmetric.

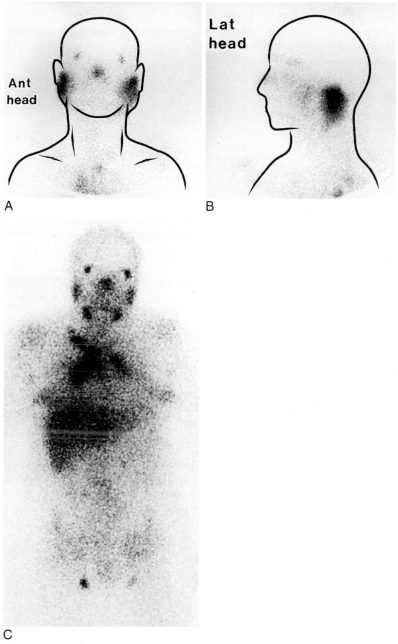

FIGURE 12–2. Sarcoidosis. (*A* and *B*) 48-hour anterior and lateral images of the head and neck from a gallium-67 (^{67}Ga) scan in this 25-year-old woman show symmetrically increased activity in the parotid glands, salivary glands, and lacrimal glands (panda sign). *C*, A ^{67}Ga scan in a different patient also shows the lambda sign of lymph nodes in the mediastinum as well as a panda sign. Either sign alone is suggestive of sarcoidosis, but together they offer high specificity for the diagnosis. Note also the active inguinal nodes.

In the later stages of sarcoid lung disease, a diffuse increase in lung activity with or without gallium-avid adenopathy is common. In this setting, gallium can be used to distinguish active parenchymal disease from inactive sarcoidosis or chronic fibrosis. Diffuse increased activity (equal or greater than liver activity) correlates with active disease, whereas normal lung activity (equal to soft-tissue background activity) is compatible with remission. Similarly, decreasing intensity of gallium activity in the lungs after steroid therapy has been shown to correlate with a favorable response. In extensive sarcoidosis, periaortic, retroperitoneal, and pelvic nodal activity may be seen, but this is more commonly found in patients with lymphoma.

RADIOLABELED LEUKOCYTES

Radiolabeled leukocytes have added an important dimension to the armamentarium of radiopharmaceuticals for infection and inflammation imaging. Because leukocytes can be separated and labeled without significant loss of function, they can be used to image inflammatory processes. Both ^{111}In-oxine leukocytes and ^{99m}Tc-hexamethylpropyleneamine oxime (HMPAO) leukocytes have been shown to retain their innate function and have demonstrated relatively high sensitivity and specificity for acute infections. However, sensitivity may be somewhat lower for chronic infections. The procedure involves removing some of the patient's own leukocytes, labeling them, and reinjecting them before scanning. As with any autologous labeled biologic agent, extreme care must be taken to maintain the integrity of the blood sample and to ensure that reinjection of the labeled leukocytes is performed only in the patient from whom the cells were taken. Clinical studies comparing ^{99m}Tc and ^{111}In-leukocytes have not shown any intrinsic differences in sensitivity for infection when standard 24-hour imaging is performed. However, some notable differences between the two radiopharmaceuticals make one or the other preferable in certain clinical situations.

Mechanism of Localization

Radiolabeled leukocytes are attracted to sites of inflammation, where they are activated by local chemotactic factors and pass from the blood stream through the vascular endothelium into the soft tissues. The leukocytes then move toward the site of inflammation in a directed migration called *chemotaxis*. If the inflammation has an infectious cause, the labeled neutrophils phagocytize and destroy any offending bacteria. External gamma camera imaging localizes these accumulations of radiolabeled leukocytes and thus reveals the site of inflammation or infection. Like gallium uptake, radiolabeled leukocyte uptake is not specific for infection and may occur in any inflammatory process that incites a leukocyte response. Occasional uptake in neoplasms may be noted.

Indium-111 Oxine Leukocytes

Compared with ^{67}Ga-citrate imaging, ^{111}In oxine–labeled leukocytes offer the following *advantages*:

- Less variable normal physiologic distribution from patient to patient
- Essentially no accumulation in the gastrointestinal tract, kidneys, or bladder, with less soft-tissue activity
- Less activity in noninfectious inflammation and tumors
- Greater concentration in abscessed tissues
- Earlier results, generally within 24 hours

There are some *disadvantages*, however:

- Tedious, expensive labeling procedure that requires precautions associated with handling blood products
- Possibility that severely leukopenic patients may not permit labeling of an adequate number of leukocytes for successful imaging
- Less success in imaging some chronic infections
- Relatively high radiation dose

Labeling Principle

Imaging leukocyte distribution in the body became possible after the development of successful methods for labeling leukocytes with ^{111}In-oxine. Indium-111 oxine labels all cell types indiscriminately, including platelets and red blood cells. Thus, the leukocytes are isolated from about 50 mL of anticoagulated blood before labeling, commonly through a process called *gravity sedimentation*, which simply consists of allowing the blood to sit for the time necessary for the red blood cells to settle to the bottom. Any red blood cells remaining in the supernatant may be either lysed by using hypotonic saline or ammonium chloride or removed by centrifugation.

Oxine forms a lipid-soluble complex with ^{111}In, which passively diffuses through the leukocyte cell membrane. Once this complex becomes intracellular, the ^{111}In separates from the oxine and binds to cytoplasmic components. The oxine then leaves the cell and is removed by washing the cells. A mixed population of leukocytes is usually labeled, although neutrophils constitute the majority. Labeling efficiencies are on the order of 95%. The patient's circulating granulocyte count should be at least 2000 cells/mL to have enough cells to label.

Minimal manipulation of the leukocytes is essential to the actual tagging procedure to avoid damage to the cells, which could diminish their viability and thus limit their effectiveness as an imaging agent. Failure to preserve normal physiologic leukocyte function may result in false-negative imaging study results.

Technique

About 0.5 to 1.0 mCi (18.5 to 37 MBq) of ^{111}In-oxine–labeled autologous leukocytes is administered intravenously. Care should be taken to avoid excessive agitation of the leukocytes because this may cause clumping, resulting in focal lung accumulation. Although some abscesses can be detected in the first few hours after the administration of labeled leukocytes, most imaging is performed 18 to 24 hours after administration. If the urgency of the clinical setting dictates, 4- to 6-hour images may be useful. A whole-body survey can be performed by using a medium-energy collimator, with gamma camera images obtained of specific areas of interest. Generally, both the 173- and 247-keV gamma emissions of ^{111}In are used.

A sample imaging protocol and radiation dosimetry are presented in Appendix E–1.

Normal Scan

In the first few hours after administration of ^{111}In-leukocytes, activity is noted in the lungs (likely due to leukocyte activation), liver, spleen, and blood pool. The lung and blood pool activity decreases during the first few hours as spleen and liver activity increases. By 18 hours, no lung or blood pool activity is detected, but bone marrow activity is noted (Fig. 12–3).

Twenty-four hours after administration, the ^{111}In-leukocyte preparation may be found in the liver, spleen, and bone marrow, with the spleen providing the most prominent accumulation, significantly more than that in the liver. No renal or bowel activity is normally present. Damaged leukocytes that remain labeled may provide increased activity in the liver if slightly damaged, and increased lung activity if severely damaged.

Clinical Applications

General Considerations. Indium-111 leukocytes are taken up nonspecifically in sites of inflammation, inciting a leukocytic response, regardless of the presence or absence of infection (Table 12–3). The sensitivity (90%) and specificity (90%) are greatest for acute pyogenic infections of less than 2 to 3 weeks' duration. Their effectiveness for detecting more chronic infections is somewhat controversial, although sensitivity with mixed cell populations, which include lymphocytes and chronic inflammatory cells as well as neutrophils, generally appears high (80% to 85%). This may also be because some common bacterial infections may demonstrate significant levels of neutrophil infiltration for months. Labeled leukocytes are of no use in the detection of viral and parasitic infections. Factors that can theoretically reduce leukocyte function, including antibiotics, steroids, chemotherapeutic agents, hemodialysis, hyperalimentation, and hyperglycemia, do not appear to diminish labeled leukocyte sensitivity for detecting infection.

Indium-labeled leukocytes are the preferred radiopharmaceutical for imaging abdominal infection, although in practice, a CT scan is usually the initial imaging study ordered for abdominal pain or suspected infection. Because of the lack of normal bowel activity, ^{111}In-labeled leukocytes have a significant advantage over ^{67}Ga- and ^{99m}Tc-labeled leukocytes in diagnosing abdominal abscesses with high sensitivity (85% to 95%). As with gallium, however, the presence of considerable hepatic and especially splenic activity may hamper detection of infection in the upper abdomen. Splenic bed abscesses with intense activity may even be confused with a normal spleen (Fig. 12–4). In this setting, ^{99m}Tc-colloid liver and spleen scans may be subtracted from the labeled leukocyte images to unmask any adjacent abnormal activity. Uncomplicated pancreatitis is usually negative, but septic complications are usually imaged successfully.

Labeled leukocyte activity in the gastrointestinal tract is nonspecific and may indicate a number of pathologies, including Crohn's disease, ulcerative colitis (Fig. 12–5), pseudomembranous colitis, diverticulitis, various gastrointestinal infections, fistulas, ischemic or infarcted bowel, and even vigorous enemazation before imaging. Increased activity in the bowel, especially the colon, may also be

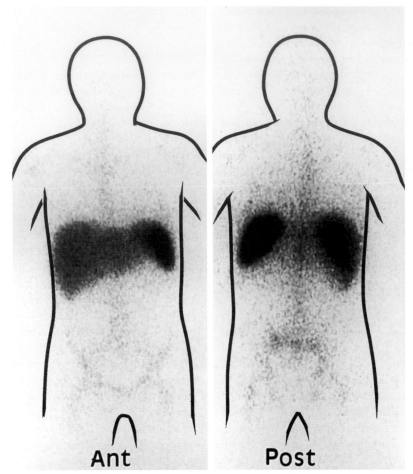

FIGURE 12–3. Normal indium-111 leukocyte scan. Anterior (*left*) and posterior (*right*) images demonstrate liver and splenic activity. The splenic activity normally is greater. A small amount of bone marrow activity is also identified.

problematic in that activity may be found in the absence of true gastrointestinal disease. False-positive results are generally caused by swallowing of leukocytes in patients with endotracheal or nasoesophageal tubes, respiratory tract infections, sinusitis, or pharyngitis or in patients with gastrointestinal bleeding of any cause. In general, the more intense the bowel activity compared with liver activity, the more likely it is to indicate a true positive study.

Normal transient physiologic lung activity on early images (1 to 4 hours) severely limits usefulness of ^{111}In-leukocytes in evaluating pulmonary abnormalities. Increased lung activity is of low specificity at 24 hours as well because it may occur in numerous infectious and noninfectious processes, including atelectasis, congestive heart failure, pul-

monary emboli, aspiration, pneumonia, and adult respiratory distress syndrome. Only one third of patients showing focal or diffuse uptake in the lungs have infectious causes, although focal uptake demonstrates a slightly better correlation with infection.

Fever of Unknown Origin (Occult Fever). In a genuine FUO, the spectrum of possible pathology is extensive, including both infectious and neoplastic causes. The value of ^{67}Ga scanning in FUO is its ability to detect any pathology rather than just infection. In occult fevers with strong suggestion of a pyogenic cause, however, leukocyte scans may be the study of choice when CT or other anatomic imaging procedures cannot localize the disease.

Immunocompromised Patients. Labeled leukocytes have significant limitations for imaging

TABLE 12–3.	Causes of Increased Activity on Labeled Leukocyte Images

CHEST
Common Causes
Adult respiratory distress syndrome
Emphysema
Pleural tubes
Noninfected intravenous lines
Pneumonia
Uncommon Causes
Aspiration
Atelectasis
Cystic fibrosis
Graft infection
Herpes esophagitis

ABDOMEN
Common Causes
Enteric tubes
Ostomies
Phlegmon
Swallowed leukocytes
Wound infection
Uncommon Causes
Acute enteritis
Bowel infarction
Colitis
Crohn's disease
Decubitus ulcer
Gastrointestinal bleeding
Graft infection
Pancreatitis
Transplant (with or without rejection)
Diverticulitis
Acute cholecystitis

MUSCULOSKELETAL AND SKIN UPTAKE
Common Causes
Intravenous site
Osteomyelitis
Sinusitis
Uncommon Causes
Lumbar puncture site
Rheumatoid arthritis
Septic arthritis

ANY BODY PART
Abscess
Cellulitis
Wound infection
Hematoma
Infected tumor

been reported in tuberculous and fungal infections. In addition, the study may be technically difficult in severely leukopenic patients. However, ^{111}In-labeled leukocytes are often useful to evaluate suspected acute pyogenic infections, including sinusitis, bowel infections, and bacterial pneumonias in this setting.

Musculoskeletal Infections. Because labeled leukocytes are taken up by the bone marrow, normal, post-traumatic, or postsurgical variations in marrow distribution may produce confusing foci of increased activity owing to regionally increased marrow uptake. Such false-positive results in the marrow-bearing skeleton can be avoided by performing simultaneous marrow imaging with ^{99m}Tc-sulfur colloid (obtained on a separate photopeak) for comparison with labeled leukocyte distribution. Techetium-99m colloid activity 1 hour after injection is compared with ^{111}In leukocyte activity at 24 hours in the area of interest. Criteria for a positive study are (1) spatial incongruence (i.e., leukocyte activity in the absence of sulfur colloid activity) or (2) incongruence of intensity of activity (i.e., leukocyte activity considerably greater than corresponding colloid activity) (Figs. 9–40 and 12–6). Throughout the skeleton, false-positive results may also be produced by nonspecific uptake in recent fractures, heterotopic bone formation, recent radiation therapy, some neoplasms, and noninfectious inflammation, including that caused by gout and rheumatoid arthritis. Simultaneous bone scans may be of value in leukocyte imaging of the hands and feet to provide anatomic detail needed to separate soft tissue from bony activity.

Osteomyelitis. In uncomplicated acute osteomyelitis, especially with normal radiographs, a positive three-phase bone scan is definitive in most settings and obviates the need for further imaging with gallium or labeled leukocytes. Indium-111 leukocytes, however, are a useful adjunctive procedure in equivocal cases and demonstrate high sensitivity for most musculoskeletal infections, in the range of 85% to 100%. Chronicity of infection does not appear to have a significant effect on sensitivity of leukocyte imaging, although false-negative results have occurred. Indium-111 leukocytes, however, have low sensitivity for spine infections, including osteomyelitis and diskitis. For uncertain reasons, more than half of spine infections appear as photopenic (cold) defects in the areas of involvement rather than as hot spots (Fig. 12–7). This focal photopenia, although suspicious

suspected infections in immunocompromised patients. They are not useful in the detection of viral or parasitic infections, demonstrate low specificity in the lungs, and are insensitive for determining active lymph node diseases such as lymphoma in these patients. False-negative examinations have

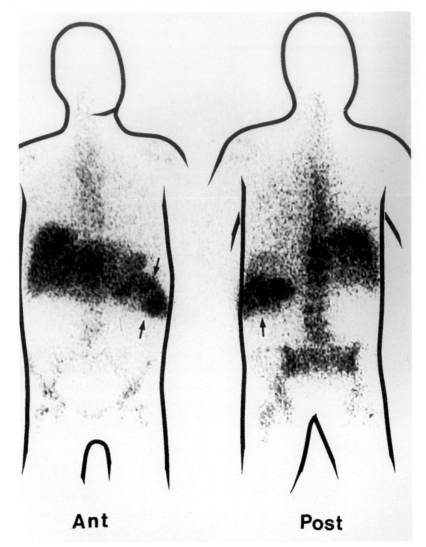

FIGURE 12–4. Postsplenectomy abscess. Anterior and posterior indium-111 leukocyte images demonstrate a focus of activity in the left upper quadrant (*arrows*) that might be mistaken for a slightly inferiorly displaced spleen, except that the spleen has been removed.

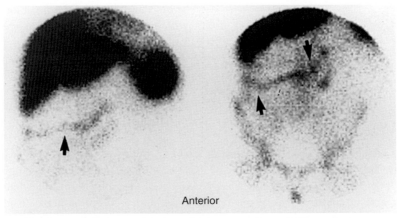

Anterior

FIGURE 12–5. Colitis. Anterior views of the upper and lower abdomen demonstrate activity in the ascending and transverse colon that is abnormal on indium-111 leukocyte scans. Remember that there is normal physiologic colonic excretion with gallium scans.

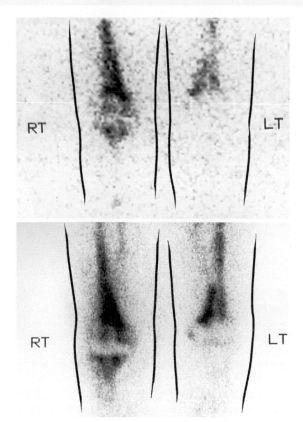

FIGURE 12–6. Expanded marrow. In this patient who has had a right knee joint replacement, there is a possibility of infection or loosening of the prosthesis. *Top,* Anterior views of an indium-111 leukocyte scan over both knees show asymmetric activity extending distal to the right knee joint. *Bottom,* Technetium-99m colloid scan over both knees demonstrates marrow activity, indicating, in this case, asymmetrically expanded marrow. The pattern of indium-111 leukocyte uptake is thus concordant with the marrow distribution and does not indicate infection.

for infection, is nonspecific and may be seen in numerous other entities, including tumor, compression fracture, avascular necrosis, radiation therapy, Paget's disease, fibrous dysplasia, and myelofibrosis. In the setting of spinal infections, ^{67}Ga may be preferred.

In the clinical circumstance of suspected osseous infection complicating disturbed or diseased bone in which radiographs and ^{99m}Tc-diphosphonate bone imaging are likely to be abnormal and nonspecific, ^{111}In-leukocytes provide an accurate tool to unmask or rule out osteomyelitis.

Post-traumatic Infections. Indium leukocyte scans may be positive for several weeks in recent fractures in the absence of superimposed infection, although the uptake is usually faint. Intense focal uptake at a site of suspected osteomyelitis is indicative of bony infection. In this setting, sensitivity and specificity exceed 90%, significantly better than the rates for gallium imaging (50% to 60%).

Prosthetic Joint Infections. Painful prosthetic joints may be due to loosening or infection. Bone scans may be falsely positive during the first year after surgery, owing to healing and bony remodeling, especially in the hip or knee. Although ^{111}In-leukocytes are very sensitive for periprosthetic infections, because labeled leukocytes may accumulate in the normal bone marrow adjacent to a prosthesis, including marrow in heterotopic bone formation, false-positive results may occur. To increase accuracy, the procedure of choice in this setting is an ^{111}In-leukocyte scan accompanied by

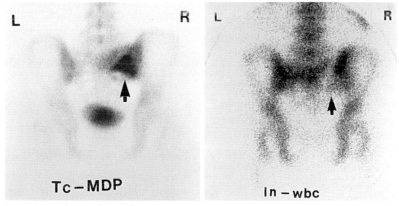

FIGURE 12–7. Osteomyelitis of the right sacroiliac joint. *Left,* A posterior view of the pelvis obtained on a bone scan demonstrates markedly increased activity (*arrow*) in the mid-portion of the right sacroiliac joint. *Right,* An indium-111 leukocyte scan in the same patient shows that the same area is relatively decreased in activity (*arrow*). This may be seen with ^{111}In leukocyte scans when the osteomyelitis is in the central portion of the skeleton, especially the spine.

^{99m}Tc-sulfur colloid marrow imaging. The sulfur colloid study provides a map of postsurgical marrow distribution, whereas the leukocytes map both the distribution of marrow and any accompanying infection. Thus, congruent images indicate that leukocyte uptake is likely related to normal marrow activity, whereas areas that concentrate leukocytes but not sulfur colloid indicate areas of infection. This combined study has a sensitivity and accuracy in excess of 90%. In the hip, labeled leukocyte activity over the head of the prosthesis is strongly suggestive of infection, whereas activity in the region of the shank is less so because of a plug of marrow that may be pushed to the tip of the prosthesis when inserted.

Diabetic Foot Infections. Labeled leukocyte activity in normal bone marrow does not usually cause a problem in interpretation of images in the peripheral skeleton. Uptake of labeled leukocytes in adjacent ulcers or cellulitis, however, along with decreased resolution of anatomic detail using the ^{111}In label, may confound separation of soft tissue from bony uptake, especially in the hands and feet. In this setting, comparison of a simultaneous bone scan (obtained on a separate photopeak) with the ^{111}In leukocyte distribution may provide the anatomic information needed to distinguish between bone and soft-tissue activity. Leukocyte scans in this setting have an overall accuracy of about 80%.

Neuropathic Joint Infections. Infections may commonly complicate neuropathic joints. However, in early, rapidly progressing sterile neuropathia, both bone scans and ^{111}In-leukocyte scans are frequently positive because of associated inflammatory and destructive bony changes. Thus, the findings on leukocyte and bone imaging may be indistinguishable from osteomyelitis. Faint, diffuse leukocyte activity that fades between the 4- and 24-hour images is suggestive of sterile disease, whereas more intense focal activity that is distinctly different in distribution from the bone scan activity and that increases over time suggests superimposed infection. In chronic forms of neuropathic osteoarthropathy, interpretation of the leukocyte and bone scans is simplified by the less avid inflammatory response and decreased soft-tissue background activity.

Active Arthritis. Arthritides, even those normally of a chronic nature, can have tremendous leukocyte responses. Thus, leukocyte scans have been applied to diagnosing and monitoring the activity of rheumatoid arthritis. In this setting,

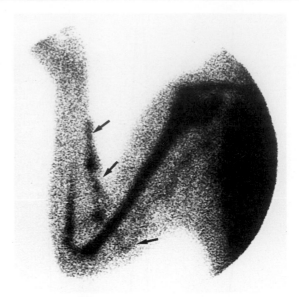

FIGURE 12–8. Graft infection. In this patient who was on renal dialysis, an infection of the dialysis graft was suspected. A technetium-99m leukocyte scan demonstrates normally expected activity in the bone marrow of the humerus and proximal forearm, but there is also markedly increased activity extending throughout and proximal to the graft site (*arrows*).

^{99m}Tc-labeled leukocytes show early positivity, improved image quality, and decreased radiation exposure compared with that of ^{111}In-labeled leukocytes.

Vascular Graft Infection. Perigraft gas on a CT scan is diagnostic of infection; however, this is only seen in 50% of cases. In the setting of a negative or equivocal CT scan, ^{111}In-leukocytes are useful in detecting vascular graft infections, including infections of dialysis access grafts. More than 90% of patients with positive scans have subsequently documented culture evidence of infection (Fig. 12–8). Causes of false-positive results are perigraft hematomas, graft thrombosis, and graft epithelialization, which occurs in the first several weeks after surgery.

Technetium-99m HMPAO Leukocytes

The role of ^{99m}Tc-HMPAO leukocytes in inflammation imaging can be better appreciated by comparison with ^{111}In leukocytes. Although they are similar in many respects, there are a few important differences:

■ The technetium label permits higher administered activity, which improves visualization of small-part anatomy, such as the hands and feet.

- The shorter, 6-hour half-life of ^{99m}Tc limits delayed imaging, which can be important for optimal accumulation of labeled leukocytes in some processes.
- Technetium-99m HMPAO leukocyte preparations display normal gastrointestinal tract, urinary tract, and gallbladder activity.
- There is faster uptake of ^{99m}Tc-HMPAO leukocytes in sites of infection, permitting earlier imaging.
- Low absorbed doses enhance suitability for imaging infants and children.

Otherwise, ^{99m}Tc-HMPAO leukocytes share most of the other advantages and disadvantages of ^{111}In leukocytes.

Labeling

The labeling process is similar in principle to that used in the ^{111}In oxine procedure. A ^{99m}Tc-HMPAO lipophilic complex enters the separated leukocytes and is converted to a hydrophilic form, which is trapped inside the cells. The efficiency of this technetium label is less than that of indium. Like the ^{111}In oxine tagging procedure, the labeling of cells is indiscriminate, and a mixed population of leukocytes is generally tagged.

Technique

Between 5 and 15 mCi (185 to 370 MBq) of ^{99m}Tc-HMPAO leukocytes is intravenously injected in adult patients. Technetium-99m leukocytes localize in sites of infection more rapidly than do ^{111}In oxine leukocytes, with a maximal sensitivity at 30 minutes. The imaging sequence depends on the clinical setting. Early images are usually acquired at 0.5 to 4 hours by using a low-energy, high-resolution collimator or a low-energy, all-purpose collimator. The abdomen and pelvis are imaged first, before interfering normal bowel activity can accumulate. For whole-body imaging, views are obtained for 300,000 to 500,000 counts of the head, chest, abdomen, and pelvis, with extremity images obtained as clinically indicated. Delayed images at 18 to 24 hours are obtained as needed, using a low-energy, all-purpose collimator if count rates are lower than expected. A sample imaging protocol is presented in Appendix E–1.

Normal Distribution

Indium-111 and ^{99m}Tc-leukocytes display identical biokinetics in the liver, spleen, and lung. Unlike ^{111}In-leukocytes, however, which show increasing bone marrow activity over 24 hours with constant activity thereafter, ^{99m}Tc leukocyte activity in bone marrow increases over the first 3 hours after injection but decreases over the next 24 hours. In addition, unbound ^{99m}Tc-HMPAO complexes from the leukocyte preparation are seen in the gastrointestinal tract, kidneys, and bladder and occasionally in the gallbladder. Bowel activity is likely related to biliary excretion. Renal activity is primarily due to urinary excretion, with a variable amount of parenchymal binding.

Clinical Applications

Thorax. Similar to their ^{111}In-labeled counterparts, ^{99m}Tc-leukocytes localize nonspecifically in lung inflammation or infection and play a limited role in chest disease. Uptake may be seen in pneumonias, systemic vasculitis, adult respiratory distress syndrome, PCP, or drug-induced pneumonitis. In bronchiectasis, preoperative ^{99m}Tc-leukocyte imaging may be used to determine which lesions noted on CT are active.

Abdomen/Pelvis. Early images for localization of abdominopelvic abscesses are sensitive because of the rapid accumulation of ^{99m}Tc-leukocytes in pyogenic foci. Sequential imaging at 1 and 4 hours is needed to differentiate abnormal leukocyte accumulations from nonspecific bowel activity and to avoid false-positive results caused by imaging only at 4 hours. For inflammatory bowel disease, 1-hour information with ^{99m}Tc is comparable to that seen on 3-hour ^{111}In images, with ^{99m}Tc providing better visualization in the small bowel. Bowel segments showing increased activity at 1 hour that increase in activity at 4 hours provide a higher specificity of diagnosis than does activity appearing for the first time at 4 hours or remaining at the same intensity. Technetium-99m leukocytes can be used to establish a diagnosis, identify diseased segments, confirm relapse, identify complications of Crohn's disease such as mural abscess, and quantify disease. The distribution of activity in the colon allows a distinction between Crohn's disease and ulcerative colitis with a high degree of certainty. Rectal sparing, small-bowel involvement, and "skip" areas suggest Crohn's disease, whereas continuous involvement from the rectum without small-bowel involvement suggests ulcerative colitis. A false-positive appearance on early images may be caused by oozing from recent anastomoses or active gastrointestinal bleeding. With ^{99m}Tc leukocytes, renal infections and hepatobiliary sepsis may be difficult to distinguish from physiologic activity, and ^{111}In-labeled leukocytes may be preferable in these settings.

RADIOLABELED ANTIBODY INFLAMMATION IMAGING

Interest in antibodies for the localization of infections has grown considerably, especially in monoclonal antibody agents capable of labeling leukocytes in vivo. Although a number of radio-pharmaceuticals have been developed, they are only now gaining entry into regular clinical usage. Radiolabeled antibodies directed against leukocyte antigens or receptors permit the imaging of collections of leukocytes in areas of inflammation or infection. Agents developed have included a murine monoclonal immunoglobulin G (Granuloscint) which binds to a cross-reactive antigen on neutrophils, and a monoclonal immunoglobulin G_1 agent (LeukoScan), which binds to a cross-reactive antigen on leukocytes. Neither of these is currently available in the United States.

The FDA–approved radiopharmaceutical ^{99m}Tc-fanolesomab (NeutroSpec) is a murine monoclonal antigranulocyte antibody that binds to cluster designation (CD15) receptors on leukoctyes (Fig. 12–9). This method has the important advantages of avoiding the expensive and labor-intensive process inherent in the in vitro labeling and reinjection of white blood cells and added risks associated with handling blood products. It also provides early sensitivity for the detection of inflammatory foci. The radiopharmaceutical has high affinity for in vivo binding to circulating white blood cells that will subsequently localize in areas of inflammation, but also presumably labels CD15 receptors on leukocytes or leukocyte debris already committed to a site of infection. Its ^{99m}Tc label is ideal for gamma camera imaging, which can be accomplished within 30 minutes to 1 hour of injection. Technetium-99m-fanolesomab has significant potential for use in a number of clinical settings in which labeled leukocytes have shown to be effective as well as appendicitis, inflammatory and ischemic bowel disease, and musculoskeletal infections, especially in the appendicular skeleton. Because CT has proved to be as sensitive as are radionuclide techniques for the detection of appendicitis, has no risk of human antimurine antibody response, and is more readily accepted by referring clinicians, it is the imaging procedure of choice for evaluation of suspected appendicitis. However, in cases of equiv-

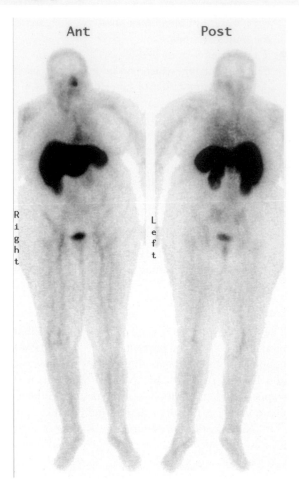

FIGURE 12–9. Monoclonal antibody infection imaging. Anterior and posterior technetium-99m fanolesomab (NeutroSpec) whole-body images performed for suspected appendicitis show normal activity in the liver, spleen, kidneys, and bladder and faint blood pool activity. Incidental note is made of left maxillary sinusitis.

ocal CT findings, ^{99m}Tc-fanolesomab imaging can be a useful adjunctive imaging technique.

MISCELLANEOUS INFLAMMATION AGENTS

Potential new inflammation imaging agents include chemotactic peptides, liposomes, and nanocolloids. A number of radiolabeled chemotactic peptides with a high affinity for inflammatory cells that bind in vivo to both circulating granulocytes and those already present at the site of inflammation have been identified as potential imaging agents. A number of these are bacterial products that initiate leukocyte chemotaxis by binding to high-affinity receptors on the surfaces of inflammatory cells.

Other interesting approaches involve the use of ^{99m}Tc multilamellar liposomes, which are phagocytized by leukocytes at sites of inflammation, and the use of ^{99m}Tc-labeled nanometer-sized human serum albumin colloids (nanocolloids), which leave the circulation and enter the extravascular spaces because of discontinuity of the vascular endothelium at sites of inflammation.

^{18}F-FDG accumulates in areas of increased metabolism. Although ^{18}F-FDG PET scans are more commonly used for neoplasm imaging, the agent also localizes in areas of active infection, including pneumonias, active granulomatous infections, and even in osteomyelitis. It may be especially useful for whole-body images in patients with FUO. However, the accumulation in infections usually is encountered as a confounding factor when a patient is being evaluated for neoplasm. In spite of their sensitivity for infection, ^{18}F-FDG positron emission tomography scans are not currently the initial imaging test used when infection is suspected. This is discussed in Chapter 13.

PEARLS & PITFALLS

Gallium-67 citrate and ^{111}In leukocyte scans are usually photon poor, and the images are coarse or grainy.

Technetium-99m leukocyte scans have more counts, and the images appear less grainy and smoother.

Gallium-67 photon energies are essentially 90, 190, 290, and 390 keV.

Gallium-67 activity is normally seen in the skeleton, lacrimal glands, nasopharynx, and liver. Liver activity is usually greater than that in the spleen. Colon activity is normal on delayed images.

Indium-111 leukocyte activity is normally seen in the bone marrow, liver, and spleen, with the spleen having more intense activity than the liver. Patchy lung activity may be due to leukocytes damaged during labeling

Colonic activity is normal on ^{67}Ga citrate and ^{99m}Tc-leukocyte scans but not on ^{111}In-leukocyte scans.

Renal activity may be seen normally on ^{67}Ga images during the first 24 hours and on ^{99m}Tc-leukocyte images, but not on ^{111}In leukocyte scans.

Focal areas of uptake on ^{67}Ga scan are nonspecific and can represent either tumor or inflammation. Indium-111-leukocytes have been reported to localize in some neoplasms, although this is an uncommon occurrence.

On ^{67}Ga imaging, sarcoidosis and lymphoma may have a similar appearance. Both may show mediastinal and lymph node involvement. Sarcoidosis is suggested by the presence of the lambda sign (increased activity in the right paratracheal and bilateral hilar regions) and the panda sign (symmetrically increased activity in the lacrimal, parotid, and salivary glands). Abdominal involvement is more common in lymphoma.

Diffuse lung activity on ^{67}Ga scan is often due to PCP in patients with AIDS.

Acute fractures and hematomas can show mildly increased activity on leukocyte scans.

Focal activity in the abdomen on a leukocyte scan may be due to an abscess or inflammatory bowel disease (such as Crohn's disease). Activity in the colon can be seen in ulcerative colitis or cytomegalovirus.

Osteomyelitis in the axial skeleton (especially the spine) produces cold defects in up to half of the cases using labeled leukocytes. The scan may also have a normal appearance. Gallium is preferred to labeled leukocytes in the setting of suspected spinal osteomyelitis or diskitis.

SUGGESTED READING

Coleman RE, Datz F: Detection of inflammatory disease using radiolabeled cells. In Sandler MP, Coleman RE, Patton JA et al. (eds): Diagnostic Nuclear Medicine, 4th ed. New York, Lippincott, Williams and Wilkins, 2003, pp 1219–1234.

Love C, Opoku-Agyemang P, Tomas MB, Pugliese PV, Bhargava KK, Palestro CJ: Pulmonary activity on labeled leukocyte images: physiologic, pathologic, and imaging correlation. RadioGraphics 22:1385–1393, 2002.

Love C, Palestro CJ: Radionuclide imaging of infection: continuing education. J Nucl Med Tech 32:47–57, 2004.

Neuman RD, McAfee JG: Gallium-67 imaging in infection. In Sandler MP, Coleman RE, Patton JA et al. (eds): Diagnostic Nuclear Medicine, 4th ed. New York, Lippincott, Williams and Wilkins, 2003, pp 1219–1234.

Palestro CJ, Love C, Tronco GG, Tomas MB: Role of radionuclide imaging in the diagnosis of postoperative infection. RadioGraphics 20:1649–1660, 2000.

Schuster DM, Alazaraki N: Gallium and other agents in diseases of the lung. Semin Nucl Med 32:193–211, 2002.

Positron Emission Tomography (PET) Imaging

13

INTRODUCTION

Although the remainder of this book is organized by subjects such as radionuclides, instrumentation, and body systems, for convenience, all information regarding positron emission tomography (PET) imaging has been included here and cross-referenced where necessary. This permits readers who may be familiar with other aspects of nuclear medicine, but not necessarily PET imaging, to review this topic as one section.

Over the past 25 years, PET imaging has developed from a research technique to the mainstream clinical imaging tool that it is today. Through

TABLE 13–1.	Characteristics of Common PET Radionuclides				
NUCLIDE (DECAY PRODUCT)	PHYSICAL HALF-LIFE	DECAY MODE	MAXIMAL AND AVERAGE POSITRON ENERGY (keV)	MAXIMUM AND MEAN RANGE IN WATER (mm)	PRODUCTION REACTION
Carbon-11 (Boron-11)	20.3 min	99.8% positron 0.2% electron capture	960, 320	4.1, 1.1	^{14}N (p,alpha)^{11}C*
Nitrogen-13 (Carbon-13)	10 min	100% positron	1198, 432	5.1, 1.5	^{16}O(p,alpha)^{13}N ^{13}C(p,n)^{13}N
Oxygen-15 (Nitrogen-15)	124 sec	99.9% positron	1732, 696	7.3, 2.5	^{15}N(p,n)^{15}O ^{14}N(d,n)^{15}O
Fluorine-18 (Oxygen-18)	110 min	97% positron 3% electron capture	634, 202	2.4, 0.6	^{18}O(p,n)^{18}F ^{20}Ne(d,alpha)^{18}F ^{16}O(^{3}He,alpha)^{18}F
Rubidium-82	1.27 min (75 sec)	96% positron 4% electron capture	3356, 1385	14.1, 5.9	^{82}Sr generator (T1/2 25.3 days)

*This symbolism means that a proton is accelerated into an atom of nitrogen-14, causing ejection of an alpha particle from the nucleus to produce an atom of carbon-11.

positron-emitting radionuclide labeling, PET allows the in-vivo imaging of physiologically and pathologically important molecules containing basic organic chemical elements such as carbon, hydrogen, and oxygen. Such data provide molecular and/or metabolic information essential to the diagnosis and evaluation of disease and thus to the effective management of patient care.

BASIC POSITRON PHYSICS

Positron-emitting radionuclides are most commonly produced in cyclotrons by bombarding a stable element with protons, deuterons, or helium nuclei. The produced radionuclides have an excess of protons and decay by the emission of positrons. The most commonly used five positron-emitting isotopes are shown in Table 13–1.

When a positron is emitted, it travels for a short distance from its site of origin, gradually losing energy to the tissue through which it moves. When most of its kinetic energy has been lost, the positron reacts with a resident electron in an annihilation reaction. This reaction generates two 511-keV gamma photons, which are emitted in opposite directions at about (but not exactly) 180 degrees from each other (Fig. 13–1). In a PET scanner, these photons interact with the detector ring at opposite sites, which defines a line along which the annihilation reaction occurred and permits localization of the reaction (Fig. 13–2). By using many such events, an image can be reconstructed.

It is important to remember that the site of origin of the positron and the site of the annihilation reaction occur at slightly different locations. Positrons are not all emitted with the same energy, and therefore, the distance the positron travels before annihilation varies for each specific radionuclide (Fig. 13–3). For example, the positrons from fluorine-18 (^{18}F; 640 keV) and carbon-11 (^{11}C; 960 keV) have a range in water of about 1 to 1.5 mm and 2.5 mm in tissue, whereas rubidium 82 (^{82}Rb; 3.15 MeV) has a range of about 10 mm in water and 16 mm in tissue before annihilation. The fact that the positron travels a distance before annihilation causes some uncertainty in determining the original location of the positron (range-related uncertainty). Further, the two resultant annihilation photons may actually be emitted up to ±0.25 degrees from the theoretical 180 degrees (Fig. 13–4). This variation in emission angles (noncolinearity) also generates some uncertainty in the original location of the annihilation reaction. Both of these issues contribute to fundamental

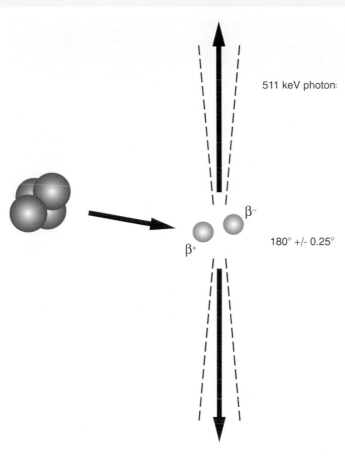

511 keV photons

β^-

180° +/- 0.25°

β^+

FIGURE 13–1. Positron decay. After the positron (β^+) is emitted from the radionuclide, it travels some distance before interacting with an electron (β^-) and undergoing annihilation, resulting in emission of two 511-keV photons at 180-degrees from each other.

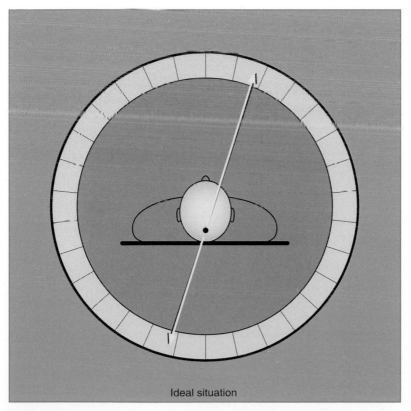

Ideal situation

FIGURE 13–2. Positron emission tomography. In the ideal situation, annihilation photons would be emitted at exactly the same point as the positron emission occurred and would travel in exactly opposite directions.

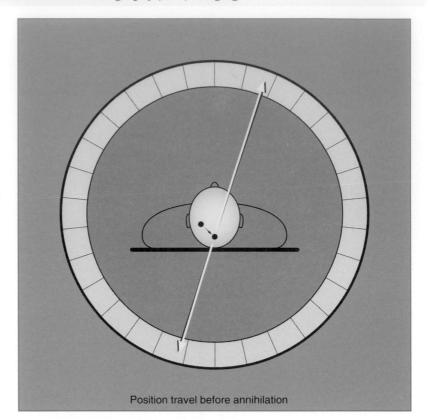

FIGURE 13–3. Image degradation due to positron travel. Positron travel after emission and before interacting with a electron results in the scanner localizing the event at some distance from the actual site of the positron emission.

Position travel before annihilation

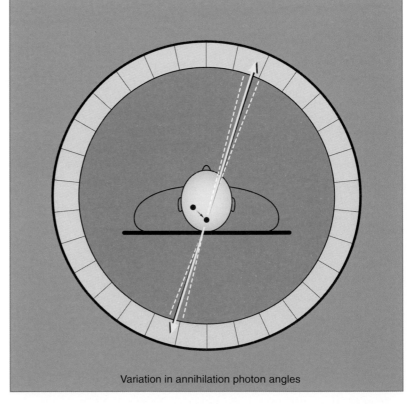

FIGURE 13–4. Image degradation due to angle of photon emission. Slight variation in angle of emission of the annihilation photons results in the scanner placing the event at some distance from where the annihilation actually occurred, causing additional loss of spatial resolution.

Variation in annihilation photon angles

degradation of spatial resolution in any PET detector system.

PET INSTRUMENTATION
Overview of PET Cameras

PET imaging is performed by using dedicated PET cameras containing multiple rings of detectors consisting of scintillation crystals coupled with photomultiplier tubes (PMTs). The ring design takes advantage of the fact that two photons detected in close temporal proximity by two opposed detectors in the ring are likely to be from a single annihilation event. Such a simultaneous detection event is called a *coincidence*. The near simultaneous detection of two photons provides localizing information in that the annihilation event can be assumed to have occurred somewhere on a line between the two detectors (the line of response, or LOR). The many coincidence events recorded by the PET scanner constitute a raw data set representing projections of the distribution of the positron radiopharmaceutical in the body. These data are then reconstructed by using a filtered back projection algorithm or an iterative algorithm to produce cross-sectional images.

Because photons travel at the speed of light, PET cameras require very fast electronics to determine if two detected photons were likely produced by a single annihilation event. In a PET scanner, each annihilation photon reaching a detector generates a single electronic pulse in the detector. For this photon to be accepted and used in the PET image, it must be in a specific energy range (ideally approaching 511 keV) and be paired with another photon reaching another detector simultaneously. Coincidence circuitry connecting the many detectors in the rings determines whether two such single pulses (representing the captured photons in opposing detectors) fall within a short *coincidence time window*, typically 6 to 12 nanoseconds. If so, they are deemed to constitute a coincidence event and are recorded in the resultant image. The actual coincidence time is typically about 1 nanosecond. However, the time window for coincidence detection varies with different camera systems and depends in large part on the speed of the electronic circuitry and detector scintillation crystal type. It is about 12 nanoseconds for bismuth germanium oxide (BGO), 8 nanoseconds for gadolinium oxyorthosilicate (GSO) and sodium iodide (NaI), and 6 nanoseconds for lutetium oxyorthosilicate (LSO) systems. Because the energy

resolution of the various crystal detectors is not precise, photons within a broad energy range ($\approx$ 250 to 600 keV) are counted as valid annihilation photons.

Because of detector ring geometry and photon attenuation through scatter and absorption, many annihilation events result in only one of the two 511-keV photons interacting with the PET camera detectors (single event). Consequently, a very large number of such single events are incident on the PET detectors. Because PET scanners use only photon pairs meeting the coincidence criterion in constructing PET images, single counts can be identified and discarded. In practice, about 99% of detected photons are rejected by the coincidence circuitry of the PET system. However, this principle of coincidence detection provides a virtual electronic collimation of the events and makes PET scanners inherently more efficient than are traditional gamma cameras, which use parallel-hole lead collimators.

Events detected by PET scanners include true, scattered, and random events, all of which may be recorded as coincidences, providing both annihilation photons are actually detected and fall within the coincidence window. True coincidences are those that result when both 511-keV photons from an annihilation reaction are detected within the coincidence time window, neither photon having undergone any form of interaction before reaching the detector. These true coincidence events provide the desired information for constructing accurate images of the distribution of a PET radiopharmaceutical in clinical imaging.

Scattered coincidences occur when one or both annihilation photons undergo Compton interaction in body tissues and are deflected away from their expected path but still reach the detectors within the time window and are recorded as a coincidence event (Fig. 13–5). Because the direction of the scattered photon has changed during the Compton interaction, the resulting coincidence event is likely to be assigned an inaccurate LOR that no longer passes though the point of annihilation, leading to erroneous localization information and decreasing image contrast.

Random coincidences arise when two photons, each originating from a different annihilation reaction, reach any detector within the time window and thus appear to represent a true coincidence (Fig. 13–6). Using detectors that allow very precise timing permits the recognition and exclusion of random events with a resultant improvement in

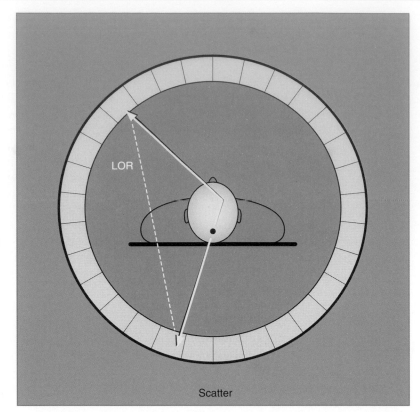

FIGURE 13–5. Image degradation due to scatter of photons. Scatter of an annihilation photon after emission can result in the scanner assuming that the positron emission took place on a line of response (LOR) very far from the actual event.

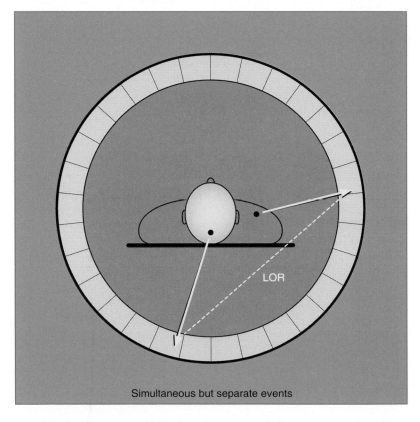

FIGURE 13–6. Image degradation due to simultaneous separate events. Photons being recorded from separate but almost simultaneous events will result in the scanner assuming that the positron emission took place on a line of response (LOR) very far from the actual event.

image quality. If left uncorrected, both scattered and random coincidences add background to the true coincidence distribution, thereby increasing statistical noise, decreasing contrast, and causing the radioisotope concentrations to be overestimated.

There are a number of methods available to reduce the image degrading impact of scattered coincidences. Most scattered photons are not detected because they are absorbed in tissues of the body, are scattered away from the detector rings, or have lost significant energy during Compton scattering. These lower-energy scattered events can be rejected by using an energy window designed to exclude photons of certain energies. The success of such rejection depends on the energy resolution characteristics of the detectors being used. Because crystal detectors have only a finite energy resolution, if one were to measure only photons approaching 511 keV and exclude scattered photons of slightly different energies, a large number of true events would also be excluded, thereby either reducing image statistics or increasing image acquisition times unacceptably. Therefore, a rather broad energy window is used that allows some scattered events to be recorded as true events.

Another method to reduce scatter from outside the plane of a detector ring is to use thin lead or tungsten septa positioned between the detector elements. Imaging with lead septa is called two-

dimensional (or slice) imaging because most of the photons counted originate in the plane of a single detector ring. Two-dimensional imaging improves image quality by reducing image noise (Fig. 13–7). It also minimizes count losses due to system dead time by incidentally reducing the very large numbers of photons reaching the detectors that may occur at high count rates. However, although this reduces the number of scattered events originating outside the field of view (FOV), it also significantly reduces the true counts and increases imaging times.

Faster detector crystals and faster electronics in new PET instruments have made imaging without septa, so-called three-dimensional (or volume) imaging possible (Fig. 13–8). This allows imaging from the volume defined by the entire FOV of the multiple detector rings of the camera and permits detection of true coincidence events that occur in different detectors on different rings. Compared with two-dimensional imaging, three-dimensional acquisitions increase sensitivity of the system by fivefold or more. However, because both true coincidence and scatter rates are increased, better temporal and energy resolutions are needed to accurately eliminate scatter and random events.

PET Scintillation Detectors

All positron systems use the principle of scintillation whereby the photon interacting with a crystal

2-D Acquisition

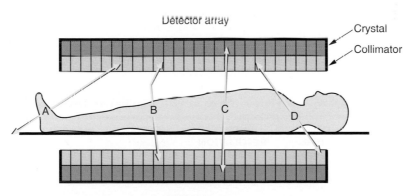

FIGURE 13–7. Two-dimensional acquisition. Two-dimensional acquisition is essentially slice acquisition performed with septae or collimation in place. The collimation results in annihilation photons occurring outside opposing detector elements (A) and scattered photons (B) being unable to reach the detector. Photons occurring in the "slice" seen by opposing detectors (C) are recorded, whereas photons emitted at steep angles (D) are not able to reach the detector elements.

3-D Acquisition

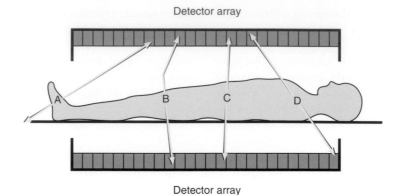

FIGURE 13–8. Three-dimensional acquisition. Three-dimensional acquisition is essentially volumetric acquisition, and collimation or septae are not used. As a result many more events are detected per unit time than with two-dimensional acquisition. Although events occurring outside the volume (A) are not recorded because the second photon is not interacting with a detector, scattered (B), central (C), and steep angle events (D) are all recorded.

produces a flash of light, which is then detected and localized by photomultiplier tubes (PMTs) coupled to the scintillation crystal. The ideal PET crystal detector would have (1) high stopping power for 511-keV photons providing high efficiency and optimum spatial resolution; (2) fast, intense light output with rapid decay of the light for decreased system dead time; and (3) good energy resolution for accurate scatter rejection. Stopping power is best for crystalline materials with high density and high effective atomic number (Z value). There are several types of crystalline detector materials used for PET imaging. These include NaI, BGO, LSO, and GSO. Some characteristics of these are shown in Tables 13–2 and 13–3.

From these tables it is evident that BGO has the poorest energy resolution, whereas NaI has the best energy resolution as a result of the highest light output. The energy resolution of BGO crystals requires that a wide energy window ($\approx$ 250 to 600 keV) be used to avoid rejecting true events and reducing the detected count rate. The use of a wide energy window means that a BGO detector system will accept more scattered events than will the other systems with better energy resolution. NaI systems use a narrower energy window than do BGO, LSO, or GSO systems.

The light signal produced by scintillation detectors is not discrete in time but occurs over a short time interval (scintillation decay time, 10 to 300

TABLE 13–2.	**Physical Properties of Various Types of PET Scintillation Detectors**					
CRYSTAL	**RELATIVE LIGHT OUTPUT (%)**	**DECAY TIME (ns)**	**ENERGY RESOLUTION AT 511 keV (%)**	**DENSITY (g/cm³)**	**EFFECTIVE Z**	**HYGROSCOPIC**
NaI (Tl)	100	230	8	3.7	51	Yes
BGO	15	300	12	7.1	75	No
LSO	75	40	10	7.4	65	No
GSO	25	60	9	6.7	59	No
BaF2	5	0.6	11	4.89	52.2	No

NaI, sodium iodide; Tl, thallium; BGO, bismuth germanate; LSO, lutetium oxyorthosilicate; GSO, gadolinium oxyorthosilicate; BaF2, Barium Fluoride.

TABLE 13–3.	Relative Properties of Various Crystalline Detector Materials			
CRYSTAL	STOPPING POWER (511-KEV PHOTONS)	LIGHT YIELD	DECAY TIME	ENERGY RESOLUTION
NaI(Tl)	Low	High	Long (slow light output)	High
BGO	High	Low	Long (slow light output)	Low
LSO	Intermediate	Intermediate	Short (fast light output)	Intermediate
GSO	Intermediate	Low	Short (fast light output)	Intermediate

NaI, sodium iodide; Tl, thallium; BGO, bismuth germanium oxide; LSO, lutetium oxyorthosilicate; GSO, gadolinium oxyorthosilicate.

nanoseconds), which includes the period over which the light fades to background. Along with the speed of processing electronics, this decay time is an important determinant of system dead time. Dead time is the brief period during which a crystal-PMT detector is busy producing and recording a scintillation event and having the scintillation light decay so that the next distinct scintillation event can be recognized and recorded. During this time additional arriving events cannot be processed and are lost. This limits the rate at which events may be detected. High count rate capability of PET instruments is particularly important in three-dimensional acquisitions and in settings requiring high activities of very short-lived radionuclides (e.g., oxygen 15). Current count rate capabilities are about 500,000 counts/second.

The relatively long decay times of both BGO and NaI crystals limit count rate capability. The shorter decay time of light output for LSO crystals can reduce scan times for comparable images to about half of the time required for BGO systems. LSO crystals probably have the best combination of properties for optimizing PET imaging, especially in three-dimensional imaging systems (without septa) with the potential for very high count rates.

PET Detector Geometry

State-of-the-art PET scanners (Table 13–4) are multidetector full ring (circular or polygonal) systems that axially surround the patient (360 degrees). These cameras have multiple adjacent detector rings that significantly increase the axial

TABLE 13–4.	Properties of a Typical PET Camera	
CHARACTERISTIC		PET SCANNER
Radionuclides imaged		PET only
Detector array		Rings (usually 18–32)
Detector (crystal material)		NaI curved
		BGO
		LSO
		GSO
Crystal number and size		Variable but in state-of-the-art ring systems with block detectors about 10,000–20,000 small crystals (about 4 × 4 × 30 mm) with 36–64 crystals per block
Counting rates		High
Algorithm for location		Specific detector
Acquisition		2 or 3 dimensional
Spatial resolution		High (5–6 mm)
Coincidence window		6–12 nsec
Energy window		≈350–650 keV
System sensitivity (cps/Bq/mL)		≈25%–35%
Axial resolution FWHM (mm) at 10 cm		≈5.5–7
Energy resolution (FWHM)		≈15%–25%

PET, positron emission tomography; NaI, sodium iodide; Tl, thallium; BGO, bismuth germanate; LSO, lutetium oxyorthosilicate; GSO, gadolinium oxyorthosilicate; FWHM, full width at half-maximum.

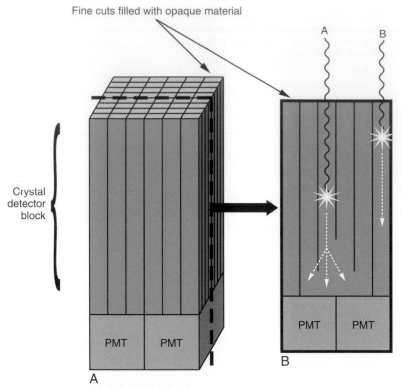

FIGURE 13–9. PET scintillation block detector. Many crystal detectors are made from a single block of material and have cuts made to different depths and filled with opaque material. There are often 8 × 8 detector elements made, and the different depths of cuts allow localization with only four photomultiplier tubes (PMTs). If a photon interacts with a central detector element (A), the shallow cut allows the light from the scintillation to be localized by several PMTs. A photon interacting with a detector element near the edge of the block (B) may have light that is only seen by one PMT.

FOV of the patient. A larger FOV allows more counts to be detected for a standardized administered radiopharmaceutical dose and a fixed scan time by allowing more time at each table position.

The most common detector arrangement used in dedicated PET cameras consists of rings of individual detector modules of small crystal arrays or cut block scintillation crystals (usually BGO or LSO) coupled with PMTs (Fig. 13–9). In crystal arrays, multiple separate very small (≈ 4-mm front surface edge) scintillation crystals are grouped together in blocks, often arranged in 6 × 6 or 8 × 8 blocks (36 to 64 "crystals" per detector block). This concept is more economically achieved by using a single crystalline block onto which deep channels have been cut, forming a matrix (8 × 8 or 64 elements) on the face of the block. The channels in the crystal are filled with opaque material so that the light from scintillation events cannot spread between sections, but travels only toward the PMTs.

This achieves the effect of multiple small crystalline detectors.

Many such blocks (hundreds) are then assembled to form a crystal ring. The light from each block is collected by PMTs (about four per block) servicing the entire block of crystals. Even though the number of PMTs per block is far less than the number of individual crystal elements, it is still possible to attribute each light pulse to a particular crystal for localization by comparing pulse heights in each of the PMTs. Most full multi-ring PET scanners have 10,000 to 20,000 "crystals" arranged in about 200 to 400 blocks and with about 500 to 1000 PMTs (Fig. 13–10). For multi-crystal PET cameras, the intrinsic spatial resolution is a function of the crystal size; thus, the small sizes of the crystal faces allowed by block design permits optimization of intrinsic resolution. Further, a large number of small independent detectors in a PET system significantly reduces dead time count losses and allows camera operation at higher count rates.

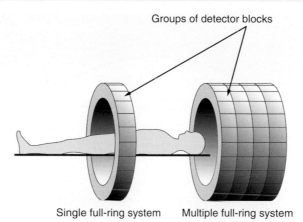

Groups of detector blocks

Single full-ring system   Multiple full-ring system

FIGURE 13–10. Ring design of PET cameras. PET cameras have rings consisting of thousands of detector elements. There may only be a single ring, but modern cameras have many rings to increase the sensitivity and speed of the system.

With ring detectors of any sort, resolution varies with location in the FOV. As an annihilation event gets closer to the edge of the FOV, more image blurring occurs because the path of an annihilation photon may traverse more than one detector element and is capable of producing a scintillation in any of them (Fig. 13–11).

Alternative detector arrangements to the small "multi-crystal" complete ring design have been available. These include an hexagonal array or a ring of large curved thallium-doped sodium iodide (NaI[Tl]), crystals, and dual opposed arcs of small detectors that rotate around the axis of the patient to acquire data. There are advantages and disadvantages to these alternative configurations. Because septa are not typically used with these systems, only three-dimensional imaging is employed.

Attenuation Correction

Attenuation is the loss of true events through photon absorption in the body or by scattering out of the detector FOV. Attenuation problems are significantly worse with PET imaging than with single-photon emission computed tomography (SPECT). Even though the energy of the annihilation photons is greater than for single-photon imaging, with PET, two photons must escape the patient to be detected and the mean photon path is longer, increasing the likelihood of attenuation. In a large person, the loss of counts due to attenuation can exceed 50% to 95%.

Loss of counts through attenuation increases image noise, artifacts, and distortion. Significant artifacts may occur on whole-body PET images obtained without attenuation correction. These include the following: (1) distortions of areas of high activity (such as the bladder) due to variable attenuation in different directions, (2) a prominent body surface edge ("hot skin"), and (3) apparently high count rates (increased activity) in tissues of low attenuation, such as the lungs. As a result, attenuation correction of these images is necessary before the true amount of radionuclide present at various locations in the body can be accurately determined. This is true both for accurate qualitative assessment of activity distribution on regional or whole-body images and for precise quantitative measurements of tracer uptake, such as standardized uptake values (SUVs).

Methods of attenuation correction include the following: (1) calculated correction, based on body contour assumptions and used primarily for imaging the head/brain where attenuation is relatively uniform; and (2) measured correction using actual transmission data, used for imaging the chest, abdomen, pelvis, and whole body where attenuation is variable. Transmission attenuation correction is performed by acquiring a map of body density and correcting for absorption in the various tissues. The amount of positron-emitting radionuclide at a specific location can then be determined. Once the correction is performed, the information is reconstructed into cross-sectional images.

One method to obtain a transmission attenuation map of the body is to use an orbiting long-lived

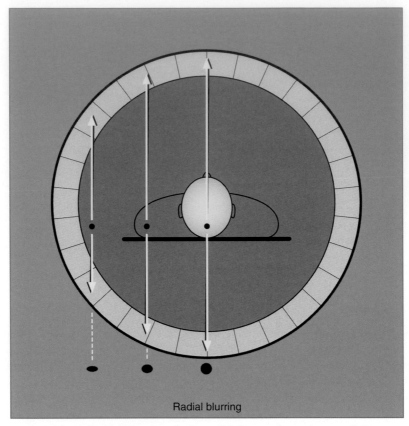

Radial blurring

FIGURE 13–11. Radial blurring. As the annihilation reaction and source of the photon emission gets closer to the edge of the field of view, the photon is more likely to traverse more than one detector element, which results in more uncertainly as to actual location of the original event and subsequent blurring of the image.

radioactive source outside the patient [typically a rod of 3–10 mCi (120 to 370 MBq) of germanium-68 (^{68}Ge)/gallium-68 (^{68}Ga) with a half-life of 9 months, or 5–20 mCi (185 to 740 MBq) of cesium-137 (^{137}Cs) with a half-life of 30 years] and measure transmission through the patient by using the same system ring detectors used for primary positron imaging. In a ^{68}Ge/^{68}Ga transmission source, the ^{68}Ge decays to ^{68}Ga, which then decays by positron emission. In general, performing the transmission scan with either of these radionuclides can take 20 to 25 minutes and account for up to 40% of total scanning time.

In PET/CT scanners, x-rays from the computed tomography (CT) scan are used for attenuation correction and for providing localizing anatomic information. Because the x-rays used are less than 511-keV, the transmission data are adjusted to construct an attenuation map appropriate for annihilation photons. Attenuation maps can be obtained

much more quickly (during a single breath-hold) with a PET/CT scanner than with external radionuclide sources, and the quality of the attenuation maps is improved. However, because the attenuation map obtained with CT is obtained much more quickly than is the PET scan, artifacts in regions of moving structures such as the diaphragm may occur.

Attenuation is more likely when the annihilation reaction occurs in the center of the patient and less likely when the event occurs at the edge of the body. Thus, in a non–attenuation-corrected image, there is less activity in the center of the body and more activity at the skin surface. Typically both attenuation-corrected and non–attenuation-corrected images are provided for interpretation. Images without attenuation correction can be recognized by the surface of the body (or "skin") and the lungs appearing to contain considerably increased activity (Fig. 13–12). On attenuation-

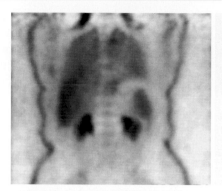
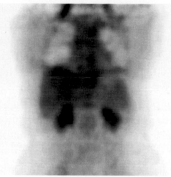

FIGURE 13–12. Unattenuated (*left*) and attenuation-corrected (*right*) images. Without attenuation correction, the surface of the body or skin appears to have an unusual amount of activity and the lungs appear dark. Once attenuation correction is applied, these effects disappear.

corrected images, the lungs have less activity than do structures nearer the surface and appear photopenic. Some lesions located near the surface of the body are more obvious on the uncorrected images, but most will be seen on the corrected images. A misalignment artifact can occur when a patient moves in between the transmission and emission scans. This can result in overcorrection on one side of the body and undercorrection on the other. In addition, an artifact may occur as a result of the bladder filling with radionuclide during the PET scan acquisition. This results in a hot area appearing around the bladder on the attenuation-corrected images but not on the non–attenuation-corrected images.

System Sensitivity and Resolution

The sensitivity is defined as the recorded true coincidence rate (i.e., without scatter and random events) divided by the activity concentration (the true emitted events from the source). Sensitivity of a PET camera is determined by multiple factors, including, but not limited to, scanner geometry, crystal efficiency, and photon attenuation in tissue. Most photons emitted from the patient (98% to 99%) are not detected because they are emitted in all directions from the patient and the detector rings cover only a fraction of the patient's body surface. And when attenuation by absorption or scatter is considered, current systems record substantially less than 0.1% of the true events. However, because state-of-the-art PET scanners typically image in three-dimensional mode (without collimators or septa), their efficiency for detecting emitted radiation is still considerably greater than

that for SPECT imaging. Further, the sensitivity of PET is such that picomolar concentrations of PET radiopharmaceuticals can be detected.

Spatial resolution in PET scanners is, in large part, a function of detector size, with smaller detectors increasing the resolving capability of the system. Because of inherent physical limitations on positron localization imposed by their movement from the site of their emission (range) and the noncolinearity of annihilation photons, submillimeter resolution, such as possible with magnetic resonance imaging (MRI), is not achieved. The ultimate limit of spatial resolution when using ^{18}F-fluorodeoxyglucose (^{18}F-FDG) is about 1 mm (see Table 13–4). However, the practical spatial resolution for clinical imaging is about 4 to 6 mm.

RADIOPHARMACEUTICALS

There are three PET radiopharmaceuticals currently in commercial production. These are ^{82}Rb-chloride, ^{13}N-ammonia (^{13}NH$_3$), and ^{18}F-FDG. Both ^{82}Rb-chloride and ^{13}NH$_3$ can be used for assessment of myocardial perfusion, but in practice they are not commonly used. Carbon-11 is also used, but the short half-life (20 minutes) requires an onsite cyclotron and rapid local radiopharmaceutical preparation.

Fluorine-18 Fluorodeoxyglucose

The most commonly used positron-emitting radiopharmaceutical in clinical imaging is the glucose analog ^{18}F-FDG. Many tumor cells use large amounts of glucose as an energy source and possess increased expression of glucose transporters (especially GLUT1) and increased hexokinase activity (especially HK2). Glucose transporters transfer glucose and fluorodeoxyglucose into the cells, where they are phosphorylated by hexokinases (Fig. 13–13). The rate-limiting step in this process is at the hexokinase level and not at glucose transport. Although phosphorylated glucose can be further metabolized, phosphorylated FDG cannot be rapidly metabolized and ^{18}F-FDG is essentially trapped within the cell in proportion to the rate of glucose metabolism. This allows sufficient time to image its distribution in normal and abnormal bodily tissues. A notable exception to the trapping of phosphorylated FDG is the liver, in which an abundance of phosphatases causes enhanced dephosphorylation of FDG-6-phosphate, which accelerates its washout from that organ.

Although ^{18}F-FDG reaches a plateau of accumulation in tumors at about 45 minutes after injection, the tumor-to-background ratio is best at 2 to 3 hours. Highest activity levels at 2 hours are seen in the brain, heart (if not fasting), and urinary system.

Other Radiopharmaceuticals

Considerable resources have and will continue to be expended in the development of promising positron-labeled molecules to expand the array of clinically relevant radiopharmaceuticals for PET imaging. The possibilities seem unlimited.

One potential tumor marker for clinical use is choline. It has been suggested that malignant transformation of cells is associated with increased activity of choline kinase. Choline is incorporated into cell membrane phospholipids via phosphorylcholine synthesis. It can be labeled with ^{11}C, but because of the short half-life other tracers may be better (e.g., ^{18}F fluoroethylcholine). Choline appears to be a potential tracer for specific tumors (such as brain and prostate). Another compound that localizes in some tumors (such as prostate) is ^{11}C-acetate. Although the localization mechanism is unclear, it may be related to enhanced lipid synthesis.

Radiopharmaceutical Quality Assurance

Product standards and quality control requirements for PET radiopharmaceuticals are provided by both the U.S. Pharmacopeia and guidance from the Food and Drug Administration (which in some instances is more restrictive). For ^{18}F-FDG injection, the Food and Drug Administration indicates that (1) the solution must be colorless and free from particulate matter when observed visually (appearance), (2) the half-life must be measured to be between 105 and 115 minutes (radionuclide identity), (3) no more than 4% of free ^{18}F$^-$ must be

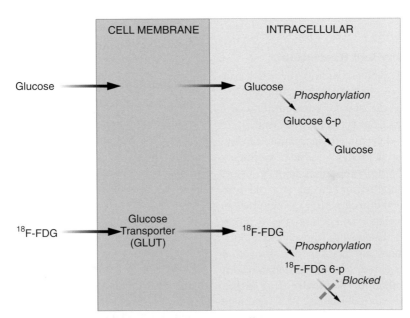

FIGURE 13–13. ^{18}F-FDG metabolism. Although ^{18}F-FDG is transported into the cell in the same manner as glucose, it cannot be dephosphorylated and remains in the cell.

present in an injection (radiochemical impurity), (4) no less than 90% of the radioactivity must locate at a specific spot on chromatography (radiochemical purity), and (5) additional tests for chemical purity must assure that various reagents, unwanted products or residual organic solvents are not present in excess. Sterility and bacterial endotoxin testing are performed in the same manner as with other radiopharmaceuticals.

Radiation Safety

With the higher energies associated with positron-emitting radionuclides, there have been concerns about the radiation safety aspects of PET scanning. Significant sources of occupational exposure may be associated with handling radiopharmaceuticals before patient injection and with repetitive close contact with patients shortly after injection. These exposures are potentially significantly higher than are those experienced with routine handling and administration of technetium-99m (^{99m}Tc) radiopharmaceuticals. Thus, review of the special radiation safety aspects of performing PET procedures is appropriate.

Occupational Considerations

When compared with 10 mCi (370 MBq) of ^{99m}Tc, the same activity of ^{18}F will result in a dose rate about sixfold higher or 35 versus 199 mR/hour (0.31 versus 1.74 mSv/hour) at a distance of 20 cm (8 inches) from the source. This is the distance corresponding to handling a vial of radionuclide with tongs. Dose rates for the same activity at 5 cm are 568 and 3189 mR/hour (5 and 28 mSv/hour) respectively. Dose rates at other distances are shown in Table 13–5. Syringe shields used for ^{99m}Tc are usually about 0.32 cm (⅛ inch) of lead or equivalent, and this is inadequate for positron emitters. Because increasing the lead thickness by a factor of 16 (to achieve the same protection) is impractical, use of tungsten, which has a higher atomic number (Z) and electron density, is preferred. It provides about 1.4 times the shielding as an equivalent thickness of lead. Dose rates from patients recently injected with ^{18}F-FDG may also be a significant source of occupational exposure.

As with other radiopharmaceuticals, the activity of positron emitters may be measured in a typical dose calibrator before administration to the patient. Although a dose calibrator (ionization chamber) cannot determine the energy of emitted photons, the amount of electrical current in the chamber produced by the photons varies directly with

TABLE 13–5.	Approximate Absorbed Dose and Exposure from a 10 mCi (370 MBq) Dose of ^{18}F-FDG
	DOSE AND EXPOSURE, mrem/hr (mSv/hr)
Surface of syringe with no shield	3000–4000 (30–40)
Surface of syringe with shield	500 (5)
Surface of patient	40 (0.4)*
1 m from patient	10 (0.1)*
2 m from patient	4 (0.04)*

*Value averaged over first hour after injection. The instantaneous dose rate immediately after injection is approximately three- to fourfold higher.

photon energy. Limits for maximum activity to be measured by dose calibrators are usually specified for ^{99m}Tc. Because the 511-keV annihilation photons are substantially more energetic than are ^{99m}Tc photons, the current produced is about three times greater. Therefore, the maximum activity limit for ^{18}F is about one third that specified for ^{99m}Tc. Consequently, a dose calibrator with relatively high specified maximum activity is preferred. In addition, more lead shielding around the dose calibrator is required. It should be at least 5 cm or greater compared with the 4- to 6-mm thickness usually supplied with a standard dose calibrator. Because of their short physical half-lives, waste disposal for most positron emitters is easily achieved by storage and decay for 1 day.

Patient Considerations

The effective dose to the patient for most ^{18}F-FDG PET scans is about 0.1 rem (1 mSv) or about 0.093 rem/mCi (0.025 mSv/MBq). Doses to various organs for ^{8}F-FDG and other PET radionuclides are shown in Tables 13–6 and 13–7.

Pregnancy and breast feeding are common concerns when administering radionuclides to women. Fetal dose estimates after administration of 13.5 mCi (500 MBq) of ^{18}F-FDG to the mother are about 1400 mrem (14 mSv) in early pregnancy and about 400 mrem (4 mSv) at term. Although ^{18}F-FDG can accumulate in breast tissue, it is not secreted to any significant degree in the milk. It is usually recommended that the mother not cuddle

TABLE 13–6. Absorbed Dose for Various Organs from ¹⁸F-FDG

ORGAN	ABSORBED DOSE, rad/mCi (mGy/MBq)
Brain	0.17 (0.046)
Heart (highly variable depending on glucose level)	0.23 (0.062)
Kidneys	0.08 (0.022)
Liver	0.09 (0.024)
Lungs	0.06 (0.016)
Pancreas	0.05 (0.014)
Red marrow	0.04 (0.011)
Spleen	0.06 (0.016)
Bladder (highly variable depending on hydration and voiding)	0.6 (0.16)
Ovaries	0.04 (0.011)
Testes	0.04 (0.011)

or breast feed the infant for about 8 hours after injection.

PET IMAGE ACQUISITION AND PROCESSING

Dedicated PET systems are most commonly used in a whole-body scanning mode. This usually entails obtaining sequential segmental views of the body by moving the scanning table stepwise to acquire multiple contiguous views. There is a need to overlap the views to get uniform counting statistics, because in multiple detector ring systems, the detector rings at the edge of the FOV have less sensitivity than do those in the middle. A whole-body scan in a dedicated PET scanner usually extends from the base of the brain to the mid-thighs using a two- or three-dimensional acquisition. Depending on the size of the patient and the scanner, overlapping images are usually obtained every 15 to 20 cm for several minutes per position.

Images on a PET scanner can be acquired by using either two-dimensional (slice) or three-dimensional (volume) technique. With two-dimensional imaging, there are thin lead or tungsten septa (axial collimators) between the detectors and the adjacent rings of detectors such that each ring of detectors accepts coincidences only between detectors in the same ring or in closely adjacent rings. This defines a single plane (slice), eliminating out-of-plane scatter. Although sensitivity is reduced, image quality is enhanced. Two-dimensional imaging is usually performed when imaging small portions of the body (such as the heart) or obese patients, when using respiratory gating or short scan times with high activity, or when obtaining higher resolution or accurate quantification.

When three-dimensional acquisition is performed, septa are not present or are retracted. This allows acquisition of a large volume defined by the FOV with coincidences recorded between the multiple detector rings in any combination. Sensitivity is about 5 to 10 times higher than with two-

TABLE 13–7. Absorbed Radiation Dose rad/mCi (mGy/MBq) and Effective Dose rem/mCi (mSv/MBq) of Administered Activity from Various PET Radiopharmaceuticals

RADIOPHARMACEUTICAL	ORGAN	ORGAN	UTERUS	EFFECTIVE DOSE
Carbon-11 acetate	Kidneys, 0.20 (0.053)		0.005 (0.0014)	0.013 (0.0035)
Nitrogen-13 ammonia	Bladder, 0.030 (0.0081)	Kidneys, 0.031 (0.0083)	0.007 (0.0019)	0.007 (0.002)
Oxygen-15 water	Heart, 0.007 (0.0019)	Kidney, 0.006 (0.0017)	0.001 (0.00035)	0.0034 (0.00093)
Fluorine-18 ion	Bladder, 0.81 (0.22)	Bone, 0.15 (0.04)	0.07 (0.019)	0.09 (0.024)
Fluorine-18 fluorodeoxyglucose	Bladder, 0.6 (0.16)	Heart, 0.23 (0.062)	0.08 (0.021)	0.07 (0.019)
Rubidium-82	Heart, 0.1 (0.0027)	Kidneys, 0.07 (0.02)		0.003 (0.00075)

dimensional acquisition due to absence of the septa and the increased FOV of each crystal. However, although the number of recorded true coincidences is increased, out-of-plane scatter and random events are also considerably increased reducing image contrast and quality. With three-dimensional acquisition as much as 30% to 60% of recorded events will be due to scatter. To compensate for increased scatter and random count rates and to minimize dead time count losses, faster detectors with significantly better energy resolution (such as LSO, GSO) are needed. Three-dimensional imaging is typically used for low-scatter studies such as imaging the brain, small patient size (pediatrics), and attempts to shorten scan times when there is low administered activity. As improvements in hardware and three-dimensional algorithms are made, the use of three-dimensional imaging, with its increased sensitivity for true coincidences, is likely to become more commonly used.

Disadvantages of three-dimensional acquisition include the following: (1) an increased number of bed positions is required; (2) more random and scatter events are detected; and (3) if too much activity is administered, the count rate limit of a three-dimensional system can be overwhelmed. Three-dimensional imaging detects more random events because in a high count rate environment the true counting rate increases linearly with activity in the FOV, whereas the random rate increases as the square of activity in or near the FOV. More bed positions are needed because the scanner has maximum sensitivity in the center of the FOV with a rapid fall in sensitivity at the edges of the FOV. As a result, there needs to be a decrease in the axial FOV to maintain a uniform count profile and hence more bed positions to cover a given length of the patient. As a general rule, if there is sufficient activity and counts to perform a study in two-dimensional mode, that is the preferred image acquisition mode.

The emission data acquired by either two- or three-dimensional technique are converted to an image format by using filtered back projection or iterative reconstruction. Filtered back projection can be used with two-dimensional reconstruction and when the data are relatively noise free. The method is simple and fast. Because of the complexity of the data from three-dimensional acquisition, iterative algorithms are used. The iterative technique involves use of several analytic processes (iterations) to reach the desired result. Compared with filtered back projection, iterative reconstruc-

tion requires substantially more time and computer power. When appropriate, iterative algorithms can also be used to reconstruct two-dimensional acquisition data.

PET IMAGE QUANTITATION

In addition to obtaining cross sectional images, it is often helpful to quantify how much radioactivity is in a voxel or volume within the patient. When a PET camera is appropriately calibrated, it is able to assess the $\mu Ci/mL$ of tissue. Although there are a number of methods for quantifying uptake, the most common is the SUV (standardized uptake value), a semiquantitative index, defined by the following equation:

$$SUV = \frac{\text{Mean ROI activity (mCi/mL)}}{\text{Administered activity}}$$
$$\text{(mCi)/body weight (g)}$$
$$= \text{grams/mL}$$

When ^{18}F-FDG is used, SUV measurements may be used to characterize a lesion with respect to its glucose metabolism. SUVs must be obtained using the attenuation-corrected (data) images. The SUV is determined by using special software by placing a region of interest (ROI) over the portion of the lesion with the greatest ^{18}F-FDG uptake and thus containing the maximum value pixel. SUVs based on maximal pixel values are recommended rather than an average pixel value. An SUV would be 1.0 if the radionuclide was uniformly distributed throughout the body. The approximate normal SUVs for ^{18}F-FDG are 2.3 in blood, 2.5 in liver, 1.9 in spleen, 0.7 in lung, and 1.0 in bone marrow. SUV measurements are typically obtained at 1-hour after injection even though activity in some lesions, such as neoplasms, may be slightly higher at 2 hours.

There are a number of factors that affect SUV measurements. Body weight and composition are obvious factors, with obese patients having higher SUVs than do thin patients for both normal and malignant tissue. SUVs based on estimated lean body mass or body surface area are generally preferred. It should be noted that when performing serial scans on oncology patients, significant weight loss between studies may well affect SUVs, and increasing severity of illness may cause significant variation in serum glucose levels from earlier studies, even in diabetics.

Because high serum glucose levels reduce tumor FDG uptake and thus SUVs, correction for glucose levels is helpful, especially when SUVs from serial studies are to be compared. The size of the ROI over an FDG-avid lesion will affect the average SUV, with smaller regions of interest resulting in higher average SUVs. However, as long as the ROI contains the maximum activity pixel, then the size of the ROI is irrelevant for determining that maximum value. Recent physical activity can elevate SUV in muscle, and inflammation in any tissue usually elevates the SUV. Because of partial volume effects, SUVs of lesions that are smaller than is the spatial resolution of the scanner will be underestimated. In addition, minor changes in scan technique can result in a change of 25% to 30% in measured SUV. When doing serial SUV measurements, it is important to standardize the time after injection because FDG accumulation in tumors, and therefore SUVs, continues to increase with time (up to at least 2 hours). SUV also depends on knowing exactly how much activity was injected and how much may have remained in the syringe. Any extravasation during injection will also affect calculated lesion SUV values. As a result of these many variables, many institutions do not actually calculate SUVs in every day practice but rather visually characterize lesions as having no visible activity or mild, moderate, or intense uptake.

It should be noted that in practice visual interpretation of the PET images often suffices and obtaining SUVs is not necessary in every patient. When they are obtained to evaluate a lesion, caution is advised, because benign lesions may be very FDG avid, rendering high SUVs, whereas some malignant lesions may demonstrate little or no FDG activity, producing low uptake values. When monitoring tumor therapy, SUVs may be requested by treating physicians as an objective index to aid in the assessment of therapeutic effects.

PET/CT IMAGING

Interpretation of PET scans has often been hampered by difficulty in determining the anatomic location of an area of increased activity. The exact location of the activity can greatly affect whether it is considered abnormal, a normal variant, or simply physiologic. For example, increased activity in a ureter or the bowel is likely normal, whereas increased activity in a lymph node is more often abnormal. Accurate localization also gives a better indication of possible causes of abnormal activity. For example, the likely etiologies may be somewhat

different if the activity is in the skeleton rather than the adjacent soft tissue. Software efforts to fuse CT images with either SPECT or PET data obtained at substantially different times are often hampered by a number of problems, such as differences in patient positioning and internal changes in organ position due to variations in breathing patterns and physiology (especially in the abdomen) between examinations. Thus, a single instrument that can acquire both PET and CT data sequentially on the same table and at close to the same time is desirable.

The addition of contemporaneous CT imaging to PET instruments yields several distinct advantages, depending on the CT protocols used. These include more efficient and accurate attenuation correction, shorter imaging times, more precise anatomic localization of lesions, and acquisition of diagnostic CT and PET scans in one effort. Recent studies have shown that PET/CT scans produce more accurate results than does CT or PET alone or side-by-side visual correlation of PET and CT scans. The primary improvement is a reduction of equivocal interpretations. Given current trends, PET/CT is likely to become the preferred technique in most clinical settings to generate images that contain both anatomic and physiologic information.

Early PET/CT scanners were two separate machines operated by different sets of software at separate consoles. Such scanners used a CT device that obtained basic anatomic and attenuation data but without sufficient spatial resolution to provide diagnostic quality images. Current PET/CT scanners may appear to be a single machine, but most are simply a CT and PET scanner placed together within a single cover. The patient table traverses the bore of both machines (Fig. 13–14). These systems obtain diagnostic quality studies with four- to sixteen-slice CT devices. For most cases it is not necessary to use a multidetector 16-slice scanner, although these may be useful for dedicated cardiac studies.

Most of the current PET/CT scanners can produce good whole-body fused or coregistered PET/CT images in less than 30 minutes. When fusing the data, matching CT and PET images is possible to within a few millimeters. However, there may still be slight differences due to the limited spatial resolution of the PET scanner as well as patient movement and/or differences in positioning occurring between the CT scan and completion of the PET scan. Because PET images

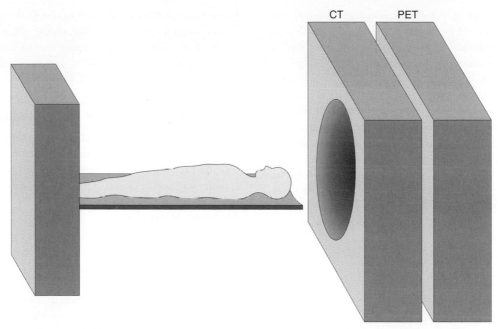

FIGURE 13–14. PET/CT scanner. The mechanical portions of these scanners are essentially separate, although they are under a single cover. They can share the same computer system, operating console, and work station.

are acquired over minutes and CT images are acquired over seconds, there are still some minor alignment problems related to the position of the diaphragm.

In addition to providing precise anatomic localization, the CT scan data are also used to perform PET attenuation correction, eliminating the need and additional time for transmission scans using ^{68}Ge or ^{137}Cs sources. The CT transmission images have less noise than do those from radionuclide sources, resulting in attenuation-corrected PET images with less noise. SUV values obtained on attenuation-corrected images using either CT or radioisotopic methods are generally comparable. However, the lower energy used in the CT scan allows more artifacts from high-density materials. Very high density (high Hounsfield units) contrast on the CT scan can cause overestimation of tissue ^{18}F-FDG concentrations, producing areas of apparent increased activity. A similar effect occurs if there are significant metallic objects (implants or dental work) in the patient.

A specific problem may occur when using bolus injection of intravenous contrast for a CT scan of the neck or chest. The attenuation-corrected images may show foci of artifactually increased ^{18}F-FDG activity in the region of venous structures first accepting the undiluted bolus. If coregistration is not perfect, this may be misinterpreted as abnormal activity in a lymph node or other structure. However, for practical purposes, most oral or intravenous contrast regimens do not cause significant artifacts, and because the high-density source of any artifacts can be recognized on the CT portion of the study, there is usually little problem in interpretation. Further, because these artifacts are the result of attenuation correction, their specious nature can be substantiated by their absence on review of the non–attenuation-corrected images. The artifacts from oral and intravenous contrast administration as well as those from metal implants have diminished as attenuation-correction algorithms have become more sophisticated and as more appropriately designed diagnostic CT protocols have become available. In addition, recent studies have shown no statistically or clinically significant spurious elevation of SUVs which may potentially interfere with the diagnostic value a PET/CT resulting from the use of intravenous iodinated contrast.

At most institutions, the CT scan is performed before the PET scan. A typical protocol with good results, uses 500 to 750 mL of oral contrast (1.3% to 2.1% barium sulfate, glucose free) 60 to 90 minutes before ^{18}F-FDG injection. High-density barium should be avoided. Another 100 to 200 mL of oral barium is given 30 minutes after the ^{18}F-FDG injection. The patient then rests quietly for an additional 30 minutes, and the CT scan is performed just before the PET scan. The CT scan uses 80 mL of intravenous contrast (300 mg I/mL) at 3 mL per second to achieve arterial contrast, followed by another 60 mL at 2 mL/second for venous and parenchymal enhancement.

Typical diagnostic CT parameters for normal weight adult patients are as follows: 80 mAs and 140 kVp, 512 × 512 matrix and a slice width of 5 mm, a pitch of 1.6 for diagnostic scans, and reconstruction increments of 2.5 mm. The mA can be reduced to 40 to 60 mA in smaller patients, and the mA can be increased to 120 to 160 for very large patients. If the CT scan is only being done for attenuation correction purposes, an mA of only 10 to 40 is necessary. The CT scan time is usually very short ($\approx$ 30 seconds) and the PET acquisition is much longer (20 to 30 minutes). For most purposes, the CT scan is usually performed from the meatus of the ear to the mid-thigh during shallow breathing. It is important to obtain the CT and PET images in the same manner, that is, with the arms up or down on both, and with shallow breathing or partial breath-hold, rather than obtaining the CT in maximum inspiration breath-hold mode. Even so, coregistration of small pulmonary, diaphragmatic, or superiorly located liver lesions, which may vary with even slight changes in position or respiration, may not be perfect.

Misregistration of CT and PET scan images by more than 1 cm can occur for peripheral or basal lung lesions or for lesions in the upper portion of the liver, if there is a difference in breathing during the two scans. If shallow breathing is used to obtain both CT and PET scans, lesions in the chest are usually registered within about 1 cm of each other, but near the diaphragm and within the superior portion of the liver, the lesions may be misregistered by up to 2 cm. In addition, if there is a liver lesion near the dome of the liver and the CT is performed with deeper inspiration than the PET scan, the lesion can erroneously appear to be in the lung base. Misregistration may be minimized by performing the CT scan during a breath-hold at normal tidal expiration and the PET scan during normal tidal breathing. A "cold" curvilinear artifact above the liver can be seen on PET scans due to respiratory motion and this particular artifact is unique to CT attenuation-corrected scans. Significant misregistration can also occur if the patient moves during the 20- to 30-minute PET scan. Many of the interpretative errors due to these and other artifacts can be avoided by examining the non–attenuation-corrected PET images.

PET SCANNER QUALITY ASSURANCE

There are a few specific quality assurance tests for dedicated PET systems. These procedures are intended to monitor system stability and maintain consistency and accuracy of performance.

Ambient Temperature

The scanning room temperature should be checked daily, because the sensitivity of the system changes with temperature. As the temperature rises, fewer visible photons are produced by the crystals. The pulse height analyzer spectrum in BGO crystals also changes with temperature, with the energy range varying inversely with room temperature (e.g., appearing lower as the temperature rises and vice versa).

Normalization Scan

Because a state-of-the-art PET camera may have thousands of crystal elements coupled to hundreds of PMTs, there are inevitable small variations in axial sensitivity among the detector units. To produce uniform images, these discrepancies must be corrected. A normalization scan is accomplished by scanning a uniform calibrated positron-emitting source placed in the FOV. This data set measures the response of each detector pair and is used to obtain a calibration factor to "normalize" the lines of response that pass through the source. These stored calibration factors can be applied to patient data sets to correct for differences in detector response so that accurate images of tracer distribution are produced. Normalization scans should be performed at least monthly, but they may be obtained weekly or more frequently as needed.

Blank Scan

This is accomplished by performing a scan by using the system transmission radiation sources with nothing in the FOV. This usually takes an hour or less. The data acquired are used with the patient transmission data to compute attenuation correction factors. Blank scans should be performed daily and, as such, are also an excellent method to monitor system stability, including significant discrepancies in individual detector sensitivities.

Some PET instruments will perform this function automatically at a specified time during the night and even compare the results to previous blank scans.

Image Plane Calibration

Calibration of each image plane by using a radioactive source is also required on multi-ring detectors. This can be done with a uniform cylinder filled with a positron-emitter and may be done weekly or monthly. This procedure is essential for the production of accurate whole-body scans.

PATIENT PREPARATION FOR ^{18}F-FDG IMAGING

The biodistribution of ^{18}F-FDG is affected by blood glucose levels. Although there can be competitive displacement of the ^{18}F-FDG by high levels of blood glucose, the primary adverse effect of elevated serum glucose is the resultant elevation of insulin levels. Patients should fast for 4 to 6 hours before a scan (preferably overnight) so that basal insulin levels will allow for optimal images. Elevated insulin levels degrade scans by increasing muscle uptake of FDG. In general, serum glucose levels should be below 150 mg/dL, but glucose levels up to 200 mg/dL are usually acceptable for satisfactory image quality. Imaging diabetic patients can be especially challenging. In type 1 diabetes, insulin is not recommended and imaging is usually performed in the morning after an overnight fast. In type 2 diabetes, short-acting insulin can be used, but this increases muscle uptake. If possible, regular insulin should not be used 2 to 4 hours before the examination. In fact, in general, the use of insulin is best avoided altogether.

Because there is significant excretion of ^{18}F-FDG via the kidneys (and ^{18}F-FDG is not reabsorbed as glucose is), good hydration is recommended. Accumulation in the bladder has prompted some to recommend catheterization of patients with suspected pelvic pathology, but in practice, this is usually unnecessary, especially if the patient has voided before beginning the scan, and if interpretation includes using a three-dimensional rotating maximum intensity projection (MIP) display. Diuretics may be helpful in some patients when clearing activity from the kidneys and ureters is crucial.

The typical administered activity for ^{18}F-FDG is in the range of 10 to 25 mCi (370–925 MBq) or about 0.14 mCi (5.5 MBq)/kg. Lower activities may be necessary on some PET scanners (such as those using NaI detectors), which cannot process the higher count rates. The injection is intravenous, and the line should be flushed with 20 to 30 mL of saline. Portacaths or indwelling catheters should not be used unless absolutely necessary, as retention in the reservoirs and catheter tips can cause errors in evaluation of the chest. If intravenous injection is not possible, ^{18}F-FDG can be administered orally. If axillary or supraclavicular lymph node involvement is a consideration (e.g., breast cancer or upper-extremity melanomas), injection should be made in the upper extremity on the opposite the side from the lesion. Imaging is typically performed 45 to 60 minutes after injection of ^{18}F-FDG. However, a longer waiting period up to 2 to 3 hours allows for better uptake in lesions, especially when imaging tumors known to have a lower avidity for FDG, including treated lesions. The patient should not talk or chew gum for 30 minutes after injection of the ^{18}F-FDG as this causes increased uptake in the muscles of the larynx and pharynx and the mastication musculature. For brain imaging the patient should be injected in a dimly lit, quiet room to avoid excess brain stimulation, which will alter FDG distribution.

The patient should wear a gown and pajama pants, and all metallic objects should be removed. With dedicated PET scanners, the patient should normally be positioned supine with the arms down and knees at rest. The scan is obtained during shallow breathing. With PET/CT scanners, the patient is usually positioned with the arms up except when the suspected pathology is in the head or neck. In this case the arms should be down. In some cases when pathology is suspected in both the neck and the chest, it may be necessary to perform scans with the arms in both positions to detect small lesions. In patients with neck muscle pain, muscle relaxants (valium, etc.) may be useful to decrease interfering activity in neck musculature.

NORMAL ^{18}F-FDG DISTRIBUTION AND VARIANTS
General

The percentage of ^{18}F-FDG distribution in the body is shown in Table 13–8 and the relative uptake in specific tissues is shown in Table 13–9. It is important to know the normal distribution and normal variants in ^{18}F-FDG accumulation so as to not confuse them with actual pathology (Fig. 13–15).

TABLE 13–8. Normal Biodistribution of ^{18}F-FDG Activity

ORGAN	% INJECTED DOSE	MEAN SUV	MEAN SUV (LEAN BODY MASS)
Blood		2.3	1.7
Brain	6.9		
Liver	4.4	2.5	1.9
Heart	3.3		
Kidneys	1.3		
Red marrow	1.7	1.0	0.8
Lungs	0.9	0.7	0.5
Spleen		1.9	1.7
Breast		0.5	0.4
Urine (second hour)	20–40		

^{18}F-FDG, fluorine-18 fluorodeoxyglucose; SUV, standardized uptake value.

TABLE 13–9. Relative ^{18}F-FDG Levels in Various Normal Tissues

HIGH TISSUE LEVEL	COMMENT
Brain	High in gray matter, low in white matter
Kidneys, ureters, bladder	Due to excretion
Ascending colon	Usually tubular in distribution
Heart	If not fasting
Skeletal muscle	If active or tense
Brown or USA fat	Frequently females and in cold environment
Uterus	During menses

MODERATE TISSUE LEVEL

Tonsils, submandibular glands	Decreases with age
Liver	
Bone marrow	Can be high after stimulating agents
Thyroid	Can be high with Graves' disease or thyroiditis

MILD TISSUE LEVEL

Heart	If fasting
Aorta	Usually band-like in thoracic aorta
Spleen	

LOW TISSUE LEVEL

Lung	
Breast	More in young women and with lactation
Esophagus	Usually diffuse distribution
Stomach	Can be focally intense
Testes and penis	

NO ACTIVITY USUALLY SEEN

Pancreas
Prostate
Lymph nodes

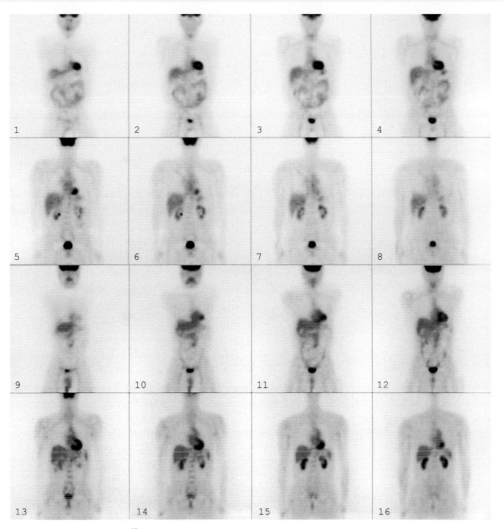

FIGURE 13–15. Normal ^{18}F-FDG PET scan. On these coronal whole-body images, normal physiologic activity is seen in the brain, heart, liver, bowel, urinary system, and to a lesser extent the marrow.

Brain

The gray matter of the brain (cortex, basal ganglia, and thalami) is always high in ^{18}F-FDG uptake, because the cells of gray matter have a high metabolic rate and use glucose as their primary substrate. When acquiring scans of the face and neck, it is important to exclude the brain from the acquisition, to be able to see abnormalities that do not have as much activity as gray matter.

Tonsils, Salivary Glands, and Thyroid

The tonsils (especially the palatine tonsils), lymphoid tissue at Waldeyer's ring, and the parotid and submandibular glands can normally accumu-
late ^{18}F-FDG. This activity usually decreases with patient age and should be symmetric. Activity also can be seen in the soft palate, vocal cords, and vocal cord muscles. The latter activity can be minimized by having the patient remain silent during injection and during the early uptake of ^{18}F-FDG. Thyroid activity is normally not seen. However, mild diffuse activity can occasionally be seen in normal glands. Significantly increased activity can occur with thyroiditis or Grave's disease (Fig. 13–16). An enlarged inhomogeneous gland should raise the possibility of a nodular goiter. An unexpected intense focal area raises the possibility of malignancy (20% to 30%), and further evaluation should be performed.

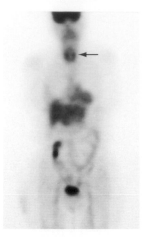

FIGURE 13–16. Thyroid activity. Coronal whole-body ^{18}F-FDG PET image shows activity in the thyroid. This can occasionally be seen in normal glands, but significantly increased activity may occur in thyroiditis or Grave's disease.

Thymus

Thymic activity can be seen normally in children but also occasionally in young adults up to the age of about 30 years. It is very uncommon in adults older than 30 years. Increased activity also can be seen as a result of thymic rebound after chemother-

apy in children and young adults, but also occasionally in older adults.

Muscle and Brown Fat

In resting skeletal muscle, ^{18}F-FDG uptake is usually low. Increased activity is often seen in the shoulder girdle (especially teres minor) and upper back if the patient was tense at the time of injection or within 30 minutes after injection. Muscle relaxants or anxiolytics may be helpful in some patients, especially when imaging the neck, where the strap muscles often demonstrate increased activity. Heavy exercise within the 24 hours before the examination can increase muscle uptake as may elevated insulin levels (Fig. 13–17).

In the neck, activity near the vocal cords is seen if the patient was talking at the time of injection (Fig. 13–18). Speaking during the uptake period may also increase ^{18}F-FDG activity in the tongue. After lingual or laryngeal surgery, asymmetric activity can often be seen in the residual intact musculature and be difficult to differentiate from residual or recurrent tumor. An intense ^{18}F-FDG focus in the lower neck just lateral to the midline may be caused by compensatory activation of an intact laryngeal muscle when the contralateral vocal cord is paralyzed due to any cause, but frequently by mediastinal tumor involvement of the recurrent

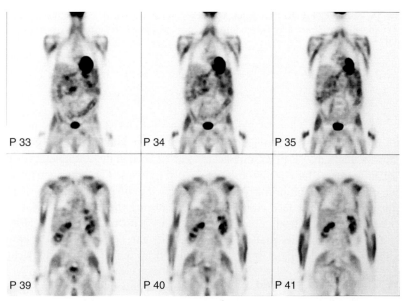

FIGURE 13–17. Muscle activity. Coronal whole-body ^{18}F-FDG PET images show abnormally increased activity in muscles of the arms and thighs due to increased insulin levels. This also can occur as a result of heavy exercise 24 hours before the examination.

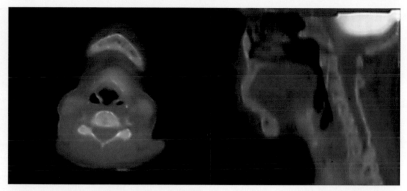

FIGURE 13–18. Larynx activity. ¹⁸F-FDG PET/CT axial and sagittal fusion images show increased activity in the larynx due to talking during or shortly after the injection.

laryngeal nerve. Activity can also be seen normally in the diaphragmatic crura, intercostal muscles, psoas muscles, thoracic paravertebral muscles, forearms, and muscles of mastication. In patients with severe dyspnea, there is often increased activity in intercostal muscles due to the increased work of breathing. At any location, symmetry and a diffuse or typical linear configuration are often helpful to distinguish normal muscle activity from pathology.

Activity in the supraclavicular region is typically due to one of three causes: muscle activity, activity in lymph nodes due to pathology, or accumulation in fat. Muscle activity is seen in about 5% of patients and is usually linear and bilateral. Activity in fat occurs in about 2% to 5% of patients (mostly female) and in about 15% of children. The reason for uptake in fat in this location is unknown but FDG is thought to accumulate in foci of brown fat (also called USA-fat; USA stands for *u*ptake in the *s*upraclavicular *a*rea). Uptake in this fat is typically symmetrical, more often multifocal than linear, and located in low Hounsfield unit areas typical of fat on PET/CT images (Fig. 13–19). SUV values can range from 2 to 20, with the mean often about 7 or more (well above the threshold value worrisome for malignancy). Uptake appears to be related to adrenergic stimulation of muscles such as during periods of anxiety or shivering in response to ambient temperature and is seen more often in the winter months or even in a cold air-conditioned room. In patients with activity in neck fat, about one third will also show focal activity in perinephric fat, in mediastinal fat, and in paravertebral and posterior intercostal patterns (Fig. 13–20).

Heart

Left ventricular ¹⁸F-FDG activity can be intense or faint (Fig. 13–21). Although the myocardium uses fatty acids as its primary substrate, it will switch to glucose if high levels are available or if the patient has been exercising. A large amount of cardiac activity often means that the patient did not fast in preparation for the examination and the heart is actively utilizing glucose. Intense cardiac activity is usually not a problem but can interfere with diagnosis of pathology located adjacent to the heart.

After 12 hours of fasting, the heart switches from glucose to fatty acid metabolism, and the activity becomes the same as the background blood pool. The switch from intense activity to faint activity is often not uniform, and the base of the heart tends to be the last section to lose glucose metabolism. It is important not to interpret lack of activity near the left ventricular apex as an infarct without additional information. It is also important not to mistake isolated activity at the base of the heart for pathology such as abnormal mediastinal lymph nodes. The right ventricle usually has faint activity when compared with that of the left ventricle, unless there is right ventricular hypertrophy. Atrial activity is not infrequently noted, especially in the right atrium. This can be spotty, and again, should not be mistaken for abnormal lymph nodes.

Aorta

¹⁸F-FDG activity is seen in the aortic wall of about 60% to 70% of older adults. The uptake can be focal or band-like and is usually more intense in the

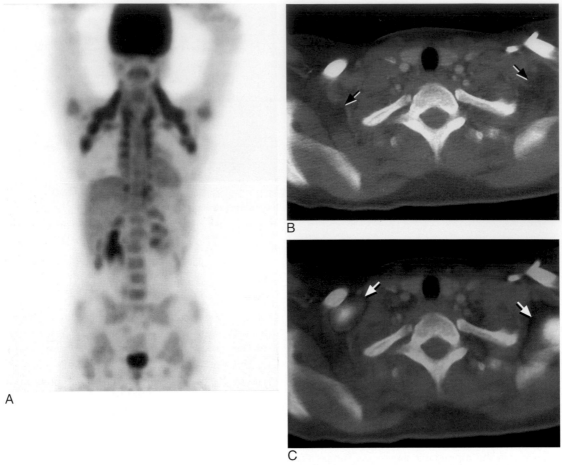

FIGURE 13–19. Brown or "USA" (uptake in the supraclavicular area) fat. *A,* Coronal whole-body ^{18}F-FDG PET image in a young female shows intense (but normal) symmetrical activity in the neck and axilla. This can be mistakenly diagnosed as lymphoma. *B,* Transaxial CT and *C,* ^{18}F-FDG PET/CT fusion images show that the increased metabolic activity is in an area that is clearly fat density.

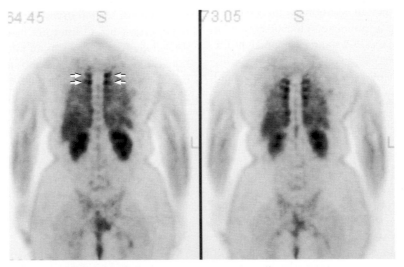

FIGURE 13–20. Paraspinous fat. Coronal whole-body ^{18}F-FDG PET images show intense (but normal) activity in paraspinous fat (*arrows*).

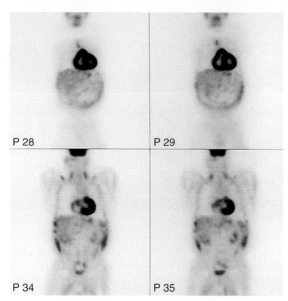

FIGURE 13–21. Cardiac activity. Coronal whole-body ^{18}F-FDG PET images show intense activity in both the left and right ventricle. Cardiac activity increases with recent glucose or caffeine ingestion. Activity is also seen in neck muscles due to tension at the time of injection.

lower descending thoracic aorta than in the ascending portion or arch. Thoracic aortic uptake appears to be more common in women and patients with hyperlipidemia. The degree of activity appears to be unrelated to calcium deposition but has been shown to correlate with macrophage content in the atherosclerotic plaques. It is possible that the uptake is depicting the metabolic activity of atherosclerotic change. Infected vascular grafts often demonstrate increased activity, conforming to the shape of the grafts. However, aortofemoral bypass grafts routinely have some mild diffuse increased activity for years even if not infected.

Lungs

The lungs have relatively low uptake, appearing photopenic on attenuation-corrected images. However, on images that are not attenuation corrected, they will appear to have increased activity. Pleural effusions from congestive failure will not accumulate activity, but empyemas and malignant effusions often do.

Breast

Breast activity slightly above that in the blood pool is normal and is more common in young women and in postmenopausal women on hormone replacement therapy. It will be greater in lactating females, but the activity is in the breast tissue and not in the milk. It is not necessary to discontinue breast feeding in these patients. However, there may be significant dose concerns to the baby from direct gamma emission from the mother, and as a result, some authors recommend that breast feeding be suspended for 8 hours after the injection. The ^{18}F-FDG activity in breast is related to the glandular volume and density. As expected, fatty breasts have less activity than do dense breasts. However, even in dense breasts the SUV is almost always less than 1.5 (much below the 2.5 value that may suggest malignant tissue).

Gastrointestinal Tract

Activity in the bowel is exceedingly variable in terms of both intensity and location. The ^{18}F-FDG activity in the bowel is located in the mucosa and not in the luminal contents. The FDG is not excreted by the liver and biliary system into the bowel. Low-level activity is sometimes seen in the normal esophagus and should be uniform throughout its length. Fusiform or focal esophageal activity should raise the possibility of pathology, including neoplasm, although esophagitis can produce a similar appearance.

Activity in the stomach is often greater than that in the liver, and a contracted normal stomach or hiatal hernia can appear very intense, causing difficulties in evaluation of gastric neoplasms or the esophagogastric junction (Fig. 13–22). Activity in the small bowel tends to be faint, but activity in the colon can normally be quite intense (Fig. 13–23). It is often essential to view the rotating three-dimensional display (MIP image) to be able to distinguish normal colonic activity from pathology. The pattern of uptake in the colon may be diffuse, segmental, or nodular. Diffuse activity is most often nonpathologic, whereas segmental uptake may imply inflammation; nodular focal uptake can occur with lesions such as polyps, villous adenomas, and carcinoma. Small-bowel activity is usually less than that seen in the colon and is commonly located in the lower abdomen or pelvis.

The liver typically has more activity than the background blood pool. The gallbladder is not usually seen, and if there is activity in this area, it should not be assumed to be normal or a normal variant. The pancreas is not normally seen.

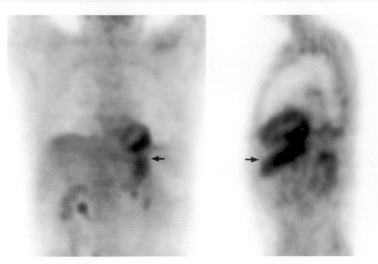

FIGURE 13–22. Normal stomach activity. Anterior (*left*) and lateral (*right*) whole-body images show diffuse normal ^{18}F-FDG activity in the stomach (*arrows*).

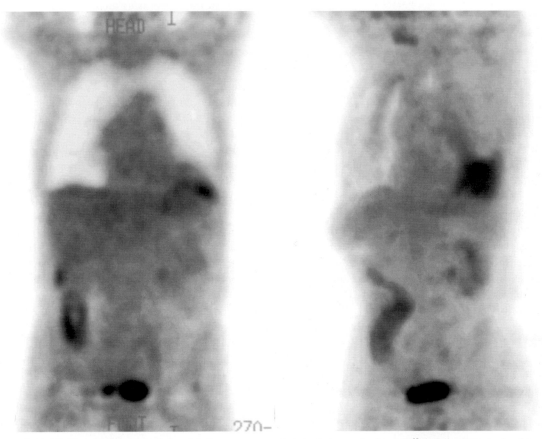

FIGURE 13–23. Normal bowel activity. *Left*, On an anterior whole-body image the focus of ^{18}F-FDG activity in the right lower quadrant may be mistaken for pathology. *Right*, An oblique view taken from the rotating whole-body image shows the area of activity to be tubular in shape.

Genitourinary Tract

Activity is almost always seen in the urinary tract because over 40% of the administered activity is excreted via the kidneys in the first 2 hours. The upper pole calyces, renal pelvis, and ureters are easily visualized on ^{18}F-FDG PET scans. Ureteral activity can be discontinuous due to peristalsis and can mimic pathologic foci. Bladder activity is intense (Fig. 13–24). In patients with suspected pelvic pathology, catheterization may be warranted to minimize or eliminate interfering bladder activity, but in practice this is usually not necessary. Activity can be present in the normal uterus (especially early in menstruation). Activity is also usually seen in the testes and to a lesser extent in the penis.

Bone Marrow, Lymph Nodes, and Spleen

Bone marrow activity is usually seen at levels that are slightly higher than the blood pool and about the same as the liver. Bone marrow activity can be increased in anemic patients or those who have had stimulatory therapy (e.g., granulocyte colony stimulation factor [G-CSF]). Increased activity will last up to a month after G-CSF therapy and may obscure marrow metastases in some cases. Marrow activity will be decreased regionally in the treated area after radiation therapy.

Normal lymph nodes have very little activity. However, if an injection of the radiopharmaceutical into an arm vein was infiltrated, there may be activity in the axillary or supraclavicular nodes on the side of injection. Splenic activity is usually low but can be increased in anemic patients or those treated with G-CSF.

IMAGE INTERPRETATION

Commonly, the attenuation-corrected PET images are displayed simultaneously in three orthogonal planes: axial, coronal, and sagittal. A three-dimensional (MIP) rotating display is also provided. Visual interpretation entails review of these images to locate areas of suspected pathology. The MIP images can be especially helpful for an overview of radiopharmaceutical distribution and for differentiating pathologic from physiologic foci.

Semiquantitative methods can also be used to aid interpretation. Suspicious or equivocal areas showing low or moderate activity can be further evaluated as needed using SUVs. A value above 2.5 should raise the possibility of malignancy. One should remember that if a lesion is small, the average measured SUV may be falsely low due to partial volume averaging. In this instance, the use

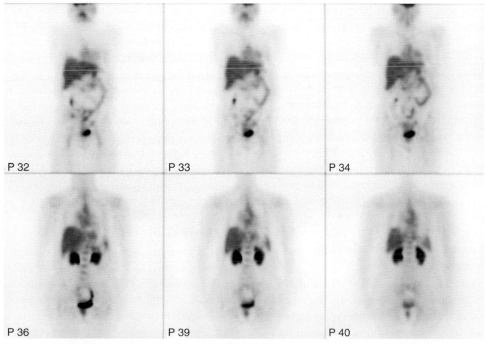

FIGURE 13–24. Normal liver, bowel, and prominent but normal kidney and bladder ^{18}F-FDG activity.

of maximum pixel value may often be more reliable and reproducible. SUVs of obviously intense lesions may also be documented for future comparison with post-treatment follow-up scans.

Finally, comparison with recent anatomical imaging, especially CT and/or MRI, should be performed. Although most lesions will be seen on the attenuation-corrected images, if a lesion is known to be present or suspected on a CT scan and is not seen on the attenuation-corrected images, review of the non–attenuation-corrected images may be helpful. This is especially true if there are artifacts due to patient motion between the time of the transmission scan and the PET scan. However, it should be noted that lesions deep within the body are often less conspicuous on uncorrected images.

A thorough knowledge of physiologic distribution, normal variants, common causes of benign radiopharmaceutical uptake, and technical artifacts is essential for accurate visual interpretation. The broad categories of benign conditions or lesions that can be associated with ^{18}F-FDG accumulation include hyperplasia, ischemia, benign tumors, and any inflammation or infection producing focal infiltration of metabolically active host cells, including granulomatous diseases and fungal infections (Table 13–10). In addition, a tailored, but rigorous clinical history is needed, including suspected or known lesion sites, tumor histology, type and timing of any treatment, as well as potentially interfering medications.

PET BRAIN IMAGING

PET with ^{18}F-FDG permits the noninvasive in vivo quantification of local cerebral metabolism and, unlike CT or MRI, provides a physiologic test that may illustrate pathologic conditions *before* morphologic manifestations are discernible. PET metabolic imaging has significant usefulness in certain discrete clinical settings and has been used to evaluate refractory seizure disorders, dementia and recurrent brain tumors.

Normal and Induced Variations in FDG Distribution

The normal distribution of ^{18}F-FDG in the brain is highest in the gray matter of the cortex, basal ganglia, and thalami. This pattern changes with aging, and significant variations in cortical uptake have been noted. Relatively decreased frontal lobe metabolism with normal aging is not uncommon.

Metabolism in the thalami, basal ganglia, cerebellum, and visual cortex is generally unchanged with normal aging.

Certain areas of the cerebral cortex can normally be focally hypermetabolic compared with the remainder of the cortex. These include the posterior cingulate cortex (anterior and superior to the occipital cortex), a focus in the posterior superior temporal lobe (Wernicke region), the frontal eye fields (anterior to the primary motor cortex and may be asymmetric), and a symmetric area of increased activity in the posterior parietal lobes. The degree of uptake in the cerebellar gray matter is significantly less on an FDG PET study than on a SPECT perfusion scan.

Areas of the brain stimulated by activity during ^{18}F-FDG injection and uptake show relatively increased metabolism. These include the visual (occipital) or auditory cortical areas in visually (eyes open) or auditorally (sound) stimulated patients, language centers in talking patients, and the motor cortex in moving patients. Thus, injection and uptake of ^{18}F-FDG are best accomplished in silent, motionless patients in a quiet, darkened room. Certain drugs may alter global and/or relative regional brain metabolism, including sedatives, antiepileptic and neuroleptic drugs, and barbiturates.

A phenomenon known as *diaschisis* may cause focal areas of hypoperfusion and hypometabolism in areas of the brain remote, but connected by neural pathways, from the location of a lesion, including neoplasm, stroke, and trauma. This reduced metabolism is often seen in the cerebellar hemisphere contralateral to a supratentorial lesion (*crossed cerebellar diaschisis*). The cerebellar metabolic depression is typically asymptomatic, and the effect frequently resolves when occurring with stroke but may persist when associated with brain tumors. Subcortical-cortical cerebral diaschisis also occurs, such as when small thalamic strokes are associated with ipsilateral depression of cortical metabolism.

Epilepsy (Seizures)

PET scanning is helpful in patients with complex partial seizures. Mesial temporal lobe epilepsy is the most common form. There is often an area of unilateral interictal temporal lobe hypometabolism in the seizure focus (Fig. 13–25), similar to the hypoperfusion seen with SPECT brain perfusion agents. Ictal studies with PET are usually not technically feasible. It is very rare to obtain scans during the

TABLE 13–10. Accumulation of ^{18}F FDG in Abnormal Conditions

TISSUE/ORGAN	ACTIVITY LEVEL	COMMENTS
BRAIN		
Ictal seizure focus	High	Very rarely done due to need to remain still and poor temporal resolution of PET
Interictal seizure focus	Low	Review temporal lobes
Radiation necrosis	Low	
Recurrent tumor	Variable	If increased activity suspect recurrence
Dementia—Alzheimer's	Low posterior temporoparietal cortical activity	Often identical pattern to Parkinson's dementia
Dementia—Pick's	Low frontal lobes	
Dementia—Multi-infarct	Scattered small areas of decreased activity	
Cerebellar diaschisis ("crossed")	Low area in one hemisphere	Low activity in cerebellum contralateral to supratentorial stroke, tumor, trauma, etc.
Huntington's disease	Low activity in caudate nucleus and putamen	
HEART		
Infarct	Low	
Hibernating	Normal or increased	
Stunned	Normal or increased	
NEOPLASM		
Head and neck	Variable: with cell type	
Brain metastases	Low	Poor sensitivity against normal high activity of gray matter
Thyroid	Moderate	Especially helpful in poorly differentiated lesions with low or absent iodine-131 uptake
Lung	Moderate	Low in bronchoalveolar cell cancer, carcinoid, well-differentiated cancer, and mucinous metastases
Breast	Moderate	
Hepatoma	Variable: often low	
Esophagus	High	Usually focal, not linear or diffuse
Stomach	Variable	Interfering normal activity
Colorectal	High	Usually focal, not tubular
Melanoma	High	
Lymphoma	Variable	Higher in aggressive forms
Renal and bladder	Variable: often low	Interfering normal activity
Skeletal metastases	Variable	
Uterine	Variable	
Cervical	Variable	
Testicular	Variable	
Prostate	Low or absent	
INFECTION		
Pneumonia	Moderate to high	
Cellulitis	Moderate	
Osteomyelitis	High	
GRANULOMAS		
Sarcoidosis	High	If active disease
Tuberculosis	High	If active disease
TRAUMA		
Recent surgery	Variable	
Fracture	Variable with age of onset	
Aortic graft	Moderate	
Radiation therapy	Moderate	May be increased for up to several months

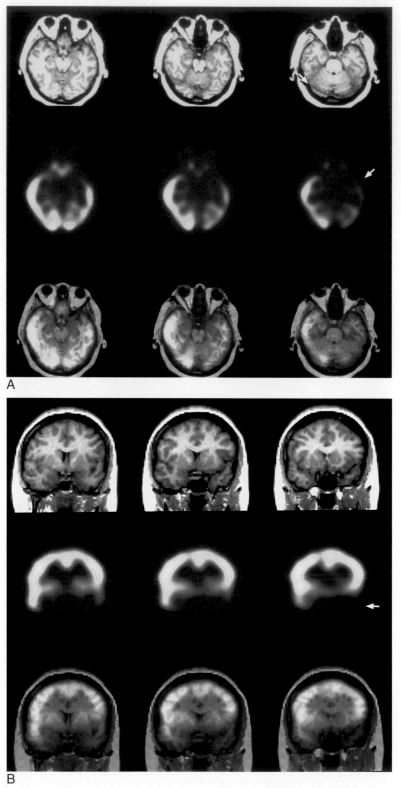

FIGURE 13–25. Epilepsy interictal study. Transaxial (*A*) and coronal (*B*) magnetic resonance imaging (MRI) (*upper row*), ¹⁸F-FDG PET images (*middle row*), and PET/MRI fusion images (*lower row*) show an area of decreased metabolism in the left temporal lobe (*arrows*).

ictal phase, and this usually occurs if a patient has an unexpected seizure during an intended interictal study. During and shortly after a seizure, a focus of increased activity should be demonstrated (Fig. 13–26). Because uptake of FDG occurs over many minutes, the area of increased activity is often diffuse and is not very reliable in precisely localizing the seizure focus. Further, unrecognized seizure activity during the FDG-uptake period may produce a relative increase on the side of the lesion, making the contralateral normal temporal lobe appear spuriously hypometabolic. Thus, EEG during administration and uptake of FDG to detect subclinical seizures may aid in preventing false localization of a presumed interictal focus in this setting. PET imaging has not proved as accurate or helpful in the localization of extratemporal seizure foci.

Dementia

In dementia, metabolic distribution patterns demonstrated on ^{18}F-FDG PET scans are broadly comparable to those seen by using SPECT brain perfusion agents, generally with greater sensitivity and overall accuracy. In Alzheimer's dementia, there is development of intracerebral senile plaques and neurofibrillary tangles with related abnormal deposition of proteins (amyloid and tau). The plaques destroy neurons by lysis of cell membranes, and the tangles fill the cytoplasm of axons and dendrites, preventing glucose transport. Thus, ^{18}F-FDG scans in patients with Alzheimer's dementia may reveal regionally decreased glucose metabolism as a result of both decreased glucose transport and neuronal loss.

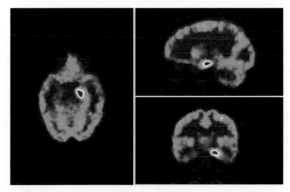

FIGURE 13–26. Epilepsy ictal study. An intense focus of metabolic activity is seen in the left temporal lobe on this ^{18}F-FDG PET scan. (Case courtesy of William Spies, M.D.)

With Alzheimer's dementia, decreased glucose metabolism is most commonly seen in the posterior temporal and parietal association cortices bilaterally with sparing of the primary sensorimotor and visual cortex, the basal ganglia, thalamus, brainstem, and cerebellum (Fig. 13–27). However, in early stages it can be significantly asymmetrical or even unilateral. One of the earliest findings is focal metabolic decrease in the posterior cingulate cortex, and frontal cortical involvement may become prominent with advanced disease. Similar findings of parietotemporal hypometabolism can be seen in dementia due to Parkinson's disease, but often with some metabolic reduction in the occipital (visual) cortex. However, ^{18}F-FDG scans cannot be used to differentiate these entities with certainty. If Parkinson dementia patients are excluded, the sensitivity and specificity for ^{18}F-FDG imaging in Alzheimer's dementia are about 90% and 70%, respectively. At present, PET scanning for Alzheimer's dementia is being used in conjunction with MR hemodynamic imaging, MR spectroscopy, and sensitive volumetric techniques.

A new investigational PET tracer, fluoro-ethyl, methyl amino-2 napthyl ethylidene malononitrile (^{18}F-FDDNP) crosses the blood brain barrier and binds to senile plaques and neurofibrillary tangles. Another approach has been development of ^{11}C-nicotine to show nicotinic (cholinergic) receptor loss in Alzheimer's disease. PET scans done by using $H_2^{15}O$ can also show reduced blood flow in areas of hypometabolism

Pick's disease is classically characterized by hypometabolism in the frontal and frontotemporal regions. Dementia with Lewy body disease demonstrates patterns similar to Alzheimer's, but with less sparing of the occipital (visual) cortex. In patients with Huntington's disease, there can be loss of ^{18}F-FDG activity in the basal ganglia, particularly the caudate and putamen nuclei.

Multi-infarct dementia can often be differentiated by its classic appearance of multiple areas of hypoperfusion scattered in cortical, subcortical, and cerebellar regions. Despite the patterns mentioned above, there remains considerable overlap in the patterns seen in various dementias (Table 13–11).

Primary Tumors and Metastases

The degree of ^{18}F-FDG uptake in primary brain tumors frequently correlates inversely with patient survival. Tumors with high FDG uptake are likely to be high-grade aggressive lesions with poor patient survival, whereas relatively hypometabolic

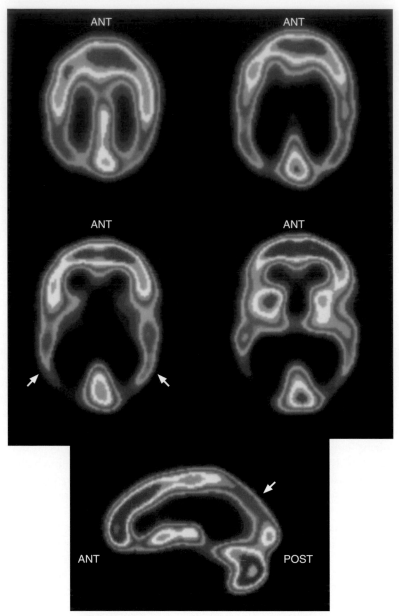

FIGURE 13–27. Alzheimer's dementia. Multiple transaxial and one sagittal image
from a ^{18}F-FDG PET scan show symmetrically decreased metabolic activity in the
posterior temporoparietal regions (*arrows*).

neoplasms generally represent lower-grade tumors.
PET can detect malignant degeneration in presumed or proven low-grade gliomas and can
increase the accuracy of stereotactic biopsy of lesions by targeting areas of focal hypermetabolism.
After therapy, PET scanning can help differentiate
recurrent tumor (increased activity) (Fig. 13–28)
from radiation necrosis (decreased activity) (Fig.
13–29). A flare response after chemotherapy of

brain neoplasms has been described, occurring a
few days after treatment. This FDG increased
activity may be related to an influx of inflammatory cells in response to tumor cell death. Detection
of brain metastases is usually poor due to the
high background activity normally present in gray
matter and the limited spatial resolution of PET
instruments. Contrast-enhanced MRI remains the
preferred imaging technique in this setting.

TABLE 13-11.   ¹⁸F-FDG PET Imaging in Dementia

DIAGNOSIS	EARLY METABOLIC DEFICITS	LATE METABOLIC DEFICITS	RELATIVE SPARING
Alzheimer's disease	Often asymmetric parietal, temporal, posterior cingulate, cortical deficits	Bilateral involvement common	Primary sensorimotor and visual cortices typical Thalamus, basal ganglia, and cerebellum sparing
Multi-infarct dementia	Scattered cerebral, cortical, subcortical, cerebellar defects		
Pick's disease (frontotemporal dementia)	Frontal, anterior, temporal, and mesiotemporal cortices	Parietal and lateral temporal cortices	Primary sensorimotor and visual cortices
Parkinson's disease	Similar to Alzheimer's disease	Similar to Alzheimer's disease	More mesiotemporal and less visual cortical sparing than in Alzheimer's disease
Huntington's disease	Caudate and lentiform nuclei	Diffuse cortical lesions	
Dementia with Lewy bodies	Similar to Alzheimer's disease	Similar to Alzheimer's disease	Less sparing of occipital cortex than in Alzheimer's disease

Adapted from Silverman DHS: Brain F-18-FDG PET in the diagnosis of neurodegenerative dementias: comparison with perfusion SPECT and with clinical evaluations lacking nuclear imaging. J Nucl Med 45:594–607, 2004.

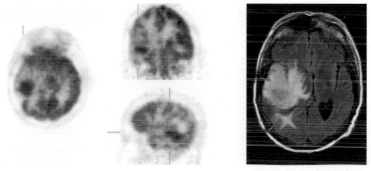

FIGURE 13–28. Recurrent glioma. *Right,* A post-treatment magnetic resonance imaging scan shows a large right hemisphere lesion. *Left,* ¹⁸F-FDG PET images show a focus of intense metabolic activity due to recurrent tumor. (Case courtesy of William Spies, M.D.)

Neuroreceptor Imaging

Imaging of neuroreceptor distribution in the brain is possible by using a number of receptor-specific radiopharmaceuticals designed to map receptors such as muscarinic cholinergic receptors, dopamine D_2 receptors, and the benzodiazepine and serotonin-2 receptors. These agents, including the dopamine receptor–seeking radiopharmaceutical, ¹¹C-N-methylpiperone, permit the mapping of neuromediator distribution in normal and pathologic states and have provided interesting informa-

tion in a number of clinical settings. However, the assessment of neurotransmitter function is complex, and the technique plays a limited role in clinical practice.

CARDIAC PET IMAGING

PET has inherent advantages that make it attractive for myocardial imaging. These include (1) better spatial resolution compared with that of SPECT; (2) higher myocardial count rates,

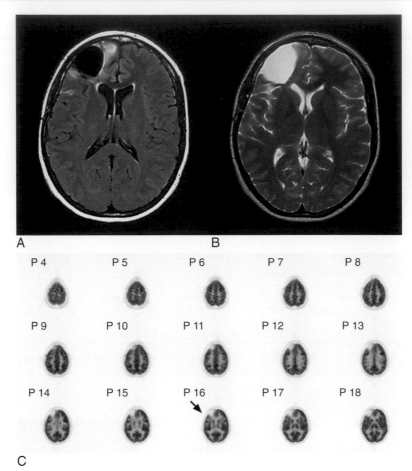

FIGURE 13–29. Radiation necrosis. A post-treatment T1-weighed (*A*) and T2-weighted (*B*) magnetic resonance imaging scans show a large right frontal lobe lesion. *C,* Axial ^{18}F-FDG PET images do not show any evidence of increased metabolic activity. (Case courtesy of William Spies, M.D.)

allowing better quality images; (3) superior quantitative capabilities; and (4) attenuation correction, which considerably reduces the false-positive studies caused by attenuation artifacts. In general, PET imaging provides assessment of myocardial perfusion or metabolism, depending on the radiopharmaceutical used.

Myocardial Perfusion

Several radiopharmaceuticals are available for PET imaging of myocardial perfusion either at rest or during pharmacologic stress. These include ^{13}N-ammonia (^{13}NH$_3$) ^{15}O-water (H$_2$^{15}O), and rubidium-82 (^{82}Rb). The first two require an on-site cyclotron, and ^{82}Rb is obtained from a generator that requires a relatively high volume of patients,

as it is very expensive. In clinical practice, these agents are not in widespread use.

^{13}NH$_3$ passively diffuses across the myocardial cell membrane with an extraction fraction approaching 100%, although some diffuses back through the cell membrane into the blood. Approximately 80% is retained in the cell through incorporation of ^{13}N into the amino acid, ^{13}N glutamine. A typical scanning dose of 15 to 30 mCi (555–1110 MBq) is used. Although the physical half-life of 11 minutes permits exercise stress to be used, pharmacological stress is preferred and is more practical.

Rubidium-82 is a potassium analog and behaves in vivo much as thallium-201 (^{201}Tl) does. Its myocardial extraction fraction is about 60% at rest and 30% at peak stress. Its short half-life of 76 seconds allows intravenous injections of doses in the range of 40 to 60 mCi (1.5–2.2 GBq).

$H_2^{15}O$ is not used for routine clinical studies but is the gold standard for visual and quanitative assessment of myocardial perfusion. It diffuses passively into and out of myocardial cells with high blood pool background, which requires correction to produce diagnostic images of the myocardium.

The physiologic principles and rationale involved in using these agents in the setting of coronary artery disease are essentially the same as in SPECT imaging with ^{99m}Tc-labeled radiopharmaceuticals. Stress-induced reversible perfusion defects represent myocardial ischemia and fixed defects are consistent with areas of scarring or hibernating myocardium. Also, ^{18}F-FDG can add specificity to these examinations by demonstrating increased FDG uptake in ischemic areas or by differentiating hibernating, viable myocardium from scar.

Comparisons of SPECT with PET stress–rest myocardial perfusion imaging have generally shown a greater sensitivity (95% versus 85%), specificity (80% versus 65%), and diagnostic accuracy (90% versus 80%) with PET for the diagnosis of coronary artery disease.

Myocardial Viability

Cardiac PET imaging with ^{18}F-FDG is considered by many to be the gold standard for assessment of myocardial viability. It is superior to delayed, reinjection, or rest thallium SPECT imaging strategies that may underestimate the amount of viable tissue. A fixed defect on SPECT myocardial perfusion studies may represent an area of prior infarction (scar), or hibernating myocardium. Hibernating myocardium presents as wall motion dysfunction in a chronically ischemic but viable segment of myocardium. Hibernating myocardium presents as a fixed perfusion defect on perfusion imaging and thus cannot effectively utilize oxidative metabolism of the preferred myocardial substrate (fatty acids) due to lack of oxygen. Consequently, a hibernating segment of myocardium switches to anaerobic metabolism of glucose and thus can be detected as metabolically viable by uptake of ^{18}F-FDG. This differentiates it from a fixed, metabolically inactive, perfusion defect caused by a postinfarction scar.

Typically, myocardial viability assessment entails combined resting perfusion and FDG imaging protocols. The resting perfusion images using PET or SPECT define the perfusion deficit in the area of suspected hibernating myocardium, whereas the ^{18}F-FDG images determine the presence of any viable myocardium (Fig. 13–30). Oral glucose loading of patients 1 to 2 hours before ^{18}F-FDG administration is commonly used. Elevated glucose levels increase insulin output, encouraging glucose uptake and metabolism by the myocardium. This optimizes FDG uptake in viable myocardium. The classic pattern of hibernating myocardium is a perfusion-metabolism mismatch with a perfusion defect in an area that exhibits preserved or increased FDG uptake. This pattern correlates with improvement in myocardial perfusion and function (regional wall motion) after revascularization and restoration of perfusion to the area. Nonviable, unsalvageable myocardium related to myocardial scarring shows no evidence of perfusion or FDG uptake.

Stunned myocardium may occur transiently after an acute episode of ischemia or after acute myocardial infarction with reperfusion therapy. It is characterized by preserved basal perfusion in a dysfunctional segment of myocardium. Stunning may also occur in patients with severe chronic coronary artery disease who experience repeated episodes of regional myocardial ischemia. Repetitive stunning may induce a more persistent wall motion abnormality. PET imaging in these patients often demonstrates an area of normal perfusion at rest and normal metabolism, indicating viable myocardium, which is expected to improve functionally after revascularization. It is important to remember that a study demonstrating normal perfusion and metabolism at rest does not exclude the presence of coronary artery disease, and a stress–rest perfusion imaging is necessary to do so.

Chronic myocardial ischemia may also be imaged on PET as diminished uptake of labeled fatty acids, the primary metabolic substrate under normal aerobic conditions. A focal myocardial defect using ^{11}C palmitate or other fatty acids, combined with increased ^{18}F FDG uptake in the same area, substantiates the shift of metabolism from fatty acids to glucose indicative of ischemic but viable myocardium.

WHOLE-BODY PET IMAGING
Inflammation

Inflammation in almost any tissue will result in increased ^{18}F-FDG accumulation. This can cause

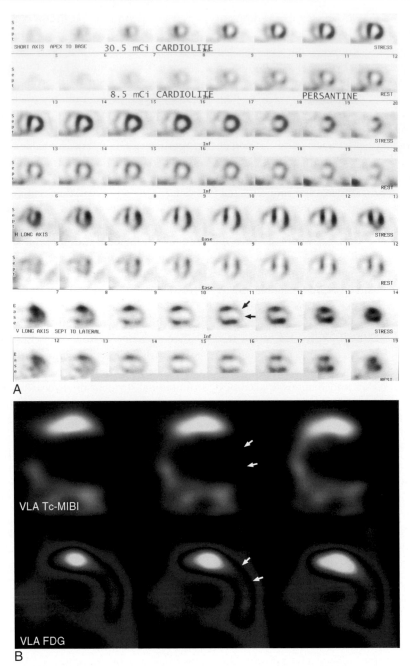

FIGURE 13–30. Hibernating myocardium. *A*, A technetium-99m (^{99m}Tc) sestamibi stress and rest SPECT scan shows a large fixed defect in the distal anterior wall and apex (*arrows*) of the left ventricle. *B*, Vertical long-axis ^{99m}Tc-sestamibi SPECT and ^{18}F-FDG PET images again show the perfusion defect but metabolic activity (*arrows*) is present.

problems in interpretation, for example, distinguishing a lung abscess or pneumonia (Fig. 13–31) from a lung cancer. Increased activity is also present in active granulomatous infections (tuberculosis and sarcoid) (Figs. 13–32 and 13–33), as well as in the lymph nodes of persons with chronic inflammatory lung disease. In addition, ^{18}F-FDG scanning can be helpful in distinguishing a noncalcified inactive granuloma (Fig. 13–34) from an active granuloma or lung cancer.

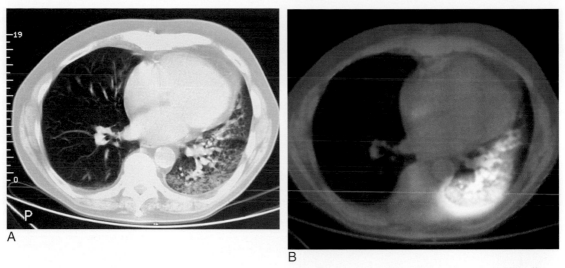

FIGURE 13–31. Pneumonia. *A*, A CT scan of the chest demonstrates an alveolar infiltrate in the left lower lobe. *B*, A ^{18}F-FDG PET/CT fusion scan shows increased metabolic activity in the pneumonia.

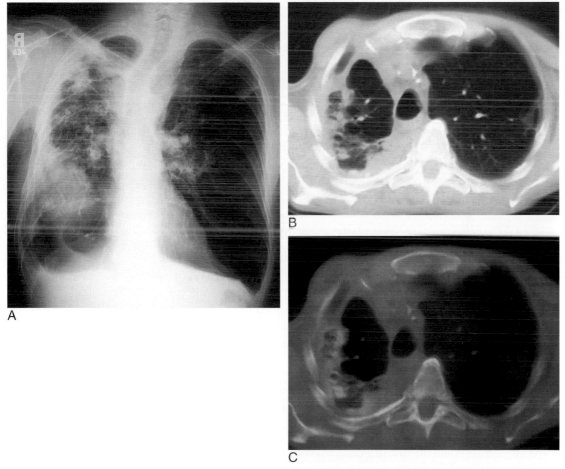

FIGURE 13–32. Active tuberculosis. *A*, A chest x-ray shows hyperinflation (chronic obstructive pulmonary disease) but also a right upper lobe cavitary infiltrate with hilar and mediastinal retraction. *B*, A chest CT confirms the findings but is unable to assess activity. *C*, ^{18}F-FDG PET/CT fusion image shows increased metabolic activity.

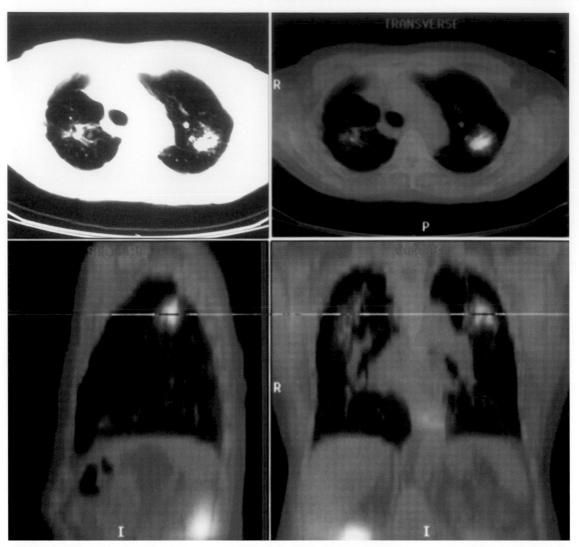

FIGURE 13–33. Sarcoidosis. ^{18}F-FDG PET/CT fusion images show increased activity in both right and left upper lung zones.

Increased ^{18}F-FDG accumulation also may be secondary to recent wounds, ostomies, infected indwelling catheters (Fig. 13–35), hematomas, thrombus, healing fractures, osteomyelitis, gastritis, thyroiditis, colitis, rheumatoid arthritis, and radiation therapy (up to 2 years). Increased activity after radiation therapy can be problematic, especially when following response to therapy. Most uptake related to radiation therapy is slightly greater than blood pool, although radiation pneumonitis can be very intense. Increased uptake has also been reported in the lymph nodes, lung, and pleura-related inflammation in patients with occupational lung disease.

With acute simple fractures, ^{18}F-FDG accumulation can be initially high, but after about 8 weeks it should resolve considerably. In chronic benign vertebral fractures, the SUV is usually less than two, whereas pathologic fractures due to neoplasm often have SUVs greater than two, usually about four. Degenerative joint disease can also result in increased ^{18}F-FDG uptake, and there can be occasional nonspecific focal uptake in anterior rib ends. Increased activity is seen in osteomyelitis, and ^{18}F-FDG scanning has been reported to be more accurate than either three-phase ^{99m}Tc-methylene diphosphonate or gallium-67 (^{67}Ga)-citrate imaging for chronic osteomyelitis (Fig. 13–36). Unfortunately, if there is a question of cellulitis versus chronic osteomyelitis, differentiation can be difficult due to the hypermetabolism associated with either entity. A negative ^{18}F-FDG

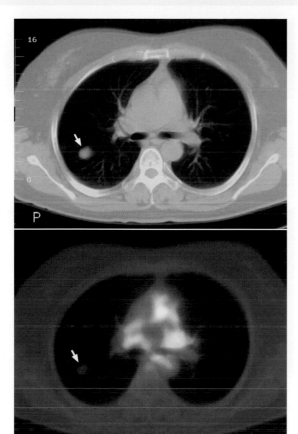

FIGURE 13–34. Inactive granuloma. *Top,* A solitary pulmonary nodule was identified on a chest X-ray. A CT scan shows the nodule to be noncalcified. *Bottom,* A ^{18}F-FDG PET/CT fusion image does not show any metabolic activity. An active granuloma can have uptake and would not be possible to differentiate from a malignancy.

scan can be very helpful in excluding chronic osteomyelitis.

As expected, there is increased activity in patients with pancreatitis, although this can be difficult to differentiate from pancreatic cancer. Vascular grafts also have been associated with increased ^{18}F-FDG uptake, but this does not necessarily indicate infection. Surgical sites will have moderately increased activity for up to about 2 months.

Neoplasms

Cancer cells exhibit a number of aberrant characteristics compared with those of normal cells, which can potentially be used to image tumors. Typically, there is increased glucose metabolism, increased DNA synthesis, increased amino acid transport, and overexpression of receptors and antigens. PET imaging with ^{18}F-FDG capitalizes on increased glucose metabolism in a wide variety of neoplasms to detect both primary lesions and their metastases.

Today, ^{18}F-FDG PET scanning has become an integral tool in management of many tumor types. It is used for diagnosis, staging, restaging, and evaluation of response to therapy. Use of PET imaging in tumor staging results in a change of therapy in as many as 25% to 50% of patients. In about 10% to 15% of patients, unsuspected distant metastases will be found. In certain settings, PET can offer some insight into tumor biology, including tumor grade and prognosis. Staging of those tumors for which PET imaging is used is presented at the end of this chapter (see Tables 13–13, 13–14, and 13–15).

Typically, the threshold for lesion detection is approximately 6 mm. Lesions greater than 1 cm are routinely detected, depending on tumor histology. In general, ^{18}F-FDG PET is more sensitive for less well differentiated cell types. Thus, high uptake in a tumor is frequently, but not always, associated with a poorer prognosis. Conversely, well-differentiated lesions may occasionally be a source of false-negative scans because of diminished ^{18}F-FDG uptake. Although the degree of initial uptake in some neoplasms and/or their metastases may correlate inversely with response to therapy, this is not always the case.

Because of the complementary information of metabolic activity and anatomy supplied by PET and CT, respectively, together they offer unique advantages in the diagnosis, staging, and monitoring of malignancy. PET may often demonstrate that lymph nodes meeting normal CT criteria (<1 cm, short-axis) do indeed harbor metastases or, conversely, that enlarged lymph nodes, residual masses, postsurgical scarring, or anatomic distortion are not metabolically active and thus not likely malignant.

Uptake of ^{18}F-FDG after treatment provides information about tumor response. To monitor therapy response, a pretreatment scan is required as well as serial scans during therapy. It is important to standardize the protocol (fasting time, glucose level, hydration, etc.) to ensure that the scans will be comparable, because evaluation involves both visual and quantitative assessment. The simplest quantitative method is the ratio of tumor to normal tissues or background, such as mediastinal blood pool, but a better method is determination of the SUV. The SUV reflects the glycolytic activity of the tumor and thus is an

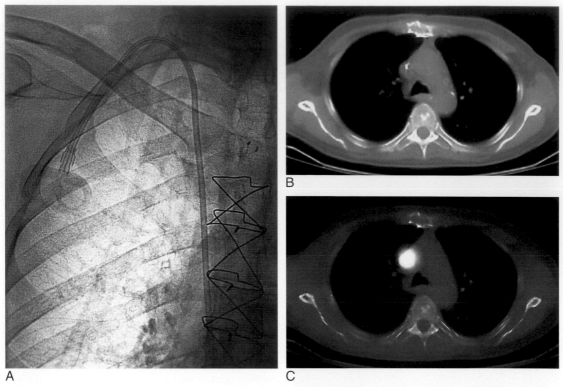

FIGURE 13–35. Infected catheter. *A,* An x-ray shows a chemotherapy catheter suspected of being infected. *B,* The chest CT shows the catheter in the superior vena cava. *C,* The ^{18}F-FDG PET/CT fusion image sows markedly increased activity around the catheter.

indirect marker of tumor growth rate. Thus, any post-treatment alteration in the SUV may provide early evidence of tumor response as well as offer prognostic information regarding the success or failure of a particular treatment, allowing a change in therapeutic approach when appropriate. It is important to remember that in order to accurately compare SUVs from different PET scans, the measurement must be performed under similar circumstances, including ROI, time after injection, and serum glucose levels.

Reduction or resolution of ^{18}F-FDG uptake is an early indicator of a favorable response. Although response to therapy using CT or MRI is based upon changes in tumor volume, residual masses may persist even after the tumor cells have been excised or eradicated. In this setting, ^{18}F-FDG imaging can determine whether the residual mass represents scar or persistent/recurrent tumor.

Although a decrease in activity in lesions after treatment is a good indication of a favorable response, the resolution or absence of ^{18}F-FDG activity in a lesion after therapy should not be interpreted as eradication, because PET cannot reliably detect residual microscopic disease. It is possible that some tumors are stunned by initiation of chemotherapy so that FDG metabolism is reduced or absent for several weeks but then returns as the tumor cells recover. This may explain the reported inaccuracy of PET in the evaluation of neo-adjuvant chemotherapy in some neoplasms. Thus, patients should continue to receive the full course of therapy. A lack of response to treatment as measured by no significant change or a measurable increase in ^{18}F-FDG uptake may indicate that alternative therapies should be tried.

Interpretation of post-therapy scans can be challenging (Table 13–12). Chemotherapy and radiation treatments can cause increased ^{18}F-FDG in both normal and neoplastic tissue. Post-treatment scans can be complicated by the presence of such inflammation, surgical site changes and wound healing, thymic rebound, or areas of infection occurring as a result of immune depression after chemotherapy. Thus, a thorough knowledge of the patient's treatment history is mandatory.

PET imaging can be of considerable value in planning radiation therapy, especially when tumor

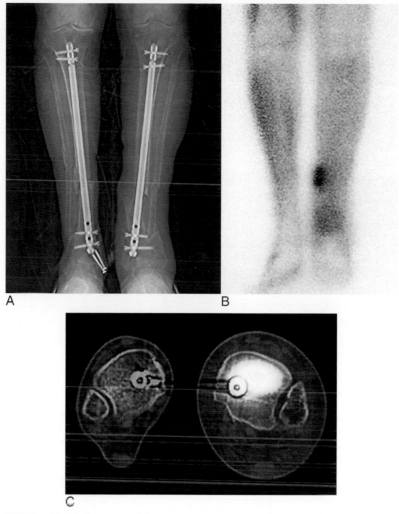

FIGURE 13–36. Osteomyelitis. *A,* An x-ray shows bilateral lower leg fractures and intramedullary fixation. *B,* Osteomyelitis was suspected, and an anterior ^{18}F-FDG image of the lower legs shows an abnormal focus of activity medially above the left ankle. *C,* A PET/CT fusion image shows that the increased activity is indeed within the bone.

anatomy and metabolism are mapped by using PET/CT. This more precise localization of disease extent, in turn, permits more accurate determination of planned treatment volumes. Irradiated neoplasms may initially show an increase in FDG uptake as well as increased uptake in the adjacent normal tissues due to inflammatory and granulation responses. In general, increased ^{18}F-FDG uptake in postirradiation regions resolves sufficiently in 2 to 3 months to permit re-evaluation by PET imaging, although significant uptake may persist for 6 months or more. Generally, a significant focus of FDG uptake more than 6 months after radiation treatment is indicative of tumor recurrence. Knowledge of the timing after therapy,

the configuration of the radiation port, and comparison with a baseline scan all greatly assist in accurately interpreting scans in this setting. Postirradiation inflammation can often be identified by its sharp demarcation, corresponding to the edges of the radiation port margins.

After chemotherapy, marrow rebound with or without G-CSF therapy, can produce intensely increased activity diffusely in the skeleton. This activity generally returns to baseline levels in 2 to 3 weeks after therapy, so that a waiting period of 2 to 4 weeks before ^{18}F-FDG PET imaging is usually sufficient to avoid interfering activity. Flare phenomena causing increased ^{18}F-FDG activity in breast cancers shortly after hormonal therapy and some

TABLE 13–12. ^{18}F-FDG PET Imaging in Oncology

ANATOMIC REGION	NORMAL DISTRIBUTION	NORMAL VARIANTS	BENIGN LESIONS THAT MAY HAVE UPTAKE POTENTIAL FALSE (+)	LOW-UPTAKE LESIONS POTENTIAL FALSE (−)
Head/Neck	**Brain:** gray matter, cortex, basal ganglia **Neck:** soft palate, tongue, vocal cords, palatine tonsils, adenoids, parotids, salivary glands, thyroid **Neck muscles:** laryngeal, masticators, genioglossus	**Head:** extraocular muscles **Neck:** brown fat	**Head:** sinusitis **Neck:** thyroiditis, Graves' disease, goiter, benign thyroid nodules, Warthin tumor, reactive lymph nodes	**Brain metastases** **Low-grade gliomas**
Chest	**Mediastinum:** heart muscle and atria, thymus in children and young adults, esophagus	**Mediastinum:** thymic rebound, base of ventricles, brown fat **Axilla:** lymph nodes (dose infiltration) **Breast:** premenopausal, hormone therapy	Aortic atherosclerosis Esophagitis, Barrett esophagus, After esophageal dilation procedure Hiatal hernia Empyema Pleurodesis Pneumonia Radiation pneumonitis **Granulomatous diseases:** tuberculosis, sarcoidosis, histoplasmosis, Aspergillosis, coccidiodomycosis, *Myobacterium avium-intracellulare,* atypical mycobacteria Reactive lymph nodes **Breast:** inflammation, biopsy site, mastitis, fibroadenomas (low), gynecomastia	**Lung:** bronchioloalveolar cancer, carcinoid, solitary pulmonary nodule <1 cm **Breast:** lobular carcinoma, carcinoma in situ, tubular carcinoma
Abdomen	Kidneys Ureters Bladder Stomach Small bowel Colon Liver Spleen (low)	**Brown fat:** perinephric	Vascular bypass grafts Colonic Adenoma/polyps Adrenal hypertrophy Pancreatitis	**MALT** **Liver:** hepatocellular cancer (40%–50%), small lesions **Kidney:** renal cell cancer

Pelvis			Ureters Bladder Bowel Uterus (menses) Testes Penis (low) Uterine fibroids Endometriosis Corpus luteum cysts Vascular bypass grafts	
Skeleton/Marrow	Skeletal muscle Brown fat: supraclavicular, paravertebral, intercostal	**Marrow:** G-CSF Tx (intense) Rad Tx (decreased)	Inflammation/infection Arthritis Phlebitis Spondylodiscitis Pigmented villonodular synovitis **Benign bone lesions:** fibrous dysplasia, Paget's disease, nonossifying fibroma, giant-cell tumor, eosinophilic granuloma, aneurysmal bone cyst, enchondroma, osteomyelitis	Chondrosarcoma Plasmacytoma Low-grade sarcomas (osseous and soft tissue) Sclerotic metastases
Skin			Inflammation/infection Wound healing	
Any location	Percutaneous lines/tubes		Inflammation/infection Granulomatous diseases Postradiation change Wound healing Reactive lymph nodes Tense musculature Resolving hematoma Ostomies Vascular grafts Atheromatous disease Healing fractures Arthritis	Small lesions, Nodal micrometastases Low-grade tumors, especially lymphomas (small lymphocytic cell) Metastases adjacent to fluorodeoxyglucose–avid primary cancer or high activity organs

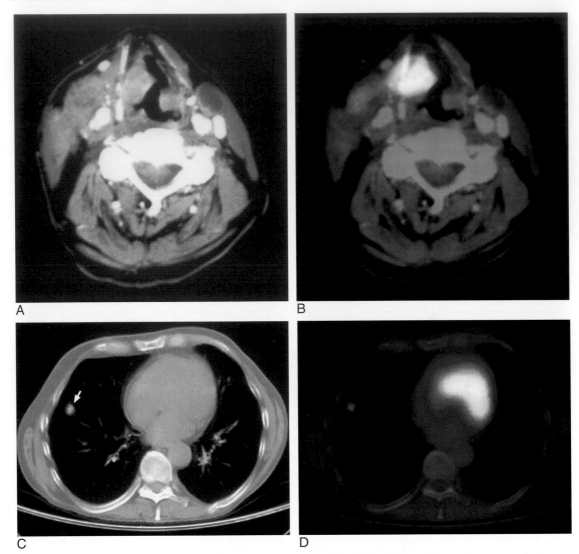

FIGURE 13–37. Laryngeal cancer. *A*, In this patient who has had a left neck dissection, a CT scan shows a mass in the right side of the larynx. *B*, A ^{18}F-FDG PET/CT fusion scan showed increased activity in the mass. *C*, A CT scan of the chest revealed a 1-cm nodule in the right lung. *D*, A PET/CT fusion image shows increased activity in this pulmonary metastasis.

brain cancers shortly after chemotherapy have been reported and should not be mistaken for exacerbation of disease.

Head and Neck Cancer

Head and neck neoplasms constitute a heterogeneous variety of lesions. Some of the more common tumors, such as squamous cell carcinomas of the nasopharynx, oral cavity, and larynx avidly accumulate ^{18}F-FDG (Fig. 13–37). Assessment of the primary lesion with PET is usually unwarranted. However, occasionally an occult lesion presents as a metastasis to cervical lymph nodes, and PET imaging can be used as an adjunct to localizing a

clinically unapparent primary tumor. However, such imaging can be challenging due to salivary gland excretion of FDG, brown fat, pharyngeal muscle uptake, inflammation at biopsy sites, complex anatomy, and the limited spatial resolution of PET scanners. In general, PET/CT has proved especially advantageous in imaging head and neck cancers and their metastases to precisely localize areas of abnormally increased activity.

A primary use of imaging is for staging head and neck cancers by identifying cervical and other regional lymph node metastases as well as distant disease, especially skeletal, hepatic, pulmonary, and distant nodal metastases. Early-stage tumors are treated and often cured by surgery or radiation therapy. Limited nodal metastases are often amenable to surgical resection, whereas more extensive regional disease usually requires radiation therapy in addition to surgery. Scanning with ^{18}F-FDG is more accurate ($\approx$ 90%) for staging than is either CT or MRI. For restaging after treatment, detection of local residual or recurrent tumor is rendered challenging for all imaging modalities because of post-therapeutic change associated with altered anatomy and inflammation. PET has been shown to be sensitive (80% to 100%) for local recurrence, but its specificity is reduced by postradiation inflammation. Radiation produces the most prominent changes in the epithelial surfaces of the oral mucosa, soft palate, paranasal sinuses, and palatine tonsils. To increase specificity, a minimum waiting period of 4 months after radiation has been recommended. At that time, there is both high sensitivity and specificity for detection of recurrent primary tumor, or development of nodal metastases.

Chemotherapy is a common first-stage treatment in advanced head and neck cancers. Scans with ^{18}F-FDG PET are useful to evaluate response during therapy. In the neoadjuvant (induction) chemotherapy setting, ^{18}F-FDG PET can identify nonresponders, and additional surgical intervention or radiation therapy can be avoided in those patients who are unlikely to benefit. A decrease in ^{18}F-FDG activity (SUV) of about 80% to 90% is often associated with complete remission. However, if the decrease is less than 40%, there is likely to be recurrent disease. The picture is somewhat complicated because in some patients the therapeutic response varies among different metastatic lymph node sites.

As mentioned earlier, false-positive ^{18}F-FDG results can occur not only as a result of recent surgery or radiation therapy but also as a result of laryngeal muscle activity, tense cervical muscles, reactive lymph nodes, and brown fat. In patients with unilateral laryngeal nerve paralysis, asymmetric laryngeal muscle (posterior arytenoid muscle) activity on the functional nonparalyzed side may mimic a metastatic lymph node. False-negative studies can result in patients with tumor deposits less than 6 mm. Small lung metastases are best identified by CT.

Thyroid Cancer

Radioiodines (iodine-131 [^{131}I] and iodine-123 [^{123}I]) are the most widely used radiopharmaceuticals used to evaluate and stage well-differentiated thyroid cancers, commonly papillary/follicular cell types. However, there are a number of thyroid cancers that do not accumulate radioiodine to a significant degree. These include poorly differentiated and medullary cancers. In addition, some thyroid cancers that are originally well-differentiated may recur as poorly differentiated cell types that do not readily accumulate radioiodines.

Patients with differentiated thyroid cancers are usually treated with thyroidectomy and ^{131}I ablation of thyroid bed remnants and regional nodal disease. Follow-up employs serum thyroglobulin levels, and whole-body radioiodine imaging if thyroglobulin levels are elevated. If radioiodine-avid lesions are identified by radioiodine whole-body imaging, then repeat ^{131}I therapy can be used. However, in some patients with elevated serum thyroglobulin levels, whole-body radioiodine scans are negative, suggesting less well differentiated, more aggressive metastases. In this setting ^{18}F-FDG PET imaging has significant value as it frequently demonstrates the recurrent lesions with an accuracy of about 90%. PET imaging is similarly useful in patients with medullary carcinoma of the thyroid treated with thyroidectomy who subsequently experience elevated serum calcitonin levels. Hürthle cell cancer, which is much more aggressive and more often metastatic than other thyroid cancers, usually has intense ^{18}F-FDG uptake, and this may be the best imaging method for evaluating this cell type.

As with cancers of the head and neck, it is often difficult to detect small nodal metastases in the neck if the patient is scanned with the arms raised; it is often necessary to scan the patient with the arms up and then again with the arms down (Fig. 13-38).

Many nonmalignant thyroid nodules accumulate ^{18}F-FDG. However, if there is a very intense focus of activity in the nodule, the probability of a malignant lesion is increased. An incidentally detected focus of increased FDG uptake in the thyroid on scans performed for unrelated reasons should be further evaluated to exclude carcinoma. Diffusely increased uptake commonly occurs in patients with thyroiditis and Grave's disease.

Solitary Pulmonary Nodules and Lung Cancer
Solitary Pulmonary Nodule

Imaging with FDG PET is a useful adjunct to CT in the evaluation of pulmonary nodules and

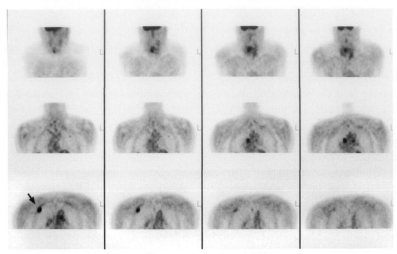

FIGURE 13–38. Thyroid cancer. ^{18}F-FDG PET coronal images of the neck and upper chest reveal asymmetric activity in the thyroid bed. The images also reveal an unexpected rib metastasis (*arrow*).

masses (Fig. 13–39). The sensitivity and specificity of ^{18}F-FDG PET for differentiating benign from malignant causes for solitary pulmonary parenchymal nodules that are greater than 1 cm is about 95% and 80%, respectively. Although CT has comparable sensitivity, its specificity is considerably lower, in the range of 50%. An SUV of 2.5 or greater usually indicates malignancy, whereas lesions with SUV's less than 2.5 have a very low likelihood of being malignant. However, SUVs are not an absolute distinguisher. False-positive studies may occur in inflammatory lesions and granulomatous diseases such a sarcoidosis, tuberculosis, and fungal infections. Such hypermetabolic lesions must be considered malignant until proved benign. Although non–FDG-avid lesions are highly unlikely to be malignant, false-negative studies may be seen in neoplasms with low metabolic activity such as carcinoid tumor, bronchioalveolar cancer, or well-differentiated adenocarcinoma. Metastasis with low cellular density, such as mucinous lesions, may also show low ^{18}F-FDG uptake. Primary lung cancers with low FDG levels usually represent stage 1 lesions with an excellent prognosis after resection.

It should be emphasized that lung nodules with suspicious CT characteristics and negative ^{18}F-FDG PET scans should be monitored with serial CT scans or biopsied. Similarly, ^{18}F-FDG negative small lung nodules less than 1 cm, especially in high-risk patients, warrant CT follow-up, because an average SUV of less than 2.5 may reflect a partial volume effect rather than the true metabolic activity of the nodule. It is important to note that if CT/PET fusion images are being performed, there may be misregistration if the scans were not both done with shallow breathing. As expected, most benign pulmonary lesions such as hamartomas, adenomas, and inflammatory nodules are not FDG avid as measured by SUV.

Primary Lung Cancer

The most common primary lung cancers are ^{18}F-FDG avid, including both small-cell and non–small-cell types. However, because small-cell carcinoma is considered to be metastatic at the time of its diagnosis and because the initial treatment is systemic chemotherapy, primary staging with PET imaging may not be warranted. Thus, PET imaging has largely been directed toward evaluation of non–small-cell lung cancer.

After a diagnosis of non–small-cell carcinoma of the lung has been made, PET imaging can play an important role in staging, treatment planning, and restaging of the disease. Although CT is the preferred method of assessing primary tumor size and invasion, ^{18}F-FDG PET can be helpful in evaluating patients presenting with pleural effusions by distinguishing malignant from benign effusions with an accuracy of 90%. PET may also aid initial CT assessment by distinguishing metabolically active primary tumor from adjacent atelectasis or postobstructive pneumonitis. Such differentiation can

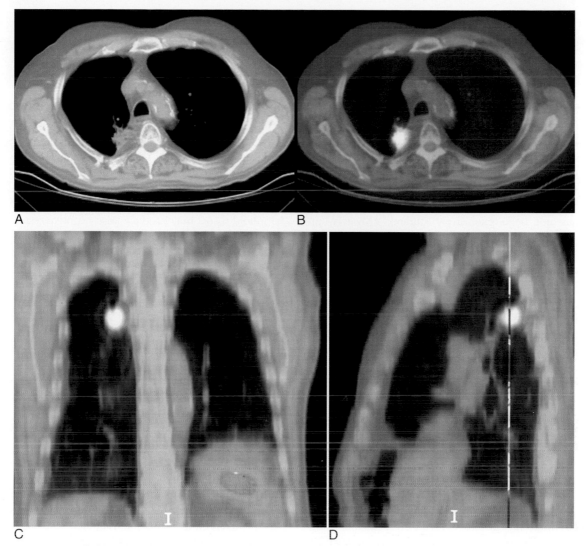

FIGURE 13–39. Non-small cell lung cancer. *A,* The CT scan demonstrates a right upper lobe soft-tissue mass. The patient did not want a needle biopsy. *B–D,* ^{18}F-FDG PET/CT fusion images show markedly increased activity in the lesion, indicating a high probability that this represents a malignancy.

greatly aid in radiation treatment planning, allowing more precise determination of treatment volumes.

Scanning with ^{18}F-FDG PET has been shown to be superior to other forms of imaging for initial staging of non–small-cell lung cancer, particularly with regard to spread to regional lymph nodes, which is an important determinant of treatment options. Surgical resection of a primary lesion is often possible with ipsilateral, hilar, and mediastinal, as well as subcarinal, lymph node involvement. But, disease in the contralateral, hilar, and mediastinal nodes usually dictates nonsurgical treatment. The CT criteria of size (>1 cm) for abnormal

lymph nodes is relatively insensitive (45% sensitivity, 85% specificity) for detecting metastatic disease to hilar and mediastinal lymph nodes. By using metabolic criteria, PET has a sensitivity and specificity of 80% to 90%. However, because the positive predictive value for mediastinal disease of an abnormal PET scan is only 65%, owing to false-positive studies caused by inflammatory lymph nodes, confirmation of metastatic disease should be sought before surgical treatment is denied. Importantly, the negative predictive value of an ^{18}F-FDG PET scan for mediastinal metastases is about 95%. Thus, surgical treatment can proceed based on a negative PET scan.

PET is an excellent technique for detecting distant metastases. About 10% of patients who have no evidence of metastatic disease on CT are subsequently shown to have metastases on ^{18}F-FDG scans. PET can reliably differentiate benign from malignant causes of abnormal body CT findings and can help distinguish benign adrenal masses from metastases. Because of the high degree of FDG uptake in normal brain tissue, PET is less sensitive for detecting small cerebral metastases and is significantly less sensitive than is MRI.

The use of PET scans to predict response to adjuvant therapies for non–small-cell lung cancer has not been extensively studied. However, an incomplete response of decreased ^{18}F-FDG uptake after radiation or chemotherapy therapy appears to have almost the same poor prognosis as those who show no decrease in ^{18}F-FDG uptake after treatment. The median survival of those patients with positive ^{18}F-FDG scans at the completion of therapy is about 1 to 2 years, whereas those with negative results have about a 80% three-year survival. Even in aggressively treated patients, the recurrence rate of intrathoracic and distant disease is high. Because of its high sensitivity and specificity, PET can be very useful in evaluating patients for suspected recurrence. In non–small-cell lung cancer, SUV has been shown to be an independent predictor of survival. Patients whose tumors exhibit high SUVs (>10 to 20) have significantly lower survival rates.

In the postsurgical patient, PET can reliably differentiate postsurgical scarring from metabolically active recurrent tumor. In patients undergoing radiation therapy, resultant radiation pneumonitis is often metabolically active, likely related to cellular inflammatory and macrophage reaction. This activity may obscure underlying persistent or recurrent viable tumor. Knowledge of the time of treatment and the position of the radiation ports is essential to accurate interpretation. Radiation pneumonitis may remain metabolically active on PET scans for 6 months after treatment and occasionally up to a year or more.

Bronchioalveolar carcinoma, carcinoid lesions less than 1 cm in diameter, and occasionally well-differentiated adenocarcinomas can have little ^{18}F-FDG uptake, resulting in false-negative scans. False-positive scans can occur as a result of benign processes with high metabolic rates including granulomas, sarcoidosis, tuberculosis, histoplasmosis, coccidiomycosis, *Mycobacterium avium intracellulare*, and simple pneumonias. Increased ^{18}F-FDG uptake

occurs in mesotheliomas. PET scanning has been reported to be superior to CT for staging this tumor, particularly in documenting extent of pleural disease and detecting small involved mediastinal lymph nodes.

Lymphomas

Both Hodgkin and non-Hodgkin lymphoma of all types accumulate ^{18}F-FDG, although low-grade lymphomas do not accumulate activity as well as intermediate- or high-grade lymphomas. Low-grade lymphomas, especially mucosa-associated lymphoid tissue, may produce false-negative results and may involve lymph nodes less than 1 cm in diameter, although these constitute about 25% of positive sites on PET scan. False-positive studies may be caused by inflammation and infections involving lymph nodes, especially granulomatous infections.

Because the anatomic distribution of active disease is a major determinant of the mode of therapy used, PET and other imaging modalities play an important role in the staging and restaging of lymphoma (Fig. 13–40). In general, ^{18}F-FDG PET is more sensitive (85% to 95%) and specific (95%) than is CT for detecting nodal disease, as well as splenic and hepatic involvement. Existing information also indicates that PET is superior to ^{67}Ga SPECT scanning for imaging lymphoma. Although marrow disease is accurately detected by using ^{18}F-FDG PET, caution should be exercised when interpreting scans of patients who have received colony stimulating factors or who may be experiencing postchemotherapy marrow rebound.

Using PET to monitor therapy response requires a baseline ^{18}F-FDG scan before treatment to compare with intra- or post-treatment images. In some settings, post-treatment scans are appropriate after one or two cycles of chemotherapy are completed. It is prudent to wait 1 to 2 weeks after therapy to avoid transient fluctuations in tumor metabolism. Scans done as early as one week after initiation of chemotherapy can show significant reduction in activity assessed both visually and using SUVs. The amount of reduction correlates with the ultimate outcome. About 80% to 90% of patients with residual activity after one cycle of chemotherapy will relapse, whereas about 80% to 90% of those with no activity at the same time will have much longer disease free periods. In the treatment setting, false-positive scans can

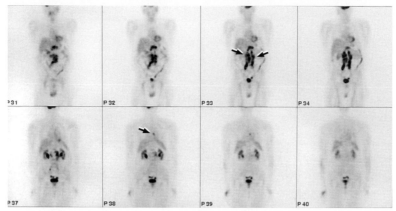

FIGURE 13–40. Recurrent lymphoma. Multiple ^{18}F-FDG whole-body images performed for restaging show abnormal activity in paraaortic nodes and a small focus in the posterior lower mediastinum. Normal bowel and renal activity is present.

result from thymic rebound, reactive bone marrow (Fig. 13–41), and inflammatory or infectious processes.

After therapy is completed, ^{18}F-FDG scanning can determine the overall response and can be very helpful in determining the significance of residual masses noted on CT (Fig. 13–42). Relapse occurs in almost all patients who have a positive PET scan after the completion of therapy, whereas relapse occurs in about 25% of patients with residual masses on CT. The absence of disease on a post-treatment PET scan correlates with a low relapse rate. However, because a negative PET scan cannot exclude minimal residual disease, about 20% will

suffer a relapse. Subsequent follow-up ^{18}F-FDG scans have a sensitivity and specificity of about 80% to 90% for detection of recurrent lymphoma. Although low-grade lymphoma initially has a low SUV, an increase in SUV on a follow-up scan suggests the possibility of transformation to a higher-grade tumor.

Even though the gray matter of the brain has high ^{18}F-FDG activity, central nervous system involvement by lymphoma in patients with human immunodeficiency virus (HIV) disease is more avid. PET has been used in this setting to distinguish central nervous system lymphoma from infections, such as toxoplasmosis.

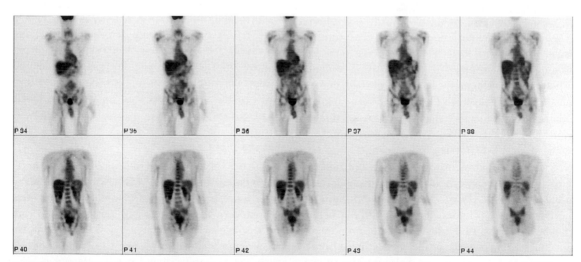

FIGURE 13–41. Postchemotherapy marrow stimulation. In this postchemotherapy lymphoma patient, use of G-CSF to help the marrow recover has resulted markedly increased ^{18}F-FDG activity in the spine, sacrum, and proximal femurs. This should not be interpreted as diffuse marrow metastases.

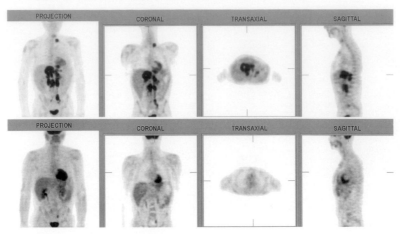

FIGURE 13–42. Lymphoma. *Top,* Multiple ^{18}F-FDG whole-body images before therapy show abnormal activity in the left neck, para-aortic nodes, and right upper quadrant. *Bottom,* Postchemotherapy images only show normal physiologic activity in the brain, heart, stomach, and urinary system.

Breast Cancer

In the setting of breast cancer, ^{18}F-FDG PET is used principally in the evaluation of locoregional recurrence, restaging, and response to therapy. However, it may occasionally be useful in the evaluation of primary breast lesions. PET can aid in evaluation of nonpalpable masses in dense breasts or when mammography is equivocal. The sensitivity and specificity for detection of primary breast cancer are both about 70% to 90%. False-negative studies may be caused by tubular and lobular carcinomas, as well as by ductal carcinomas in situ and small lesions. For lesions less than 2 cm in diameter, ^{18}F-FDG scanning has a negative predictive value of only 50%, and therefore, it cannot reliably be used to defer or delay biopsy of a mammographically suspicious lesion. Benign breast tumors usually have very low ^{18}F-FDG uptake and are usually not a source of false-positive studies, although approximately 10% of fibroadenomas may show uptake of FDG. However, benign inflammatory processes may demonstrate significant FDG uptake.

Because ^{18}F-FDG scanning cannot reliably detect small nodal metastases, it does not replace sentinel node biopsy or axillary node dissection for initial staging of breast cancer. For detection of metastatic disease beyond the axilla, PET is better than is CT. Thus, PET may be used as an adjunct to initial staging of large or locally advanced breast cancers to find distant disease. False-positive results can occur due to inflammatory changes shortly after biopsy or surgery.

PET can be used to monitor response to therapy. Shortly after initiation of therapy with tamoxifen in patients with ER-positive breast cancers, there can be a "flare" phenomenon, during which uptake of ^{18}F-FDG actually increases even though the tumor is responding favorably to therapy. When PET imaging is used to monitor early response of breast cancer to cytotoxic chemotherapy, favorable results can often be identified as early as a week or so after commencing treatment. As with other tumors, persistence of ^{18}F-FDG activity after therapy carries a poor prognosis. A negative scan at the end of therapy is still associated with about a 25% recurrence rate. This may be due to nonvisualization of lesions less than 0.6 to 1.0 cm in size or when the lesion is well-differentiated. For restaging, ^{18}F-FDG PET has a relatively high sensitivity (90%) and specificity (80%) for the detection of recurrent disease, both locoregionally and at distant sites. It is especially useful to distinguish mature postsurgical scarring and fibrosis seen on CT from locally recurrent cancer.

Esophageal Cancer

Normal ^{18}F-FDG uptake in the esophagus should be uniform. Because ^{18}F-FDG will accumulate in both esophageal adenocarcinoma and squamous cell cancers, focally-increased activity should raise the suspicion of malignancy (Fig. 13–43). However, focal activity can also be due to benign processes such as esophagitis, hiatal hernia, Barrett esophagus, postprocedural changes from balloon dilatation procedures, and inflammatory changes from

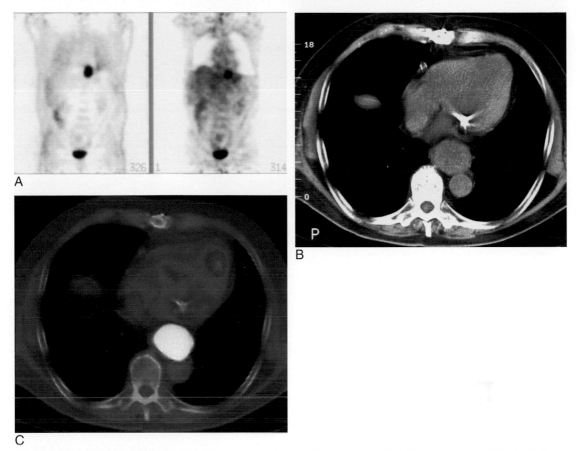

FIGURE 13–43. Esophageal cancer. *A,* Uncorrected and attenuation-corrected ¹⁸F-FDG anterior images of the body show an intense focus of activity at the gastroesophageal junction. *B,* A CT scan shows a soft-tissue mass in the same area. *C,* The PET/CT fusion image shows markedly increased ¹⁸F-FDG activity in the mass.

radiation therapy, which reduces the specificity of such esophageal activity.

The limited resolution of PET scans compromises the evaluation of local invasion or regional lymph node metastases, so that PET does not appear to be accurate enough to be consistently used for presurgical staging. The insensitivity for detecting regional nodal disease is likely related to the proximity of involved nodes to the primary lesion, which makes differentiation difficult, and to the often microscopic nature of the nodal disease. However, when present, the finding of a discrete positive periesophageal or regional focus on PET imaging is highly predictive of metastatic nodal disease, with a specificity of about 90%.

PET scanning is primarily used to evaluate the possibility of stage 4 disease (distant metastases) and to identify those patients who are not candidates for surgical resection. PET is more accurate (80% to 90%) than is CT for the evaluation of cervical and upper abdominal nodal disease and

spread to liver, lung, or bone. In patients treated by resection of the primary lesion, PET is very sensitive, but not specific for recurrence at the anastomotic site. However, for the detection of distant recurrence outside the surgical field, PET is both sensitive (95%) and specific (80%). Thus, in restaging esophageal cancer after surgery, a multimodality approach including both PET and CT is advisable.

In unresectable esophageal cancer treated with adjuvant therapy, a decrease in ¹⁸F-FDG activity is associated with a favorable response to chemotherapy. Those who are nonresponsive to adjuvant chemotherapy can be spared additional ineffective treatment. Follow-up scans should not be performed less than 4 to 6 weeks after surgery and less than 8 to 12 weeks after completion of radiation therapy. Activity in the primary lesion may increase during the early course of radiation treatments, but responding lesions will ultimately show a decrease in FDG uptake later in the course. Further,

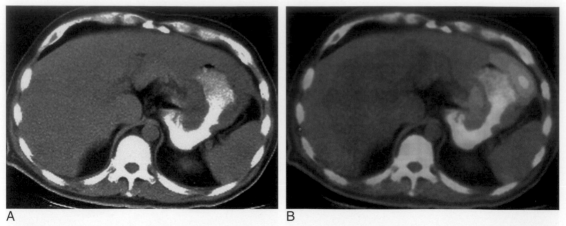

FIGURE 13–44. Gastric cancer. *A*, A CT scan shows a markedly thickened stomach wall. *B*, A ¹⁸F-FDG PET/CT fusion scan shows increased activity in the neoplasm.

esophagitis related to recent radiation therapy may cause interfering activity, which usually resolves after 4 to 6 weeks. False-positive results can occur also as a result of significant uptake in gastric mucosa near the esophagogastric junction or from reflux esophagitis. False-negative studies occur when the lesion is small or located in close proximity to other structures that avidly accumulate ¹⁸F-FDG, such as the heart.

Gastric Cancer

In contrast to ¹⁸F-FDG–avid esophageal carcinomas the detection rate of ¹⁸F-FDG for gastric cancer depends on the cell type (Fig. 13–44). Mucinous tumors, diffuse tumors, and intestinal type tumors typically have low ¹⁸F-FDG uptake.

Gastrointestinal Stromal Tumors

This uncommon tumor represents about 5% of all sarcomas. It most frequently occurs in the stomach, less often in the small intestine, and rarely in the colon. The sensitivity and positive predictive value are very high (85% to 100%) for both CT and ¹⁸F-FDG PET. These tumors typically have high peripheral activity with central cold areas. Compared with CT, ¹⁸F-FDG PET is somewhat better at predicting response after therapy.

Colorectal Cancer

Although ¹⁸F-FDG PET is very sensitive in the identification of primary colorectal adenocarcinomas (90% to 100%), the specificity (40% to 60%) is limited by the presence of physiologic bowel activity as well as activity accumulation in inflammatory lesions and benign colonic polyps (Fig. 13–45). As

was noted with stomach cancers, mucinous cell type lesions and their metastases tend to have relatively low ¹⁸F-FDG uptake.

The initial staging of colon cancer is predicated on surgical and pathological findings. Because PET has serious limitations in spatial resolution and anatomic detail, it has a minor role in local and regional staging. Further, sensitivity (≈ 30%) is reduced by the presence of small quantities of malignant cells in pericolic lymph nodes and by the close proximity of the nodes to the primary tumor. However, when nodes are detected as FDG positive, the specificity of the study is high (95%).

In detecting distant metastases, both nodal (internal iliac and retroperitoneal) and extranodal, PET is superior to CT in both sensitivity and specificity, at 95% and 75%, respectively. In the liver, both modalities are limited in detecting lesions less than 1 cm in size (Fig. 13–46). However, PET can play an important role in the selection of patients for curative resection or ablation of isolated hepatic metastases by determining the presence or absence of coexisting extrahepatic metastases. In this respect, PET offers significant incremental value to CT imaging, by identifying 10% to 20% additional extrahepatic sites of involvement than with CT alone. With respect to evaluation of treatment success after local ablative therapy of liver metastases from colorectal carcinoma, including cryotherapy, hepatic artery chemotherapy, and radiofrequency ablation, metabolic imaging with PET has been shown to be more accurate than is CT in differentiating post-therapy change from residual or recurrent tumor.

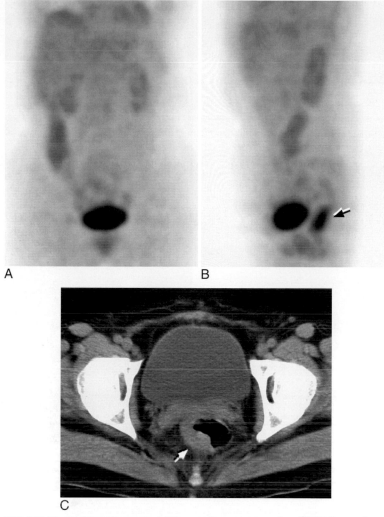

FIGURE 13–45. Rectal cancer. *A,* The anterior projection of an ¹⁸F-FDG scan does not show any obvious abnormality. *B,* Inspection of the rotating whole-body images shows that on the lateral view, there is an abnormal focus in the pelvis that was obscured by physiologic bladder activity. *C,* The CT scan shows the irregular mass in the rectum.

After initial treatment of colorectal carcinoma, PET offers significant information for restaging the disease: ¹⁸F-FDG PET has been shown to be more sensitive than is CT or carcinoembryonic antigen (CEA) levels, and equally as specific as CEA levels for detecting recurrence. In this setting, PET is particularly useful for differentiating postsurgical and radiation change from recurrent disease, especially in the pelvis and presacral space. The ¹⁸F-FDG scans are also valuable in cases in which there is a rising CEA titer and no obvious abnormality on CT. Positive ¹⁸F-FDG follow-up scans should be correlated with CT findings to avoid false-positive etiologies such as sigmoid diverticulitis or even bladder diverticula. Both during and after radio-

therapy and chemotherapy, tumor uptake of ¹⁸F-FDG may increase even though the lesion is responding. This is somewhat similar to the flare phenomenon described for breast cancer. Follow-up scans are not usually performed during therapy, and post-therapy scans are usually delayed for about 2 months after the completion of therapy.

Hepatocelluar Carcinoma (Hepatoma)

Although frequently hypermetabolic, hepatocellular caricinomas may contain high levels of phosphatases (as do normal hepatocytes), which can dephosphorylate FDG, permitting it to diffuse out of the tumor cells. Thus, ¹⁸F-FDG activity in

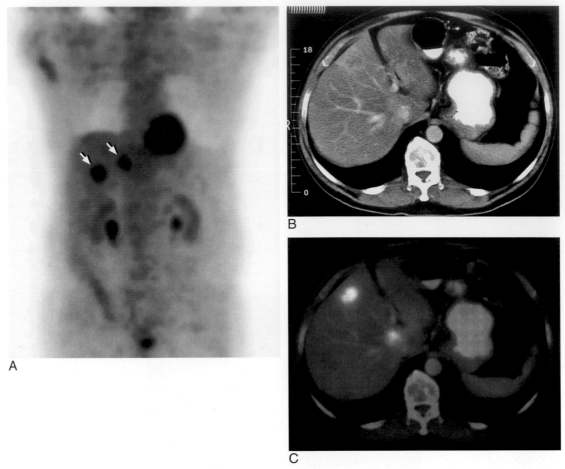

FIGURE 13–46. Hepatic metastases. *A,* A ^{18}F-FDG PET scan in a patient with treated colon cancer and a rising carcinoembryonic antigen titer shows two abnormal foci in the liver. *B,* A contrasted CT scan shows one peripheral lesion. *C,* The PET/CT fusion image accurately localized both lesions.

hepatomas is variable, and only about 50% of hepatocellular carcinomas can be imaged with ^{18}F-FDG. Therefore, ^{18}F-FDG PET is not useful as a screening tool to detect small hepatocellular carcinomas or distant disease. Some authors have examined the potential utility of [11]C- acetate for evaluation of hepatomas. Although the sensitivity is not as high as for ^{18}F-FDG, ^{11}C-acetate may accumulate in those well-differentiated tumors that ^{18}F-FDG does not. In general, for a hepatic lesion, if it accumulates both ^{18}F-FDG and ^{11}C-acetate, a diagnosis of hepatoma should be favored. However, if the lesion accumulates only FDG and not acetate, a lesion other than hepatoma is likely.

Pancreatic Cancer

PET is sensitive and specific for detection of primary pancreatic carcinoma. Thus, it may be a useful adjunct to equivocal CT or ERCP examina-

tions to establish the presence of a significant lesion. However, a role for PET in staging and restaging pancreatic carcinoma or in directing management of patients awaits further definition.

Malignant Bone Tumors

Scanning with ^{18}F-FDG PET is useful in evaluating the metabolic rate of osteosarcomas, their response to adjuvant and aggressive chemotherapy, and location of residual viable tumor. Because osteosarcomas are often heterogeneous, the maximum SUV is a better indicator of the true malignant potential than is average tumor SUV. In general, a higher maximum SUV correlates with a poorer prognosis. PET has been used to monitor response to therapy in both osteosarcoma and Ewing's tumor. Decline in ^{18}F-FDG uptake after therapy has been associated with an improved prognosis. For differentiation of residual masses after therapy, ^{18}F-FDG PET is more reliable than either CT or MRI, and it is sensitive for the detection and evaluation of pulmonary metastases. A variety of benign and malignant bone neoplasms will accumulate FDG, and it should be noted that aggressive benign bone tumors (e.g., giant cell tumors) can have SUVs as high or higher than that of osteosarcomas.

Malignant Melanoma

Scanning with ^{18}F-FDG is of limited use in initial staging of patients for spread to region lymph nodes or in patients with primary lesions less than 1 mm in thickness and no evidence of metastases. Although melanoma typically exhibits marked FDG avidity, minimal nodal metastases may simply be too small to be detected. The sensitivity for detecting melanoma lesions greater than 1 cm is about 95%; for lesions 6 to 10 mm, about 80%; and for lesions less than 5 mm, less than 20% (Fig.

13–47). Thus, ^{18}F-FDG scanning cannot replace lymphoscintigraphy to identify sentinel nodes for staging biopsy of regional lymph nodes.

However, PET has proved to be very useful in detecting distant metastases. Because of the wide variety of sites to which melanoma can metastasize, PET is an efficient examination to detect such spread throughout the body. It is more accurate than is CT in this setting, with sensitivity and specificity for melanoma metastases of approximately 90%. In addition, detection of unsuspected distant metastases at initial staging or restaging has been shown to alter patient management in a significant percentage of patients, particularly those who are at a high risk for distant disease based on extent of locoregional disease or those who have distant disease and are considering aggressive therapy. Because of the normally high uptake of ^{18}F-FDG in the brain, evaluation of central nervous system metastases is best done with MRI.

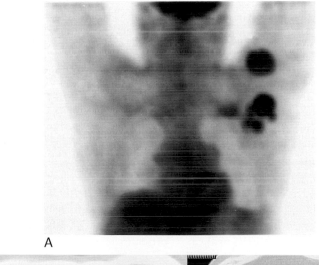

A

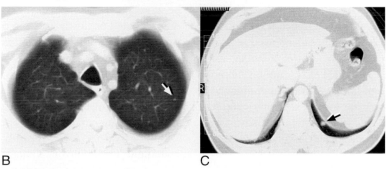

B   C

FIGURE 13–47. Melanoma. *A*, A ^{18}F-FDG PET scan of the chest shows multiple foci of increased activity in left auxiliary nodes but no obvious abnormality in the lungs. *B* and *C*, CT images of the chest show multiple small pulmonary nodules that are below the resolution of the PET scan.

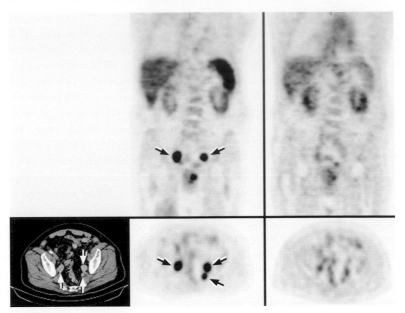

FIGURE 13–48. Prostate cancer. Carbon-11 acetate. PET scan and CT images demonstrate functional and anatomic abnormalities (*arrows*) due to metastases. (Case courtesy of Thomas Miller, M.D.)

Gynecologic Cancers

For ovarian cancer located inside the pelvis, adding ^{18}F-FDG PET scan to a CT scan does not improve accuracy of diagnosis even though the PET sensitivity and positive predictive values are about 80% to 90%. However, ^{18}F-FDG PET does add to the accuracy for lesions outside the pelvis (such as the diaphragm, liver surface, omentum, and lymph nodes). For peritoneal carcinomatosis, sensitivity with ^{18}F-FDG is only about 60%, but it is still higher than that with CT (≈ 45%). If either a nodular or diffuse pattern is seen in the peritoneum, the positive predictive value with PET is about 90%.

The value of PET scanning in cervical cancer or endometrial cancers is yet to be fully defined. Cervical cancer can accumulate ^{18}F-FDG with a sensitivity of about 70% and specificity of about 90%. Unfortunately, there is significant difficulty in differentiating tumor and nodal metastases from ^{18}F-FDG activity in nearby bowel, bladder, and ureters. In these cases PET/CT can be helpful. Uterine myomas can have relatively high uptake of FDG and be a cause for false-positive results. Leiomyosarcomas of the uterus usually have intense ^{18}F-FDG uptake.

Renal and Bladder Cancer

Renal and bladder cancers are both difficult to evaluate with ^{18}F-FDG PET. There is great variability of FDG uptake by renal cell cancers. Only 50% to

70% have sufficient ^{18}F-FDG uptake to be imaged successfully. Interpretation can also complicated by occasional normal variant increase of ^{18}F-FDG in the perirenal fat and in benign renal lesions, such as angiomyolipomas. However, the most significant issue is the large amount of urinary excretion of ^{18}F-FDG, which can easily mask a tumor in the kidney or bladder. Further, activity in ureters segmented by peristalsis can mimic pathologic retroperitoneal nodes. FDG is not a useful tracer for the detection of primary bladder cancer.

Prostate and Testicular Cancer

The sensitivity of ^{18}F-FDG for detection of prostate cancer is poor (≈ 50% to 65%). Even aggressive prostate cancers can be ^{18}F-FDG negative. This may be due to the low glucose metabolism of well-differentiated or slowly growing cells. An additional problem is the marked urinary excretion and accumulation in the bladder of the ^{18}F-FDG, obscuring nearby minimal or moderate uptake. A major problem is that ^{18}F-FDG uptake is not specific and cannot distinguish between benign prostatic hyperplasia, prostate cancer, or postoperative scarring.

Other tracers have recently been proposed, including ^{11}C choline or ^{11}C acetate (Fig. 13–48). In early studies, ^{11}C-acetate appears to be significantly more sensitive than is ^{18}F-FDG but less specific because acetate accumulates substantially in hyperplasic tissue. Carbon-11 choline is known to be

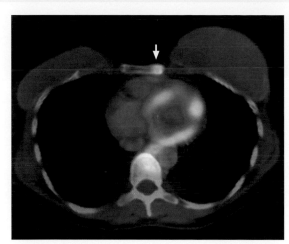

FIGURE 13–49. Skeletal metastases. A ^{18}F-FDG PET/CT fusion scan done in a patient with breast cancer shows a focus of increased activity (*arrow*) in a sternal metastasis.

more sensitive than is FDG-PET for imaging prostate carcinoma and shows promise in a number of clinical settings, especially for the detection of local recurrence. These tracers have the potential to notably impact therapy planning and assessing response to treatment.

The normal testes can show variable accumulation of FDG with SUVs ranging from about 1 to 6 and a mean of about 2.2. In testicular cancer, seminomas avidly use FDG, whereas other non-seminomatous germ-cell tumors can have variable uptake. Teratomas may demonstrate low FDG uptake, especially mature teratomas, and PET using FDG cannot reliably differentiate post-treatment scar tissue from residual disease in mature lesions.

Miscellaneous Tumors
Multiple Myeloma

Disease status in myeloma is often difficult to assess. Radionuclide bone scans are frequently insensitive to focal lesions. Although CT and MRI can identify lesions, they cannot differentiate active disease from inactive disease, post-treatment scarring, fractures, or benign lesions. Scans with ^{18}F-FDG can impact patient management by detecting sites of radiographically occult disease, recognizing disease progression, identifying extramedullary disease that worsens the patient's prognosis, and assessing success of localized skeletal radiation therapy. PET has shown to be useful in evaluating early-stage plasma cell dyscrasias (monoclonal gammopathy of undetermined significance), which may progress to multiple myeloma, to exclude the presence of more extensive disease.

Neuroblastoma

Neuroblastomas and their metastases often accumulate ^{18}F-FDG. However, radioiodine-labeled MIBG is still felt to be superior, particularly for detection of residual disease. Bone marrow involvement with neuroblastoma is often difficult to detect due to mild uptake and the presence of normal marrow activity.

Pheochromocytoma

PET agents, such as ^{18}F-fluorodopamine, ^{18}F-dihydroxyphenylalanine, and ^{11}C-hydroxyephedrine, have been shown to localize in pheochromocytomas.

Sarcomas

Soft-tissue sarcomas, Ewing's sarcomas, and rhabdomyoscarcomas show variable degrees of ^{18}F-FDG uptake.

Bone Metastases

Scans with ^{18}F-FDG PET have at least as good, if not better, sensitivity for detection of bone metastases (Fig. 13–49) as do ^{99m}Tc diphosphonates. The scans can be somewhat difficult to interpret because of variation in normal marrow activity and diffusely enhanced marrow activity after the administration of granulocyte-stimulating factors. False-positive studies can be caused by focal benign processes such as vertebral compression fractures or sacral insufficiency injuries. If the SUV is above two, malignancy should be suspected. Excellent quality images can also be obtained using sodium fluoride-^{18}F (Na^{18}F, not FDG) which has excellent sensitivity for detecting skeletal metastases.

Screening for Occult Tumors or Unknown Primary Tumors

The incidence of unknown primary tumors in oncologic patients is 0.5% to 7% at the time of initial diagnosis. In these cases the primary tumor is detected in less than 40% of patients by using conventional diagnostic procedures. Scanning with ^{18}F-FDG PET has been used to evaluate the origin of these neoplasms and can detect the primary tumor in about 40% of cases. Overall, ^{18}F-FDG PET has an intermediate specificity and high sensitivity in this setting. This is expected because although the procedure can easily identify many tumor types, there are a few common lesions (such as prostate cancer) that are not readily detected.

TABLE 13–13.   TNM Classification and Staging of Tumors Commonly Evaluated with PET ^{18}FDG Imaging*

STAGE	LARYNX	NASOPHARYNX	LUNG	BREAST	ESOPHAGUS	COLON/RECTUM	MELANOMA[†]
Primary tumor							
TX	Cannot be assessed	Same	Same	Same	Same	Same	Same
T0	No evidence of primary tumor	Same	Same	Same	Same	Same	Same
Tis	Cancer in situ	Same	Same	Same	Same	Same	Same or Clark's level I ≤0.75 cm (Clarks level II)
T1	Limited to one subsite of supraglottis with normal vocal cords	Limited to one subsite of nasopharynx	Tumor < 3 cm, surrounded by lung without evidence of invasion into main bronchus	≤2 cm	Invades Lamina propria or submucosa	Invades submucosa	
T1a	NA	NA	NA	≤0.5 cm	NA	NA	NA
T1b	NA	NA	NA	>0.5 but <1 cm	NA	NA	NA
T1c	NA	NA	NA	>1 cm but not > 2 cm	NA	NA	NA
T2	Limited to pharynx with vocal cord fixation or invades locally	Invades more than one subsite	>3 cm or involves main bronchus >2 cm from carina, invades pleura, or associated with atelectasis or pneumonia not involving entire lung	>2 cm but not >5 cm	Invades muscularis propria	Invades muscularis propria	>0.75 cm and not >1.5 mm or invades papillary-reticular dermal interface (Clark's level III)

T3	Limited to larynx with vocal cord fixation	Invades nasal cavity or oropharynx	Any size that invades chest wall, diaphragm, pericardium, mediastinal pleura, associated atelectasis, or pneumonia of entire lung or is <2 cm from but not involving carina	>5 cm	Invades adventitia	Invades through muscularis propria	>1.5 cm but not >4 cm in thickness and invades reticular dermis (Clark's level V)
T4	T4a, tumor invades through thyroid cartilage, into soft tissues, muscles, esophagus, thyroid T4b, tumor involves carotid, prevertebral space, or mediastinum	Invades skull or cranial nerves	Any size that invades mediastinum, heart, great vessels, trachea, esophagus, vertebral body, carina, or presents with malignant pleural effusion	Any size with extension to chest wall	Invades adjacent structures	Invades other organs or structures or peritoneum	>4 cm in thickness or invades subcutaneous tissue or satellites within 2 cm of primary tumor
Lymph nodes							
NX	Regional nodes cannot be assessed	Same	Same	Same	Same	Same	Same
N0	No nodal metastases	Same	Same	Same	Same	Same	Same
N1	Single ipsilateral node <3 cm	Same	Ipsilateral peribronchial or hilar lymph node involved	Metastases to movable ipsilateral axillary nodes	Regional nodal metastases	Metastases to 1–3 pericolic or perirectal nodes	Metastases ≤3 cm in any regional nodes

Continued

TABLE 13–13. TNM Classification and Staging of Tumors Commonly Evaluated with PET ^{18}FDG Imaging*—cont'd

STAGE	LARYNX	NASOPHARYNX	LUNG	BREAST	ESOPHAGUS	COLON/RECTUM	MELANOMA[†]
N2	Nodal involvement >3 but <6 cm	Same	Ipsilateral mediastinal or subcarinal nodes	Metastases to ipsilateral nodes fixed to other structures	NA	Metastases in four or more pericolic or perirectal nodes	Metastases >3 cm in regional nodes or in-transit metastases
N2a	Multiple ipsilateral nodes <6 cm	Same	NA	NA	NA	NA	Metastases >3 cm in regional node
N2b	Multiple contralateral nodes <6 cm	Same	NA	NA	NA	NA	In-transit metastases
N2C	Node >6 cm	Same	NA	NA	NA	NA	Both N2a and N2b
N3	NA	NA	Metastases in contralateral, mediastinal, or hilar nodes; scalene nodes; or supraclavicular nodes.	Metastases or ipsilateral internal mammary nodes	NA	Metastasis to any node along named vascular trunk or to apical node.	NA
Distant metastases							
MX	Cannot be assessed	Same	Same	Same	Same	Same	Same
M0	No distant metastases	Same	Same	Same	Same	Same	Same
M1	Distant metastases	Same	Same	Same	Same M1a, celiac or cervical nodes M2b, nonregional nodes or other distant sites	Same	Same M1a, metastases in skin, subcutaneous tissue, or beyond regional nodes M1b, visceral metastases

*Size refers to greatest dimension.
[†]Melanoma uses pathological classification (p).
NA, not applicable.

TABLE 13–14.   Staging of Solid Cancers

STAGE	LARYNX	NASOPHARYNX	LUNG	BREAST	ESOPHAGUS	COLON/RECTUM	MELANOMA
0	Tis N0M0	Tis N0M0	Tis N0M0	Tis N0M0	Tis N0M0	Tis N0M0	pTis N0M0
I	T1N0M0	T1N0M0		T1N0M0	T1N0M0	T1-2N0M0	pT1N0M0
IA			T1N0M0				pT1aN0M0
IB			T2N0M0				pT1aN0M0 pT2aN0M0
II	T2N0M0						
IIA		T2aN0M0	T1N1M0	T0N1M0 T1N1M0 T2N0M0	T2-3N0M0	T3N0M0	pT2bN0M0 pT3aN0M0
IIB		T1N1M0 T2aN1M0 T2bN0,N1,M0	T2N1M0 T3N0M0	T2N1M0 T3N0M0	T1-2N1M0	T4N0M0	pT3bN0M0 pT4aN0M0
IIC							pT4bN0M0
III	T1,T2N1M0 T3N0,N1,M0	T1N2M0 T2a,T2bN2M0, T3N0-2M0			T3N1M0 T4, any N, M0		Any pT N1,N2,N3,M0
IIIA			T1-2N2M0, T3N1-2M0 Any T, N3M0 T4, any N, M0	T0-3N2M0 T3N1-3M0		T1-2N1M0	pT1a-4a,N1a, N2a,M0
IIIB				T4N0-2M0		T3-4N1M0	pT1a-4a,N1b, 2b,2cM0 pT1b-4bN1a,2b,2c,M0
IIIC				Any T, N3M0		Any T, N2M0	pT1b-4b,N1b, 2b,M0
IV			Any T, any N, M1	Any T, any N, M1	Any T, any N, M1	Any T, any N, M1	Any pT, N3M0 Any pT, any N, M1
IVA	T1,T2,T3, N2M0 T4aN0,N1,N2,M0	T4N0-2M0			Any T, any N, M1a		
IVB	T4b, any N, M0 any T, N3M0	Any T, N3M0			Any T any N, M1b		
IVC	Any T, any N, M1	Any T, any N, M1					

TABLE 13–15.	Staging of Hodgkin's and Non-Hodgkin's Lymphoma		
STAGE	**EXTENT**	**STAGE**	**EXTENT**
I	Single lymph node region (I) or localized involvement of extralymphatic organ or site (I$_E$)		accompanied by localized involvement of an extralymphatic organ or site (III$_E$), by involvement of the spleen (III$_S$), or both
II	Two or more lymph node regions on the same side of the diaphragm (II) or localized involvement of a single extralymphatic organ or site and its regional nodes with or without involvement of other node regions on the same side of the diaphragm (II$_E$).	IV	Disseminated multifocal involvement of one or more extralymphatic organs or sites with or without associated lymph node involvement, or isolated extralymphatic organ involvement with distant (nonregional) nodal involvement
III	Lymph node regions on both sides of the diaphragm (III), may also be		

From Sobin LH and Wittekind C (eds): TNM Classification of Malignant Tumors, 6th Ed. New York, Wiley-Liss, 2002.

PEARLS & PITFALLS

With FDG scans of the brain, the cerebellum does not have the intense activity seen on SPECT perfusion scans.

Glucose metabolism patterns seen in dementias are nonspecific, although symmeticially decreased activity in temporoparieotal regions should suggest Alzheimer's, decreased frontal activity Pick's disease, and scattered decreased areas multi-infarct dementia.

With temporal lobe epilepsy, during a seizure there is a significant increase in glucose metabolism, and in between seizures there is hypometabolism.

Cardiac PET perfusion imaging is performed with ^{13}N-ammonia or ^{82}Rb, and metabolic or viability imaging is performed with ^{18}F-FDG.

Myocardial activity of ^{18}F-FDG decreases with fasting and increases with glucose or caffeine ingestion. The left ventricle switches back to fatty acid metabolism first at the apex, and this should not be mistaken for an apical infarct.

Abnormal ^{18}F-FDG activity may represent malignancy but is not pathognomonic and may represent inflammation, infection, or granulomatous disease.

Diffuse FDG activity may be seen in the thyroid, but focal activity should raise the suspicion of thyroid cancer.

Cancers that avidly accumulate FDG are larynx, esophagus, non–small-cell lung, colorectal cancer, melanoma and lymphoma.

Conversely, some malignancies do not accumulate ^{18}F-FDG well, such as prostate, carcinoid, and mucinous cancers.

An SUV above 2.5 is suggestive of malignancy but is not specific and should be used with caution.

Well-differentiated or mucinous tumors, carcinoid, and bronchoalveolar cell lung tumors may not be FDG-avid or may have SUVs well below 2.5.

Focal, often symmetric ^{18}F-FDG activity in the neck, supraclavicular, and axillary regions should raise the suspicion of brown fat, particularly in females and during cold weather. Linear areas in the neck and shoulders may be from tense muscles.

The limit of spatial resolution for PET scans is about 5 to 8 mm. Thus, primary or metastatic FDG-avid lesions smaller than this may be present but not visualized.

Diffusely increased bone marrow activity may occur following G-CSF therapy. Increased activity is often seen for months in body areas that received radiation therapy.

SUGGESTED READINGS

Aoki J, Watanabe H, Shinozaki T, et al.: FDG PET of primary benign and malignant bone tumors: SUV in 52 lesions, Radiology 219:774–777, 2001.

Bar-Shalom R, Yefremov N, Haim N, et al.: Camera-based FDG PET and ^{67}Ga SPECT in Evaluation of Lymphoma: Comparative Study. Radiology 227:353–360, 2003.

Blodgett TM, Fukui MB, Snyderman CH, Branstetter BF, McCook BM, Townsend DW, Metzler CC: Combined PET-CT in head and neck, part 1. physiologic, altered physiologic, and artifactual FDG uptake. RadioGraphics 25:897–912, 2005.

Crymes WB, Demos H, Gordon L: Detection of musculoskeletal infection with ^{18}F-FDG PET: Review of the current literature. J Nucl Med Technol 32:12–15, 2004.

Czernin J (ed): PET/CT: Imaging function and structure. J Nucl Med 45(Supplement 1), 2004.

Eubank WB, Mankoff DA, Vesselle HJ, Eary JF, et al.: Detection of Locoregional and Distant Recurrences in Breast Cancer Patients by Using FDG PET. RadioGraphics 22:5–17, 2002.

Ferdinand P, Gupta P, Kramer EL: Spectrum of Thymic Uptake at ^{18}F-FDG PET. RadioGraphics 24:611–1616, 2004.

Fukui MB, Blodgett TM, Snyderman CH, Johnson JJ, Myers EN, Townsend DW, Metzler CC: Combined PET-CT in head and neck, part 2. diagnostic uses and pitfalls of diagnostic usage. RadioGraphics 25:913–930, 2005.

Kapoor V, McCook BM, Torok FS: An Introduction to PET-CT Imaging. RadioGraphics 24:23–543, 2004.

Katrin D, Stumpe M, Notzli H, et al.: FDG PET for differentiation of infection and aseptic loosening in total hip replacements: comparison with conventional radiography and three-phase bone scintigraphy. Radiology 231:333–341, 2004.

Kazama T, Faria SF, Varavithya V, Phongkitkarun S, Ito H, Macapinlac HA: FDG PET in the Evaluation of Treatment for Lymphoma: Clinical Usefulness and Pitfalls. RadioGraphics 25:91–207, 2005.

Kostakoglu L, LAgress Jr H, Goldsmith SJ: Clinical Role of FDG PET in Evaluation of Cancer Patients. RadioGraphics 23:315–340, 2003.

Kostakoglu L, Goldsmith SJ: ^{18}F-FDG PET Evaluation of the Response to Therapy for Lymphoma and for Breast, Lung, and Colorectal Carcinoma. J Nucl Med 44:224–239, 2003.

Kostakoglu L, Hardoff R, Mirtcheva R, Goldsmith SJ: PET-CT Fusion Imaging in Differentiating Physiologic from Pathologic FDG Uptake. RadioGraphics 24:411–1431.

Langleben DD, Segall GM: PET in Differentiation of Recurrent Brain Tumor from Radiation Injury. J Nucl Med 41:1861–1867, 2000.

Positron Emission Tomography: part I. Semin Nucl Med 34:83–163, 2004.

Positron Emission Tomography: part II. Semin Nucl Med 34:164–240, 2004.

Positron Emission Tomography: part III. Semin Nucl Med 34:241–329, 2004.

Rohren E, Turkington T, Coleman R: Clinical applications of PET in oncology. Radiology 231:305–332, 2004.

Silverman DHS: Brain ^{18}F-FDG PET in the Diagnosis of Neurodegenerative Dementias: Comparison with Perfusion SPECT and with Clinical Evaluations Lacking Nuclear Imaging. J Nucl Med 45:594–607, 2004.

Skehan SJ, Brown AL, Thompson M, Young JEM, Coates G, Nahmias C: Imaging Features of Primary and Recurrent Esophageal Cancer at FDG PET. RadioGraphics 20:713–723, 2000.

Turkington T: Introduction to PET instrumentation. J Nucl Med Technol 29:4–11, 2001.

Wahl RL, Buchanan JW (eds): Principles and Practice of Positron Emission Tomography. Philadelphia, Lippincott, Williams & Wilkins, 2002.

Yat-Yin Y, et al.: Application of intravenous contrast in PET/CT: Does it really introduce significant attenuation correction error? J Nucl Med 46:283–291, Feb. 2005.

Legal Requirements and Radiation Safety

14

INTRODUCTION

Legal and regulatory requirements are important in daily operation of a nuclear medicine section or department. In 2002 there were revised federal regulations and rules regarding a number of issues but particularly required training and the content of that training. These regulations, which become final in 2005, are presented in this chapter. For most uses of nuclear medicine, 700 hours (4 months) of training is required. This is in contrast to the previous requirement of 6 months. The reader can review recent changes to legal requirements on the Web site reference at the end of this chapter.

Patient dosimetry from specific procedures can be found in Appendix E. Issues related to pregnancy and breast feeding are in Appendix G. Items related to release of radionuclide therapy patients are in Appendix H and emergency procedures for radioactive spills can be found in Appendix I.

REGULATORY AGENCIES

Radioactive materials and radioactive exposure are regulated by the U.S. Nuclear Regulatory Commission (NRC), other federal agencies, and the states. The NRC regulates special nuclear material (enriched uranium and plutonium), source material (uranium and thorium), and by-products. By-products are materials made radioactive by exposure to radiation in a nuclear reactor or from the

425

decay products of uranium and thorium. The NRC authority does not cover naturally-occurring radionuclides (such as radium) or accelerator-produced radioactive material; the individual states are responsible for possession and use of these materials. The states are also responsible for radiation-producing instrumentation such as x-ray machines and particle accelerators.

NRC regulations govern most nuclear medicine operations and include the Code of Federal Regulations (10 CFR Parts 20 and 35). Part 20 is concerned with standards for protection against radiation, including permissible dose limits, levels, concentrations, precautionary procedures, waste disposal, posting in radiation areas, and reporting theft of radioactive materials. Part 35 is concerned with the medical use of by-product material, including the ALARA (*as low as reasonably achievable*) program, licensing, required surveys, instrumentation, and training requirements.

Many states have an agreement with the NRC and accept the responsibility of regulating by-product, source, and special nuclear materials within their jurisdiction. These are "agreement states" (Fig. 14–1), and their regulations are at least as strict as those of the NRC. The agreement states regulate all sources of radiation in the state (with the exception of federally controlled sites, such as the Department of Veterans Affairs (VA) facilities and military bases).

The philosophy of a radiation protection program required by the NRC is that of ALARA. This is designed to keep radiation doses *as low as reasonably achievable*. To satisfy requirements of ALARA, administrative personnel, the radiation safety officer (RSO), and all authorized users must participate in an ALARA program as requested by the facility's radiation safety committee (RSC) or RSO. The program must also include notice to the workers of the program's existence and the worker's responsibility to participate in this philosophy.

TYPES OF LICENSES

NRC regulations describe two types of specific licenses for the medical use of by-product materials. There are specific licenses of broad-scope and specific licenses of limited scope. Broad-scope licenses are described in NRC regulations Part 33.11 and are usually reserved for large hospitals and academic institutions. There are type A, B, and C broad-scope licenses, depending on the amount of by-product material in possession. Type A broad-scope licensees are typically the largest licensed programs. Broad-scope licensees have significant decision-making authority and are not normally issued to a new licensee.

Part 35–specific licenses of limited scope are usually for small hospitals and office practices.

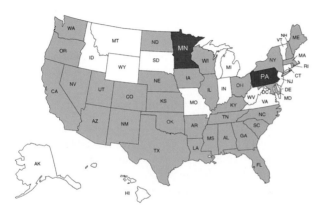

NRC States (15) □

Agreement States (33) ▨

NRC States that have expressed intent to sign Agreement (2) ■

* Idaho Agreement terminated April 26, 1991

FIGURE 14–1. Agreement states.

Human research is usually conducted under a broad-scope license but is also possible with a limited scope license. Specific Part 35 licenses are related to the particular use or uses of by-product materials, as addressed in the specific sections of the regulations as follows:

CFR 35.100—the use of radiopharmaceuticals for uptake, dilution, and excretion studies.

CFR 35.200—the use of radiopharmaceuticals, generators, and reagent kits for imaging and localization studies.

CFR 35.300—the use of radiopharmaceuticals for unsealed radiopharmaceutical therapy.

CFR 35.400—the use of radioisotope sealed sources in brachytherapy and for teletherapy.

CFR 35.500—the use of radioisotope sealed sources for diagnosis. This includes iodine-125 (^{125}I), americium-241 (^{241}Am), and gadolinium-153 (^{153}Gd) as a sealed source for bone mineral analysis and iodine-124 (^{124}I) for use in a portable imaging device.

There is also an NRC "Master Materials" license. Formerly the NRC issued individual licenses to VA medical centers. Under the master materials license, the VA is authorized to issue individual permits to each of its VA medical centers replacing the previous NRC licenses. The license requires use of NRC licensing and inspection criteria. Finally, there is a general in-vitro license for clinical or laboratory tests not involving administration of by-product material to humans.

DOSE LIMITS

NRC dose limits are shown in Table 14–1.

Occupational

Occupational dose is that received in the course of employment in which the individual's assigned duties involve exposure to radiation or radioactive material from licensed and unlicensed sources of radiation whether in the possession of the licensee or other person. Occupational dose does not include doses from natural background radiation, from medical exposures of the individual, from exposure to persons who have been administered radioactive material and released, from voluntary participation in medical research, or as a member of the public.

TABLE 14–1. **Nuclear Regulatory Commission Dose Limits (2004)**

A. Occupational exposures (annual)	
1. Whichever is more limiting:	
a. Total effective dose equivalent, or	5 rem (50 mSv)
b. Sum of deep dose equivalent and committed dose equivalent to any organ/tissue except lens of the eye (nonstochastic)	50 rem (500 mSv)
2. Eye dose equivalent	15 rem (150 mSv)
3. Shallow dose equivalent to skin/extremity	50 rem (500 mSv)
4. Minors (occupational under the age of 18 years)	10% of the above
B. Public exposure	
1. Total effective dose equivalent (annual)	0.1 rem (1 mSv)
2. Dose in unrestricted area (in any 1 hr)	2 mrem/hr (0.02 mSv/hr)
C. Embryo/fetus exposures	
1. Total dose equivalent (after pregnancy declared)	0.5 rem (5 mSv)
D. Planned special occupational exposure	
1. In any year	as in A, above
2. In individual's lifetime	5 × A, above
E. Required notification of NRC*	
1. Immediate (telephone)	
a. Total effective dose equivalent	25 rem (0.25 Sv)
b. Eye dose equivalent	75 rem (0.75 Sv)
c. Shallow dose equivalent	250 rem (2.5 Sv)
2. Within 24 hours (telephone)	
a. Total effective dose equivalent	5 rem (0.05 Sv)
b. Eye dose equivalent	15 rem (0.15 Sv)
c. Shallow dose equivalent	50 rem (0.5 Sv)
3. 30 days	any doses in excess of occupational, public, or embryo/fetus limits

*If in a Nuclear Regulatory Commission state. If in agreement state, reporting to the state may vary but is usually very similar.

A licensee must demonstrate that unmonitored individuals are not likely to receive, in 1 year, a radiation dose in excess of 10% of the allowable limits or they must monitor external and/or internal occupational radiation exposure.

Public

Public dose is that received by a member of the public from exposure to radiation or to radioactive material released by a licensee. Public dose does not include occupational exposure, any medical exposure the individual has received, exposure to natural background radiation, any medical exposure from another person who has received radioactive material and been released, or voluntary participation in biomedical research.

Embryo/Fetus

An embryo/fetus is subject to a dose equivalent limit of less than 0.5 rem (<5 mSv) during the entire pregnancy, due to occupational exposure of a woman who has declared her pregnancy. This is true even though the mother may be subject to higher occupational exposure limits in her employment. If the dose equivalent to the fetus is found to have exceeded 0.5 rem (5 mSv) or is within 0.05 rem (0.5 mSv) of this dose by the time the woman declares the pregnancy to the licensee, the licensee is in compliance as long as the additional dose equivalent to the embryo/fetus does not exceed 0.5 rem (5 mSv) during the remainder of the pregnancy.

Family and Caregivers

In 1997 the NRC amended its regulations for the release of patients receiving treatment with radioactive materials from an activity-based limit to a dose-based limit. The regulation was based on the maximally-exposed individual not being likely to exceed an effective dose equivalent of 0.5 rem (5 mSv) (see Appendix H). Compliance with the dose limit is demonstrated by using a default table for activity or dose rate or performing a patient-specific dose calculation. There is no specific guidance with regard to exposure of pregnant women, but it does indicate that written instructions have to be provided if a nursing child is likely to exceed an effective dose of 100 mrem (1 mSv).

RADIATION SAFETY OFFICER

With either a type A or B broad scope license, a radiation safety officer (RSO) is required who is responsible for implementing the radiation safety program and who ensures that activities are being performed in accordance with approved procedures and regulatory requirements.

The RSO must meet the training requirements (10 CFR Part 35.50) A, B or C and D and E listed below however an individual identified as a RSO on a broad scope permit or license before April 29, 2005 need not comply with these training requirements.

(A) Be certified by a specialty board whose certification process has been recognized by the NRC or Agreement State and who meets the requirements listed in (D) and (E) below. To have its certification process recognized, the specialty board must require that the candidate

(1)(i) Hold a bachelor's or graduate degree from an accredited college or university in physical science or engineering or biological science with a minimum of 20 college credits in physical science.

(ii) Have 5 or more years of professional experience in health physics (graduate training may be substituted for no more than 2 years of the required experience) including at least 3 years in applied health physics.

(iii) Pass an examination administered by diplomates of the specialty board, which evaluates knowledge and competence in radiation physics and instrumentation, radiation protection, mathematics pertaining to the use and measurement of radioactivity, radiation biology and radiation dosimetry.

or require that the candidate

(2)(i) Hold a master's or doctor's degree in physics, medical physics or other physical science, engineering or applied mathematics from an accredited college or university.

(ii) Have 2 years of full-time practical training and/or supervised experience in medical physics under the supervision of a certified medical physicist or in a clinical nuclear medicine facility under the direction of an authorized user physician.

(iii) Pass an examination administered by diplomates of the specialty board that assesses knowledge and competence in clinical diagnostic radiological or nuclear medicine physics and in radiation safety.

(B) Have completed a structured education program consisting of both 200 hours of classroom and laboratory training in radiation physics and instrumentation, radiation protection, radiation biology, mathematics pertaining to the use of measurement of radioactivity, radiation biology and radiation dosimetry *and* one year of full-time experience under an RSO including shipping, receiving, radiation surveys, using and performing checks for proper operation of instruments to determine the activity of dosages, survey meters and instruments used to measure radionuclides, securing and controlling byproduct material, using administrative controls to avoid mistakes in the administration of byproduct material, preventing contamination and using decontamination techniques, using emergency procedures to control byproduct material and disposing of byproduct material.

(C) (1) Is a medical physicist who has been certified by a specialty board whose certification process has been recognized by the Commission or an agreement state and has experience in radiation safety for similar types of use of byproduct material for which the licensee is seeking the approval of the RSO and who meets the requirements listed in (D) below or

(2) Is an authorized user, authorized medical physicist or authorized nuclear pharmacist identified on the license and has experience with the radiation safety aspects of similar types of use of byproduct material for which the individual has RSO and responsibilities.

and

(D) Has obtained written attestation signed by a preceptor RSO that the individual has completed the requirements in (E) and in paragraphs (A)1 i and ii or (B)1 or (C1) and has achieved a level of radiation safety knowledge sufficient to function independently as an RSO for a medical use licensee

and

(E) Has training in the radiation safety, regulatory issues and emergency procedures for the types of use for which a licensee seeks approval. This training requirement may be satisfied by completing training that is supervised by a RSO, authorized medical physicist, authorized nuclear pharmacist or authorized user who is authorized for the types of use for which the licensee is seeking approval.

The training and experience specified must have been obtained within 7 years preceding the date of application or the individual must have related continuing education and experience since the required training and experience was completed.

The licensee also needs to provide the RSO sufficient authority, organizational freedom, time, resources and management prerogative to 1) identify radiation safety problems, 2) initiate, recommend or provide corrective actions 3) stop unsafe operations and 4) verify implementation of corrective actions.

Duties of the RSO include investigating overexposures, accidents, and other mishaps and collecting or establishing written policies and procedures relative to purchasing, receipt and opening, storage, inventory, use, and disposal of by-product material. The RSO is also responsible for taking emergency action if control of by-product material is lost, disposing of by-product material, performing checks of survey instruments and other safety equipment, training personnel, performing radiation surveys, keeping copies of reports and policies, briefing management once each year, and establishing investigational levels of personnel exposure, which when exceeded initiate an investigation by the RSO. For up to 60 days each year a licensee may permit one or more authorized users or individuals qualified to be a RSO to function as an RSO.

AUTHORIZED MEDICAL PHYSICIST

An authorized medical physicist is an individual who is predominantly involved with high energy external beam radiotherapy, brachytherapy and stereotactic radiosurgery and who has little involvement with most diagnostic nuclear medicine operations. Specific training requirements can be found in 10 CFR Part 35.51.

AUTHORIZED NUCLEAR PHARMACIST

An authorized nuclear pharmacist is an individual who meets specific requirements and is so identified on the license or permit. The individual must (10 CFR Part 35.55)

A) Be certified by a specialty board whose certification process has been recognized by the NRC or Agreement State and who meet the requirements in (B)2 listed below. To have its certification process recognized, the specialty board must require that the candidate

1) Have graduated from a pharmacy program accredited by the American Council on Pharmaceutical Education of have passed the Foreign Pharmacy Graduate Examination Committee examination.

2) Hold a current, active license to practice pharmacy.

3) Provide evidence of having acquired at least 4000 hours of training/experience in nuclear pharmacy practice. Academic training may be substituted for no more than 2000 hours of the required training and experience and

4) Pass an examination in nuclear pharmacy administered by diplomates of the specialty board that assesses knowledge and competency in procurement, compounding, quality assurance, dispensing, distribution, health and safety, radiation safety, provision of information and consultation, monitoring patient outcomes, research and development or

B) 1) Have completed 700 hours in a structured educational program consisting of both a) 200 hours of classroom and laboratory training in radiation physics and instrumentation, radiation protection, mathematics pertaining to the measurement of radioactivity, chemistry of byproduct material for medical use, radiation biology and b) supervised practical experience in nuclear pharmacy involving shipping, receiving and performing radiation related surveys, using and performing checks for proper operation of instruments used to determine activity of dosages, survey meters and, if appropriate, instruments to measure alpha or beta emitting radionuclides, calculating, assaying and safely preparing dosages, using administrative controls to avoid medical events and minimizing contamination and

2) Has written attestation from a preceptor who is an authorized nuclear pharmacist that the individual has satisfactorily completed the requirements in section (A) 1-3 and (B)1 above.

The training and experience specified must have been obtained within 7 years preceding the date of application or the individual must have related continuing education and experience since the

required training and experience was completed. An individual identified as a nuclear pharmacist on a broad scope permit or license before April 29, 2005 need not comply with the above training requirements.

AUTHORIZED USER

An authorized user is a licensed physician (medical or osteopathic), dentist or podiatrist who meets specific requirements and is so identified on the license or permit. Other persons may work with byproduct material under the supervision of an authorized user. Training requirements for an authorized user vary depending on the type of procedure and are covered below. The training and experience specified must have been obtained within 7 years preceding the date of application or the individual must have related continuing education and experience since the required training and experience was completed. A physician, dentist or podiatrist identified as an authorized user on a broad scope permit or license before April 29, 2005 need not comply with the new training requirements as long as they perform only those medical uses for which they were authorized on that date.

RADIATION SAFETY COMMITTEE

Under NRC regulations, each medical institution with a type A broad-scope license is required to have a radiation safety committee (RSC). The committee membership must include an authorized user of each type of use permitted by the licensee—the RSO, a representative of the nursing service, and a representative of management who is not an authorized user or a RSO. Other members may be included as appropriate. Institutions with type B or C broad-scope licenses or those with program-specific licenses are not required to have an RSC.

The committee must meet at intervals not to exceed 6 months, and at a minimum at least half the members (including the RSO and management representative) must be present. Minutes must include the date of the meeting; a listing of those present and absent; summary of deliberations, discussions, and recommended actions; as well as ALARA program review. The committee is required to maintain a copy for the duration of the license.

The committee also reviews for approval or disapproval those who wish to become authorized users, the RSO, and or other staff members requiring approval. They also review audits, reviews, and inspections; evaluate the results; and specify necessary corrective actions. The committee must review every 6 months the summary of occupational radiation dose records and any health and safety issues or possible radiation safety program deviations from regulatory compliance or required practices. There must be an annual review of the radiation safety program. Other duties include review and approval of changes to training, equipment, physical plant or the facilities, radiation safety procedures, or practices. The RSC also has duties relative to research. They must evaluate human subject research and coordinate with the institutional review board to ensure that for research requiring ionizing radiation, the informed consent process has been followed.

TECHNICAL REQUIREMENTS
Dose Calibrators and Survey Instruments

If radiopharmaceuticals are prepared on-site, split or modified, the licensee must possess and use instrumentation to measure the activity of unsealed by-product material before it is administered to each patient. The instrument must also be calibrated according to nationally-recognized standards or manufacturer's recommendations. Survey instruments must also be calibrated before first use, annually and after repair. All scales with readings up to 1000 mrem (10 mSv) must be checked for accuracy by obtaining two separate readings on each scale, and the indicated exposure must be within 20% of the calculated exposure. Dates of calibration must be indicated on the instrument. Records of the above, including serial number of instruments, names of those performing the calibration, and dates, must be kept for 3 years.

Determination and Records of Dosages

The licensee needs to determine and record the administered activity of each dosage before medical use. For unit doses supplied by a commercial radiopharmacy, there must be direct measurement or a decay correction based on the activity determined by the licensed preparer. For other than unit doses, determination of activity must be made by direct measurement, combination of measurement and mathematical calculations, or combinations of volumetric measurements and mathematical calculations. Unless specified by the authorized user, a licensee may not use a dosage if it falls outside the prescribed dosage range or differs from the prescribed dosage by more than 20%.

Records of dosage determination must be retained for a period of 3 years and must contain the name of the radiopharmaceutical, patient's or subject's name or identification number, the prescribed dosage or a notation that the total activity is less than 30 µCi (1.1 MBq), date and time of administration of the dosage, and the name of the individual who determined the dosage.

Calibration, Transmission and Reference Sources

Any person authorized for medical uses of by-product material may receive, possess, and use by-product material for check, calibration, transmission, and reference use. This includes sealed sources not exceeding 30 mCi (1.11 GBq) provided or redistributed in original packing by a licensed manufacturer. Possession also includes by-product material with a half-life of not longer than 120 days in individual amounts not to exceed 15 mCi (0.56 GBq) or by-product material with a half life of longer than 120 days not to exceed the smaller of 200 µCi (7.4 MBq) or 1000 times the quantity in Appendix B of Part 30 of 10 CFR. One can also possess technetium 99m (^{99m}Tc) for these purposes in amounts as needed.

Labeling of Vials and Syringes

Each vial or syringe that contains unsealed by-product material must be labeled to identify the radiopharmaceutical. Each syringe shield and vial shield must also be labeled unless the label on the syringe or vial is visible when shielded.

Survey of Ambient Exposure Rate

The licensee is required to perform surveys with a radiation detection survey instrument at various intervals but at least once a month. Surveys must be done weekly in areas of radionuclide use or storage and waste storage. A daily survey must be done of all areas where by-product material requiring a written directive was prepared or administered. A daily survey is not required if the patient is confined to a hospital room. Records must include the instrument used, the name of the individual making the survey, and the date; these records must be retained for 3 years

Release of Individuals Containing Unsealed By-product Materials

A patient may be released if the total effective dose equivalent to any other individual is not likely to exceed 0.5 rem (5 mSv). If the total effective dose to any other individual is likely to exceed 0.1 rem (1 mSv), then the patient must be given instructions (including written) on actions to maintain doses to others following ALARA principles. If the total effective dose equivalent to a nursing infant or child is likely to exceed 0.1 rem (1 mSv), assuming there were no interruption of breast feeding, then instructions must also include guidance on discontinuation of breast feeding and potential consequences. See also Appendix G for further information.

Because of the threat of terrorism, radiation detectors have been installed in many airports, border crossings, public buildings, and even subways. These devices are very sensitive and can easily detect most nuclear medicine patients for several days (e.g., bone and thyroid scans), weeks (e.g., thallium-201 [^{201}Tl] cardiac scans), or even several months (e.g., therapies containing iodine-131 [^{131}I]) after the procedure. As a result the NRC has recommended that nuclear medicine patients be advised that they may set off alarms and that they receive written information for law enforcement use. It should contain (1) patient identification, (2) nuclear medicine facility contacts, and (3) a statement that the radiation received by the patient is allowed by NRC medical use regulations and poses no danger to the public with specifics to include the name and date of the nuclear medicine procedure, the radionuclide, its half-life, and administered activity.

TRAINING REQUIRED FOR USE OF UNSEALED BYPRODUCT MATERIAL
Uptake, Dilution and Excretion Studies: Written Directive Not Required

Except for quantities that require a written directive a licensee may use any unsealed byproduct material for uptake, dilution or excretion studies if it is obtained from a licensed manufacturer, prepared by an authorized nuclear pharmacist, is used by a physician who is an authorized user or used in accordance with a radioactive drug research committee or investigational new drug protocol accepted by the FDA.

An authorized user for these purposes is a physician who meets the specific requirements of (10 CFR Part 35.190)

A) Is certified by a medical specialty board whose certification process has been recognized by the NRC or an Agreement State and who meets the requirements listed in paragraph C) below. To have

its certification process recognized the specialty board shall require all candidates to have completed 60 hours of training and experience in applicable basic radionuclide handling techniques and radiation safety and passed an passed an examination of the specialty board or

B) Be an authorized user for imaging or therapeutic studies before October 24, 2005 or

C) Have completed 60 hours of training and experience, including a minimum of 8 hours of classroom and laboratory training in radionuclide handling techniques applicable to the use. The training must training in radiation physics and instrumentation, radiation protection, mathematics pertaining to the measurement of radioactivity, chemistry of byproduct material for medical use, radiation biology. There must also have been supervised work experience in ordering, receiving and unpacking radioactive materials and making necessary surveys, performing quality control procedures on instruments to determine activity of dosages and operation of survey meters, calculating, measuring and safely administering dosages, prevention of medical events and cleanup of spills and written attestation from a preceptor authorized user regarding fulfillment of requirements and the individual's ability to function independently for these uses.

Imaging and Localization Studies: Written Directive Not Required

Except for quantities that require a written directive a licensee may use any unsealed byproduct material for imaging and localization studies if it is obtained from a licensed manufacturer, prepared by an authorized nuclear pharmacist, or by a physician who is an authorized user for imaging or therapeutic studies that require a written directive before October 29, 2005 or who meets those requirements or an individual under the supervision of an authorized nuclear pharmacist or physician authorized user. The material also may be used in accordance with a radioactive drug research committee or investigational new drug protocol accepted by the FDA.

Training for this category requires that the authorized user be a physician who meets one or more of the following criteria (10 CFR Part 35.290)

A) Is certified by a medical specialty board whose certification process has been recognized by the NRC or an agreement state and who meets the requirements listed in paragraph C) below. To have its certification process recognized the specialty board shall require all candidates to have completed 700 hours of training and experience in applicable basic radionuclide handling techniques and radiation safety and passed an passed an examination of the specialty board which assesses knowledge and competence in radiation safety, radionuclide handling and quality control or

B) Was an authorized user of procedures requiring a written directive before October 24, 2005 and has experience with radiopharmaceutical preparation or

C) Has completed 700 hours of training and experience, including a *minimum* of 80 hours of classroom and laboratory training in basic radionuclide handling techniques applicable to use of unsealed byproduct material for medical use not requiring a written directive. The training must include at a minimum a) classroom and laboratory training in radiation physics, instrumentation, radiation protection, mathematics pertaining to the measurement of radioactivity, chemistry of byproduct material for medical use, radiation biology and b) supervised work experience under an authorized user of at least this level, in ordering, receiving and unpacking radioactive materials and making necessary surveys, calibrating instruments to determine activity of dosages and operation of survey meters, calculating, measuring and safely administering doses, prevention of medical events and cleanup of spills, elution of generator systems, testing the cluate for radionuclidic purity, preparing reagent kits with the eluate, administering radioactive materials to patients or research subjects *and* written attestation from a preceptor authorized user regarding fulfillment of requirements and the individual's ability to function independently for these uses.

Written Directive Required

A written directive is a written order by an authorized user for the administration of byproduct material or radiation from byproduct material to a specific patient or human research subject. A written directive must be dated and signed by an authorized user before the administration of ^{131}I sodium iodide greater than 30 µCi (1.11 MBq), any therapeutic dosage of unsealed byproduct material or any therapeutic dose of radiation from byproduct material. If the patient's life is in danger, the written directive can be delayed up to 48 hours. The written directive must include the patient's name, the dosage and route of administra-

tion. Copies of written directives must be retained for 3 years.

A licensee may use any unsealed byproduct material for medical use and for which a written directive is required if it is obtained from a licensed manufacturer, prepared by an authorized nuclear pharmacist, is used by a physician who is an authorized user or in accordance with a radioactive drug research committee or investigational new drug protocol accepted by the FDA.

Training for this category requires that the authorized user be a physician who meets one or more of the following criteria (10 CFR Part 35.390)

A) Is certified by a medical specialty board whose certification process has been recognized by the NRC or an agreement state and who meets the requirements listed in paragraph C) below. To have its certification process recognized the specialty board shall require all candidates to have successfully completed residency training in radiation therapy or nuclear medicine training program or in a related medical specialty. These programs must include 700 hours of training as described in paragraph C) and must be accredited by appropriate U.S. or Canadian authorities or

B) Was an authorized user of procedures requiring a written directive before October 24, 2005 or

C) Has completed 700 hours of training and experience, including a *minimum* of 200 hours of classroom and laboratory training in basic radionuclide handling techniques applicable to use of unsealed byproduct material for medical use requiring a written directive. The training must include at a minimum a) classroom and laboratory training in radiation physics, instrumentation, radiation protection, mathematics pertaining to the measurement of radioactivity, chemistry of byproduct material for medical use, radiation biology and b) supervised work experience under an authorized user of at least this level, in ordering, receiving and unpacking radioactive materials and making necessary surveys, calibrating instruments to determine activity of dosages and operation of survey meters, calculating, measuring and safely administering doses, prevention of medical events and cleanup of spills, administering of radioactive drugs to patients or research subjects *and* written attestation from a preceptor authorized user regarding fulfillment of requirements and the individual's ability to function independently for these uses.

The training (under item C above) also requires training in administering doses to a minimum of three patients/subjects in each of the following categories for which the user is requesting user status 1) oral administration of less than or equal to 33 mCi (1.22 GBq) of sodium iodide-131 for which a written directive is required, 2) administration of greater than 33 mCi (1.22 GBq) of sodium iodide-131, 3) parenteral administration of any beta emitter or photon emitting radionuclide with an energy of less than 150 keV; for which a written directive is required and or 4) parenteral administration of any other radionuclide for which a written directive is required. There also must be written attestation regarding competency from a preceptor authorized user who meets all the training requirements or was an authorized user of this type before October 24, 2005.

For those procedures requiring a written directive, the licensee must have procedures to assure with high confidence that the patient's or subject's identity is verified, that the administration is in accordance with the patient's treatment plan and that manual and/or computer generated dose calculations have been performed prior to dosage administration.

Safety instruction also must be provided initially and at least annually to personnel caring for patients or research subjects who cannot be released in the guidance contained in Appendix G. The training must include issues related to patient and visitor control, contamination and waste control and notification of the RSO. Records of this training must be kept for 3 years. When patients cannot be released due to the amount of radioactivity or ambient dose rate, the patient must be in a private room with a private sanitary facility. Two such patients however, may be in the same room. The door to the room must have a radioactive materials sign and there must be an indication as to how long visitors may stay. The RSO must be notified if the patient has a medical emergency or dies.

Oral Administration of ^{131}I-sodium Iodide

These sections refer to those users (such as endocrinologists) who only wish to use ^{131}I for therapeutic purposes and who are not engaged in other nuclear medicine practice. In the first section, the use would be for treatment of hyperthyroidism, and the second section would be predominantly for those who wish to treat thyroid cancer.

Less than or equal to 33 mCi (1.22 GBq) iodine-131

The training requirements (10 CFR Part 35.392) are similar to those described above to be an authorized user for procedures requiring a written directive except that the required training is only 80 hours, and except for the general categories of training curriculum subjects, the training is specific to ^{131}I-sodium iodide. Oral administration to three patients or research subjects of less than or equal to 33 mCi (1.22 GBq) ^{131}I are required as a part of the training.

Greater than 33 mCi (1.22 GBq) iodine-131

Training (10 CFR Part 35.394) for users in this category is as specified in the preceding paragraph except that the training must include three patients or research subjects who have been orally administered more than 33 mCi (1.22 GBq) ^{131}I.

TRAINING FOR SEALED SOURCES FOR DIAGNOSIS

An authorized user of sealed sources for diagnosis must be a physician, dentist, or podiatrist who (1) is certified by a specialty board that includes the following as part of the training or (2) has had 8 hours of classroom and laboratory training in handling techniques specific to the device to be employed. Training must include radiation physics and instrumentation, radiation protection, mathematics pertaining to the use and measurement of radioactivity, radiation biology, and training in the use of the device for the uses requested.

PERMISSIBLE MOLYBDENUM CONCENTRATION

A licensee may not administer a radiopharmaceutical that contains more than 0.15 µCi (55 kBq) of molybdenum-99 (^{99}Mo) per mCi (MBq) of ^{99m}Tc. Persons using ^{99}Mo/^{99m}Tc generators are required to measure the ^{99}Mo concentration in the first eluate after receiving the generator. Records must include the ^{99}Mo/^{99m}Tc ratio, time and date of the measurement, and the name of the individual who made the measurement. The record must be retained for 3 years.

MEDICAL EVENTS AND REQUIRED REPORTING

Medical events occur when a patient intervention using by-product material results in unintended radiation exposure. Formerly the term "misadministration" was used, although it was defined some-what differently. A medical event must be reported if it is:

A.
   1. A dose that differs from the prescribed dose or dose that would have resulted from the prescribed dose by more than
   5 rem (0.05 Sv) effective dose equivalent, or
   50 rem (0.5 Sv) to an organ, tissue or
       shallow dose equivalent to the skin
       and
       the total dose delivered differs from the prescribed dose by 20% or more, or
       the total dosage delivered differs from the prescribed dosage by 20% or more or falls outside the prescribed dose range, or
       the fractionated dose delivered differs from the prescribed dose, for a single fraction by 50% or more
   2. A dose that
   exceeds 5 rem (0.05 Sv) effective dose equivalent, or
   50 rem (0.5 Sv) to an organ, tissue, or shallow dose equivalent to the skin
   from any of the following:
       —an administration of a wrong radioactive drug containing by-product material,
       —an administration of a radioactive drug containing by-product material by the wrong route of administration,
       —an administration of a dose or dosage to the wrong individual or research subject,
       —an administration of a dose or dosage by the wrong mode of treatment, or
       —a leaking sealed source
   3. A dose to the skin or an organ or tissue other than the treatment site that exceeds by 50 rem (0.5 Sv) to an organ or tissue and 50% or more of the dose expected from the administration defined in the written directive.
B. Any event resulting from intervention of a patient or human research subject in which the administration of by-product material or radiation from by-product material results or will result in unintended permanent functional damage to an organ or a physiological system, as determined by a physician.

For any of the above, the licensee in an NRC state must notify by telephone the NRC operations center no later than the next calendar day after the discovery of the medical event. In addition, a written report must be submitted to the NRC regional office within 15 days after the discovery of the medical event. The report must include the licensee's and prescribing physician's name; a description of the event; what effect occurred if any; why the event occurred and subsequent actions taken; and certification that the individual or relative was notified and, if not, why not. The name or identifying information of the exposed individual is not to be included. The referring physician and the exposed individual also must be notified within 24 hours or as soon as possible unless the referring physician indicates that he or she will inform the person or responsible relative or guardian unless the referring physician based on medical judgment feels that telling the individual would be harmful. A copy of the report to the NRC with the patients names added must be provided to the referring physician no later than 15 days after discovery of the event. A record of the medical event is not required to be retained, although it is probably a good idea. If a licensee is in an agreement state, the report is made to appropriate regulatory agency in that state. In the VA, reports are made by the hospital to the central VA office under their Master Materials license.

Reports and notification must also be made in circumstances of an unintended dose to an embryo/fetus or a nursing child that is greater than 5 rem (0.05 Sv) dose equivalent, resulting from administration of a by-product material to the mother or from external radiation from a by-product material. Notification and reports are not required if the dose was specifically approved in advance by the authorized user. Reporting requirements are almost identical to those described for a medical event.

MAINTENANCE OF RECORDS

Required records must be kept for various specified periods of time and are specified in 10 CFR Part 35, subpart K. They must be legible for the entire period, and there must be provisions to prevent loss or tampering. Records may be kept in electronic format. A copy of the authorities, duties and responsibilities of the RSO (with signatures of the RSO and management), and records of procedures for administrations requiring a written directive must be kept for the duration of the license. Records of actions taken by management relative to the radiation protection program need to be kept for 5 years. Most other records need to be kept for 3 years.

TRANSPORTATION OF RADIOACTIVE MATERIALS

Interstate transportation of radioactive materials usually is controlled by regulations of the Department of Transportation (DOT). The NRC requires that DOT regulations be observed when radiopharmaceuticals are returned to a manufacturer or transported between offices, laboratories, or hospitals, with the exception of materials transported by a physician for medical practice.

The DOT has assigned hazard levels to radionuclides based on their toxicity. Transport group I is reserved for very hazardous radionuclides, such as plutonium-239 (^{239}Pu) and americium-241 (^{241}Am), whereas transport group VI includes radionuclides of very low hazard, such as uncompressed krypton-85 (^{85}Kr) gas. Radionuclides used in nuclear medicine are in transport groups III and IV.

The type and amount of radionuclide determine the hazard level of the material and therefore the type of packaging required. Packaging of medical radionuclides is of two common forms: type A packaging is designed to prevent loss or disbursement of a limited amount of radioactive material under normal conditions during transport. Type B packaging is for higher-activity radioactive material and is more accident-resistant than is type A packaging.

Packages of radioactive materials must be labeled according to one of the three following categories:

Radioactive-white I. No special handling is required. Surface dose rate must not exceed 0.5 mrem/hour (5 μSv/hour).

Radioactive-yellow II. Special handling is required. Surface dose rate may not exceed 50 mrem/hour (0.5 mSv/hour), and dose rate may not exceed 1 mrem/hour (10 mSv/hour) at 3 feet from any external surface.

Radioactive-yellow III. Surface dose rate may not exceed 200 mrem/hour (2 mSv/hour), and dose rate may not exceed 10 mrem/hour (100 mSv/hour) at 3 feet from any external surface.

The transportation index is the number of millirems per hour measured at 3 feet from the package. Thus, any package with a transportation index from greater than 1 to 10 would be required to have a radioactive-yellow III label.

RECEIPT OF RADIOACTIVE SHIPMENTS

When any package of radioactive material is received, it should be checked for contamination and leakage. Its receipt should be noted in a log, and then the package should be stored in an appropriate shielded area. Although many materials being received at a nuclear medicine laboratory are not required to be monitored, it is certainly a good idea to do so. Packages that require radioactive labels must be monitored. Dose rate and contamination monitoring are required if activities are greater than Type A amounts or if there has been degradation of package integrity. Most packages being received in nuclear medicine departments are not in excess of Type A activities. These are typically in the range of curies (TBq). If such a package is received, it must be monitored within 3 hours of receipt or within 3 hours of the next business day.

To perform a contamination survey, absorbent paper is usually wiped over an area of about 300 cm^2 and counted. Removable contamination in excess of 6600 disintegrations/minute over 300 cm^2 requires notification of the appropriate agency. An external measurement also should be made, and for transportation index greater than 10 (yellow III label), the dose rate at the surface cannot exceed more than 200 mrem/hour (2 mSv/hour). A shipment of arriving radioactive material should be recorded in both a receiving report and the radionuclide logbook. The receiving report should indicate the shipment identification, including supplier, radionuclide and lot number, measured radiation level, results of surface and internal package wipes for removable contamination, and amount and type of radionuclide as indicated by the manufacturer, as well as the nuclear medicine laboratory confirmation of this. Each entry into the logbook should be recorded on a separate page. The inventory record (radiopharmaceutical logbook) should indicate all records of bulk dilutions, use, and disposal, so that all of the radionuclide may be accounted for.

PREPARATION AND ADMINISTRATION OF RADIOPHARMACEUTICALS

Unshielded radioactive materials should never be picked up directly with the fingers because very high doses may result. Instead, these materials should be handled with clamps, forceps, or other holding devices. When time and distance are not adequate or practical for radiation protection, shielding must be used. It is important to remember that when dealing with beta radiation, a shield should be made of a low-atomic-number material. If a high-atomic-number material, such as lead, is used, the interaction between the beta particles and the lead may cause the emission of bremsstrahlung radiation, which is highly penetrating.

When using ^{99m}Tc, lead shielding is sufficient. The half-value layer, which is the amount of lead required to reduce the radiation exposure by half, is 0.2 mm of lead for ^{99m}Tc. A thickness of 2.5 mm of lead attenuates radiation from ^{99m}Tc by a factor of about 1000. Radionuclides with more energetic gamma rays may require much more shielding.

Shielding is of two general types: (1) benchtop shields and (2) syringe or vial shields. Benchtop shields are frequently constructed of lead bricks and usually have a viewing portal of lead glass to shield the face and eyes. Direct handling of unshielded thin-walled plastic syringes containing short-lived radionuclides can cause skin exposure in the range of 500 to 1000 mrad/hour/mCi (0.14 to 0.27 mGy/hour/MBq). Although brief handling of unshielded radionuclides is usually well within permissible limits, syringe shields reduce exposure levels by a factor of at least three.

Syringe shields should be used when preparing a radiopharmaceutical kit or performing a radiopharmaceutical injection unless the use of the shield is contraindicated for that patient. It is not necessary to use a syringe shield for drawing up a dose. If vials are used, the vials must be kept in radiation shields, and the shield must be labeled with the radiopharmaceutical name.

Because the basis of imaging procedures is the detection of radiation emanating from the patient, the patient is by definition a source of exposure. Estimates of typical exposure to technologists from standard imaging procedures range from 0.4 mrem to 3 mrem (4 to 30 μSv)/hr (Table 14–2). Between 50% and 90% of the dose technologists receive usually comes from being with the patient while the patient is imaged rather than from the radiopharmaceutical preparation, assay, or injection. Although radiation from the patient constitutes a measurable level, these levels are not high enough to be used as an excuse to keep the technician and physician from providing the patient with the best medical care.

For diagnostic clinical procedures, it is not necessary to follow the package inserts in the use of a radiopharmaceutical. The only restriction is that the chemical form must not be changed. This allows the authorized user to administer an approved radiopharmaceutical to patients in a different physical state, such as gas instead of liquid; by a different route of administration; or in a different administered activity without filing a notice of claimed investigational exemption for a new drug.

RESTRICTED AREAS, RADIATION AREAS, AND POSTING

Nuclear medicine laboratories are generally divided into restricted and nonrestricted areas. Examples of unrestricted areas are offices, file space, patient waiting areas, and nonradiation laboratory space. These areas must have dose rates of less than 2 mrem/hour (20 μSv/hour) and of less than 100 mrem (1 mSv) over 7 consecutive day's total. If these limits are exceeded, control of the area is required. A restricted area is one in which the occupational exposure of personnel is under the supervision of a person in charge of radiation protection. Access to the area is restricted, and working conditions within it are regulated. Restricted areas are not accessible to the general public. Examples of restricted areas are those dedicated to radiopharmaceutical preparation, dispensing, administration, and storage areas, as well as the imaging area.

A "radiation area" is one that has levels that could result in dose equivalent in excess of 0.005 rem or 5 mrem (0.05 mSv) in 1 hour at 30 cm from the radiation source. A "high radiation area" is one in which there are levels that could result in dose equivalent of over 0.1 rem or 100 mrem (1 mSv) in 1 hour at 30 cm from the source. All radiation areas require posting with a conspicuous sign. Posting is also required for areas where there is likely to be airborne radioactivity. Areas where licensed radioactive material is used or stored must have a "caution radioactive materials" sign. If a patient who has received radioactive material is in a hospital room and that patient could have been legally released (based on activity or dose rate levels) posting is not required.

SURVEYS

Typical radiation detection instruments generally measure either beta or gamma radiation. Only a

TABLE 14–2.   Approximate Radiation Dose Rates at 1 m from Nuclear Medicine Patients

STUDY	RADIOPHARMACEUTICAL	ADMINISTERED ACTIVITY, mCi (MBq)	TIME AFTER ADMINISTRATION, hr	DOSE RATE, mrad/hr (μGy/Hr)
Bone	^{99m}Tc-MDP	20 (740)	0	0.9 (9)
		20 (740)	3	0.35 (3.5)
Blood pool	[99m]Tc red blood cells	20 (740)	0	1.4 (14)
CSF	^{111}In-DTPA	(18.5)	0	0.08 (0.8)
Heart	^{201}Tl-chloride	20 (740)	0	2 (20)
	^{99m}Tc-sestamibi	20 (740)	0	0.9 (9)
Liver	[99m]Tc sulfur-colloid	4 (148)	0	0.2 (2)
Tumor/Infection	[67]Ga citrate	3 (111)	0	0.35 (3.5)
Tumor	^{18}F-FDG	10 (370)	0	30 (300)
	^{18}F-FDG	10 (370)	1	5 (50)
Thyroid cancer therapy	^{131}I-sodium-iodide	100 (3700)	0	22 (220)
	^{131}I-sodium-iodide	100 (3700)	12	12 (120)
	^{131}I-sodium-iodide	100 (3700)	24	11 (110)
	^{131}I-sodium-iodide	100 (3700)	72	1.8 (18)

[99m]Tc, technetium-99m; MDP, methylene diphosphonate; ^{111}In, indium-111; DTPA, diethylenetriaminepenta acetate; ^{201}Tl, thallium-201; ^{67}Ga, gallium-67; ^{18}F-FDG, fluorine-18 fluorodeoxyglucose.

Adapted from Sources and magnitude of occupational and public exposures from nuclear medicine procedures, report no. 124. Bethesda, Maryland, National Council on Radiation Protection and Measurements, 1996.

very sophisticated and expensive piece of equipment can measure alpha particles. The most common piece of survey equipment found in a nuclear medicine department is a Geiger-Müeller counter. These survey instruments are usually capable of measuring absorbed dose rates from about 1 to 500 mrad (10 μGy to 5 mGy) per hour. They are useful for detecting small amounts of contamination on people or on laboratory surfaces. These instruments also can be used to provide an estimate of dose rate at a particular distance from a patient who has received a radionuclide. If dose rates in excess of 500 mrad (5 mGy) per hour are expected, an ionization chamber, such as a "cutie pie," is necessary. Such an instrument is most useful in monitoring patients who have received higher levels of radionuclides, such as for therapeutic purposes.

A licensee possessing sealed sources must leak test the source every 6 months. If more than 0.005 μCi (185 Bq) of removable activity is on a wipe sample, the source is said to be leaking. This procedure is not required if the materials (1) have less than a 30-day half-life, (2) are gases, or (3) consist of less than 100 μCi (3.7 MBq) of beta- or gamma-emitting radionuclide. It is also not required of alpha-emitting radionuclides of less than 10 μCi (0.37 MBq) or sources stored and not being used. Semiannual inventory of all sealed sources and survey of all stored materials in sealed sources are required.

Surveys for contamination and ambient radiation exposure are covered in NRC guidelines CFR 20.1101, 20.1402, and 35.70. A licensee is required to survey all areas in which radiopharmaceuticals requiring a written directive are prepared and administered at the end of each day (except where patients are confined and cannot be legally released). In addition, for procedures requiring a written directive, if the patient is kept in the hospital, items removed from a patient's room must either be monitored or treated as radioactive waste.

Survey records must also contain the instrument used to make the survey and the initials of those persons performing such a survey. In addition, if a licensee uses radioactive gases, there is a requirement to check the operation of the traps or collecting systems each month and to measure ambient ventilation rates in areas of use every 6 months. Areas in which radioactive gas is used must be designed to provide negative pressure, and the licensee must calculate and post the time needed after a spill of radioactive gas to reduce the concentration in the room to the occupational limit. A record of the calculations and assumptions must be retained as long as the area is utilized.

WASTE DISPOSAL

The following methods are available for radioactive waste disposal:

Transfer to an authorized commercial facility for burial. Waste must be packaged and shipped according to appropriate regulations.

Burial. Burial in the soil may be approved by the NRC or an agreement state. This method is usually not available to nuclear medicine laboratories.

Return to Supplier. Some nuclear medicine laboratories return residual spent dosages, contaminated syringes, and multidose vials to the supplying commercial radiopharmacy for disposal. In this case the hospital should have a written agreement with the supplier that they will accept the responsibility of being the shipper for the return. If this is not done, the hospital will be held responsible for all DOT and NRC shipping requirements.

Release into sewer system. If the material is readily soluble or dispersible in water, it may be released in the following amounts:

Ten times the limit specified in Appendix C of 10 CFR 20, or the quantity of radioactive material that, when diluted by the average daily amount of liquid released by the hospital into the sewer system, results in an average concentration not greater than the amount specified in Appendix B, table 3, column 2 of 10 CFR 20. The greater of these two values is permitted.

Monthly. The amount of radioactive material that when diluted by the average monthly total amount of liquid released into the sewer system results in an average concentration of not greater than the amount specified in Appendix B, table 1, column 2 of 10 CFR 20.

Yearly. A total of not more than 1 Ci (37 GBq) of NRC-licensed or other accelerator-produced materials.

Excreta from people who have received radioactive materials for medical diagnosis or therapy is not regulated by the NRC.

Decay in Storage. A licensee may hold by-product material with a physical half-life of less than 120 days for decay in storage before disposal without regard to the amount of radioactivity if (1) monitoring at the surface cannot distinguish any difference from natural background, and (2) labels are removed or obliterated and a record of each disposal is maintained for 3 years.

Venting. Many nuclear medicine laboratories use xenon-133 (^{133}Xe) for pulmonary ventilation studies. Although direct venting into the atmosphere of certain amounts of this material is permissible (for limits, see CFR Part 20.1101d) and gives the least dose to the technologists, it often requires physical plant remodeling for adequate air flow. Another means of disposing of ^{133}Xe is storage and decay using commercially available, activated charcoal traps. Radioactive gases can only be administered in rooms that are at negative pressure compared to the surrounding rooms.

Other Disposal Methods. Methods such as incineration may be approved by the NRC for disposal of research animals or organic solvents containing radioactive materials. Such disposal must comply with existing applicable state and local regulations.

PEARLS AND PITFALLS

All packages with radioactive labels must be monitored for surface contamination upon receipt. If the package is damaged or contains very large activities (in excess of Type A DOT amounts) both contamination and dose rate monitoring are necessary.

The amount of activity in a diagnostic unit dose from a radiopharmacy does not need to be measured and can be calculated from the labeled activity and decay time. If doses are prepared in-house or unit doses are modified or split, the activity must be measured in a dose calibrator.

Typical dose rates to the hands from holding radiopharmaceutical syringes range from 0.5–1.0 rad/hr/mCi (0.14–0.27 mGy/hr/MBq). Syringe shields are recommended and usually reduce the dose by a factor of about 3. All vials, syringes and syringe shields must be labeled with the radiopharmaceutical name unless the label can be seen through the shield.

Typical doses from patients soon after injection of most diagnostic radiopharmaceuticals at 1 meter are about 1 mrem (10 µSv)/hr but for ^{18}F-FDG patients the dose rate is 5–30 mrem (50–300 µSv)/hr. From iodine-131 therapy patients, the dose rates are about 5–30 mrem (50–300 µSv)/hr for hyperthyroidism and cancer respectively.

Annual occupational dose limits are 5 rem (50 mSv) effective dose, 50 rem (0.5 Sv) to any organ or tissue and 15 rem to (150 mSv) the eye. Public dose limits are 0.1 rem (1 mSv) annually or 2 mrem (20 µSv)/hr. The fetal dose limit is 0.5 rem (5 mSv) after the pregnancy is declared.

Personal dosimeters need to be used on individuals who are likely to receive in excess of 10% of the allowable occupational dose limits.

A written directive is not required for most diagnostic procedures. A written directive is required for diagnostic procedures exceeding 30 µCi (1.1 MBq) of iodine-131 and all therapy procedures. Daily surveys are required in areas where written directive procedures are administered and performed.

A medical event refers to a patient intervention that results in unintended radiation exposure. For nuclear medicine this generally means that there was an effective dose in excess by 5 rem (50 mSv) or an absorbed dose in excess by 50 rem (0.5 Sv) to a tissue or organ *and* 1) which differs from the prescribed dose by 20% or more *or* 2) that the excess dose was caused by administration of the wrong radiopharmaceutical, the wrong route of administration or to the wrong patient. The NRC must be notified of a medical event and a written report filed.

Release of nuclear medicine patients can be done under NRC regulations based upon a certain amount of administered activity or dose rate (e.g. 33 mCi [1.2 GBq] or less of iodine-131 or 7 mrem [70 µSv]/hr or less at 1 meter for iodine-131). Patients also can be can be released with much higher activities based on patient specific calculations and if the effective dose to a maximally exposed other person is not likely to exceed 0.5 rem (5 mSv).

Breast-feeding cessation is not regulated but there are guidelines. Cessation is not needed for ^{18}F-FDG and cessation times for technetium radiopharmaceuticals range from 0–24 hours. Breast feeding is usually discontinued for a week or more for thallium-201, gallium-67 and indium-111 pharmaceuticals. Breast feeding is contraindicated for several months after radioiodine therapy (see appendix G).

PEARLS & PITFALLS—cont'd

Major radiation spills are based on activity released (greater than 100 mCi [3.7 GBq] of ^{99m}Tc or ^{210}Tl, 10 mCi [370 MBq] of ^{67}Ga and ^{111}In and 1 mCi [37 MBq] of ^{131}I). For minor spills efforts should be directed at containment, decontamination and notification of the RSO. All major spills require the presence of the RSO (see Appendix I).

Radioactive materials can be stored and decayed. If the material no longer can be distinguished from background radiation it may be disposed of as in-house waste. Any generators or other material being returned to the supplier must meet DOT packaging and labeling requirements.

SUGGESTED READING

http://www.nrc.gov/reading-rm/doc-collections/cfr/.

http://www.doseinfo-radar.com/RADARDoseRiskCalc.html.

Radiation Protection for Medical and Allied Health Personnel, report no. 105. Bethesda, Maryland, National Council on Radiation Protection and Measurements, 1989.

Sources and magnitude of occupational and public exposures from nuclear medicine procedures, report no. 124. Bethesda, Maryland, National Council on Radiation Protection and Measurements, 1996

U.S.NRC. Consolidated Guidance about materials Licenses. Program-Specific Guidance About Medical Use Licenses NUREG-1556, Vol 9, Revision 1, May 2005 Washington D.C. This has model procedures and is available at www.nrc.gov.

Unknown Case Sets

The following case sets have been designed to test your overall knowledge in nuclear imaging. Each set contains 10 cases, and almost all sets have an example of central nervous system, thyroid, cardiac, respiratory, gastrointestinal, musculoskeletal, tumor, or abscess and positron emission tomography (PET) cases. This is a common testing format. You should be able to recognize most of the examinations, know the radiopharmaceutical used, understand the technique, give a differential diagnosis of one to three entities, and, in some cases,

discuss management. Table 1 in this Set may help you differentiate and recognize different types of whole body scans. You should be able to complete a set in about 20 to 25 minutes. By testing yourself on all the case sets, you will have covered many of the most common entities in nuclear medicine. Answers to all the cases and additional questions are given after case set 7. If you have trouble with a case, go back to the chapter and specific text on that topic and review it. Good luck.

| **TABLE 1.** | **Normal distribution of activity on various types of whole body scans** | | | | | | | |

RADIOPHARMACEUTICAL	LIVER	SPLEEN	GU	BOWEL	BONE MARROW	SALIVARY	THYROID	OTHER
^{18}F-FDG	+	+	+++	++ usually colon	+	+	+/−	Brain+++ Heart ++/− Larynx +/− Muscle +/−
^{111}In-WBC	++	+++			+			
^{99m}Tc WBC	++	+++	+	+	+			
^{67}Ga-citrate	++	+	+ 0 1 day	+++ usually colon	+	+		Lacrimal +/−
^{123,131}I sodium iodide	+		++	++ stomach, colon		+	If present or remnant	Nasal +
^{111}In-octreotide	++	+++	+++	+			+	
^{123,131}I-MIBG	+		+ +	+		+	+	Heart +, nasal +, lung +
^{99m}Tc-sulfur colloid	+++	++			+			
^{99m}Tc-sestamibi	+	+	+	++			+	Heart ++ Gallbladder
^{201}Tl-chloride	++	++	+	++		+		Muscle ++ Heart ++ Testis ++
^{99m}Tc-Neutrospec	+++	+++	+++		+			
^{131}I-NP-59	++			++				Gallbladder
^{111}In-Zevalin	++	++	+	+	+ 2–3 days			Blood pool 0–1 days

Adapted from table of Harry Agress Jr., M.D.

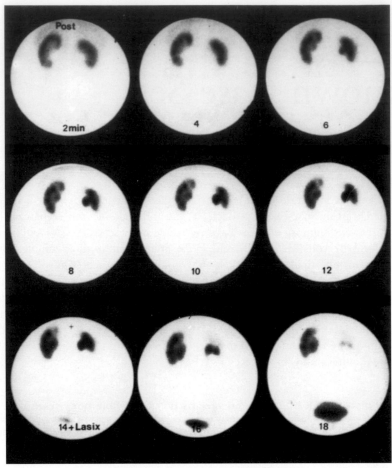

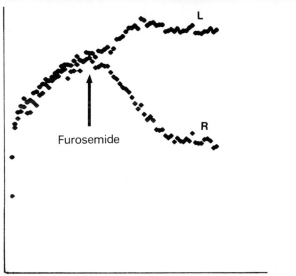

CASE 1–1.   Bilaterally dilated collecting system seen on ultrasound. Question obstruction.

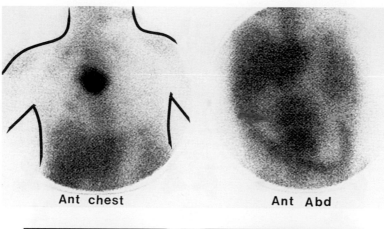

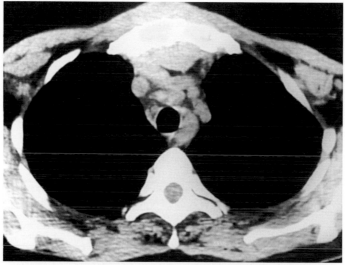

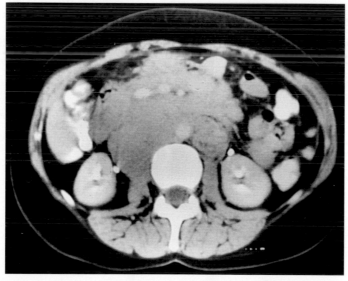

CASE 1–2.   Fever of unknown origin in a 14-year-old male.

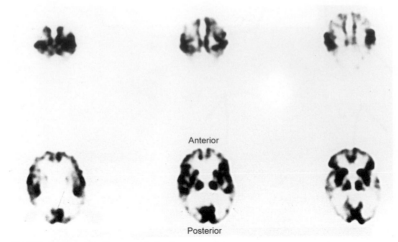

CASE 1–3.   Patient with dementia.

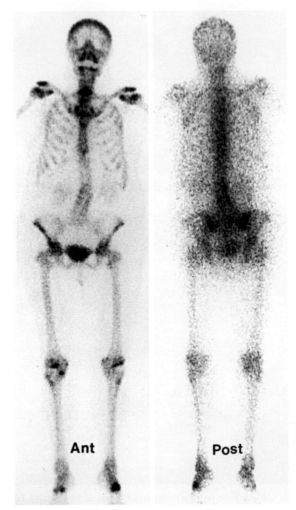

CASE 1–4.   Rule out metastatic disease.
Examination performed on a dual headed
gamma camera.

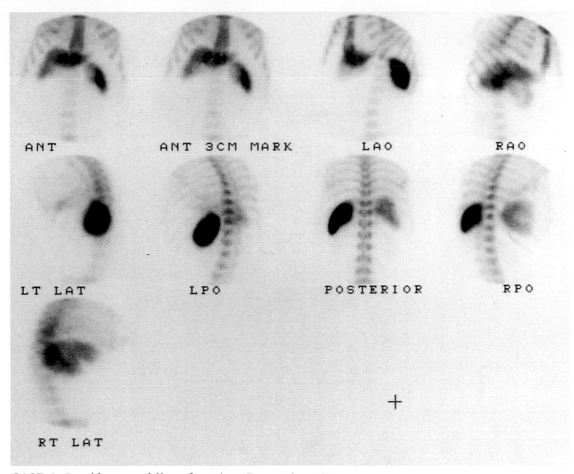

ANT   ANT 3CM MARK   LAO   RAO

LT LAT   LPO   POSTERIOR   RPO

RT LAT

CASE 1–5.   Abnormal liver function. Suspect hepatitis.

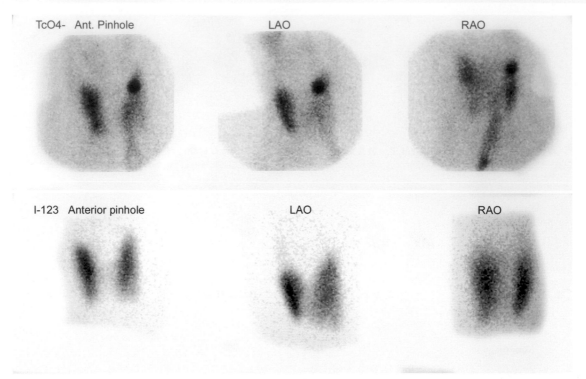

CASE 1–6. Suspected thyroid nodule palpated on annual physical examination.

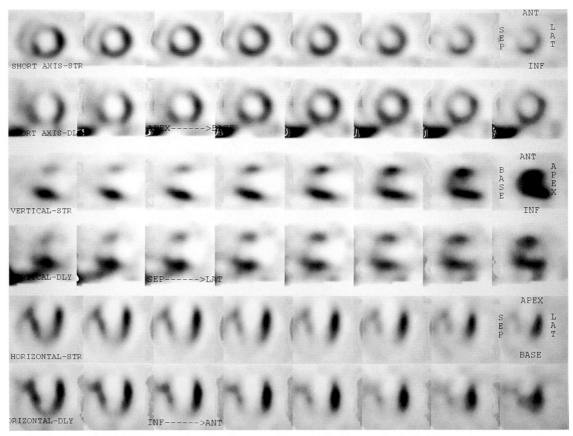

CASE 1–7. Man, 51 years, who is short of breath and has chest pain.

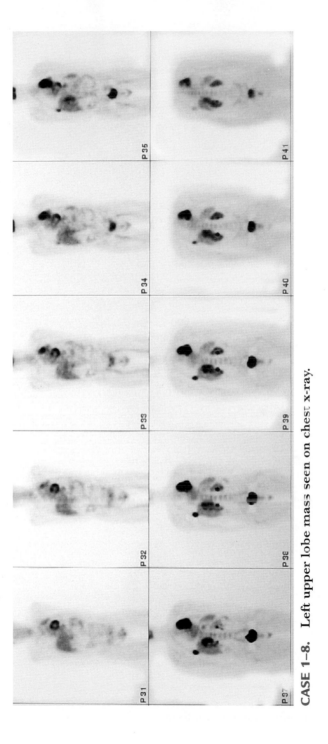

CASE 1–8.   Left upper lobe mass seen on chest x-ray.

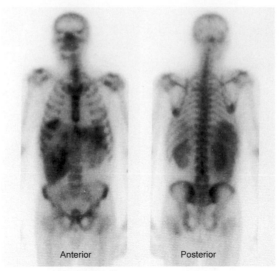

Anterior   Posterior

**CASE 1–9.   Rule out metastases in this
41-year-old woman.**

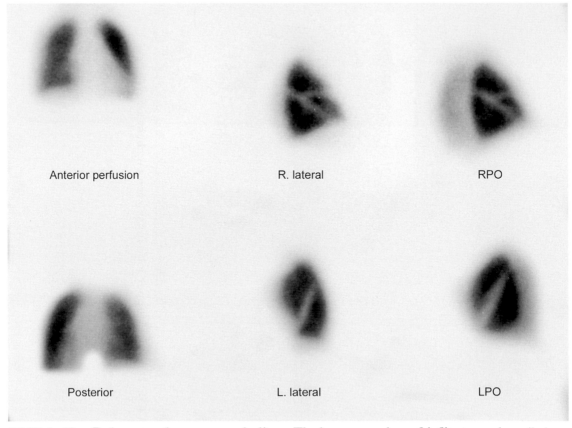

Anterior perfusion   R. lateral   RPO

Posterior   L. lateral   LPO

CASE 1–10.   Rule out pulmonary embolism. The lungs were clear of infiltrates and ventilation
scan was normal.

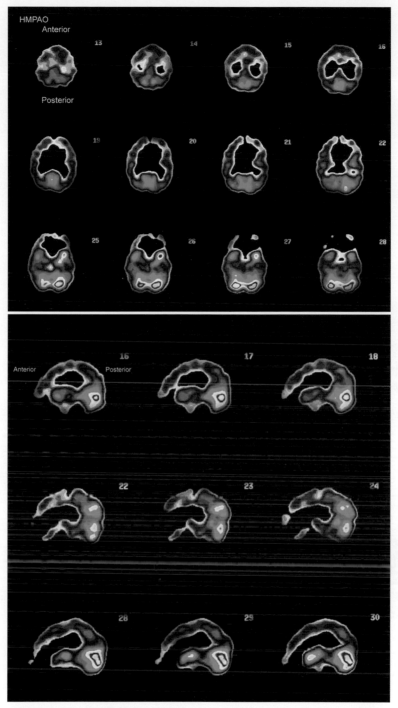

CASE 2–1. Radiology department chairman, 45 years old, with dementia.

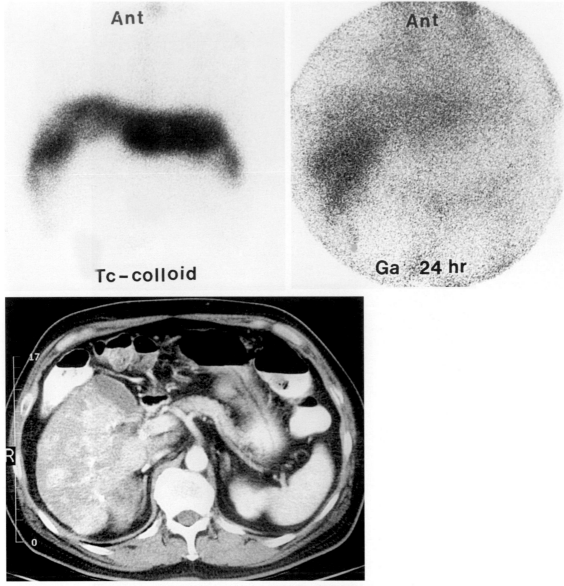

CASE 2–2.   Liver mass incidentally found on computed tomography. Additional images from technetium-99m sulfur colloid and gallium-67 citrate scans.

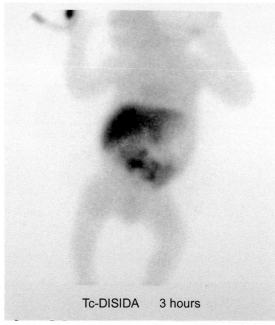

Tc-DISIDA   3 hours

CASE 2–3.   Jaundice? Supply likely etiology.

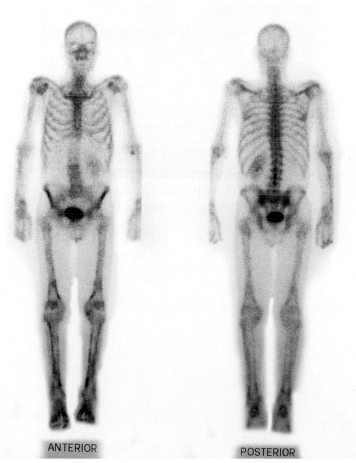

ANTERIOR   POSTERIOR

CASE 2–4.   Prior history of renal cancer now with lung cancer. Rule out metastases.

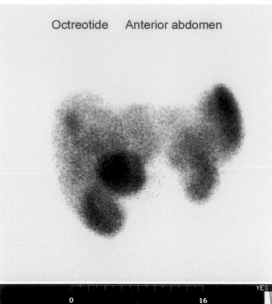

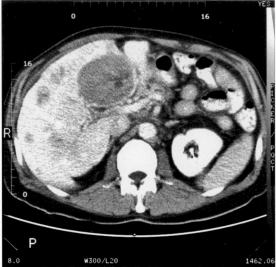

CASE 2–5. Patient with episodes of flushing, wheezing and diarrhea.

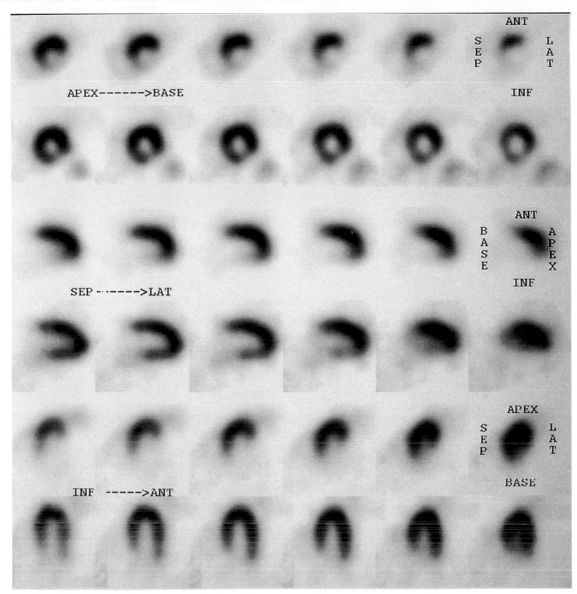

APEX------>BASE

SEP ------->LAT

INF -----> ANT

ANT
SEP   LAT
INF

ANT
BASE   APEX
INF

APEX
SEP   LAT
BASE

CASE 2-6. Smoker, 65 years old, with suspected coronary artery disease.

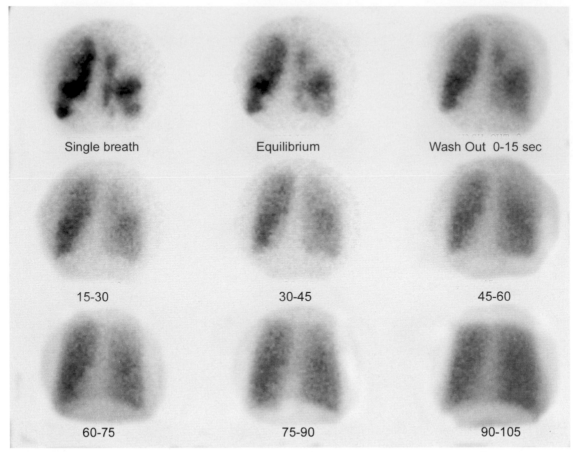

CASE 2–7.   Postoperative for hip replacement. Rule out pulmonary embolism. Chest x-ray normal except for hyperinflation.

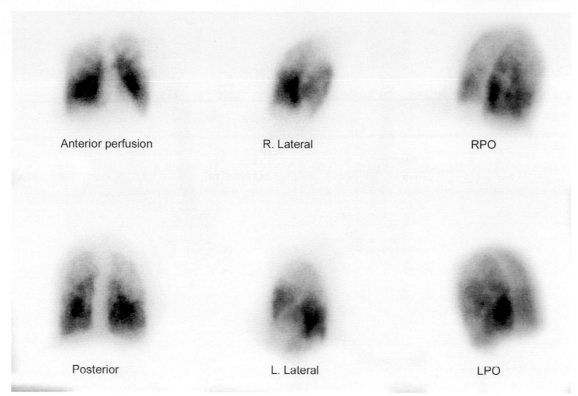

Anterior perfusion   R. Lateral   RPO

Posterior   L. Lateral   LPO

CASE 2–7, cont'd
For legend see opposite page

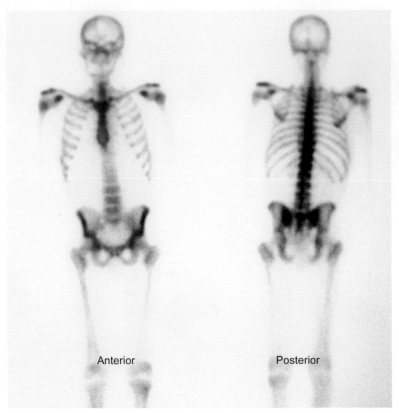

Anterior   Posterior

CASE 2–8.   Prostate cancer. Rule out metastases.

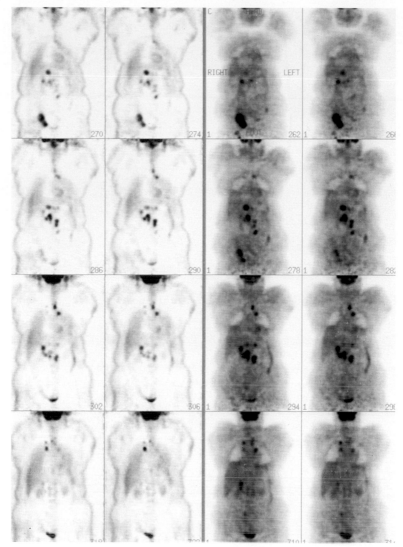

CASE 2–9.   Hilar adenopathy seen on chest x-ray.

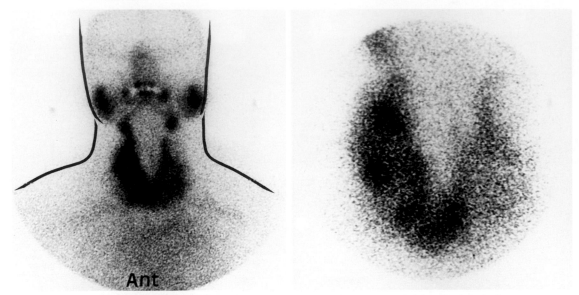

CASE 2–10.   Enlarged thyroid on physical examination. Large field and pinhole images.

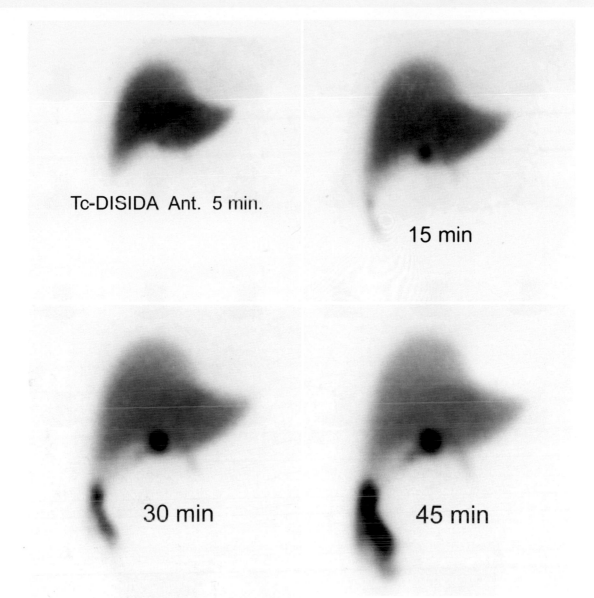

Tc-DISIDA Ant. 5 min.

15 min

30 min

45 min

CASE 3–1.   Right upper quadrant pain.

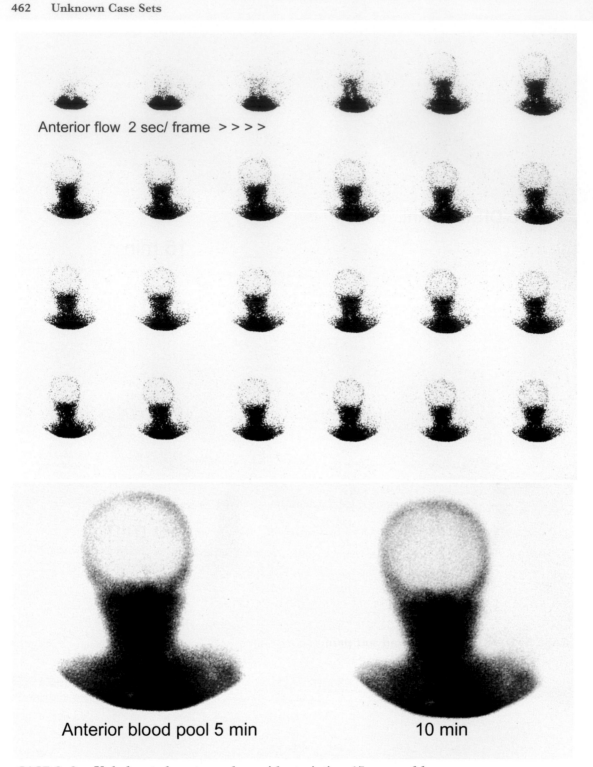

Anterior flow 2 sec/ frame > > > >

Anterior blood pool 5 min   10 min

CASE 3–2.   Unhelmeted motorcycle accident victim, 17 years old.

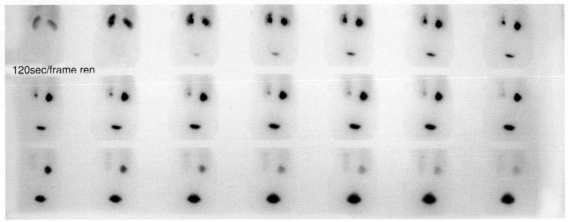

120sec/frame ren

RENOGRAM CURVE RESULTS

Curves in percent	Left
Peak time in min:	4.0
Peak counts:	109406
T 1/2 in min:	9.0
Differential (%):	52.6%
Diff time in min:	3 min
Lasix time min:	29 min

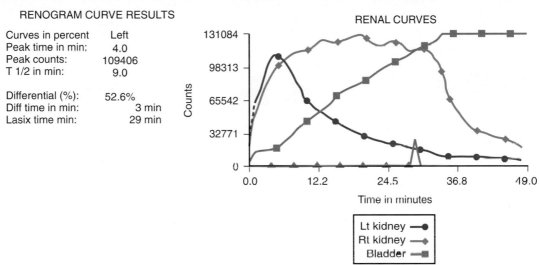

CASE 3–3. Rule out obstruction. Hydronephrosis. Lasix administered at 28 minutes.

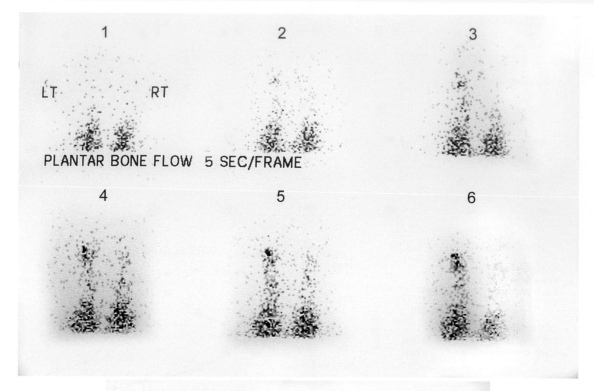

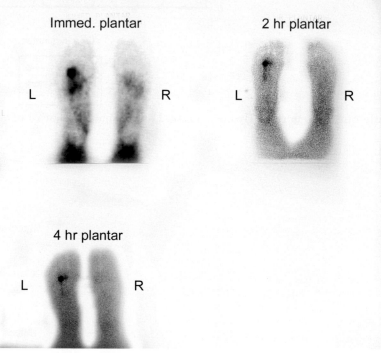

CASE 3–4. Pain and swelling of left foot.

24 hour MIBG

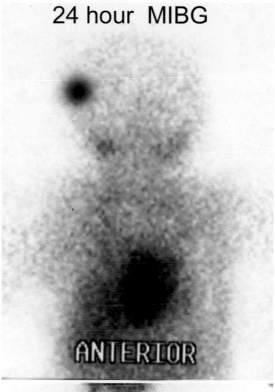

ANTERIOR

Tc-MDP

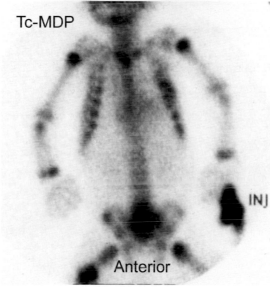

INJ

Anterior

CASE 3–5.   Child, 2 years old, with
mediastinal mass.

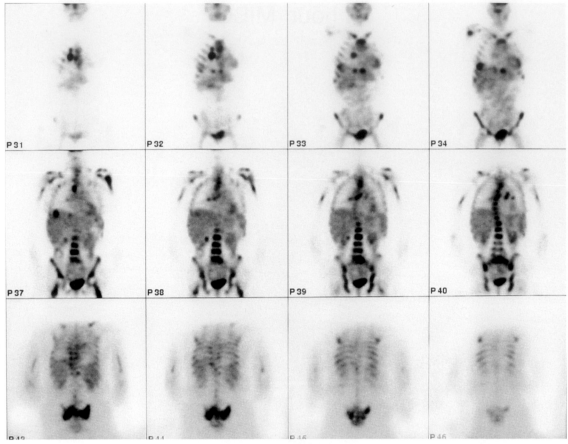

CASE 3–6.   Patient with history of treated cancer.

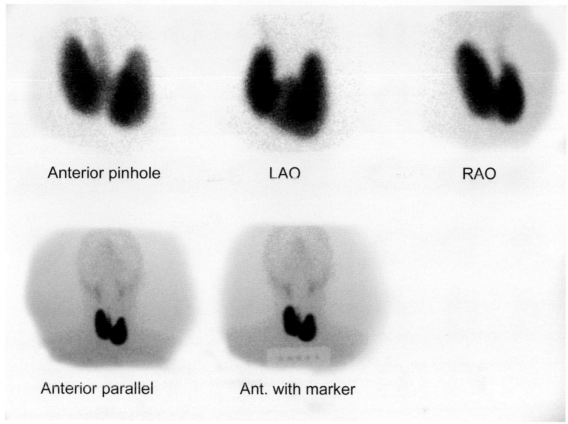

Anterior pinhole   LAO   RAO

Anterior parallel   Ant. with marker

CASE 3–7. Suspected hyperthyroidism.

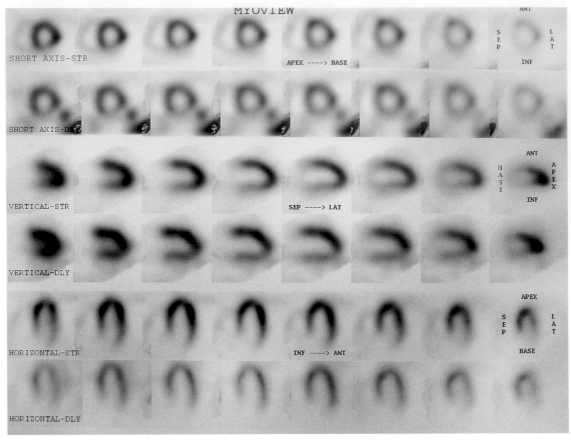

CASE 3–8. **Chest pain.** Rule out coronary artery disease.

Rotating display images

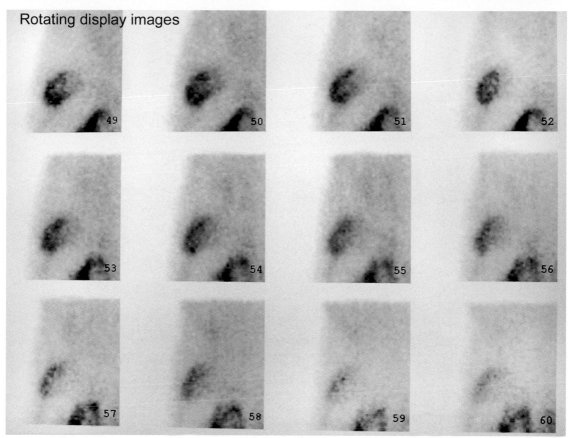

CASE 3–8, cont'd
For legend see opposite page

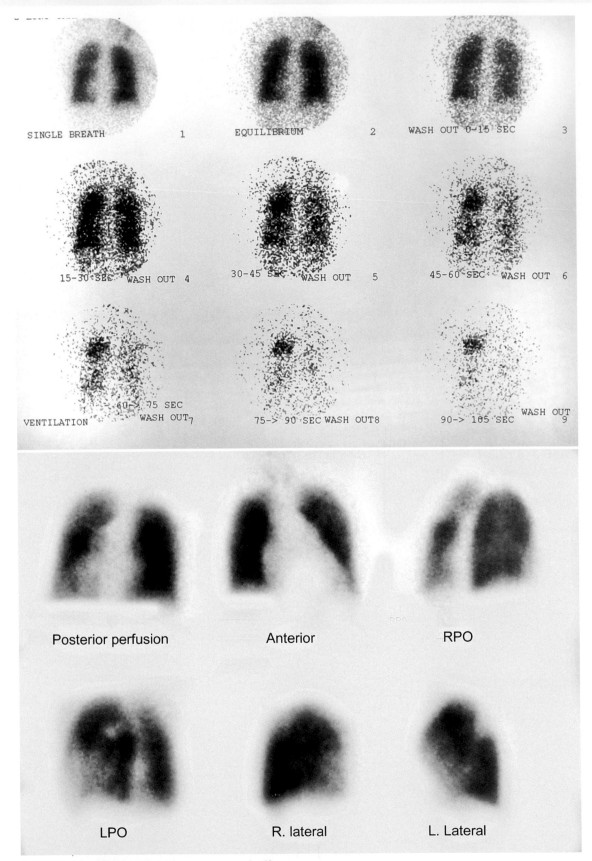

SINGLE BREATH   1   EQUILIBRIUM   2   WASH OUT 0–15 SEC   3

15–30 SEC WASH OUT 4   30–45 SEC WASH OUT   5   45–60 SEC WASH OUT 6

VENTILATION   60→ 75 SEC WASH OUT 7   75→ 90 SEC WASH OUT 8   90→ 105 SEC WASH OUT 9

Posterior perfusion   Anterior   RPO

LPO   R. lateral   L. Lateral

CASE 3–9.   Rule out pulmonary embolism.

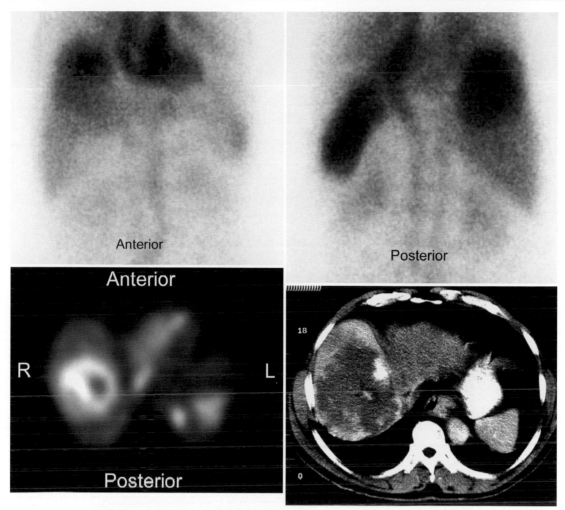

Anterior

Posterior

Anterior

R   L

Posterior

CASE 3–10. Hepatic lesion seen on computed tomography scan in this young female on birth control pills.

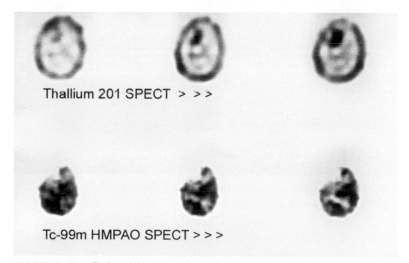

Thallium 201 SPECT > > >

Tc-99m HMPAO SPECT > > >

CASE 4–1. Prior history of brain tumor and radiation therapy. Suspected radiation necrosis.

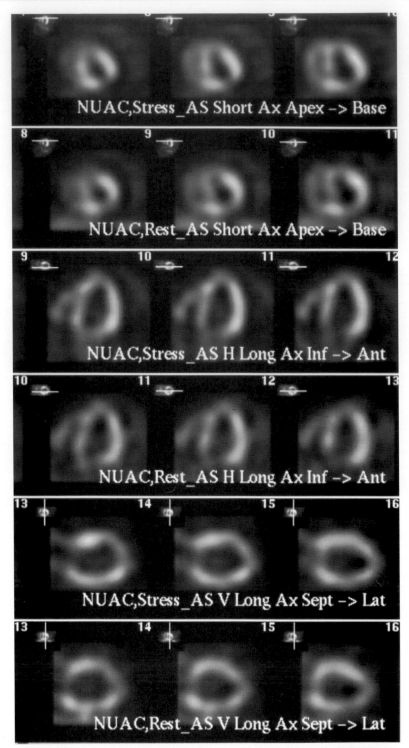

CASE 4–2.   Rule out coronary artery disease. Left ventricle
end diastolic volume is 320 mL.

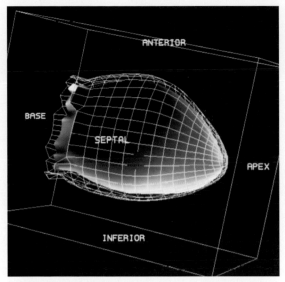

CASE 4–2, cont'd
For legend see opposite page

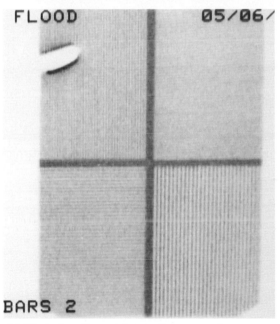

**CASE 4–3.   Image brought to you by a
technologist before scanning patients.**

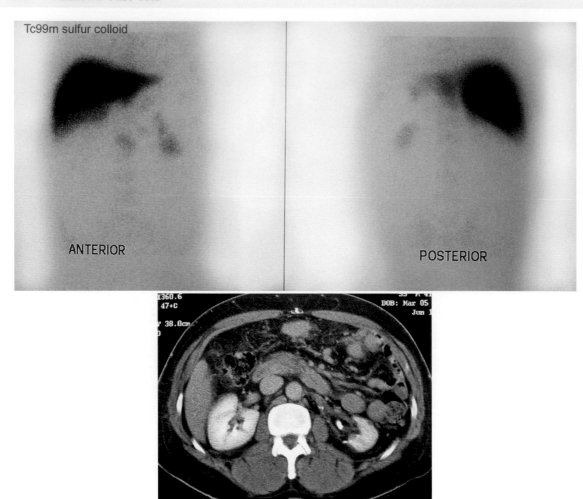

CASE 4–4.   Abnormal mass seen on computed tomography. Remote history of trauma.

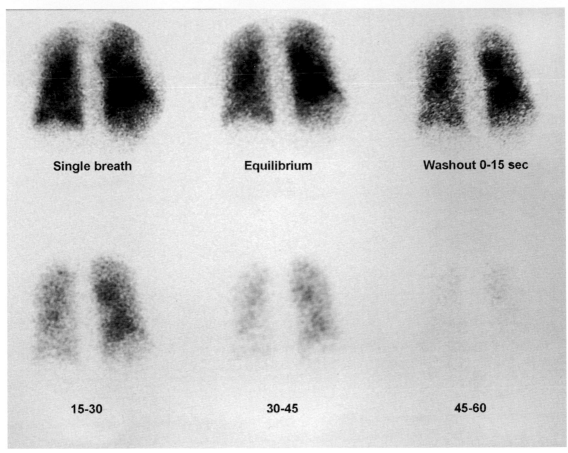

Single breath   **Equilibrium**   **Washout 0-15 sec**

15-30   **30-45**   **45-60**

CASE 4–5. Rule out pulmonary embolism.

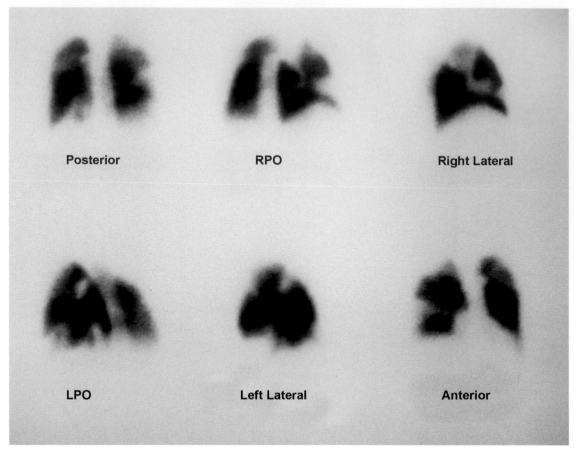

CASE 4–5, cont'd
For legend see p. 475

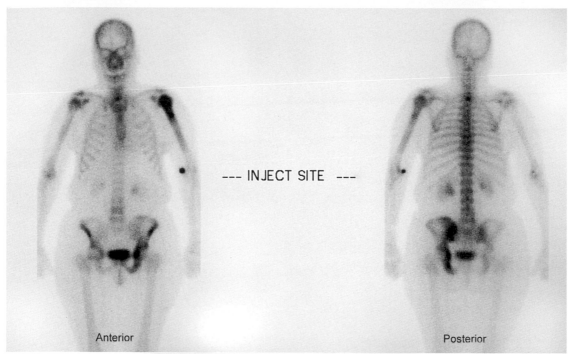

--- INJECT SITE ---

Anterior

Posterior

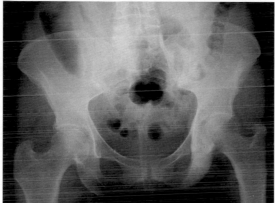

CASE 4–6. Rule out metastases in this 65-year-old man with prostate cancer.

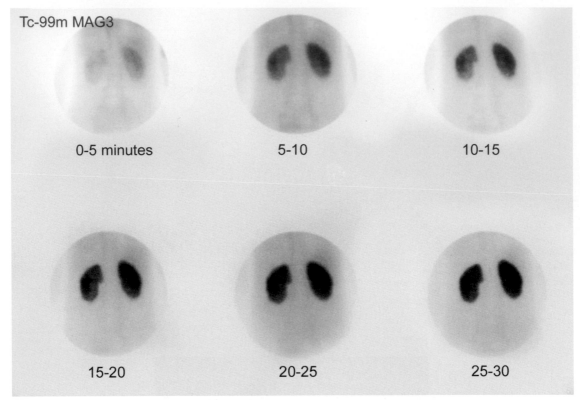

Tc-99m MAG3

0-5 minutes   5-10   10-15

15-20   20-25   25-30

CASE 4–7.   **Renal failure?** Supply etiology.

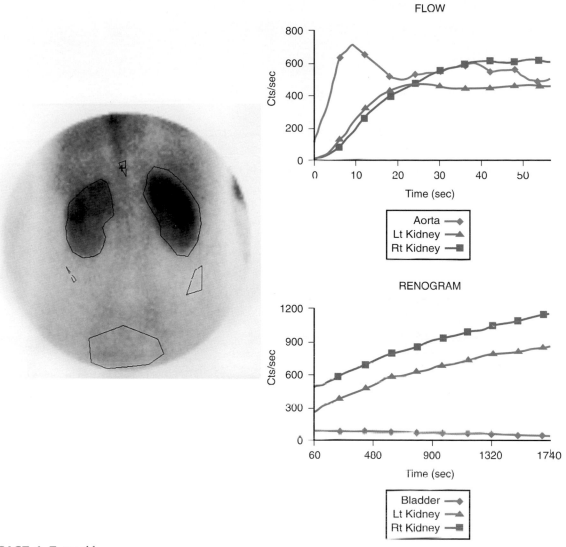

FLOW

RENOGRAM

CASE 4–7, cont'd
For legend see opposite page

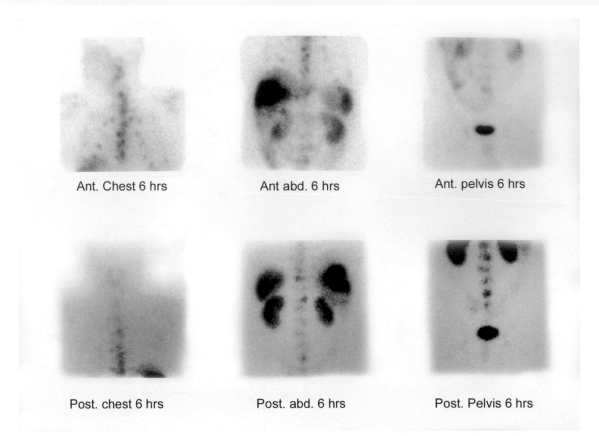

Ant. Chest 6 hrs   Ant abd. 6 hrs   Ant. pelvis 6 hrs

Post. chest 6 hrs   Post. abd. 6 hrs   Post. Pelvis 6 hrs

CASE 4–8.   Senior-level radiology resident, 30 years old, with hypertension, tachycardia, headaches, and sense of impending doom.

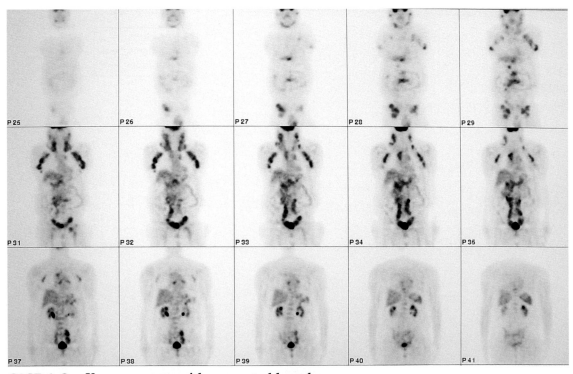

CASE 4–9.   Young woman with suspected lymphoma.

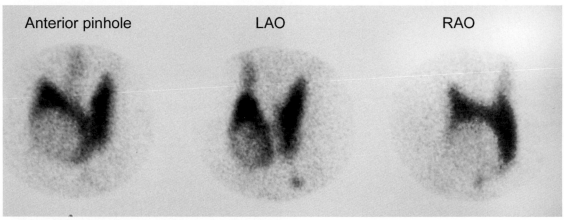

Anterior pinhole   LAO   RAO

CASE 4–10.   Palpable thyroid mass.

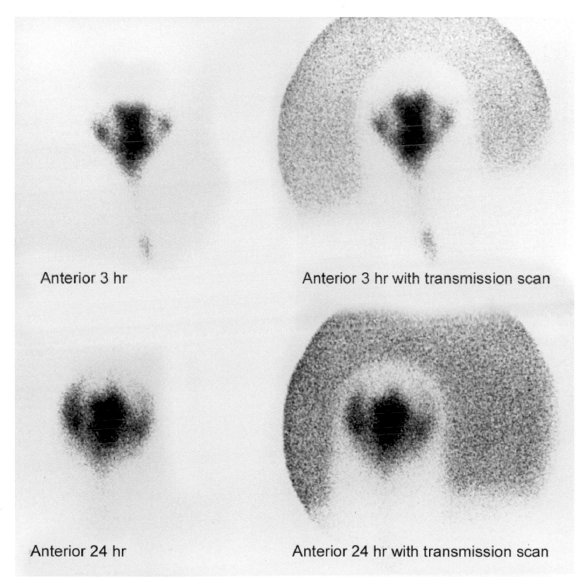

Anterior 3 hr   Anterior 3 hr with transmission scan

Anterior 24 hr   Anterior 24 hr with transmission scan

CASE 5–1.   Dilated lateral ventricles identified on computed tomography scan of the head.

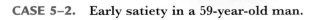

Ga-67 72 hrs

ANTERIOR

CASE 5–2.   Early satiety in a 59-year-old man.

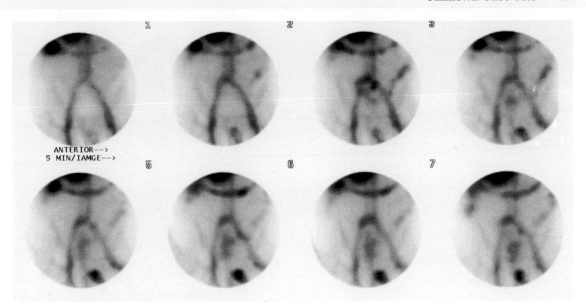

CASE 5–3.   Rectal bleeding.

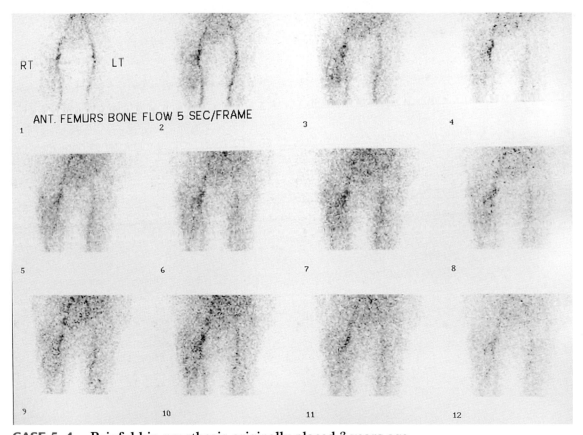

CASE 5–4.   Painful hip prosthesis originally placed 3 years ago.

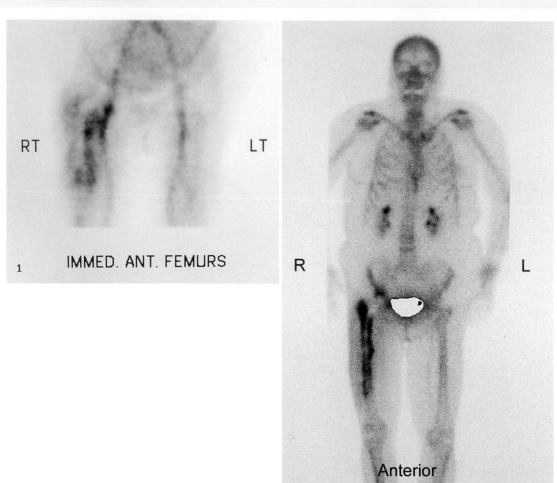

CASE 5–4, cont'd
For legend see p. 483

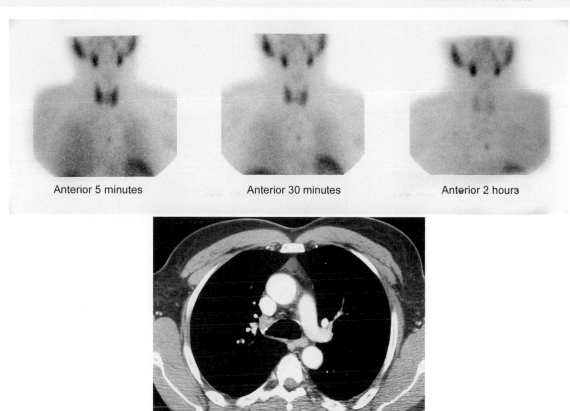

Anterior 5 minutes   Anterior 30 minutes   Anterior 2 hours

CASE 5–5. Previously unknown small mass found on annual screening chest computed tomography scan.

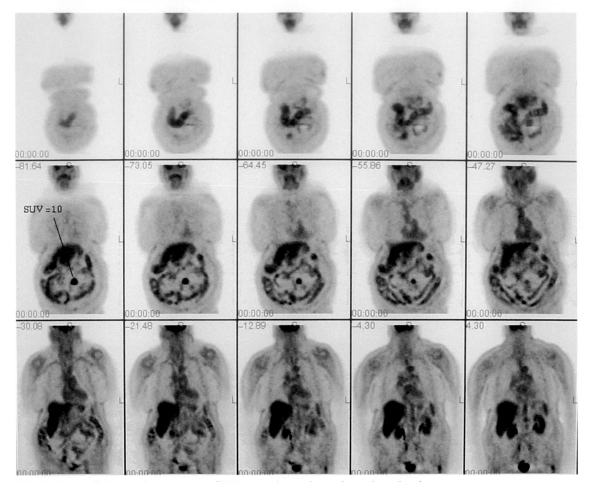

CASE 5–6.   Prior colon cancer. Rising carcinoembryonic antigen level.

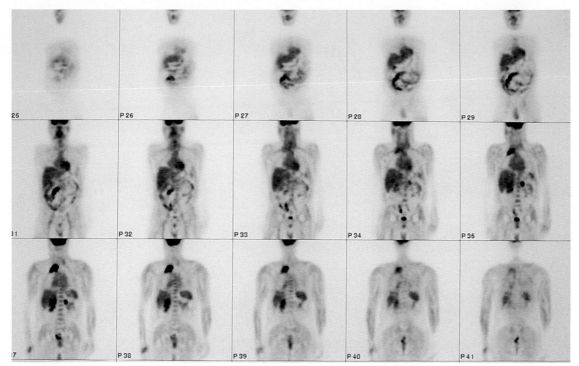

CASE 5–7. Lung cancer restaging. Please stage.

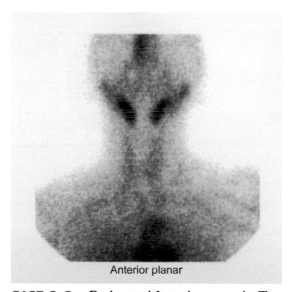

Anterior planar

CASE 5–8.   Patient with an increase in T_3 and T_4 with a decrease in thyroid-stimulating hormone. The 24-hour iodine uptake is 0.1%.

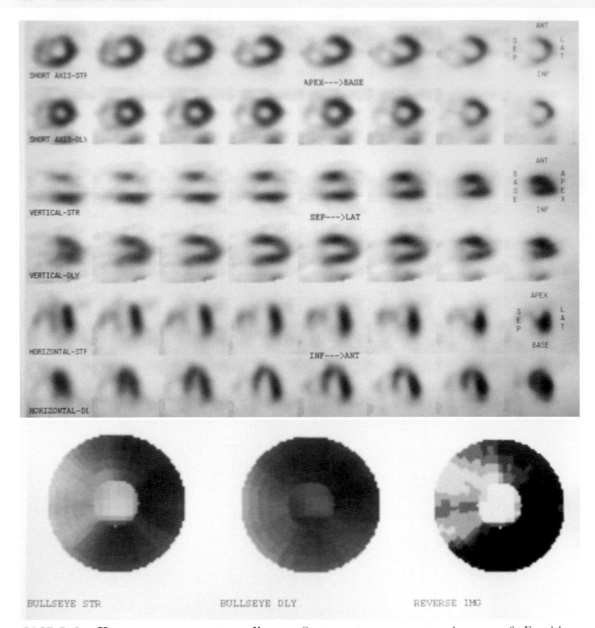

CASE 5–9.   Known coronary artery disease. Status post coronary artery bypass graft. For risk stratification.

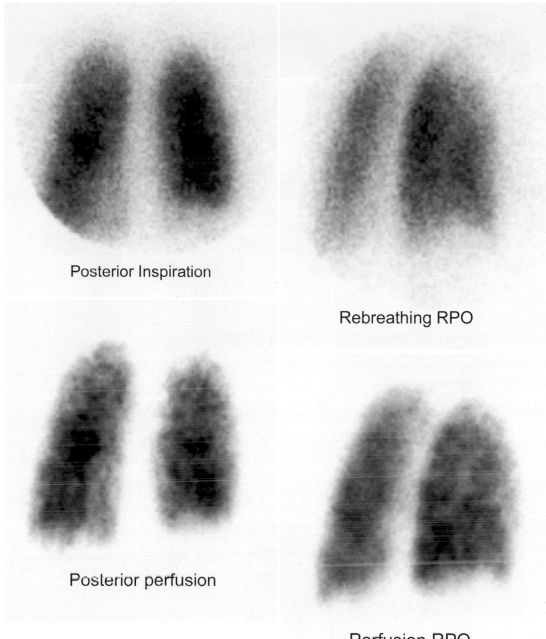

Posterior Inspiration

Rebreathing RPO

Posterior perfusion

Perfusion RPO

CASE 5–10. Woman, 41 years old, with shortness of breath.

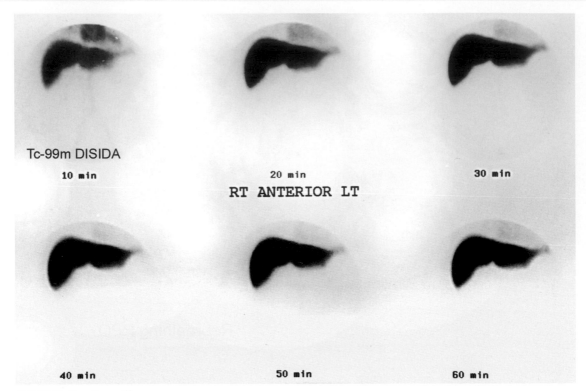

CASE 6–1. Jaundice.

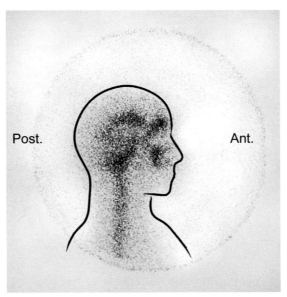

CASE 6–2. Prior head injury. Patient now has headaches.

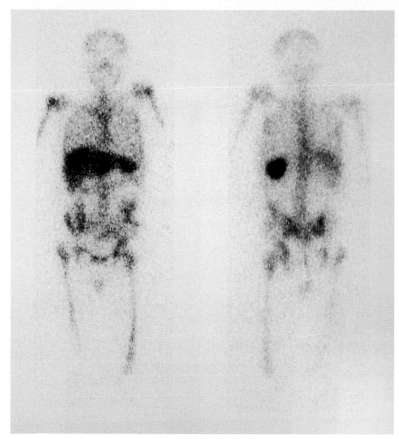

CASE 6–3.   Automobile accident 4 weeks ago. Status post splenectomy, now with fever.

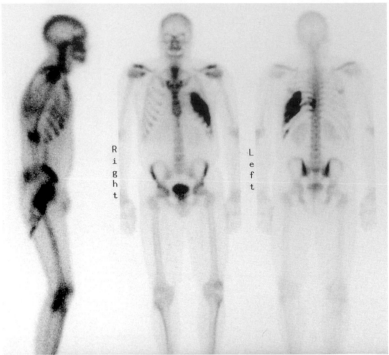

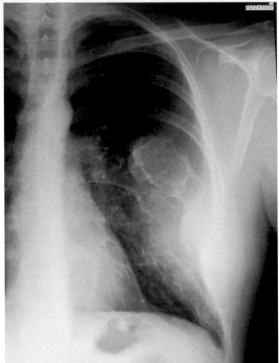

CASE 6–4.   Abnormal chest x-ray. Rule out metastases.

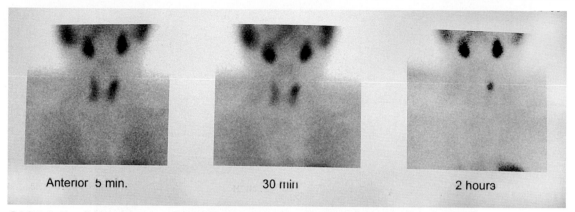

Anterior 5 min.   30 min   2 hours

CASE 6–5.   Man, 34 years old, with pain in large joints and known renal stones.

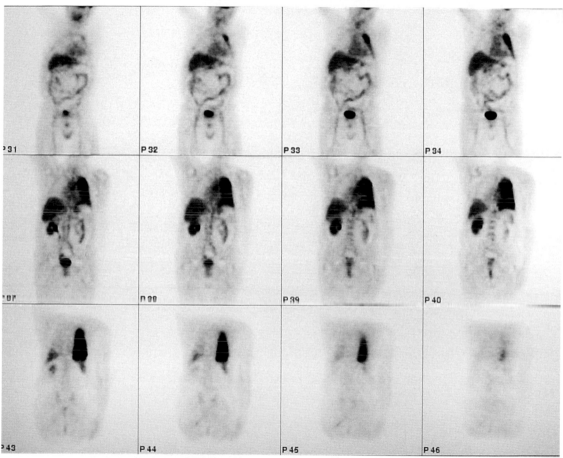

CASE 6–6.   Abnormal chest x-ray.

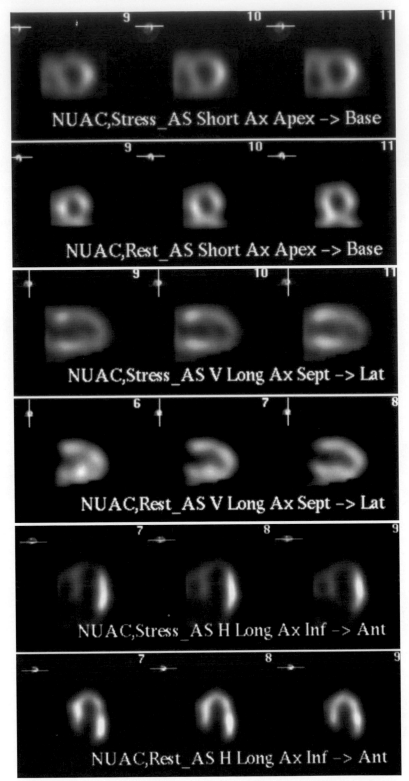

CASE 6–7. Known coronary artery disease.

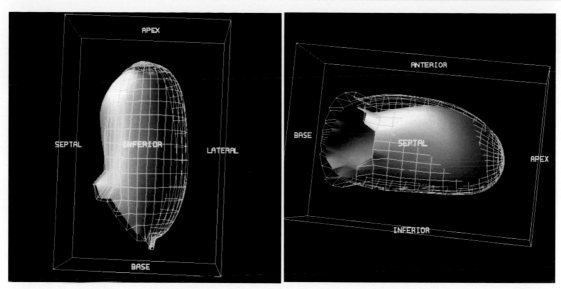

CASE 6–7, cont'd
For legend see opposite page

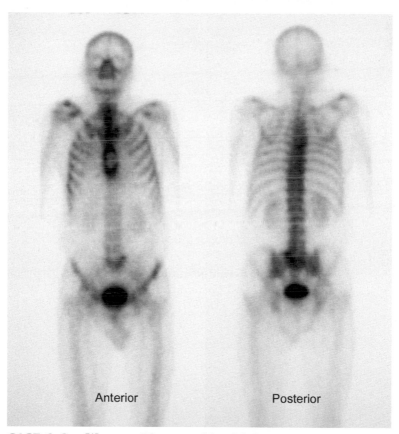

Anterior   Posterior

CASE 6–8.   Woman, 56 years old, with breast cancer.

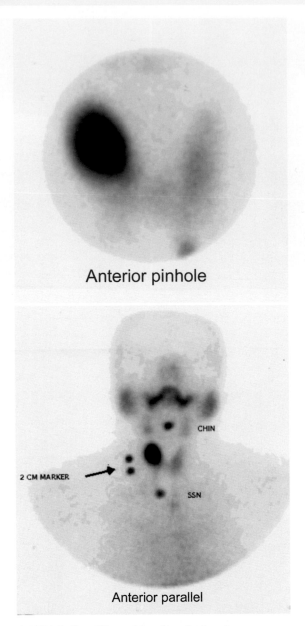

Anterior pinhole

Anterior parallel

CASE 6–9.   Thyroid-stimulating hormone of 0.1 μU/mL and radioiodine uptake of 60% at 24 hours.

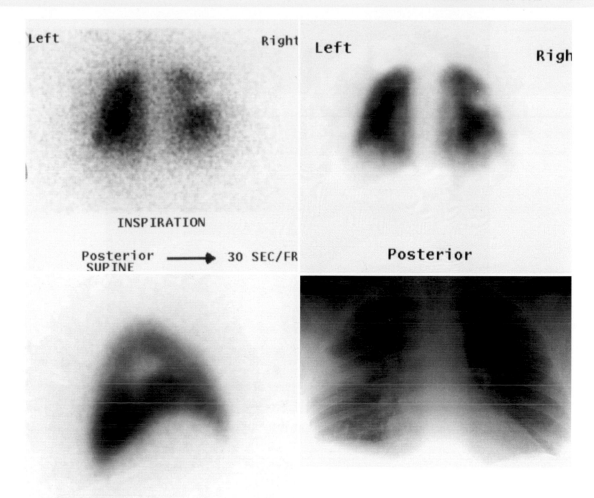

Rt Lat

CASE 6–10.   Rule out pulmonary embolism.

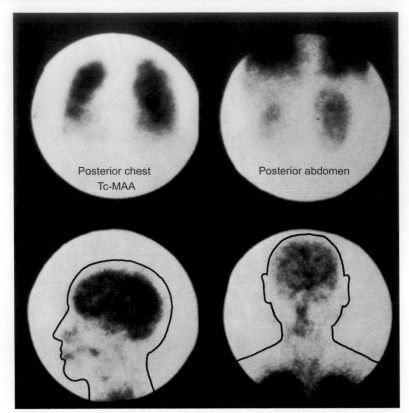

CASE 7–1. Images obtained at the end of a perfusion lung scan.

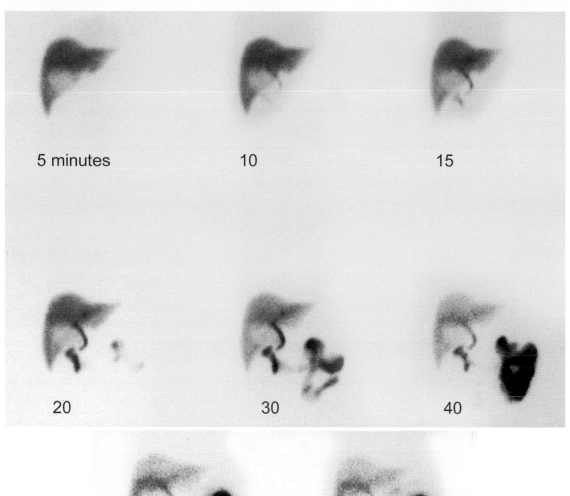

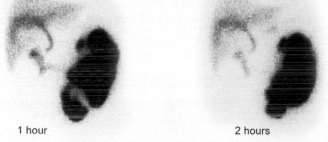

CASE 7–2. Woman, 34 years old, with right upper quadrant pain.

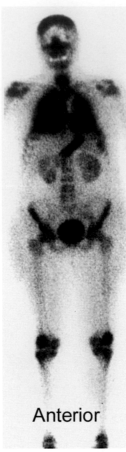

Anterior

CASE 7–3.   Woman, 60 years old, with
weakness, fatigue, loss of appetite, and
constipation.

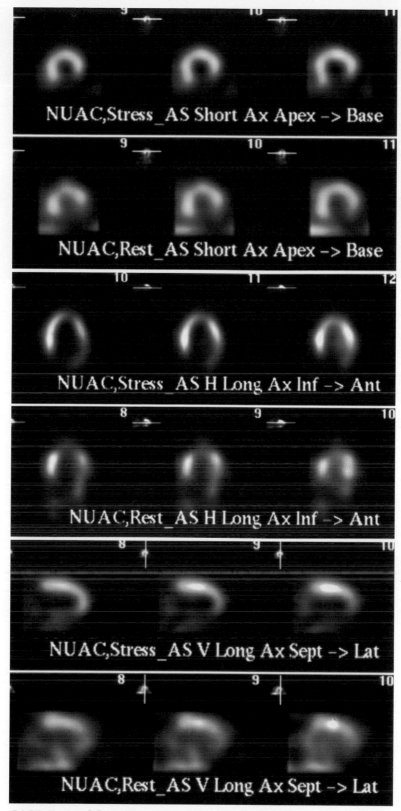

CASE 7–4. Man, 72 years old, with chest pain.

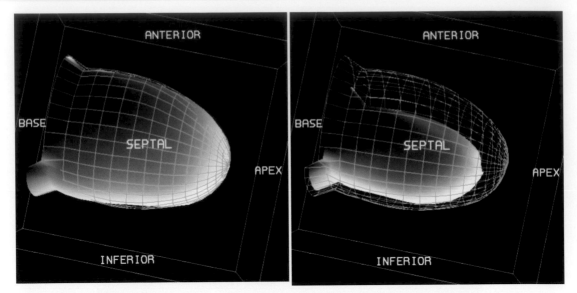

CASE 7–4, cont'd
For legend see p. 501

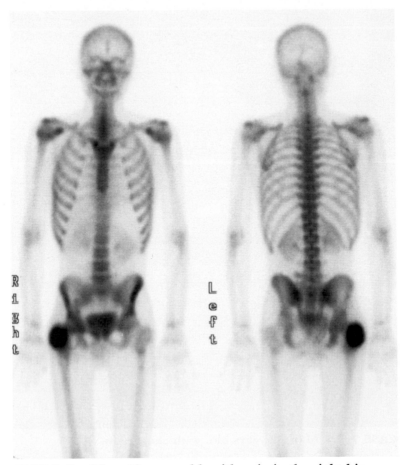

CASE 7–5.   Man, 18 years old, with pain in the right hip.

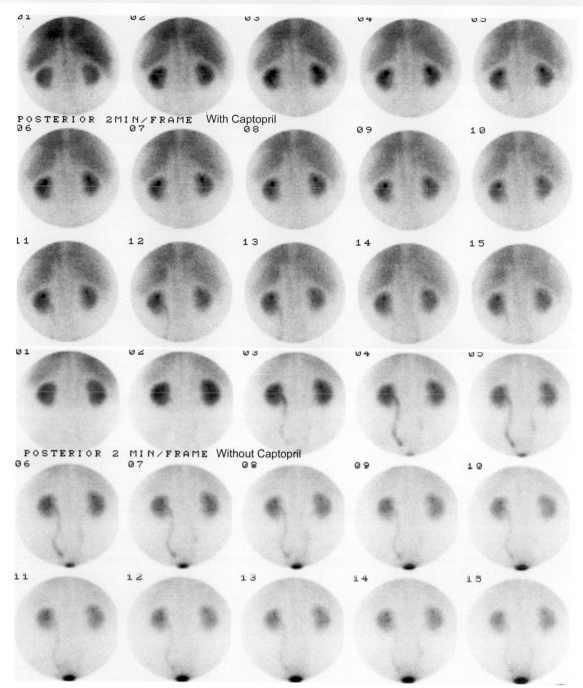

POSTERIOR 2MIN/FRAME   With Captopril

POSTERIOR 2 MIN/FRAME   Without Captopril

CASE 7–6.   Woman, 48 years old, with hypertension.

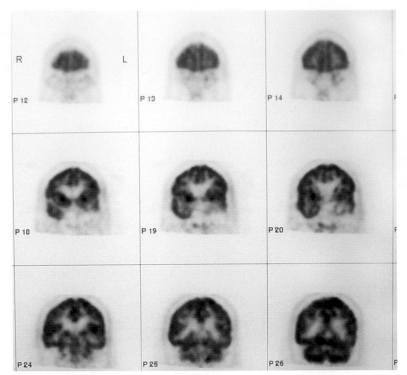

CASE 7–7.   History of seizures.

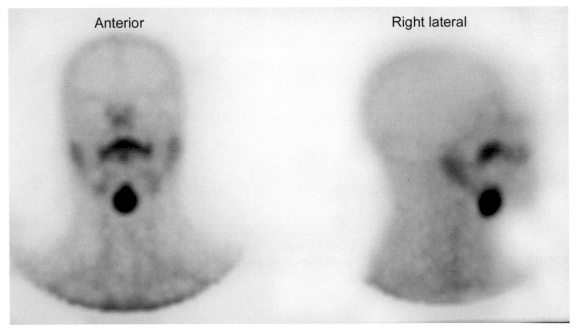

CASE 7–8.   Elevated thyroid-stimulating hormone.

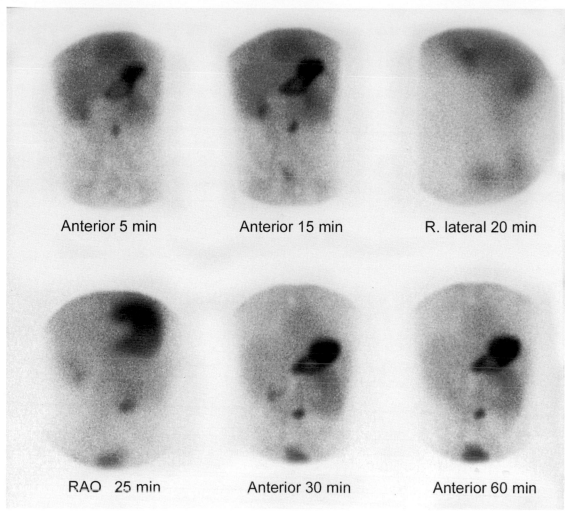

Anterior 5 min   Anterior 15 min   R. lateral 20 min

RAO   25 min   Anterior 30 min   Anterior 60 min

CASE 7–9.   Rectal bleeding.

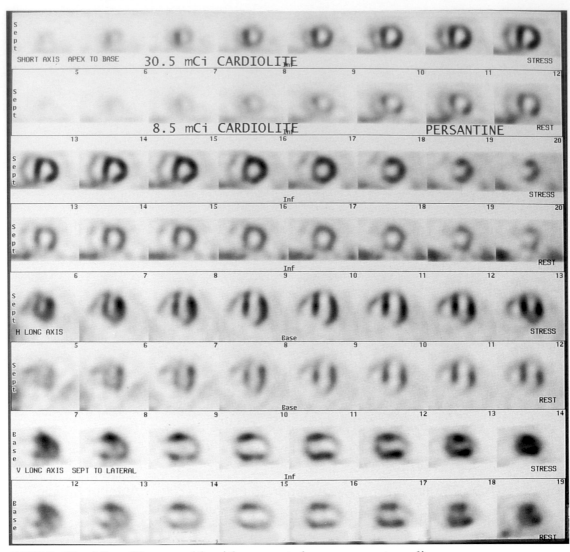

CASE 7–10. Man, 67 years old, with suspected coronary artery disease.

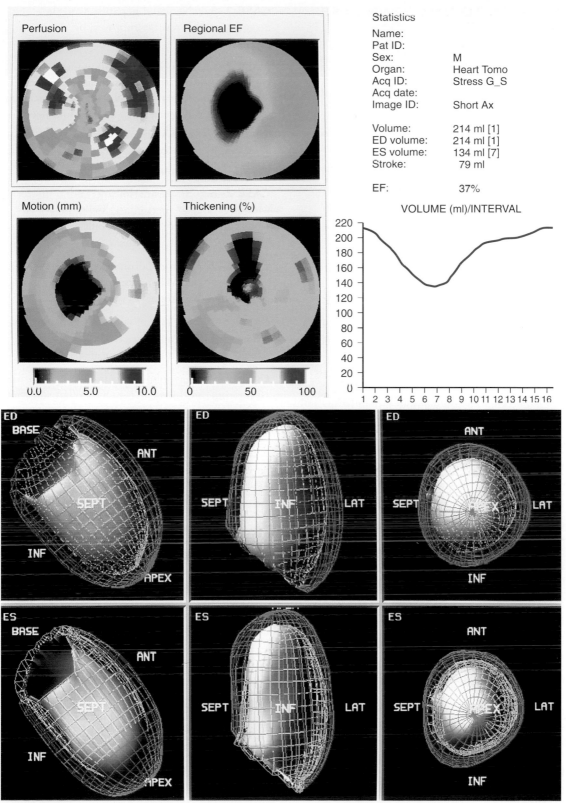

CASE 7–10, cont'd

For legend see opposite page

ANSWERS TO UNKNOWN CASE SETS

CASE 1–1. Lasix renogram and time-activity curves demonstrating high-grade obstruction of the left kidney and a nonobstructed extra-renal pelvis on the right.

CASE 1–2. Lymphoma. Gallium scan showing accumulation in both mediastinal and abdominal nodal masses. How did you know this was a gallium scan? What stage is the lymphoma?

CASE 1–3. Positron emission tomography (PET) scan in an Alzheimer's patient. Is it possible to distinguish a PET fluorine-18 fluorodeoxyglucose (^{18}F-FDG) scan from a technetium-99m hexamethylpropyleneamine oxime (^{99m}Tc-HMPAO) scan?

CASE 1–4. Degenerative disease but no evidence of metastatic disease. Technetium-99m (^{99m}Tc) methylene diphosphonate (MDP) bone scan with loss of resolution on posterior image. This was caused by the posterior camera head being off-peak (not set for the correct energy window). What energy window should be used?

CASE 1–5. Cirrhosis with ascites. How did you know there was ascites?

CASE 1–6. Thyroid discordant nodule. What does this likely represent?

CASE 1–7. Large anterior-apical infarct with ventricular walls diverging toward apex. What is the significance of this finding (trumpet sign)?

CASE 1–8. Lung cancer with contralateral lung and right adrenal metastases. What are the staging criteria for lung cancer?

CASE 1–9. Diffuse hepatic metastases. What tumors have metastases that calcify and may be seen on bone scans?

CASE 1–10. Ventilation/perfusion (V/Q) fissure sign. Very low probability for pulmonary embolism. What are the PIOPED II criteria for very low probability category?

CASE 2–1. Picks disease on a technetium 99m hexamethylpropyleneamine oxime (^{99m}Tc-HMPAO) scan.

CASE 2–2. Hepatoma. What other liver lesions may accumulate gallium?

CASE 2–3. Neonatal hepatitis. Can the accuracy of this test be improved by premedication?

CASE 2–4. Hypertrophic pulmonary osteoarthropathy. If the bone imaging radiopharmaceutical had been delivered as a unit dose from a radiopharmacy what would need to be done upon receipt of the package and dose?

CASE 2–5. Carcinoid hepatic metastasis. What other tumors accumulate octreotide?

CASE 2–6. Small inferior and lateral infarct with large area of peri-infarct ischemia. What vessels are involved? How is a bull's eye image generated?

CASE 2–7. Chronic obstructive pulmonary disease (COPD). What category is this according to PIOPED II criteria?

CASE 2–8. Superscan with diffuse metastases. Under what circumstances would you treat a patient with strontium-89 chloride?

CASE 2–9. Lymphoma accumulating fluorine-18 fluorodeoxyglucose (^{18}F-FDG). What stage is this? What do you know about radioimmunotherapy for lymphoma? Which set of images is non-attenuation corrected?

CASE 2–10. Multinodular goiter. How does treating a toxic multinodular goiter with radioiodine differ from treating Graves' disease?

CASE 3–1. Bile leak with activity in the portahepatis and right paracolic gutter.

CASE 3–2. Brain death with no intracranial perfusion on the technetium-99m (^{99m}Tc) pertechnetate study. Can this study be done with ^{99m}Tc hexamethylpropyleneamine oxime (HMPAO)?

CASE 3–3. Unobstructed patulous collecting system of the right kidney. If ^{99m}TcO$_4^-$ had been administered inadvertently would this constitute a "medical event"?

CASE 3–4. Stress fracture of third metatarsal. Would osteomyelitis look different?

CASE 3–5. Neuroblastoma with activity in the lower chest on both iodine-131 metaiodobenzylguanidine (^{131}I-MIBG) and technetium-99m methylene diphosphonate (^{99m}Tc-

MDP) scans. A skull metastasis is also present. Could the tumor have been imaged with indium-111 pentetreotide?

CASE 3–6. Metabolically active metastases in a patient with marked marrow activity due to stimulation with colony stimulating factors.

CASE 3–7. Graves' disease. How would you determine how much radioiodine-131 to administer to the patient?

CASE 3–8. Fixed inferior wall diaphragmatic attenuation artifact. What type of artifact is caused by breast attenuation or left bundle branch block?

CASE 3–9. Left upper lobe mucous plug. Where does the xenon go when the patient exhales? Are there special requirements for imaging room design?

CASE 3–10. Hepatic hemangioma. What radiopharmaceutical was used in this examination and how was it prepared?

CASE 4–1. Recurrent brain tumor. How would the pattern differ with radiation necrosis?

CASE 4–2. Dilated cardiomyopathy with global hypokinesia. What are the normal left ventricle (LV) end-diastolic volume, LV end-systolic volume, cardiac output, and cardiac index?

CASE 4–3. Cracked crystal. How was this image obtained? Is it necessary to obtain this type of image daily? What would a photomultiplier tube defect look like?

CASE 4–4. Splenosis. What radiopharmaceutical besides technetium-99m sulfur colloid can be used to make this diagnosis?

CASE 4–5. High probability for pulmonary embolism. What is the approximate number and size of particles administered?

CASE 4–6. Paget's disease. What are the findings on the pelvis x-ray that distinguish this from metastatic disease?

CASE 4–7. Acute tubular necrosis. Could severe dehydration produce the same pattern?

CASE 4–8. Pheochromocytoma with osseous metastases. What radiopharmaceutical is used to image pheochromocytoma?

CASE 4–9. Lymphoma and brown fat or USA fat. How does one distinguish between the two entities? Approximately what is the absorbed radiation dose involved in handling a syringe with ^{18}F-FDG or standing near the patient after injection?

CASE 4–10. Cold thyroid nodule. What is the differential diagnosis? What is the next step in management.

CASE 5–1. Normal pressure hydrocephalus. What characteristics differentiate this from a normal study? Point out the anatomy.

CASE 5–2. Lymphoma with gallium accumulation. What is the current role of gallium versus fluorine-18 fluorodeoxyglucose (^{18}F-FDG) positron emission tomography scanning in patients with lymphoma?

CASE 5–3. Gastrointestinal bleed at the hepatic flexure. What bleeding rate is necessary to detect the bleeding? If the study had been negative, what would be the next step in management?

CASE 5–4. Infected prosthesis on three-phase bone scan. What other nuclear medicine techniques could have been used to confirm this diagnosis?

CASE 5–5. Ectopic mediastinal parathyroid adenoma. What radiopharmaceutical was used for this study?

CASE 5–6. Colon cancer recurrence centrally in the abdomen. What radiopharmaceutical was used? What does the term SUV refer to, and what is the importance of it?

CASE 5–7. Lung cancer with adrenal metastasis on positron emission tomography (PET) ^{18}F-FDG scan. What size do metastases need to be in order to be reliably detected on most PET scans?

CASE 5–8. Subacute thyroiditis. Are there other scintigraphic patterns of thyroiditis? Could this pattern be due to an organification defect?

CASE 5–9. Anterior wall and septal ischemia. What would be the implications if the left ventricle dilated on the stress images?

CASE 5–10.   Vasculitis. What PIOPED probability category would this be? Would fat or tumor emboli have a similar appearance?

CASE 6–1.   Liver scan sign on a hepatobiliary study due to intrahepatic cholestasis. Could this pattern be secondary to acute common duct obstruction?

CASE 6–2.   Cerebrospinal fluid rhinorrhea. How is the patient prepared for this procedure?

CASE 6–3.   Splenic bed abscess. What are the advantages/disadvantages of technetium-99m (^{99m}Tc) white blood cells compared with indium-111–labeled leukocytes?

CASE 6–4.   Fibrous dysplasia. Why is this not likely to be metastatic disease? Are multiple enchondromas typically "hot" on a bone scan?

CASE 6–5.   Parathyroid adenoma. How would the appearance of a thyroid adenoma or thyroid cancer differ from parathyroid adenoma on the serial images?

CASE 6–6.   Malignant effusion on an ^{18}F-FDG scan. Could this represent an empyema?

CASE 6–7.   Reversible ischemia of the septum, anterior wall, apex, and distal inferior wall with septal dyskinesia. Are the gated images usually obtained at rest or stress?

CASE 6–8.   Lytic sternal metastases. What tumors often produce lytic metastases?

CASE 6–9.   Toxic thyroid adenoma. What dose of I-131 would you use to treat this patient? What are the criteria upon which any patient can be released from the hospital after radioiodine therapy?

CASE 6–10.   Pneumonia. What is meant by the term "triple match," and what probability category does that indicate?

CASE 7–1.   Right-to-left shunt. If you suspected such a shunt was present, should you have done this procedure at all or modified the procedure?

CASE 7–2.   Rim sign of acute cholecystitis. Does this finding indicate the potential of anything other than simple acute cholecystitis? What is the significance of a gallbladder ejection fraction measurement?

CASE 7–3.   Hyperparathyroidism with activity in lungs, thyroid, kidneys, and stomach. What is the other common bone scan presentation?

CASE 7–4.   Inferior wall myocardial wall infarction with severe hypokinesis. Could this pattern be seen with stunned or hibernating myocardium? What is the difference between the two entities? What artifact may occur when there is a large amount of gastrointestinal activity?

CASE 7–5.   Chondroblastoma. What would a septic hip look like on bone scan?

CASE 7–6.   Bilateral renal artery stenosis. What is the mechanism by which captopril works?

CASE 7–7.   Interictal temporal lobe epilepsy positron emission tomography fluorodeoxyglucose scan. How are ictal studies performed? What pattern would be seen with mesial temporal sclerosis?

CASE 7–8.   Lingual thyroid. What is the usual thyroid function status in these patients?

CASE 7–9.   Meckel's diverticulum. What radiopharmaceutical was used? What premedication can increase the sensitivity of this procedure?

CASE 7–10.   Multivessel coronary artery disease. Large anteroapical infarct with akinesis, small inferior infarct, reduced left ventricle (LV) ejection fraction and dilated LV. What are the adverse reactions associated with dypridamole and how are they treated?

Characteristics of Radionuclides for Imaging and Therapy

NUCLIDE	SYMBOL	HALF-LIFE	DECAY MODE	MAJOR EMISSIONS (MeV)*
Carbon-11	$^{11}_{6}C$	20.3 min	β+	γ 0.511 (200%)
Cesium-137	$^{137}_{55}Cs$	30 yr	β−	γ 0.660 (85%)
Chromium-51	$^{51}_{24}Cr$	27.8 day	E.C.	γ 0.320 (10%)
Cobalt-57	$^{57}_{27}Co$	270 day	E.C.	γ 0.122 (86%)
				γ 0.136 (11%)
Cobalt-58	$^{58}_{27}Co$	71.3 day	E.C. and β+	γ 0.811 (99%)
				γ 0.511 (31%)
Cobalt-60	$^{60}_{27}Co$	5.26 yr	β−	γ 1.173 (100%)
				γ 1.332 (100%)
Fluorine-18	$^{18}_{9}F$	109 min	E.C. and β+	γ 0.511 (194%)
Gadolinium-153	$^{153}_{64}Gd$	240 day	E.C.	γ 0.100 (55%)
				γ 0.040
				γ 0.048†
Gallium-67	$^{67}_{31}Ga$	78.1 hr	E.C.	γ 0.093 (38%)
				γ 0.184 (24%)
				γ 0.296 (16%)
				γ 0.388 (4%)
Gallium-68	$^{68}_{31}Ga$	68.3 min	E.C. and β+	γ 0.511 (178%)
				γ 1.077 (3%)
Indium-111	$^{111}_{49}In$	67 hr	E.C.	γ 0.172 (90%)
				γ 0.247 (94%)
Iodine-123	$^{123}_{53}I$	13 hr	E.C.	γ 0.159 (83%)
Iodine-125	$^{125}_{53}I$	60 day	E.C.	γ 0.027 (76%)
Iodine-131	$^{131}_{53}I$	8.06 day	β−	γ 0.284 (6%)
				γ 0.364 (82%)
				γ 0.637 (7%)
				β 0.192 (90%)
Krypton-81m	$^{81m}_{36}Kr$	13 sec	I.T.	γ 0.191 (66%)
Molybdenum-99	$^{99}_{42}Mo$	66.7 hr	β−	γ 0.181 (8%)
				γ 0.740 (14%)
				γ 0.778 (5%)
Nitrogen-13	$^{13}_{7}N$	10 min	β+	γ 0.511 (200%)
Oxygen-15	$^{15}_{8}O$	124 sec	β+	γ 0.511 (200%)
Phosphorus-32	$^{32}_{15}P$	14.3 day	β−	β 0.695 (100%)
Rhenium-186	$^{186}_{75}Re$	90 hr	E.C.	γ 0.137
				β 0.349
Rubidium-82	$^{82}_{37}Rb$	1.3 min	E.C. and β+	γ 0.511 (189%)
				γ 0.777 (13%)

NUCLIDE	SYMBOL	HALF-LIFE	DECAY MODE	MAJOR EMISSIONS (MeV)*
Samarium-153	$^{153}_{62}$Sm	46.3 hr		γ 0.103 (30%) β 0.640 (30%) β 0.710 (50%) β 0.810 (20%)
Strontium-87m	$^{87m}_{38}$Sr	2.8 hr	I.T. and E.C.	γ 0.388 (83%)
Strontium-89	$^{89}_{38}$Sr	50.5 day	β−	γ 1.463 (100%)
Technetium-99m	$^{99m}_{43}$Tc	6.03 hr	I.T.	γ 0.140 (88%)
Thallium-201	$^{201}_{81}$Tl	73 hr	E.C.	γ 0.135 (2%) γ 0.167 (8%) (Hg daughter x-rays 0.069–0.081)
Xenon-127	$^{127}_{54}$Xe	36.4 day	E.C.	γ 0.145 (4%) γ 0.172 (25%) γ 0.203 (68%) γ 0.375 (18%)
Xenon-133	$^{133}_{54}$Xe	5.3 day	β−	γ 0.081 (36%)

*Mean energy. Information in parentheses refers to the percentage of emissions of that type that occurs from disintegration. For example, carbon-11 gives off a gamma ray of 0.511 MeV 200% of the time; i.e., two gamma rays are emitted per disintegration.
†From Europium 153.
β+, positron (beta plus) decay; β−, beta decay; E.C., electron capture; I.T., isomeric transition.
Adapted from Dillman LT, Von der Lage FC: Radionuclide Decay Schemes and Nuclear Parameters for Use in Radiation Dose Estimation. New York, Society of Nuclear Medicine, 1975.

Radioactivity Conversion Table for International System (SI) Units (Becquerels to Curies)

0.05 MBq = 1.4 µCi	90.0 MBq = 2.43 mCi	875.0 MBq = 23.7 mCi
0.1 MBq = 2.7 µCi	100.0 MBq = 2.70 mCi	900.0 MBq = 24.3 mCi
0.2 MBq = 5.4 µCi	125.0 MBq = 3.38 mCi	925.0 MBq = 25.0 mCi
0.3 MBq = 8.1 µCi	150.0 MBq = 4.05 mCi	950.0 MBq = 25.7 mCi
0.4 MBq = 10.8 µCi	175.0 MBq = 4.73 mCi	975.0 MBq = 26.4 mCi
0.5 MBq = 13.5 µCi	200.0 MBq = 5.41 mCi	1.0 GBq = 27.0 mCi
0.6 MBq = 16.2 µCi	225.0 MBq = 6.08 mCi	1.1 GBq = 29.7 mCi
0.7 MBq = 18.9 µCi	250.0 MBq = 6.76 mCi	1.2 GBq = 32.4 mCi
0.8 MBq = 21.6 µCi	275.0 MBq = 7.43 mCi	1.3 GBq = 35.1 mCi
0.9 MBq = 24.3 µCi	300.0 MBq = 8.11 mCi	1.4 GBq = 37.8 mCi
1.0 MBq = 27.0 µCi	325.0 MBq = 8.78 mCi	1.5 GBq = 40.5 mCi
2.0 MBq = 54.1 µCi	350.0 MBq = 9.46 mCi	1.6 GBq = 43.2 mCi
3.0 MBq = 81.1 µCi	375.0 MBq = 10.1 mCi	1.7 GBq = 46.0 mCi
4.0 MBq = 108 µCi	400.0 MBq = 10.8 mCi	1.8 GBq = 48.7 mCi
5.0 MBq = 135 µCi	425.0 MBq = 11.5 mCi	1.9 GBq = 51.3 mCi
6.0 MBq = 162 µCi	450.0 MBq = 12.2 mCi	2.0 GBq = 54.1 mCi
7.0 MBq = 189 µCi	475.0 MBq = 12.8 mCi	2.2 GBq = 59.5 mCi
8.0 MBq = 216 µCi	500.0 MBq = 13.5 mCi	2.4 GBq = 64.9 mCi
9.0 MBq = 243 µCi	525.0 MBq = 14.2 mCi	2.6 GBq = 70.3 mCi
10.0 MBq = 270 µCi	550.0 MBq = 14.9 mCi	2.8 GBq = 75.7 mCi
15.0 MBq = 405 µCi	575.0 MBq = 15.5 mCi	3.0 GBq = 81.1 mCi
20.0 MBq = 541 µCi	600.0 MBq = 16.2 mCi	3.2 GBq = 86.5 mCi
25.0 MBq = 676 µCi	625.0 MBq = 16.9 mCi	3.4 GBq = 91.9 mCi
30.0 MBq = 811 µCi	650.0 MBq = 17.6 mCi	3.6 GBq = 97.3 mCi
35.0 MBq = 946 µCi	675.0 MBq = 18.2 mCi	3.8 GBq = 103 mCi
40.0 MBq = 1.08 mCi	700.0 MBq = 18.9 mCi	4.0 GBq = 108 mCi
45.0 MBq = 1.22 mCi	725.0 MBq = 19.6 mCi	5.0 GBq = 135 mCi
50.0 MBq = 1.35 mCi	750.0 MBq = 20.3 mCi	6.0 GBq = 162 mCi
55.0 MBq = 1.49 mCi	775.0 MBq = 20.9 mCi	7.0 GBq = 189 mCi
60.0 MBq = 1.62 mCi	800.0 MBq = 21.6 mCi	8.0 GBq = 216 mCi
70.0 MBq = 1.89 mCi	825.0 MBq = 22.3 mCi	9.0 GBq = 243 mCi
80.0 MBq = 2.16 mCi	850.0 MBq = 23.0 mCi	10.0 GBq = 270 mCi

Radioactivity Conversion Table for International System (SI) Units (Curies to Becquerels)

1.0 µCi = 0.037 MBq	450.0 µCi = 16.7 MBq	17.0 mCi = 629 MBq
2.0 µCi = 0.074 MBq	500.0 µCi = 18.5 MBq	18.0 mCi = 666 MBq
3.0 µCi = 0.111 MBq	600.0 µCi = 22.2 MBq	19.0 mCi − 703 MBq
4.0 µCi = 0.148 MBq	700.0 µCi = 25.9 MBq	20.0 mCi = 740 MBq
5.0 µCi = 0.185 MBq	800.0 µCi = 29.6 MBq	21.0 mCi = 777 MBq
6.0 µCi = 0.222 MBq	900.0 µCi = 33.3 MBq	22.0 mCi − 814 MBq
7.0 µCi = 0.259 MBq	1.0 mCi = 37.0 MBq	23.0 mCi = 851 MBq
8.0 µCi = 0.296 MBq	1.5 mCi = 55.5 MBq	24.0 mCi = 888 MBq
9.0 µCi = 0.333 MBq	2.0 mCi = 74.0 MBq	25.0 mCi = 925 MBq
10.0 µCi = 0.370 MBq	2.5 mCi = 92.5 MBq	30.0 mCi = 1.11 GBq
15.0 µCi = 0.555 MBq	3.0 mCi = 111 MBq	35.0 mCi − 1.30 GBq
20.0 µCi = 0.740 MBq	3.5 mCi = 130 MBq	40.0 mCi = 1.48 GBq
25.0 µCi = 0.925 MBq	4.0 mCi = 148 MBq	45.0 mCi = 1.67 GBq
30.0 µCi = 1.11 MBq	4.5 mCi = 167 MBq	50.0 mCi = 1.85 GBq
35.0 µCi = 1.30 MBq	5.0 mCi − 185 MBq	60.0 mCi = 2.22 GBq
40.0 µCi = 1.48 MBq	5.5 mCi = 204 MBq	65.0 mCi − 2.41 GBq
45.0 µCi = 1.67 MBq	6.0 mCi = 222 MBq	70.0 mCi = 2.59 GBq
50.0 µCi = 1.85 MBq	6.5 mCi = 241 MBq	80.0 mCi = 2.96 GBq
60.0 µCi = 2.22 MBq	7.0 mCi = 259 MBq	90.0 mCi = 3.33 GBq
70.0 µCi = 2.59 MBq	7.5 mCi = 278 MBq	95.0 mCi = 3.52 GBq
80.0 µCi = 2.96 MBq	8.0 mCi = 296 MBq	100.0 mCi = 3.70 GBq
90.0 µCi = 3.33 MBq	8.5 mCi = 315 MBq	110.0 mCi = 4.07 GBq
100.0 µCi = 3.70 MBq	9.0 mCi = 333 MBq	120.0 mCi = 4.44 GBq
125.0 µCi = 4.63 MBq	9.5 mCi = 366 MBq	130.0 mCi = 4.81 GBq
150.0 µCi = 5.55 MBq	10.0 mCi = 370 MBq	140.0 mCi = 5.18 GBq
175.0 µCi = 6.48 MBq	11.0 mCi = 407 MBq	150.0 mCi = 5.55 GBq
200.0 µCi = 7.40 MBq	12.0 mCi = 444 MBq	175.0 mCi = 6.48 GBq
250.0 µCi = 9.25 MBq	13.0 mCi = 481 MBq	200.0 mCi = 7.40 GBq
300.0 µCi = 11.1 MBq	14.0 mCi = 518 MBq	250.0 mCi = 9.25 GBq
350.0 µCi = 13.0 MBq	15.0 mCi = 555 MBq	300.0 mCi = 11.1 GBq
400.0 µCi = 14.8 MBq	16.0 mCi = 592 MBq	400.0 mCi = 14.8 GBq

Technetium-99m Decay and Generation Tables

The table below may be used to determine the amount of technetium-99m (^{99m}Tc) remaining in a sample after a given period of time using the following formula: original activity (mCi or Bq) at time T multiplied by the fraction remaining. Time is given in hours and minutes.

The table to the right may be used to determine the yield of Technetium-99m from a Mo-99/Tc-99m generator when eluted at a particular time interval after the previous elution.

Molybdenum-99/^{99m}Tc Generator Yield

HOURS SINCE PREVIOUS ELUTION	^{99M}TC YIELD (PERCENTAGE OF PREVIOUS ELUTION)
1	9
2	18
3	26
4	33
5	39
6	45
7	50
8	54
10	62
12	69
18	80
24	87

^{99m}Tc activity reaches maximum in 22.9 hr (transient equilibrium).

^{99m}Tc Decay Chart

TIME	FRACTION REMAINING	TIME	FRACTION REMAINING
0:00	1.000	3:00	0.707
0:10	0.981	3:10	0.694
0:20	0.962	3:20	0.680
0:30	0.944	3:30	0.667
0:40	0.926	3:40	0.655
0:50	0.908	3:50	0.642
1:00	0.891	4:00	0.630
1:10	0.874	4:10	0.618
1:20	0.857	4:20	0.606
1:30	0.841	4:30	0.595
1:40	0.825	4:40	0.583
1:50	0.809	4:50	0.572
2:00	0.794	5:00	0.561
2:10	0.779	5:10	0.551
2:20	0.764	5:20	0.540
2:30	0.749	5:30	0.530
2:40	0.735	5:40	0.520
2:50	0.721	5:50	0.510

Other Radionuclide* Decay Tables

Flourine-18

TIME (HOURS)	FRACTION REMAINING
0.25	0.910
0.50	0.827
0.75	0.753
1.00	0.685
1.25	0.623
1.50	0.567
1.75	0.515
2.00	0.469
2.50	0.387
3.00	0.321
4.00	0.219
5.00	0.150
6.00	0.109
12.00	0.011

Gallium-67

TIME (HOURS)	FRACTION REMAINING
0	1.00
6	0.95
12	0.90
18	0.85
24	0.81
36	0.73
48	0.65
60	0.59
72	0.53
90	0.45
120	0.35
168	0.23

Indium-111

TIME (DAY)	FRACTION REMAINING
0	1.000
1	0.781
2	0.610
3	0.476
4	0.372
5	0.290

Iodine-123

TIME (HOURS)	FRACTION REMAINING
0	1.00
3	0.854
6	0.730
12	0.535
15	0.455
18	0.389
21	0.332
24	0.284
30	0.207

* A decay calculator for many radionuclides is available on the web at http://www.mcgill.ca./ehs/radiation/basics/decay

Iodine-131

TIME (DAY)	DECAY FACTOR
0	1.000
1	0.918
2	0.841
3	0.771
4	0.707
5	0.648
6	0.595
7	0.545
8	0.500
9	0.458
10	0.421
11	0.386
12	0.354
13	0.324
14	0.297
15	0.273
16	0.250
17	0.229
18	0.210
19	0.193
20	0.177

Strontium-89

TIME (DAY)	DECAY FACTOR
0	1.00
6	0.92
8	0.90
10	0.87
12	0.85
14	0.83
16	0.80
18	0.78
20	0.76
22	0.74
24	0.72
26	0.70
28	0.68

Injection Techniques and Pediatric Dosage

INJECTION TECHNIQUES

Each of the two commonly used rapid bolus injection techniques, when properly executed, provides a high-quality bolus of radiopharmaceutical, assuming patent venous pathways and adequate cardiac function.

Oldendorf Tourniquet Method

In the Oldendorf method, first the blood pressure is taken to determine diastolic and systolic pressures in the arm to be used for injection. The blood pressure cuff is then inflated to a level above diastolic pressure but less than systolic pressure. The pressure in the cuff is left at this level for 1 to 2 minutes to allow engorgement of the venous system in the lower arm, thereby building up a considerable back pressure that will constitute the forward momentum of the injected bolus. The cuff is then inflated above systolic pressure to prevent further entry of blood into the veins. At this point, a venipuncture of an antecubital vein (preferably a basilic vein) is performed, if not already done. Next, the radiopharmaceutical, in a volume of less than 1 mL, is injected, and the cuff is removed from the arm with a single swift motion. It is important to leave the needle in place until the dynamic images are complete so that no pressure on the venipuncture site is instituted.

Intravenous Push Method

The intravenous push technique is simpler than is the Oldendorf method and is in general more commonly used. The technique requires a special tubing set-up with an additional intravenous entry site for the introduction of the radiopharmaceutical. Antecubital venipuncture is performed in the usual way, preferably by using a large-bore needle. The end of the intravenous push tubing is connected to a syringe containing 25 to 30 mL of normal saline. Once the needle is in place, the radiopharmaceutical is injected into the distal tubing through the rubber entry portal, immediately followed by rapid injection of the saline, which propels the bolus to the right heart.

PEDIATRIC DOSAGE

Pediatric doses of radiopharmaceuticals ideally should be kept as low as possible. A balance must be achieved between the smaller doses needed in a small patient and the minimum dose needed to get a statistically valid examination in a reasonable time period. Simple reduction of an adult dose per unit weight necessitates an extremely long imaging time, and the image may be compromised by patient motion. Some authors use formulas based on either body surface area or weight. The former method requires consulting published nomograms. A modified Young's rule or Webster's rule is one method commonly used to estimate pediatric doses. In this case, the adult dose is multiplied by the following fraction:

$$(\text{age in years} + 1)/(\text{age in years} + 7)$$

For example, if the adult dose of technetium-99m (^{99m}Tc) phosphate for a bone scan is 20 mCi (740 MBq), then the dose for a 5-year-old child would be as follows:

$$[5+1]/[5+7] = 6/12 = 1/2, \text{ or}$$
$$20 \text{ mCi}(740 \text{ MBq}) \times 1/2 = 10 \text{ mCi}(370 \text{ MBq})$$

The minimum pediatric doses needed for various examinations are seen in the Table D–1.

TABLE D-1.	Minimum Pediatric Administered Activity for Various Examinations	
EXAMINATION	**RADIOPHARMACEUTICAL**	**DOSE**
Gastroesophageal reflux	^{99m}Tc-sulfur colloid	0.5 mCi (18.5 MBq) p.o.
Brain death scan	^{99m}TcO$_4^-$, ^{99m}Tc-DTPA, or ^{99m}Tc-hexamethyl-propyleneamineoxime	2 mCi (74 MBq)
Meckel's diverticulum scan	^{99m}TcO$_4^-$	2 mCi (74 MBq)
Angiocardiogram	^{99m}TcO$_4^-$	2 mCi (74 MBq)
Thyroid uptake	^{123}I	10 µCi (0.37 MBq)
Thyroid scan	^{99m}TcO$_4^-$	1 mCi (37 MBq)
	^{123}I	30 µCi (1.1 MBq) (newborn)
	^{123}I	60 µCi (2.2 MBq) (to 1 yr)
	^{123}I	90 µCi (3.3 MBq) (1–5 yr)
	^{123}I	120 µCi (4.6 MBq) (5–10 yr)
	^{123}I	170 µCi (6.4 MBq) (10–15 yr)
Bone scan	^{9m}Tc-phosphate	2 mCi (74 MBq)
Lung scan	^{99m}Tc-macroaggregated albumin	500 µCi (18.5 MBq)
	^{133}Xe	Ventilation xenon 2.0 mCi/L or 74 MBq/L
Liver scan	^{99m}Tc-sulfur colloid	750 µCi (27.8 MBq)
Renal scan	^{99m}Tc-DTPA, ^{99m}Tc-MAG3, or ^{99m}Tc-DMSA	500 µCi (18.5 MBq)
Cisternogram	^{111}In-DTPA	25 µCi (0.93 MBq)
Gallium scan	^{67}Ga citrate	500 µCi (18.5 MBq)
Hepatobiliary scan	^{99m}Tc-IDA	1 mCi (37 MBq)

^{99m}Tc, Technetium-99m; ^{99m}TcO$_4^-$, pertechnetate; DTPA, diethylene triamine pentaacetic acid; ^{123}I, iodine-123; ^{133}Xe, xenon-133; MAG3, mertiatide; DMSA, dimercaptosuccinic acid; ^{111}In, indium-111; ^{67}Ga, gallium-67; IDA, iminodiacetic acid.

Sample Techniques for Nuclear Imaging

This appendix is provided as a guide to the technical aspects of various imaging procedures. Some of the less common procedures have not been included, and the procedures described herein may need to be adjusted, depending on the equipment available. Each nuclear medicine laboratory should have a standardized procedures manual; this appendix may be used as a beginning point for the development of such a manual. The reader is also referred to procedure guidelines in the practice management section of the Society of Nuclear Medicine Web site (http://www.snm.org).

BRAIN DEATH OR CEREBRAL BLOOD FLOW SCAN

Procedure imaging time
  20 to 30 minutes
Radiopharmaceutical
  Technetium-99m (^{99m}Tc) diethylene triamine pentaacetic acid (DTPA), or glucoheptonate. Brain specific agents such as ^{99m}Tc hexamethylpropyleneamine oxime (HMPAO) single-photon emission computed tomography (SPECT) scan and ^{99m}Tc ethyl cysteinate dimer (ECD), also called Tc-Bicisate, can be used, but there is no clear evidence that they are more accurate. They do obviate the need for a very good bolus injection.
Method of administration
  Bolus IV injection
Normal adult administered activity
  15 to 30 mCi (555 MBq to 1.11 GBq)
Injection-to-imaging time.
  Immediate
Conflicting examinations and medications
  None
Patient preparation

None necessary, although some institutions put a rubber band or tourniquet around the head just above ears to help diminish scalp blood flow. This should not be done in patients with a history of head trauma. Patient should be normally ventilated.
Technique
  Collimator
    High-resolution or ultrahigh-resolution; field of view (FOV) should include from the level of the common carotids to the skull vertex.
  Dynamic flow imaging time
    Blood flow images: 1 to 3 seconds/frame for at least 60 seconds. Flow images should start before the arrival of the bolus in the neck.
  Routine views
    Immediate blood pool anterior and anterior image at 5 minutes each. Many institutions also obtain posterior and both lateral views. Note: If brain specific images are obtained, initial images as described above are obtained as well as planar and SPECT images obtained after 20 minutes.
  Patient positioning
    Sitting or supine
  Photopeak selection
    140-keV (15% to 20% window)
Dosimetry: rads/mCi (mGy/MBq) of administered activity
  DTPA
    Effective dose   0.02 (0.005)
    Bladder wall   0.19 (0.05)
  HMPAO (also called Ceretec or exametazime)
    Effective dose   0.034 (0.009)
    Kidneys   0.126 (0.034)
  ECD (Bicisate or Neurolite)
    Effective dose   0.041 (0.020)
    Kidneys   0.27 (0.073)
    Bladder wall   0.21 (0.057)

SPECT BRAIN IMAGING

Procedure imaging time
30 to 60 minutes

Instrumentation
SPECT camera

Radiopharmaceutical
^{99m}Tc-HMPAO (Exametazime unstabilized or stabilized), ^{99m}Tc-ECD
For unstabilized ^{99m}Tc-HMPAO, inject no sooner than 10 minutes after preparation and not more than 30 minutes after preparation. For seizure disorders, inject within 1 minute after reconstitution. For stabilized ^{99m}Tc-HMPAO, inject no sooner than 10 minutes after preparation and no more than 4 hours after preparation. For ^{99m}Tc-ECD, inject no sooner than 10 minutes after preparation and no more than 4 hours after preparation.

Method of administration
Place patient in a quiet, dimly lit room and instruct him or her to keep eyes and ears open. The patient should be seated or reclining comfortably. IV access should be placed at least 10 minutes before injection. The patient should not speak or read, and there should be little or no interaction before, during or up to 5 minutes after injection.

Normal administered activity
15 to 30 mCi (555 MBq to 1.11 GBq), children 0.2 to 0.3 mCi/kg (7.4 to 11.1 MBq/kg). Minimum dose, 3 to 5 mCi (111 to 185 MBq).

Injection-to-imaging time
90 minutes or later for stabilized or unstabilized ^{99m}Tc-HMPAO, although images obtained after 40 minutes will be interpretable; 45-minute delay for ^{99m}Tc-ECD, although images obtained after 20 minutes will be interpretable. If possible, all imaging should be obtained within 4 hours of injection.

Conflicting examinations and medications
None

Patient preparation
Patient should be instructed, if possible, to avoid caffeine, alcohol, or other drugs known to affect cerebral blood flow. If sedation is required, it should be given after the injection. Patient should void before study for maximum comfort.

Technique
Collimator
Low-energy, high- or ultrahigh-resolution, or fan beam; all-purpose
Acquisition
128 × 128 or greater acquisition matrix; 3-degree or better angular sampling. Acquisition pixel size should be one third to one half of the expected resolution. Low-pass Butterworth filters should be used for processing in all three dimensions. Attenuation correction should be performed.

Routine views
360-degree arc of rotation single head camera; however, multiple head detectors may produce better images.

Patient positioning
Supine

Photopeak selection
140-keV ^{99m}Tc (20% window)

Dosimetry: rads/mCi (mGy/MBq) administered.

HMPAO (also called Ceretec or exametazime)	
Effective dose	0.034 (0.009)
Kidneys	0.126 (0.034)
ECD (Bicisate or Neurolite)	
Effective dose	0.041 (0.020)
Kidneys	0.27 (0.073)
Bladder wall	0.21 (0.057)

Comments
Vasodilatory challenge with acetazolamide (Diamox) may be ordered for evaluation of cerebrovascular reserve in transient ischemic attack, completed stroke, or vascular anomalies. Known sulfa allergy is a contraindication, and the procedure is usually avoided within 3 days of an acute stroke. The challenge study is usually done first, and if normal, the baseline study may be omitted. The dosage is 1000 mg in 10 mL sterile water by slow IV push (over 2 minutes) and 14 mg/kg for children. Wait 10 to 20 minutes before injecting tracer. The patient should void immediately before acquisition.

CISTERNOGRAM

Procedure imaging time
30 minutes for each set

Instrumentation
Planar gamma camera

Radiopharmaceutical
Indium-111 (^{111}In)-DTPA

Method of administration
Spinal subarachnoid space injection

Normal adult administered activity
0.5 mCi (18.5 MBq)

Injection-to-imaging time
2 hours, 6 hours, 24 hours, 48 hours, and 72 hours (as needed)

Conflicting examination and medications

Acetazolamide (Diamox) can cause false-positive results

Patient preparation

If the clinical diagnosis is cerebrospinal fluid (CSF) rhinorrhea or otorrhea, the patient's nose and ears should be packed with pledgets before injection for later counting.

Technique

Collimator

Low-energy, all-purpose, parallel-hole

Counts

1. 50 to 100 k counts for ^{111}In
2. Cobalt (^{57}Co) for 50-k counts transmission scan (if useful for anatomic definition)

Routine views

1. Anterior transmission scan: position patient's head between ^{57}Co sheet source and collimator surface. Peak in ^{57}Co by after photopeak determination. Set intensity, but collect only 50-k counts. Do not advance film or image. Remove sheet source from behind patient. Peak detector for ^{111}In. Collect 100-k counts.
2. Lateral transmission scan
3. Anterior head
4. Lateral head (same lateral as transmission scan)

Patient positioning

Supine. If a large CSF leak is suspected in a specific area, the patient may be positioned with that portion dependent.

Photopeak selection

^{57}Co (for transmission images); ^{111}In-DTPA 173-keV (20% window)

Dosimetry: rads/mCi (mGy/MBq) of administered activity

Effective dose	0.6 (0.162)
Spinal cord	12.0 to 20.0 (3.2 to 5.4)

Comments

For CSF rhinorrhea or otorrhea, count all pledget samples in well counter after removal from nose and ears. Note: Remove the pledgets and place each in a separate counting vial at time of removal, labeling each vial with its location.

THYROID SCAN (^{99M}TC-PERTECHNETATE)

Procedure imaging time

15 minutes

Radiopharmaceutical

^{99m}Tc-sodium pertechnetate

Method of administration

IV injection

Normal administered activity

2 to 10 mCi (75 to 370 MBq). For 5-year-old child, 15 to 70 µCi/kg (1 to 5 MBq/kg)

Injection-to-imaging time

15 to 30 minutes

Conflicting examinations and medications

None

Patient preparation

None

Technique

Collimator

Low-energy parallel and pinhole

Counts

100- to 250-k counts per image or 5 minutes

Patient positioning

1. Supine
2. Extend neck forward by placing a positioning sponge under back of neck

Routine views

1. Anterior view of the thyroid to include salivary glands, using parallel collimator
2. Pinhole views of thyroid only, in anterior and both anterior oblique positions (positioned so that the thyroid gland fills two thirds of the FOV)

Photopeak selection

140-keV (20% window)

Dosimetry: rads/mCi (mGy/MBq) of administered activity

Effective dose	0.05 (0.01)
Gonads	0.01 to 0.04 (0.003 to 0.011)
Thyroid	0.12 to 0.20 (0.04 to 0.06)
Stomach and colon	0.10 to 0.30 (0.03 to 0.08)

Comments

Remind the patient not to swallow while the camera is imaging. Drinking water is sometimes useful to eliminate confusing esophageal activity.

THYROID SCAN AND UPTAKE (IODINE-123)

Procedure imaging time

1 hour

Radiopharmaceutical

Iodine-123 (^{123}I) sodium iodide

Method of administration

Oral

Normal administered activity

200 to 600 µCi (7.4 to 25 MBq). For 5-year-old child, 3 to 10 µCi/kg (0.1 to 0.3 MBq/kg)

Administration-to-imaging time

3 to 24 hours

Conflicting examinations and medications

1. Radiographic procedures using IV iodine contrast media (e.g., IV pyelogram, computed tomography [CT] scan with contrast)
2. Other radiographic procedures using iodine contrast media (e.g., myelogram, oral cholecystogram)
3. Exogenous T_3 or T_4 (liothyronine, levothyroxine)
4. Thyroid-blocking agents such as propylthiouracil, perchlorate, and methimazole
5. Oral iodides in medications containing iodine (e.g., kelp preparations, vitamins, Lugol's solution)
6. If necessary, do a pertechnetate ($^{99m}TcO_4^-$) scan.

Patient preparation

Scanning dose to be administered 3 to 24 hours before scanning. Patient should be NPO overnight before examination. If patient is pregnant or lactating consider using $^{99m}TcO_4^-$

Technique

Collimator
  Pinhole
Counts
  50- to 100-k counts per image or 10 minute/image
Routine views
  Anterior, right and left anterior oblique
Patient positioning
  Supine, neck extended
Photopeak selection
  159-keV (20% window)

Dosimetry: rads/mCi (mGy/MBq) of administered activity

Effective dose	0.6 (0.2)
Gonads	0.01 to 0.03 (0.003 to 0.008)
Thyroid	16.6 (4.5) assuming 35% uptake
Stomach	0.22 (0.06)

Comments

1. Iodine uptake is normally measured at 24 hours, although rarely it is also measured at 6 hours. It is measured with a sodium iodide probe.
2. Patient's thyroid should be palpated by physician.

THYROID CANCER SCAN

Procedure imaging time
  1 to 2 hours

Radiopharmaceutical
  ^{131}I-sodium iodide or ^{123}I-sodium iodide
Method of administration
  Oral
Normal adult administered activity
  1 to 5 mCi (37 to 185 MBq) ^{131}I-sodium iodide
  1 to 2 mCi (37 to 74 MBq) ^{123}I-sodium iodide
  10 to 20 mCi (370 to 740 MBq) ^{99m}Tc-sestamibi
Injection-to-imaging time
  72 hour (96 h, if needed) ^{131}I sodium iodide
  24 hour for ^{123}I sodium iodide
  15 minutes for ^{99m}Tc-sestamibi
Conflicting examinations and medications
  Iodine-containing medications and contrast agents
Patient preparation
  For radioiodine 2 weeks off T_3 replacement or 4 to 6 weeks off T_4 replacement. In some patients, the use of rTSH (thyrogen) may be useful to supplement thyroid hormone withdrawal. Some institutions use a low iodine diet 3 to 10 days before administration of tracer.
Technique
  Whole-body scan or spot views of head, neck, chest, and other clinically suspect areas
  Collimator
    Medium- or high-energy-^{131}I-sodium iodide or low-energy for ^{123}I-sodium iodide or ^{99m}Tc
  Counts
    200-k counts or 10-minute spot views
  Routine views
    Anterior and posterior whole-body views
  Patient positioning
    Supine
  Photopeak selection
    364-keV (20% window) for ^{131}I-sodium iodide or 159-keV (20% window) ^{123}I-sodium iodide
    Absorbed dose with thyroid removed or ablated.

Dosimetry: rads/mCi (mGy/MBq) of administered activity

^{123}I	Effective dose	0.50 (0.135)
	Bladder wall	0.33 (0.09)
^{131}I	Whole body	0.27 (0.073)
	Bladder wall	2.3 (0.62)
^{99m}Tc sestamibi (Cardiolite)		
	Effective dose	0.03 (0.008)
	Gallbladder	0.14 (0.038)

Comments

1. This scan for metastatic disease is done only after ablation of normal thyroid tissue.

2. Serum thyroid-stimulating hormone (TSH) levels should be above 40 mU/mL before start.
3. Scanning can also be done 7 to 10 days after a cancer therapy treatment with [131]I.
4. Scanning with ^{123}I may prevent stunning of thyroid remnant or metastases.
5. Occasionally scans are done by using ^{99m}Tc-sestamibi or thallium-201 (^{201}Tl) chloride to locate nonfunctioning metastases.

PARATHYROID SCAN (DUAL-PHASE STUDY)

Procedure imaging time
  2 hours
Radiopharmaceutical
  ^{99m}Tc-sestamibi
Method of administration
  IV administration
Normal adult administered activity
  20 mCi (740 MBq)
Injection-to-imaging time
  5 minutes
Conflicting examinations and medications
  None
Patient preparation
  None
Technique
  Collimator
    Low-energy, high resolution, or pinhole
  Counts/time
    Acquire image for 10 minutes, and if digital acquisition use a 128 × 128 or larger matrix.
  Routine views
    Anterior images of the neck at 5, 20, and 120 minutes after injection. A single anterior large-FOV image should also be obtained that includes the mediastinum.
  Patient positioning
    Supine
  Photopeak selection
    140-keV (20% window)
Dosimetry: rads/mCi (mGy/MBq) of administered activity
  Effective dose 0.03 (0.008)
  Gallbladder   0.14 (0.04)
Comments
  There are a number of dual-isotope methods that are more complicated and require computer subtraction.

REST GATED EQUILIBRIUM VENTRICULOGRAPHY*

Procedure imaging time
  30 minutes
Radiopharmaceutical
  ^{99m}Tc-labeled red blood cells (RBCs). See RBC labeling procedures at the end of this appendix. We prefer the modified in vivo method for this examination.
Method of administration
  IV injection
Normal adult administered activity
  15 to 30 mCi (555 MBq to 1110 MBq)
Injection-to-imaging time
  Immediate
Conflicting examinations and medications
  None
Patient preparation
  Fasting for 3 to 4 hours before the study is preferred
Technique
  Collimator
    Low-energy, all-purpose, or high-resolution parallel-hole
  Counts
    3 to 7 million counts with a minimum of 16 and preferably 32 to 64 frames per second
  Patient positioning
    Supine or upright
  Photopeak selection
    140-keV (20% window)
Dosimetry: rads/mCi (mGy/MBq) of administered activity
  Effective dose   0.026 (0.007)
  Heart   0.085 (0.023)
Comments
  In vivo RBC labeling.
    1. Take a vial of cold pyrophosphate and dilute with 1 to 3 mL of *sterile* saline (not bacteriostatic). Shake the mixture, and let it stand 5 minutes. Without injecting air into the vial, withdraw the contents into a 3-mL syringe, avoiding inclusion of an air bubble.
    2. Inject patient with cold pyrophosphate (0.8 to 1 mg stannous chloride).
    3. After 20 minutes, inject the radiopharmaceutical.
    4. Connect electrocardiogram leads to patient 5 to 10 cm below the axilla bilaterally. Remember to abrade the skin well enough so that the leads have good contact.

5. Place the patient in the supine position on an imaging table with left side toward the camera.

*Stress study and computer operation vary widely and are not presented here.

SPECT MYOCARDIAL PERFUSION IMAGING

Procedure imaging time
    30 minutes for each set of images
Instrumentation
    SPECT camera
Radiopharmaceutical
    ^{99m}Tc-sestamibi, ^{201}Tl-chloride, ^{99m}Tc-teboroxime, or ^{99m}Tc-tetrofosmin
Method of administration
    IV injection
Normal adult administered activity

^{99m}Tc-sestamibi	20 to 30 mCi (750 to 1100 MBq)
^{201}Tl-chloride	3 to 5 mCi (111 to 185 MBq)
^{99m}Tc-teboroxime	30 to 50 mCi (1110 to 1850 MBq)
^{99m}Tc-tetrofosmin	20 to 40 mCi (750 to 1500 MBq)

Injection-to-imaging time
    For poststress images, immediate for thallium, 30 to 90 minutes for sestamibi.
Conflicting examinations and medications
    Discontinue calcium antagonists, β-blockers, and nitrates, if possible.
    With thallium, increased myocardial uptake has been reported with dipyridamole, furosemide, isoproterenol sodium bicarbonate (IV), and dexamethasone; decreased myocardial uptake with propranolol, digitalis, doxorubicin, phenytoin (Dilantin), lidocaine, and minoxidil.
Patient preparation
    NPO for 4 hours; exercise, if required. In patients with severe coronary disease, it may be advisable to administer nitroglycerin sublingually about 3 minutes before rest injection of the radiopharmaceutical.
Technique
    Collimator
        Low-energy, all-purpose
    Counts and time
        30 to 32 stops for 40 seconds each for ^{201}Tl and 10 seconds for ^{99m}Tc sestamibi
    Routine views

180 or 360 degree arc of rotation; 180 degrees is preferred from right anterior oblique to left posterior oblique. Either step and shoot acquisition with 32 or 64 stops separated by 3 to 6 degrees or continuous acquisition may be used. The duration for each stop varies but is generally 40 seconds per image for thallium and 25 seconds for technetium radiopharmaceuticals.
Patient positioning
    Supine, left arm overhead
Photopeak technetium
    85-keV (15% window) and possibly 135- to 160-keV for thallium and 140-keV (20% window) for technetium
Dosimetry: rads/mCi (mGy/MBq) of administered activity

^{201}Tl-chloride	
Effective dose	0.60 (0.16)
Kidneys	1.7 (0.46)
Thyroid	2.3 (0.62)
^{99m}Tc-sestamibi	
Effective dose	0.03 (0.008)
Gallbladder	0.14 (0.038)
^{99m}Tc-teboroxime	
Effective dose	0.041 (0.011)
Colon	0.13 (0.035)
^{99m}Tc-tetrofosmin (Myoview)	
Effective dose	0.025 (0.007)
Gallbladder	0.13 (0.035)

Comments
1. Process for short- and long-axis views.
2. Parametric images such as "bull's eye" maps can be used to map perfusion and motion and to quantitate washout.
3. Use 64 × 64 matrix, Butterworth filter, 0.4 cutoff.
4. Attenuation correction significantly reduces artifacts.

EXERCISE PROTOCOL USING A BRUCE MULTISTAGE OR MODIFIED BRUCE TREADMILL EXERCISE PROTOCOL

Patient preparation
    Initial imaging
    Within 10 to 15 minutes after injection, perform SPECT imaging. Time should be long enough to permit clearance of liver activity when using ^{99m}Tc-sestamibi or ^{99m}Tc-tetrofosmin. This is usually 15 to 30 minutes after a stress injection.
    After exercise instructions
        Only light food intake; minimal physical exertion

Redistribution imaging
   3 to 4 hours after injection
Contraindications
   Unstable angina with recent (<48 h) angina or congestive heart failure, documented acute myocardial infarction within 2 to 4 days of testing, uncontrolled systemic (systolic >220 mmHg, diastolic >120 mmHg) or pulmonary hypertension, untreated life-threatening arrhythmias, uncompensated congestive failure, advanced atrioventricular block (without a pacemaker), acute myocarditis, acute pericarditis, severe mitral or aortic stenosis, severe obstructive cardiomyopathy, and acute systemic illness. Relative contraindications to exercise stress include conditions that may interfere with exercise such as neuralgic, arthritic, or orthopedic conditions or severe pulmonary or peripheral vascular disease.

DIPYRIDAMOLE PHARMACOLOGIC STRESS PROCEDURE*

Patient preparation
   NPO 4 to 6 hours; withhold caffeine-containing beverages for at least 12 hours and preferably 24 hours.
Drug administered
   IV infusion of dipyridamole in antecubital vein with patient supine; rate, 0.5 mg/kg over 4 minutes in 20 to 40 mL of normal saline.
Radiopharmaceutical administered
   IV administration of any of the radiopharmaceutical listed above 3 minutes after dipyridamole infusion, with patient supine or upright.
Imaging
   Begin 3 to 4 minutes after thallium injection; SPECT imaging; repeat in 3 to 4 hours. For technetium radiopharmaceuticals, postinjection imaging time is not as critical and may be done at 30 to 60 minutes.
Comments
   Side effects may be reversed by IV administration of 100 to 200 mg of aminophylline over 1 minute. No caffeine or theophylline for 12 hours before procedure.
*Possibly reinject before delayed imaging.

ADENOSINE PHARMACOLOGIC STRESS PROCEDURE

Patient preparation
   Contraindicated in patients with second- or third-degree atrioventricular block, sinus node disease, or asthma. Withhold dipyridamole for 12 to 24 hours before adenosine.
Drug administered
   Adenosine, 140 µg/kg/minute peripheral IV infusion over 6 minutes (total dose, 0.84 mg/kg) or 50 µg/kg/minute increased to 75, 100, and 140 µg/kg/minute each minute to 7 minutes.
Radiopharmaceutical administered
   Administered at the midpoint (3 minutes) of the infusion.
Imaging
   As for dipyridamole
Comments
   Side effects of hypertension, flushing, chest discomfort, dyspnea, headache, dizziness, or gastrointestinal discomfort may occur and usually resolve quickly, although theophylline (50 to 125 mg slow IV injection) may be necessary in rare cases.

PULMONARY VENTILATION SCAN (XENON)

Procedure imaging time
   5 minutes
Instrumentation
   Large-FOV camera, if available
Radiopharmaceutical
   ^{133}Xe
Method of administration
   Gas is inspired through an enclosed ventilation system with appropriate mouthpiece or face mask.
Normal adult administered activity
   4 to 20 mCi (185 to 740 MBq). (If done after perfusion scan, dose may have to be 20 mCi [740 MBq]).
   Dose for children, 0.3 mCi/kg (10 to 12 MBq/kg) with a minimum of 3 mCi (100 to 120 MBq)
Conflicting examination and medications
   None
Patient preparation
   None
Technique
   Collimator
      Low-energy, all-purpose, parallel-hole
   Counts
      All images are taken for 10 to 15 seconds.
   Routine views
      All views are performed in the posterior position unless otherwise specified by the physician.

1. Begin ^{133}Xe and obtain 10-second inspiration image (1000-k counts).
2. Record three equilibrium images (300-k counts).
3. Exhaust ^{133}Xe and record 10- to 40-second images until the bulk of the gas has left the lungs.

Patient positioning
  Sitting, preferably. Supine is also acceptable.
Photopeak selection
  81-keV (25% window)
Dosimetry: rads/mCi (mGy/MBq) of administered activity

Effective dose	0.003 (0.0008)
Lung	0.004 (0.001)

Comments
  An exhaust system or xenon trap should be available for expired xenon. Room must be negative pressure.

PULMONARY VENTILATION SCAN (DTPA AEROSOL)

Procedure imaging time
  15 minutes
Instrumentation
  Large-FOV camera, if available
Radiopharmaceutical
  ^{99m}Tc-diethylene triamine pentaacetic acid (DTPA) aerosol
Method of administration
  Nebulizer connected to a mouthpiece. The nose should be occluded. Patient performing tidal breathing in the upright position if possible.
Normal adult administered activity
  25 to 35 mCi (900 to 1300 MBq) in the nebulizer from which the patients receives about 0.5 to 1.0 mCi (20 to 40 MBq).
Conflicting examination and medications
  None
Patient preparation
  None
Technique
  Collimator
    Low-energy, all-purpose, parallel-hole
  Photopeak selection
    140-keV (20% window)
  Counts
    When the camera sees 1000 counts per second, discontinue nebulizer and then do images for 100-k counts per image
  Routine views
  Anterior, posterior, and four obliques

Patient positioning
  Sitting, preferably. Supine is also acceptable.
Dosimetry: rads/mCi (mGy/MBq) of administered activity

Effective dose	0.026 (0.007)
Bladder	0.17 (0.046)

Comments
  Should usually be performed before the ^{99m}Tc-macroaggregated albumin (MAA) perfusion scan.

PULMONARY PERFUSION SCAN

Procedure imaging time
  30 minutes
Radiopharmaceutical
  ^{99m}Tc-macroaggregated albumin (MAA), about 300,000 particles; however, this can be reduced to 100,000 to 200,000 in persons with known right to left shunts, infants, and children.
Method of administration
  Before injection the patient should, if possible, cough and take several deep breaths. Invert syringe immediately before injection to resuspend particles. With the patient supine, or as close to supine as possible, begin slow IV injection in antecubital vein during three to five respiratory cycles.
Normal adult administered activity
  5 mCi (185 MBq); reduce to 3 mCi (111 MBq) if expecting to do xenon study afterward.
Injection-to-imaging time
  Immediate
Conflicting examinations and medications
  None
Patient preparation
  None
Technique
  Collimator
    Low-energy, all-purpose, parallel-hole
  Counts
    500-k counts
  Routine views
  1. Posterior
  2. Left posterior oblique
  3. Left lateral
  4. Left anterior oblique
  5. Anterior
  6. Right anterior oblique
  7. Right lateral
  8. Right posterior oblique
  Patient positioning
    Preferably sitting although supine is acceptable

Photopeak selection

140-keV (20% window)

Dosimetry: rads/mCi (mGy/MBq) of adminis-tered activity

Effective dose	0.044 (0.012)
Lung	0.25 (0.068)

Comments

If blood is introduced into the syringe con-taining the radiopharmaceutical, the injection must be completed immediately or small blood clots entrapping the radiopharmaceutical may cause hot spots in the lung. If the injected par-ticles are too small, they will accumulate in the liver and spleen.

In patients with right-to-left shunts, young chil-dren, and patients with pulmonary hyperten-sion, reduce the number of particles to about 60,000 to 100,000.

A chest x-ray is used for correlation. It should be obtained within an hour or so but be no more than 24 hours.

A well flushed indwelling line can be used. Do not administer in the distal port of a Swan-Ganz catheter or any indwelling line or port that con-tains a filter (e.g., chemotherapy line).

LIVER AND SPLEEN SCAN

Procedure imaging time

30 minutes

Radiopharmaceutical

^{99m}Tc-sulfur or albumin colloid

Method of administration

IV injection; bolus injection in antecubital vein for dynamic imaging. Invert syringe before injecting to resuspend particles.

Normal adult administered activity

4 to 6 mCi (148 to 222 MBq)

Injection-to-imaging time

20 minutes

Conflicting examinations and medications

1. Recent upper gastrointestinal series or barium enema with retained barium
2. Increased bone marrow uptake will occur with nitrosoureas or if the colloid size is too small
3. Increased spleen uptake will occur with nitrosoureas, recent halothane or methylcel-lulose.

    Decreased spleen uptake can occur as a result of chemotherapy, epinephrine, and anti-malarials
4. Lung uptake can be increased as a result of aluminum antacids, iron preparations, viril-

izing androgens, Mg^{2-} preparations, niacin, colloid size too large, Al^{3-} in preparation, and particle clumping.

Patient preparation

None

Technique

Collimator

Low-energy, all-purpose, parallel-hole

Counts

1. 1000-k counts: anterior supine
2. 500-k counts: all other views

Routine views

1. Anterior supine
2. Anterior supine with lead marker
3. Anterior erect, if possible
4. Right anterior oblique
5. Right lateral
6. Right posterior oblique
7. Posterior
8. Left lateral

Optional views

In patients who require supine imaging, obtain anterior erect view whenever possible.

Patient positioning

Supine

Photopeak selection

140-keV (20% window)

Dosimetry: rads/mCi (mGy/MBq) of adminis-tered activity

Effective dose	0.034 (0.009)
Spleen	0.27 (0.07)

Comments

1. Breast-shadow artifact is often seen in women. Eliminate artifact by moving right breast away from liver in anterior and right anterior oblique views.
2. Selective splenic imaging can be performed by using an ultratag kit for red cells and injecting 1 to 3 mCi (40 to 110 MBq) of heat damaged ^{99m}Tc-labeled RBCs. Cells are typ-ically damaged by heating to 49°C to 50°C in a water bath for 20 minutes.
3. Blood pool imaging is done for evaluation of cavernous hemangioma after red cell label-ing and administration of 20 to 25 mCi (740 to 925 MBq). SPECT imaging is very helpful.

SPECT LIVER AND SPLEEN IMAGING

Procedure imaging time

30 minutes

Instrumentation

SPECT camera

Radiopharmaceutical

^{99m}Tc-sulfur or albumin colloid
Method of administration
    IV injection
Normal adult administered activity
    6 mCi (222 MBq)
Injection-to-imaging time
    20 minutes
Conflicting examinations and medications
    Retained barium
Patient preparation
    None
Technique
    Collimator
        Low-energy, high-resolution
    Counts and time
        60 to 64 stops for 30 seconds each
    Routine views
        360-degree arc of rotation
    Patient positioning
        Supine; both arms over head
    Photopeak selection
        140-keV (20% window)
Dosimetry: rads/mCi (mGy/MBq) of administered activity

Effective dose	0.034 (0.009)
Spleen	0.27 (0.07)

Comments
    128 × 128 matrix, if available

HEPATOBILIARY SCAN

Procedure imaging time
    1 to 4 hours
Radiopharmaceutical
    ^{99m}Tc-diisopropyl iminodiacetic acid (DISIDA; disofenin) or bromotrimethyl IDA (BrIDA; mebrofenin)
Method of administration
    IV injection; bolus injection in antecubital vein for dynamic imaging
Normal administered activity
    1.5 to 5 mCi (50 to 185 MBq). Higher activities may be needed in patient with hyperbilirubinemia 5 to 10 mCi (185 to 370 MBq). For infants and children, the administered activity is 0.05 to 0.2 mCi/ kg (2 to 7 MBq/kg) with a minimum of 0.4 to 0.5 mCi (15 to 20 MBq)
Injection-to-imaging time
    5 minutes
Conflicting examinations and medications
    1. Retained barium.
    2. Serum bilirubin level above 20 mg/dL may cause a nondiagnostic examination owing to poor hepatocellular function.

3. Delayed biliary-to-bowel transit will occur in patients who have received narcotic analgesics.
4. Liver uptake and excretion will be decreased by chronic high-dose nicotinic acid therapy, and phenobarbital will enhance hepatic excretion.
Patient preparation
    NPO for 2 hours and preferably 4 hours before procedure. If the patient has fasted for more than 24 hours or is on total parenteral nutrition, the gallbladder may not fill. In these cases, it may be necessary to pretreat with sincalide (see below).
Technique
    Collimator
        Low-energy, all-purpose, parallel-hole, or high-resolution
    Counts
        1. Three images (at 5, 10, and 15 minutes) at 500-k counts
        2. Record time of third (15-minute) image
        3. Remaining images for preset time, taken at 5-minute intervals for 45 minutes
    Routine views
        Optional views
            Serial images with continuous computer acquisition in anterior position (1 frame per minute for 30 to 60 minutes) reformatted at 5- to 15-minute images for filming.
            If visualization of gallbladder is questionable, obtain right lateral view.
    Patient positioning
        Supine
    Photopeak selection
        140-keV (20% window)
Dosimetry: rads/mCi (mGy/MBq) of administered activity

Effective dose	0.06 (0.016)
Gallbladder	0.41 (0.11)

Comments
    1. If gallbladder is not seen by 45 minutes, delayed images should be taken at 15-minute intervals until 2 hours after injection, and then hourly until 4 hours. An alternative is to administer morphine (0.04 mg/kg in 10 mL saline IV over 5 to 10 minutes) at 1 hour and continue imaging for 45 minutes or until gallbladder visualizes.
    2. If gallbladder is visualized but activity is not seen in the small bowel by 1 hour after injection, or a gallbladder ejection fraction is needed, consider using sincalide (0.02 μg/kg

in 10 mL of normal saline IV over 3 to 10 minutes). This can also be used for evaluation of the gallbladder ejection fraction by administering sincalide when the gallbladder is filled (usually at 1 hour).

3. If duodenal activity is confusing, have the patient drink water; wait 10 minutes and take another view. A left anterior oblique image may also separate duodenal loop activity from the gallbladder.

4. Delayed imaging at 24 hours may be necessary in infants with suspected biliary atresia.

MECKEL'S DIVERTICULUM SCAN

Procedure imaging time
$\frac{1}{2}$ to 1 hour
Radiopharmaceutical
^{99m}Tc-sodium pertechnetate
Method of administration
IV injection
Normal administered activity
10 mCi (370 MBq) or 200 to 300 µCi/kg (7.4 to 11.1 MBq/kg) in children and at least 2.0 mCi (74 MBq)
Injection-to-imaging time
Immediate
Conflicting examinations and medications
1. Increased gastric will be caused by Pentagastrin and Cimetidine. Decreased gastric mucosa activity will be caused by Al^{3-} ion (antacids) and perchlorate.
2. Recent upper gastrointestinal series can leave attenuating barium in abdomen.
3. Recent in vivo RBC labeling study with IV administration of stannous ion.
Patient preparation
See comments below
Technique
Collimator
Low-energy, all-purpose, parallel-hole
Counts
All static images: 500-k counts in the lower mid-abdomen above the bladder
Routine views
1. Sequential anterior abdominal images at 30- to 60-second intervals that can be reformatted at 5-minute intervals for 30 to 60 minutes.
2. Right lateral mid-abdomen at 45 minutes.
Patient positioning
Supine
Photopeak selection
140-keV (20% window)

Dosimetry: rads/mCi (mGy/MBq) of administered activity

Effective dose	0.048 (0.013) in an adult, 0.15 (0.04) in a 5-year-old child
Colon	0.23 (0.06) in an adult, 0.78 (0.21) in a 5-year-old child

Comments
Premedication may increase the sensitivity of the study but is not necessary for a high-quality study. Cimetidine (20 mg/kg in children or 10 to 20 mg/kg in neonates) given orally for 2 days before the study is the most common method. In adults Cimetidine should be administered at a rate of 300 mg in 100 mL of dextrose 5% in water (D5W) over 20 minutes, with imaging starting 1 hour later. It may also be given 300 mg orally four time a day before the study. Ranitidine may be substituted for cimetidine. Ranitidine dosage is 1 mg/kg IV for infants children and adults infused over 20 minutes, with imaging starting 1 hour later, or 2 mg/kg/dose PO for children and 150 mg/dose for adults. Pentagastrin (6 µg/kg given subcutaneously 5 to 15 minutes before the study) can be used, but because it increases peristalsis, glucagon (30 µg/kg for an adult [maximum 0.5 mg] and 5 µg/kg for a child, IV 10 minutes before the study) is also necessary.

GASTROINTESTINAL BLEEDING SCAN

Procedure imaging time
1 to 2 hours
Radiopharmaceutical
^{99m}Tc-labeled RBCs
Method of administration
IV injection (see RBC labeling procedures at end of this appendix). We prefer the ultratag method for this study.
Normal adult administered activity
20 mCi (740 MBq) IV
Injection-to-imaging time
Immediate
Conflicting examinations and medications
1. Recent upper gastrointestinal series
2. Recent barium enema
Patient preparation
None
Technique
Collimator
Low-level, all-purpose, parallel-hole
Counts
Collect 500-k counts per image with camera.

Routine views

Sequential anterior abdominal images taken at 5- to 10-minute intervals for 1 hour or continuous dynamic acquisition for 1 to 2 hours. Computer acquisition 128 × 128 matrix, 10 to 60 seconds per frame and cine replay at 1-minute frames ×60 is often helpful.

Optional views

Oblique images may be helpful in locating an abnormality.

Patient positioning

Supine

Photopeak selection

140-keV (20%) window)

Dosimetry: rads/mCi (mGy/MBq) of administered activity

Effective dose	0.026 (0.007)
Heart	0.085 (0.023)

Comments

Delayed images over 24 hours may be needed to document an intermittent bleed.

ESOPHAGEAL TRANSIT

Procedure imaging time

20 minutes

Radiopharmaceutical

^{99m}Tc-sulfur colloid in 15 mL of water

Method of administration

Oral

Normal adult administered activity

150 to 300 μCi (5.6 to 11.1 MBq)

Ingestion-to-imaging time

Immediate

Conflicting examinations and medications

None

Patient preparation

NPO for 4 hours

Technique

Collimator

Low-energy

Counts

Computer acquisition, 0.8-second frames ×240, 64 × 64 matrix

Routine views

Anterior, swallow radiopharmaceutical as a bolus, dry swallow at 30 seconds three or four times

Patient positioning

Sitting

Photopeak selection

140-keV (20% window)

Dosimetry: rads/mCi (mGy/MBq) of administered activity

Effective dose	0.089 (0.024)
Colon	0.48 (0.13)

Comments

1. Computer required
2. In a normal person, 90% of activity should have transversed esophagus in 15 seconds.

GASTROESOPHAGEAL REFLUX

Procedure imaging time

1 to 2 hours

Radiopharmaceutical

^{99m}Tc-sulfur or albumin colloid in 150 mL of orange juice and 150 mL of 0.1 N HCl

Method of administration

Oral

Normal adult administered activity

300 μCi (11.1 MBq)

Administration-to-imaging time

Immediate

Conflicting examinations and medications

None

Patient preparation

NPO for 6 hours

Technique

Collimator

Low-energy

Counts

30-second images; computer acquisition mandatory, 5 to 10 seconds per frame for 60 minutes

Routine views

Anterior; image with Valsalva maneuver and then with abdominal binder at 0, 20, 40, 60, 80, and 100 mmHg. Do not use a binder on infants or children.

Patient positioning

Upright, supine, or both as needed.

Photopeak selection

140-keV (20% window)

Dosimetry: rads/mCi (mGy/MBq) of administered activity

Effective dose	0.089 (0.024)
Colon	0.48 (0.13)

Comments

1. More than 4% reflux is abnormal.
2. A nasogastric tube may be used in young children for insertion of sulfur colloid.
3. To look for pulmonary aspiration in infants, use 5 μCi/mL (0.19 MBq) in milk or formula

(for a total of 500 μCi or 18.5 MBq). Image over lungs at 4, 6, and 12 hours as needed.

GASTRIC EMPTYING

Procedure imaging time
   1½ to 2 hours
Radiopharmaceutical
   Liquid phase, ^{111}In-DTPA (diethylene triamine pentaacetic acid) or ^{99m}Tc-DTPA in 300 mL water, orange juice, or milk
   Solid phase, ^{99m}Tc-sulfur colloid in scrambled eggs, egg whites, beef stew, or oatmeal
Method of administration
   Oral. The meal should be optimally be ingested within 10 minutes
Normal adult administered activity
   Liquid phase, 0.1 to 0.2 mCi (3.7 to 7.4 MBq) of ^{111}In-DTPA in 300 mL
   Solid phase, 0.2 to 0.4 mCi (7.4 to 14.8 MBq) of ^{99m}Tc-sulfur colloid;
Administration-to-imaging time
   Immediate
Conflicting examinations, conditions, and medications
   Drugs affecting gastric motility. Delayed gastric emptying is caused by aluminum hydroxide, narcotics, and propantheline. Gastric emptying enhanced by Reglan.
   Optimally premenopausal women should be studied on days 1 through 10 of their menstrual cycle to avoid effects of hormonal variation on gastrointestinal motility.
Patient preparation
   NPO for 8 hours. Diabetics need to be instructed to bring insulin with them. The dose of insulin is to be adjusted when the meal is given.
Technique
   Collimator
      Low-energy for ^{99m}Tc; medium-energy for [111]In
   Counts
      500-k counts in images at 5, 10, 15, 30, 60, and 90 minutes, or continuous dynamic acquisition for 90 minutes
   Routine views
      Left anterior oblique only or anterior and posterior sequentially for geometric mean method
   Patient positioning
      Sitting between images, supine for imaging
   Photopeak selection

172 and 246-keV (20% windows) for [111]In
140-keV (20% window) for [99m]Tc
Dosimetry: rads/mCi (mGy/MBq) of administered activity
   [99m]Tc nonabsorbable solid or liquid
      Effective dose   0.089 (0.024)
      Colon   0.41 to 0.48 (0.11 to 0.13)
   [111]In nonabsorbable solid or liquid
      Effective dose   1.1 (0.3)
      Colon   7.4 to 7.8 (2.0 to 2.1)
Comments
   1. Normally, for eggs or oatmeal, half of the activity leaves the stomach in 60 to 120 minutes. For liquids only, the half-emptying time is normally less than 20 minutes.
   2. Computer acquisition is essential. Half-time for emptying is done by drawing a region of interest around the stomach and determination of the time it takes to reach half the peak counts or a least-squares fit method to derive a half-emptying time to reach 50% of the peak counts.

LEVEEN SHUNT PATENCY

Procedure imaging time
   1 hour
Radiopharmaceutical
   ^{99m}Tc-macroaggregated albumin (MAA)
Method of administration
   Intraperitoneal
Normal adult administered activity
   1 to 2 mCi (37 to 74 MBq)
Injection-to-imaging time
   Immediate
Conflicting examinations and medications
   None
Patient preparation
   Void before examination; local anesthesia at injection site
Technique
   Collimator
      Low-energy
   Counts
      2-second dynamic images. If flow is slow, use 2-minute static images. Image as soon as lower portion of tube is seen. At 1 hour, image lungs.
   Routine views
      Anterior abdomen and chest
   Patient positioning
      Supine
   Photopeak selection
      140-keV (20% window)

Comments
1. Flush needle with 3 to 5 mL saline.
2. Abdominal ballotment may facilitate mixing with ascitic fluid.
3. If tube does not appear, delaying views up to 5 hours may be necessary.

BONE SCAN

Procedure imaging time
  30 to 60 minutes
Radiopharmaceutical
  ^{99m}Tc-labeled phosphates and phosphonates
Method of administration
  IV injection
Normal administered activity
  Adults 20 to 30 mCi (740 MBq to 1.11 GBq)
  Markedly obese adults, 300 to 350 μCi/kg (11 to 13 MBq/kg)
  Children, 250 to 300 μCi/kg (9 to 11 MBq/kg), with a minimum of 0.5 to 1.0 mCi (20 to 40 MBq)
Injection-to-imaging time
  Immediate to 3 hours (see comments)
Conflicting examinations and medications
1. Renal uptake can be increased by amphotericin B, aluminum antacids, iron preparations, Al^{3-} ions in preparation, radiation therapy, recent radiographic contrast sodium diatrizoate, dextrose, gentamycin, and chemotherapy agents, particularly, vincristine, doxorubicin, and cyclophosphamide.
2. Breast uptake can be increased by gynecomastia-producing drugs, digitalis, estrogens, cimetidine, spironolactone, and diethylstilbestrol.
3. Stomach uptake can be caused by isotretinoin.
4. Liver uptake can be caused by aluminum antacids, iron preparations, Al^{3-} ions in preparation, excess Sn^2 ions in preparation, recent radiographic contrast, sodium diatrizoate, and alkaline pH.
5. Spleen uptake can be increased by phenytoin and aluminum preparations.
6. Excessive blood pool activity can be the result of aluminum preparations, iron dextran, or too few Sn^2 ions in preparation.
7. Focal soft tissue or muscle uptake can result from ion dextran injections, calcium gluconate injections, heparin injections, or meperidine injections.

Patient preparation
1. If not contraindicated, the patient should be hydrated, IV or PO (two or more 8-ounce glasses of water).
2. Patient should void before imaging.
Technique
  Collimator
    Low-energy, high-resolution, or ultrahigh-resolution parallel-hole
  Counts
1. 500-k to 1 million counts over the chest with other axial skeletal images for the same time
2. 150- to 250-k counts in extremities
3. Minimum of 1000-k counts per view for whole-body imaging systems
4. Whole-body images usually obtained with a $256 \times 256 \times 16$ or greater matrix and spot images with a $128 \times 128 \times 16$ or $256 \times 256 \times 16$ matrix. The scanning speed should be adjusted so that routine anterior or posterior whole-body delayed images contain more than 1.5 million counts.
  Routine views
    Anterior and posterior skeleton, lateral skull
  Patient positioning
    Supine, prone, or sitting
  Photopeak selection
    140-keV (20% window)
Dosimetry: rads/mCi (mGy/MBq) of administered activity

Effective dose	0.02 (0.005)
Bone surface	0.23 (0.06)

Comments
1. Differential diagnosis of cellulitis from osteomyelitis requires flow study of 30 frames ($64 \times 64 \times 16$ or greater matrix at 1 to 3 seconds per frame) and a 3- to 5-minute blood pool image ($128 \times 128 \times 16$ or greater matrix and 200- to 300-k counts /image) within 10 minutes of injection over the region of interest. Delayed images at 3 to 4 hours are also necessary.
2. Prevent cold spot artifacts by having patient remove metal objects (e.g., money, lighter, jewelry).
3. Identify region of interest to be imaged before selecting injection site to prevent injection in area of interest.
4. Urine contamination is the most common hot spot artifact. Decontaminate patient, and image again.

SPECT BONE IMAGING

Procedure imaging time
    30 minutes
Instrumentation
    SPECT camera
Radiopharmaceutical
    ^{99m}Tc-phosphates or diphosphonates
Method of administration
    IV injection
Normal administered activity
    Same as for standard bone scan
Injection-to-imaging time
    3 hours
Conflicting examinations and medications
    Retained barium
Patient preparation
    None
Technique
    Collimator
        High-resolution
    Counts and time
        60 to 120 stops, 64 × 64 × 16 or greater
        matrix and 10 to 40 seconds per stop
    Routine views
        360-degree arc of rotation
    Patient positioning
        Supine
    Photopeak selection
        140-keV (20% window)
Dosimetry: rads/mCi (mGy/MBq) of administered activity
    Effective dose   0.02 (0.005)
    Bone surface   0.23 (0.06)

BONE MARROW SCAN

Procedure imaging time
    1 hour
Radiopharmaceutical
    ^{99m}Tc-sulfur colloid
Method of administration
    IV injection
Normal adult administered activity
    8 to 10 mCi (296 to 370 MBq)
Injection-to-imaging time
    20 minutes
Conflicting examinations and medications
    None
Patient preparation
    None
Technique
    Collimator
        Low-energy, all-purpose, parallel-hole

Counts
    All images: 250-k count in bone marrow
Routine views
    1. Anterior: shoulders, sternum, ribs, pelvis,
       thighs
    2. Posterior: thorax, lumbar spine, pelvis
Patient positioning
    Supine or prone or sitting
Photopeak selection
    140-keV (20% window)
Dosimetry: rads/mCi (mGy/MBq) of administered activity
    Effective dose   0.035 (0.009)
    Spleen   0.27 (0.07)
Comments
    1. Overlap spot images of regions of interest to
       prevent loss of information.
    2. Liver and spleen require lead shielding if
       within region of interest.

RENAL BLOOD FLOW SCAN

Procedure imaging time
    5 minutes
Radiopharmaceutical
    ^{99m}Tc-diethylene triamine pentaacetic acid
    (DTPA), glucoheptonate, or mercaptoacetyl-
    triglycine (MAG3)
Method of administration
    IV injection; bolus injection in antecubital vein
Normal adult administered activity
    10 mCi (370 MBq)
Injection-to-imaging time
    Immediate
Conflicting examinations and medications
    None
Patient preparation
    None
Technique
    Collimator
        Low-energy, all purpose, parallel-hole
    Counts
        500-k count for static image
    Routine views
        1. Dynamic (anterior: transplant; posterior:
           retroperitoneal): 2 to 3 seconds per frame
           for 30 seconds
        2. Static (immediate) image
    Patient positioning
        Sitting or supine
    Photopeak selection
        140-keV (20% window)
Dosimetry: rads/mCi (mGy/MBq) of administered activity

DTPA
    Effective dose   0.02 (0.005)
    Bladder   0.19 (0.05)
MAG3
    Effective dose   0.026 (0.007)
    Bladder   0.41 (0.11)
Glucoheptonate
    Effective dose   0.089 (0.024)
    Bladder   0.56 (0.15)

RENAL SCAN (A) CORTICAL IMAGING

Procedure imaging time
    20 minutes
Radiopharmaceutical
    ^{99m}Tc-DMSA (cortical agent) if not available ^{99m}Tc-glucoheptonate
Method of administration
    IV administration: bolus injection in antecubital vein in less than 0.5 mL volume using a 22-gauge needle
Normal administered activity
    5 mCi (185 MBq) ^{99m}Tc-DMSA for adults, and a minimum of 0.3 mCi ($\approx$ 11 MBq) in children with a maximum of 3.0 mCi ($\approx$ 110 MBq)
    10 to 20 mCi (370 to 740 MBq) ^{99m}Tc-glucoheptonate for adults, and a minimum of 0.5 mCi (18 MBq) for children
Injection-to-imaging time
    Immediate and at 2 to 4 hours for DMSA
    Immediate for glucoheptonate
Conflicting examinations and medications
    None
Patient preparation
    None
Technique
    Collimator
        Low-energy, high-resolution, or ultrahigh-resolution
    Counts
        500-k counts for static image on 128 × 128 or 256 × 256 matrix
    Routine views
        1. Dynamic (anterior: transplant; posterior: retroperitoneal), 2 to 3 seconds per frame for 30 seconds
        2. Static imaging immediately after flow study
        3. Static imaging 2 hours after flow study
    Patient positioning
        Supine (or prone for pinhole)
    Photopeak selection
        140-keV (20% window)

Dosimetry for children: rads/mCi (mGy/MBq) of administered activity
    DMSA
        Effective dose   0.03 (0.008)
        Kidneys   0.66 (0.18)
    Glucoheptonate
        Effective dose   0.089 (0.024)
        Bladder   0.56 (0.15)
Comments
    SPECT imaging is very helpful with either 180- or 360-degree sampling on a 128 × 128 matrix

RENAL SCAN (B) GLOMERULAR FILTRATION

Procedure imaging time
    45 minutes
Radiopharmaceutical
    ^{99m}Tc–diethylene triamine pentaacetic acid (DTPA) or glucoheptonate
Method of administration
    IV injection: bolus injection in antecubital vein
Normal adult administered activity
    10 mCi (370 MBq)
Injection-to-imaging time
    Immediate
Conflicting examination and medications
    None
Patient preparation
    None
Technique
    Collimator
        Low-energy, all-purpose, parallel-hole
Counts
    1. First dynamic study: 2 seconds per frame
    2. Second dynamic study: 120 seconds per frame
    3. Static image for 500-k counts
Routine views
    1. A flow study at 2 seconds per image in the anterior position for a transplanted kidney and the posterior position for a retroperitoneal kidney (perfusion study).
    2. On completion of the initial flow study, a second phase of dynamic study is performed at 3 minutes per frame with the patient in the same position. The second phase is carried out for 20 minutes after injection (excretion study).
    3. A delayed image may be taken in the same position as the previous studies. An upright postvoid image may be useful to assess collecting system drainage.

Patient positioning
Supine or sitting
Photopeak selection
140-keV (20% window)
Dosimetry: rads/mCi (mGy/MBq) of adminis-
tered activity
DTPA

Effective dose		0.02 (0.005)
Bladder		0.19 (0.05)

RENAL SCAN (C) TUBULAR FUNCTION

Procedure imaging time
30 minutes
Radiopharmaceutical
^{99m}Tc-mercaptoacetylglycine (MAG3)
Method of administration
IV injection
Normal adult administered activity
8 mCi (296 MBq)
Injection-to-imaging time
Immediate
Conflicting examinations and medications
None
Patient preparation
None
Technique
Collimator
Low-energy, all-purpose, or high-resolution
Counts
15 dynamic images of 2 minutes each are
obtained.
Views
Anterior for transplant evaluation; posterior
for native kidneys
Patient positioning
Supine
Photopeak selection
140-keV (20% window)
Dosimetry: rads/mCi (mGy/MBq) of adminis-
tered activity
MAG3

Effective dose		0.026 (0.007)
Bladder		0.41 (0.11)

Comments
Erect posterior images may be obtained after the
patient has ambulated if ureteral obstruction is
suspected.

DIURETIC (LASIX) RENOGRAM

Procedure imaging time
30 to 60 minutes

Radiopharmaceutical
^{99m}Tc-DTPA (glomerular agent) or MAG3
(tubular secretion)
Method of administration
Bolus IV injection in antecubital vein
Normal administered activity
10 mCi (370 MBq) for adults. For children, at
least 0.5 mCi (18.5 MBq).
Injection-to-imaging time
Immediate
Conflicting examinations and medications
IV iodine contrast media should not be used
on the same day that this examination is
performed.
Patient preparation
1. See requisition because some patients may
require an indwelling bladder catheter
placed before this procedure.
2. Patient should be hydrated unless
contraindicated.
3. Patient must void before imaging.
Technique
Collimator
Low-energy, all-purpose, parallel-hole
Counts and time
15 to 60 seconds per frame computer acqui-
sition 64 × 64 or 128 × 128 matrix and filmed
as 2-minute images for at least 30 minutes
Routine views
Posterior
Patient positioning
Sitting, if possible
Photopeak selection
140-keV (20% window)
Dosimetry: rads/mCi (mGy/MBq) of adminis-
tered activity
DTPA

Effective dose		0.020 (0.005)
Bladder		0.19 (0.05)

MAG3

Effective dose		0.026 (0.007)
Bladder		0.41 (0.11)

Comments
1. Furosemide (for adults 0.3 mg/kg body
weight IV or 20 to 40 mg) is given about 10
to 15 minutes into the study if there appears
to be delay in excretion. Note frame number
of administration. For children, 1.0 mg/kg
with a usual maximum of 40 mg IV over
1–2 min.
2. A region of interest can be drawn around the
dilated collecting system and a t$\frac{1}{2}$ calculated
after administration of furosemide. A t$\frac{1}{2}$ less

than 10 minutes usually means the absence of obstruction, and a t½ of more than 20 minutes identifies obstruction. t½ value of 10 to 20 minutes is equivocal.

CAPTOPRIL RENOGRAM FOR DIAGNOSIS OF RENOVASCULAR HYPERTENSION

Procedure imaging time
  1 hour
Radiopharmaceutical
  99mTc-DTPA, or 99mTc-MAG3
Method of administration
  Radionuclide administered 1 hour IV after 25 to 50 mg captopril given as single oral dose.
Normal adult dose
  1 to 10 mCi (37 to 370 MBq), 99mTc-DTPA or 99mTc-MAG3
Injection-to-imaging time
  Immediate; however, injection of radiopharmaceutical should be done 60 minutes after administration of captopril or 15 minutes after enalaprilat administration.
Conflicting examinations and medications
  Short-acting angiotensin-converting enzyme (ACE) inhibitors, such as captopril, should be withheld 3 days before the study, and longer-acting ACE inhibitors should be withheld for 5 to 7 days before the study. If this is not done, the study still can be performed but with some reduction in sensitivity. The study should not be initiated if systolic blood pressure is below 140 mmHg.
Patient preparation
  Patient should be hydrated orally. Patients on an oral ACE inhibitor should drink only water and should not eat a solid meal within 4 hours of the study. The recommended dose of captopril is 25 to 50 mg PO. Enalaprilat can also be used at 40 µg/kg administered intraveneously over 3 to 5 minutes with a maximum dose of 2.5 mg.
Technique
  Collimator
    Low-energy or general all-purpose
  Counts and time
    Flow study at 1 or 2 seconds obtained for 1 minute, followed by sequential imaging every 2 to 3 minutes on film or every 30 seconds on computer for 20 minutes. A postvoid image is obtained.
  Routine views

Posterior blood flow and sequential imaging. In some protocols, patients may receive furosemide (40 mg) 3 minutes after administration of the MAG3.
Patient positioning
  Supine
Photopeak selection
  140-keV (20% window)
Dosimetry: rads/mCi (mGy/MBq) of administered activity
  DTPA
    Effective dose   0.020 (0.005)
    Bladder   0.19 (0.05)
  MAG3
    Effective dose   0.026 (0.007)
    Bladder   0.41 (0.11)
Comments
  Patients may become seriously hypotensive with this procedure. It is advisable to establish IV infusion of normal saline before administration of captopril; blood pressure should be recorded every 15 minutes. Many patients who become hypotensive respond to IV fluids without the need for vasopressive drugs.

RADIONUCLIDE CYSTOGRAM IN CHILDREN

Procedure imaging time
  20 minutes
Radiopharmaceutical
  99mTc-pertechnetate (preferred). 99mTc-sulfur colloid or 99mTc-DTPA are nonabsorbable and can also be used.
Method of administration
  Sterile urethral catheterization. Radiopharmaceutical mixed in 250 to 500 mL of saline or irrigating solution, with shielded bag hung 100 cm above the table or introduced directly into the catheter. Filling usually ends when the patient voids spontaneously; the estimated bladder volume of the bladder is reached or the flow from the hung solution stops due to back pressure.
Normal administered activity
  0.5 to 1.0 mCi (18.5 to 37 MBq)
Infusion-to-imaging time
  Immediate
Conflicting examinations and medications
  None
Patient preparation
  Sterile uretheral catheterization
Technique

Collimator

Low-energy, high-resolution, or general-purpose

Routine views

30-second anterior pre- and postvoid image

5-second images during filling and voiding on 128×128 matrix with camera positioned under the table.

Patient positioning

Supine

Photopeak selection

140-keV (20% window)

Dosimetry for children: rads/mCi (mGy/MBq) of administered activity

^{99m}Tc-pertechnetate, ^{99m}Tc-sulfur colloid, or ^{99m}Tc-DTPA

Effective dose	0.009 (0.0024)
Bladder	0.10 (0.027)

Comments

1. Bladder volume in an individual patient can be approximated in mL by the formula (age in years + 2) × 30 mL = bladder volume

2. Residual postvoid volume can be quantitated with regions of interest drawn over the bladder on pre- and postvoid images and requires recording voided volume as follows: RV (mL) = [Voided volume (mL) × postvoid bladder counts (ROI)] / [Initial bladder counts (ROI) − post-void bladder counts (ROI)]

3. Another method requires an empty bladder and uses the following formula: RV (mL) = [Post void bladder counts (ROI) × volume infused] / [Initial bladder counts (ROI)]

TESTICULAR SCAN

Procedure imaging time

30 minutes

Radiopharmaceutical

^{99m}Tc-sodium pertechnetate

Method of administration

Bolus IV injection in an antecubital vein

Normal adult administered activity

30 mCi (1.11 GBq)

Injection-to-imaging time

Immediate, followed by 15-minute delayed image

Conflicting examinations and medications

None

Patient preparation

None

Technique

Collimator

Converging low-energy

Counts

1. Anterior blood flow: 2 seconds per frame
2. Static image: 500-k counts

Routine views

1. Anterior blood flow study
2. Static anterior immediately after blood flow study
3. Delayed anterior 15 to 20 minutes after injection

Patient positioning

Supine

Photopeak selection

140-keV (20% window)

Dosimetry: rads/mCi (mGy/MBq) of administered activity

^{99m}Tc-pertechnetate

Effective dose	0.05 (0.01)
Colon	0.10 to 0.30 (0.03 to 0.08)

Comments

It is important to record which side the pain or mass is on.

GALLIUM SCAN FOR TUMOR OR INFECTION

Procedure imaging time

30 minutes

Radiopharmaceutical

^{67}Ga-citrate

Method of administration

IV injection

Normal administered activity

In adults, 4 to 6 mCi (150 to 220 MBq) for infection; 5 to 10 mCi (185 to 370 MBq) for neoplasm

In children, 0.04 to 0.07 mCi/kg (1.5 to 2.6 MBq/kg) with a minimum dose of 0.25 to 0.5 mCi (9 to 18 MBq)

Injection-to-imaging time

6 and 24 hours for abscess; 48 and 72 hours for tumor imaging

Conflicting examinations and medications

1. Retained barium can cause attenuation.
2. Excessive bone uptake can result from iron preparations, chemotherapy, hemodialysis.
3. Excessive liver uptake can result from iron dextran or phenobarbital.
4. Excessive renal uptake can occur from chemotherapy, furosemide, phenytoin, allopurinol, ampicillin, erythromycin, cephalosporin, ibuprofen, sulfonamides, rifampin, pentamidine, phenylbutazone, and phenobarbital.

Stomach uptake also can be increased by chemotherapy and breast uptake increased by reserpine, phenothiazine, metoclopromaide, estrogens, and oral contraceptives. Colon uptake will be increased in antibiotic-induced pseudomembranous colitis, especially from clindamycin, cephalosporins, and ampicillin.

Prolonged whole-body clearance can occur as a result of vincristine, steroid treatment, or mechlorethamine.

8. Mediastinal and hilar lymph node uptake has been reported in patients taking phenytoin (Dilantin).

9. Lung uptake can be increased as a result of cyclophosphamide, amiodarone, bleomycin, busulfan, and *Bacillus* calmette-guerin (BCG).

10. Thymus activity can be increased as a result of radiation therapy, chemotherapy, or antibiotics.

Patient preparation

Bowel preparation after initial images may occasionally be helpful

Technique

Collimator

Medium-energy, parallel-hole, large FOV

Counts

Usually about 10 to 20 minutes per view for planar images. At least 500-k counts per image and 1.5 to 2 million counts for images of the chest, abdomen, and pelvis. For whole-body images, a scanning speed to achieve an information density of 450 counts/cm^2 or greater than 1,500,000 counts for each view.

Patient positioning

Supine

Photopeak selection

93, 184-keV (20% windows). Other photopeaks (296 and 388-keV) can be used.

Routine views

1. Anterior and posterior whole-body images with scanning gamma camera

2. Spot views (optional)

Dosimetry: rads/mCi (mGy/MBq) of administered activity

Effective dose 0.44 (0.12)

Bone surface 2.2 (0.6)

Comments

1. Subtraction views with ^{99m}Tc-sulfur colloid may be considered.

2. SPECT scanning may be useful.

SOMATOSTATIN RECEPTOR SCAN WITH INDIUM-111 PENTETREOTIDE

Procedure imaging time

1 hour

Radiopharmaceutical

^{111}In-pentetreotide (Octreoscan). Should be used within 6 hours of preparation.

Method of administration

IV Administration

Normal administered activity

6 mCi (222 MBq) for adults. 0.14 mCi/kg (5 MBq/kg) for children.

Injection-to-imaging time

4 and 24 hours; 48 hours may be needed when there is significant bowel activity at 24 hours.

Conflicting examinations and medications

Consideration should be given to discontinuing octreotide therapy 24 hours before administration of the radiopharmaceutical

Radiotracer should not be injected into IV lines for, or together with, solutions for total parenteral nutrition

Patient preparation

Void before imaging

Technique

Collimator

Medium-energy, large FOV

Routine views

Anterior and posterior views of head, chest, abdomen, pelvis

Counts

10 to 15 minutes per image using 512 × 512 or 256 × 256 word matrix. For dual-headed cameras, anterior and posterior whole-body images from head to upper femurs in a 1024 × 512 or 1024 × 256 word matrix for a minimum of 30 minutes (speed 3 cm/minute)

Patient positioning

Supine

Photopeak selection

173 and 247-keV (symmetrical 20% window)

Dosimetry: rads/mCi (mGy/MBq) of administered activity

Effective dose   0.4 (0.11)

Spleen   2.4 (0.65)

Comments

1. In patients suspected of having insulinoma, an IV infusion of glucose should be available because of the potential for inducing severe hypoglycemia

2. SPECT imaging may be very helpful, and images are usually obtained at 24 hours with 3-degree angular sampling. 128 × 128 matrix, 360-degree rotation and 20 to 30 seconds per stop.

LYMPHOSCINTIGRAPHY (SENTINEL NODE LOCALIZATION)

Procedure imaging time
   30 minutes
Radiopharmaceutical
   Filtered (0.22 micron millipore filter) ^{99m}Tc-sulfur colloid
Method of administration
   Intradermal or peritumoral, 4 to 8 injections within 1 cm that surround the biopsy or tumor site. Finger massage at each site may promote drainage. High pressure of intradermal injection can cause leakage upon needle removal, and site should be covered with bandage or cotton ball.
Normal administered activity
   100 μCi (3.7 MBq)
Injection-to-imaging time
   Immediate
Conflicting examination and medications
   None
Patient preparation
   None
Technique
   Collimator
      Low-energy, all-purpose, parallel-hole
   Counts/time
      Sequential or continuous imaging after injections for 30 to 60 minutes. Continuous images of 30 seconds per frame or sequential images every 5 minutes.
   Routine views
      Over area of injection and with FOV to include expected drainage direction. Injection site may need to be covered with a piece of lead to discern lymphatic drainage. Transmission and oblique views are often helpful for localization.
   Patient positioning
      Usually supine or prone
   Photopeak selection
      140-keV (20% window)
Dosimetry: rads/mCi (mGy/MBq) of administered activity (local radiation dose has been ignored and effective dose is calculated assuming 20% of administered activity is absorbed

Effective dose	0.0071 (0.002)
Spleen	0.057 (0.015)

Comments
   1. Skin is usually marked over the sentinel node.
   2. For trunk lesions, axillary as well as inguinal view should be included; for lesions of the head and neck anterior, posterior and oblique images should be obtained; and for extremity lesion, in-transit nodes around the knee or elbow should also be imaged.
   3. Use of a gamma probe in the operating room can be done 0.5 to 3 hours after injection to help localize the node, and a sentinel node typically has 10 times the background counts taken at a location remote from the injection site.

LEUKOCYTE (WHITE BLOOD CELL) SCAN

Procedure imaging time
   1 hour
Radiopharmaceutical
   ^{111}In autologous oxine-labeled or ^{99m}Tc-HMPAO (Ceretec, Amersham) leukocytes
   Only the unstabilized form of HMPAO should be utilized.
Method of administration
   IV administration
Normal administered activity
   In adults, 500 μCi (18.5 MBq) of ^{111}In; in children, 7.5 to 15 μCi/kg (0.25 to 0.5 MBq/kg), with a minimum administered activity of 50 to 75 μCi (1.85 to 2.3 MBq)
   In adults, 10 to 20 mCi (370 to 740 MBq) for ^{99m}Tc HMPAO; in children, 0.1 to 0.2 mCi/kg (3.7 to 7.4 MBq/kg) for HMPAO, with a minimum of 0.5 to 1.0 mCi (18 to 37 MBq).
Injection-to-imaging time
   1 to 4 hours and 16 to 24 hours for ^{111}In oxine leukocytes
   0.5 to 4 hours for ^{99m}Tc-HMPAO (exametazime). With HMPAO, early imaging of the abdomen and pelvis is essential because of hepatobiliary excretion and bowel transit, and 15-minute images at 8 hours after injection may be needed for pulmonary infection or osteomyelitis.
Conflicting examinations and medications
   Patients on antibiotics or with altered chemotaxis may have false-negative examination results.
Patient preparation
   None

Technique
Collimator
Medium-energy for ^{111}In, and low-energy all-purpose for [99m]Tc. 500-k counts per view
Routine views
Anterior and posterior views of head, chest, abdomen, pelvis
Counts
10 to 20 minutes per image for ^{111}In oxine leukocytes
800 k or 5 to 10 minutes per view for ^{99m}Tc-HMPAO
Patient positioning
Supine
Photopeak selection
Dual: 173- and 247-keV (20% window) for [111]In
140-keV (20% window) for [99m]Tc
Dosimetry: rads/mCi (mGy/MBq) of administered activity
[111]In leukocytes

Effective dose	1.3 (0.35)
Spleen	20.0 (5.4)

[99m]Tc-exametazime (HMPAO)

Effective dose	0.063 (0.017)
Spleen	0.56 (0.15)

Comments
1. Leukocytes are obtained from 20 to 80 mL of venous blood in adults. The minimum volume of blood needed for a child is about 10 to 15 mL.
2. It is difficult to obtain enough cells to label in leukopenic (<4000 cells/μL) patients.
3. Labeled cells should be reinjected as soon as possible and no later than 3 to 4 hours after obtaining the sample.
4. Gallium scintigraphy is usually preferred for patients with neutropenia, fever of unknown origin, or nonsuppurative, granulomatous, or lymphocyte-mediated infections.

POSITRON EMISSION TOMOGRAPHY TUMOR IMAGING WITH FLUORINE-18 FLUORO-2-DEOXYGLUCOSE

Procedure imaging time
30 to 60 minutes
Radiopharmaceutical
Fluorine-18 fluoro-2-deoxyglucose (^{18}F-FDG)
Method of administration
IV administration. For brain imaging, for several minutes before FDG administration and for 30 minutes after, the patient should be in a quiet and darkened room.
Normal adult administered activity
10 to 20 mCi (370 to 740 MBq)
Injection-to-imaging time
30 to 60 minutes. Void before imaging
Conflicting examination and medications
High serum glucose level will reduce tumor uptake
Patient preparation
Patients should fast at least 4 hours; this will reduce serum insulin levels to near basal levels and diminish uptake by some organs such as the heart.
Some institutions will check the blood glucose level, but many do not.
Technique
Collimator
None in three-dimensional acquisition. Present in two-dimensional acquisition
Counts/time
Routine views
Whole body. Usually from just below the brain to the knees. This may require up to 10 bed positions with overlap fields by one or more of the acquisition slices.
Patient positioning
Supine. For neoplasms of the head or neck, the arms should be down, and for lesions of the chest, the arms should be up. For lesions of the neck that may have mediastinal or pulmonary involvement, it may be necessary to do imaging twice with the arms in both positions
Photopeak selection
300- or 350- to 650-keV for BGO, 435- to 590- or 665-keV for NaI (CPET).
Dosimetry: rads/mCi (mGy/MBq) of administered activity

Effective dose	0.07 (0.019)
Bladder	0.60 (0.16)

Comments
Attenuation correction can be performed with or with cesium, germanium, or CT.
IV and oral contrast can be used with positron emission tomography (PET)/CT; however, the barium should be oral glucose-free 1.3% to 2.1% barium sulfate 500–750 mL 60 to 90 minutes before FDG injection. High-density barium should be avoided. Another 100 to 200 mL of oral barium is given 30 minutes after the FDG injection. The patient then sits or lies

quietly, and the CT scan is performed just before the PET scan and uses IV contrast (300 mg I/mL) 80 mL at 3 mL/second achieve to arterial contrast, followed by another 60 mL at 2 mL/second for venous and parenchymal enchancement.

POSITRON EMISSION TOMOGRAPHY CARDIAC IMAGING WITH FLUORINE-18 FLUORO-2 DEOXYGLUCOSE

Procedure imaging time
  30 to 60 minutes
Radiopharmaceutical
  ^{18}F-FDG
Method of administration
  IV administration. Normal adult administered activity
  10 to 20 mCi (370 to 740 MBq)
Injection-to-imaging time
  30 to 60 minutes. Void before imaging
Conflicting examination and medications
  Caffeine will increase cardiac uptake
Patient preparation
  Patient should eat a light, nonfat, high-carbohydrate breakfast or lunch or have a glucose solution (1 to 3 hours before FDG injection) to change the heart from fatty acid to glucose metabolism. Some institutions will check the blood glucose level, but many do not.
Technique
  Collimator
    None in three-dimensional acquisition. Present in two-dimensional acquisition
  Counts/time
    20 minute static acquisition
  Routine views
    Chest
  Patient positioning
    Supine with arms raised
Photopeak selection
  300- or 350- to 650-keV for BGO, 435- to 590- or 665-keV for NaI (CPET).
Dosimetry: rads/mCi (mGy/MBq) of administered activity

Effective dose	0.07 (0.019)
Bladder	0.60 (0.16)

Comments
  Attenuation correction can be performed with or with cesium, germanium, or CT.
  Compare to myocardial perfusion images

POSITRON EMISSION TOMOGRAPHY BRAIN IMAGING WITH FLUORINE-18 FLUORO-2-DEOXYGLUCOSE

Procedure imaging time
  30 to 60 minutes
Radiopharmaceutical
  ^{18}F-FDG
Method of administration
  IV administration. For brain imaging, for several minutes before FDG administration and for 30 minutes after, the patient should be in a quiet and darkened room.
Normal adult administered activity
  10 to 20 mCi (370 to 740 MBq)
Injection-to-imaging time
  60 minutes. Void before imaging
Conflicting examination and medications
  High serum glucose level will reduce tumor uptake
Patient preparation
  Patients should fast at least 4 hours; this will reduce serum insulin levels to near basal levels and diminish uptake by some organs such as the heart.
  Some institutions will check the blood glucose level, but many do not.
Technique
  Collimator
    None in three-dimensional acquisition. Present in two-dimensional acquisition
  Counts/time
    6-minute static acquisition in the three-dimensional mode or 20-minute acquisition in the two dimensional mode
  Routine views
    Head
  Patient positioning
    Supine with arms down
  Photopeak selection
    300- or 350- to 650-keV for BGO, 435- to 590- or 665-keV for NaI (CPET).
Dosimetry: rads/mCi (mGy/MBq) of administered activity

Effective dose	0.07 (0.019)
Bladder	0.60 (0.16)

Comments
  Attenuation correction can be performed with or with cesium, germanium, or CT
  Fusion with CT or MRI images is desirable

POSITRON EMISSION TOMOGRAPHY CARDIAC REST/STRESS IMAGING WITH RUBIDIUM-82 OR NITROGEN-13 AMMONIA

Procedure imaging time

30 minutes with rubidium-82 (^{82}Rb), 90 minutes with nitrogen-13 (^{13}N)-ammonia

Radiopharmaceutical

^{82}Rb from strontium-82 (^{82}Sr) generator system or ^{13}N-ammonia

Method of administration

IV administration.

Normal adult administered activity

With rubidium 50 mCi (1850 MBq) at rest and 50 mCi (1850 MBq) for stress

With ^{13}N-ammonia, 10 to 20 (370 to 740 MBq) at rest and 10 to 20 mCi (370 to 740 MBq) at stress

Injection-to-imaging time

70 seconds with the patient at rest

6-minute rest emission scan performed

Transmission scan for attenuation correction (when using ^{13}N-ammonia, there must be 45 minutes between rest and stress injections to allow for radioactive decay due to the longer half-life of ^{13}N)

3 to 4 minutes dypyridamole infusion

Reinject for stress

6-minute stress emission scan performed

Conflicting examination and medications

None

Patient preparation

Technique

Collimator

None in three-dimensional acquisition. Present in two-dimensional acquisition

Counts/time

20 to 40 million counts for each 6 minute emission scan

Routine views

Chest

Patient positioning

Supine arms down

Photopeak selection

300- or 350- to 650-keV for BGO, 435- to 590- or 665-keV for NaI; CPET.

Dosimetry: rads/mCi (mGy/MBq) of administered activity

^{82}Rb

Effective dose   0.013 (0.004)

^{13}N-ammonia

Effective dose   0.007 (0.002)

Comments

1. Cost for a ^{82}Rb from ^{82}Sr generator system is about $20,000 or more for a month.

2. ^{13}N-ammonia requires an on-site cyclotron.

RED BLOOD CELL LABELING TECHNIQUES

1. In vitro commercial kit (Ultratag, Mallinckrodt): Results in 98% labeling. Add 1 to 3 mL of blood (heparin or ACD as an anticoagulant) to reagent vial (stannous chloride sodium citrate and dextrose). Allow to react for 5 minutes. Add syringe 1 (sodium hypochlorite) and mix by gently inverting four to five times. Add syringe 2 (citric acid, sodium citrate, and dextrose) and mix. Add 10 to 100 mCi (370 to 700 MBq) of ^{99m}Tc-pertechnetate to vial. Mix and allow to react for 20 minutes.

2. In vivo: Add 3 mL saline to Mallinckrodt stannous pyrophosphate kit. Wait 5 minutes and inject intravenously. Wait 10 to 20 minutes and inject 20 mCi (740 MBq) ^{99m}TcO$_4^-$. Results in 60% to 80% labeling, with remaining activity in kidneys, bladder, stomach, thyroid, and salivary glands.

3. Modified in vivo: Results in about 85% to 90% labeling. Add 3 mL of normal sterile saline to Mallinckrodt stannous pyrophosphate kit. Wait 5 minutes and then inject 1 mL intravenously. Wait 20 minutes. Using a 20-gauge needle, draw 10 mL of patient's blood into a syringe containing 20 mCi (740 MBq) of ^{99m}TcO$_4^-$ and 0.5 mL of heparin. Allow this mixture to incubate for 10 minutes at room temperature before reinjecting into the patient. Patients with low hematocrit counts may need more than 10 minutes of incubation.

Reduced RBC labeling efficiency in patients on heparin, methyldopa, hydralazine, quinidine, digoxin, prazosin, propranolol, doxorubicin, and recent iodinated contrast media.

Abnormal Radiopharmaceutical Distribution Due to Medications and Other Extrinsic Factors

FINDINGS	CAUSE
BONE IMAGING ^{99m}Tc DIPHOSPHONATES	
Renal uptake	Amphotericin B
	Aluminum antacids
	Iron preparations
	Al^{3+} ions in preparation
	Radiation therapy
	Radiographic contrast—sodium diatrizoate
	Chemotherapy agents
	Vincristine
	Doxorubicin
	Cyclophosphamide
	Gentamicin
	Dextrose
Breast uptake	Gynecomastia-producing drugs
	Digitalis
	Estrogens
	Cimetidine
	Spironolactone
	Diethylstilbestrol
Stomach uptake	Isotretinoin
Liver uptake	Aluminum antacids
	Iron preparations
	Al^{3+} ions in preparation
	Excess Sn^{2+} ions in preparation
	Radiographic contrast—sodium diatrizoate
	Alkaline pH
Spleen uptake	Phenytoin
	Aluminum preparations
Excessive blood pool activity	Iron dextran
	Aluminum preparations
	Too few Sn^{2+} ions in preparation

FINDINGS	CAUSE
Myocardial activity	Doxorubicin
	Recent electrocardioversion
Excessive soft tissue uptake	Iron dextran injections (focal)
	Iodinated antiseptics
	Calcium gluconate injections
	Heparin injections (focal)
	Meperidine injections (focal)
Muscle activity	ε-Aminocaproic acid
	Intramuscular injections
Decreased skeletal uptake	Corticosteroids
	Etidronate therapy
	Iron compounds
	Phospho-Soda
	Recent cold diphosphonate (hours)
	Vitamin D_3
Increased calvarial activity ("sickle sign")	Cytotoxic chemotherapy
	Calcium carbonate antacids
Regionally increased skeletal uptake	Regional chemoperfusion
	Melphalan
	Actinomycin

LABELED LEUKOCYTE IMAGING—[111]In

Reduced or absent abscess uptake (false-negative results) Antibiotics	Lidocaine
	Procainamide
	Corticosteroids
	Hyperalimentation
Lung activity	Cell clumping due to excessive agitation
Colon activity	Antibiotic-induced pseudomembranous colitis

LIVER AND SPLEEN IMAGING—[99m]Tc SULFUR COLLOID

Increased bone marrow uptake	Nitrosoureas
	Colloid size too small
Increased spleen uptake	Nitrosoureas
	Halothane
	Methylcellulose
Decreased spleen uptake	Chemotherapy
	Epinephrine
	Antimalarials
	Thorium dioxide (Thorotrast)
Lung uptake	Aluminum antacids
	Iron preparation
	Virilizing androgens
	Mg^{2+} preparation
	Niacin
	Colloid size too large
	Al^{3+} in preparation
	Particle clumping
Focal areas of decreased liver activity	Estrogens

HEPATOBILIARY IMAGING—[99m]Tc IDA DERIVATIVES

Delayed biliary-to-bowel transit	Narcotic analgesics
	Morphine
	Demerol
	Phenobarbital
Decreased liver uptake and excretion	Chronic high-dose nicotinic acid therapy
Enhanced hepatobiliary excretion	Phenobarbital
Nonvisualization of the gallbladder (false-positive results)	Hepatic artery chemotherapy infusion

FINDINGS	CAUSE
Prolonged gallbladder activity and decreased contractile response to stimulation	Atropine

18F-FDG PET IMAGING

FINDINGS	CAUSE
Decreased tumor uptake	Elevated glucose levels
	Elevated insulin levels
Increased muscle uptake (generalized)	Elevated insulin levels
	Elevated glucose levels
Increased cardiac uptake	Elevated insulin levels
	Elevated glucose levels
	Caffeine and possibly nicotine
Decreased cardiac uptake	Fasting
Focally increased brain uptake	External stimulation (light and noise during of shortly after injection)

67Ga CITRATE IMAGING

FINDINGS	CAUSE
Excessive bone uptake	Iron preparation
	Gadopentetate
	Chemotherapy
	Methotrexate
	Cisplatin
	Vincristine
	Mechlorethamine
	Hemodialysis
Excessive liver uptake	Iron dextran
	Phenobarbital
Excessive renal uptake	Doxorubicin
	Bleomycin
	Cisplatin
	Vinblastine
	Furosemide
	Phenytoin
	Allopurinol
	Cephalosporin
	Ampicillin
	Ibuprofen
	Sulfonamides
	Methicillin
	Erythromycin
	Rifampin
	Pentamidine
	Phenylbutazone
	Phenobarbital
	Phenazone
Stomach uptake	Chemotherapy
	Doxorubicin
	Bleomycin
	Cisplatin
	Vinblastine
Breast uptake	Estrogens
	Diethylstilbestrol
	Oral contraceptives
	Reserpine
	Phenothiazine
	Metoclopramide
Colon uptake	Antibiotic-induced pseudomembranous colitis, especially:
	Clindamycin
	Cephalosporins
	Ampicillin
Decreased abscess uptake	Prior treatment with iron dextran, deferoxamine

FINDINGS	CAUSE
Prolonged whole-body clearance	Vincristine
	Steroid treatment
	Mechlorethamine
Mediastinal and hilar lymph node uptake	Phenytoin (Dilantin)
Lung uptake	Cyclophosphamide
	Amiodarone
	Bleomycin
	Busulfan
	BCG
Thymus activity	Chemotherapy/Radiation therapy
	Antibiotics

BLOOD POOL IMAGING—^{99m}Tc-LABELED RED BLOOD CELLS

Reduced red blood cell labeling efficiency	Heparin
	Methyldopa
	Hydralazine
	Quinidine
	Digoxin
	Prazosin
	Propranolol
	Doxorubicin
	Iodinated contrast media

MYOCARDIAL PERFUSION IMAGING—^{201}Tl CHLORIDE

Increased myocardial uptake	Dipyridamole
	Furosemide
	Isoproterenol
	Sodium bicarbonate (IV)
	Dexamethasone
Decreased myocardial uptake	Propranolol
	Digitalis
	Doxorubicin
	Phenytoin (Dilantin)
	Lidocaine
	Minoxidil

MECKEL'S DIVERTICULUM IMAGING—^{99m}Tc PERTECHNETATE

Increased gastric mucosa activity	Pentagastrin
	Climetidine
Decreased gastric mucosa activity	Al^{3+} ion (antacids)
	Perchlorate

LUNG PERFUSION IMAGING—^{99m}Tc-LABELED MAA

Focal hot spots or patchy distribution in lungs	Mg^{2+} sulfate therapy/Clot formation
Increased liver uptake	Particles too small

THYROID UPTAKE AND IMAGING RADIONUCLIDES (^{131}I, ^{123}I)

See Chapter 5 Tables 5–1 and 5–2

GASTRIC EMPTYING STUDIES—ANY RADIOPHARMACEUTICAL

Delayed gastric emptying	Aluminum hydroxide
	Narcotics
	Propantheline
Shortened gastric emptying	Reglan

CEREBRAL CISTERNOGRAPHY—^{111}In DTPA

Ventricular entry and stasis (false-positive results)	Acetazolamide (Diamox)

Nonradioactive Pharmaceuticals in Nuclear Medicine*

PHARMACEUTICAL	INDICATION	ADULT DOSE
Acetazolamide (Diamox)	Brain perfusion	1 g in 10 mL sterile water, IV over 2 min for adults (14 mg/kg for children) 10–20 minutes before injecting tracer
Adenosine (Adenocard)	Cardiac stress	140 μg/kg/min for 6 min, or 50 μg/kg/min increased to 75, 100, and 140 μg/kg/min each min to 7 min
Bethanechol (Urecholine)	Gastric emptying	2.5–5 mg subcutaneously
Captopril (Capoten)	Renovascular hypertension evaluation	25–50 mg orally before study
Cholecystokinin (Sincalide or Kinevac)	Hepatobiliary imaging	0.02 μg/kg in 10 mL saline IV over 3–10 min
Cimetidine (Tagamet)	Meckel's diverticulum imaging	Adult 300 mg/four times daily, pediatric 20 mg/kg in 20 mL saline IV over 20 min
Dipyridimole (Persantine)	Cardiac stress	0.57 mg/kg IV over 4 min in 20–40 mL of normal saline
Dobutamine (Dobultex)	Cardiac stress	Incremental dose rate of 15 μg/kg/min up to 40 μg/kg/min every 3 min
Enalaprilat (Vasotec IV)	Renovascular hypertension evaluation	0.04 mg/kg in 10 mL saline IV over 3–5 min maximum dose 2.5 mg
Furosemide (Lasix)	Renal imaging	Adult 20–40 mg, pediatric 1.0 mg/kg given IV over 1–2 min
Glucagon	Meckel's diverticulum imaging	Adult 0.5 mg, pediatric 5 μg/kg given IV or IM
Morphine (Astramorph, Duramorph)	Hepatobiliary imaging	0.04 mg/kg diluted in 10 mL saline, IV over 3–5 min (range, 2.0–4.5 mg)
Pentagastrin (Peptavalon)	Meckel's diverticulum imaging	6 μg/kg 5–15 min before study
Phenobarbital (Luminal)	Hepatobiliary imaging	5 mg/kg/day for 5 days

*Many of these drugs can cause hypotension, dizziness, nausea, vomiting, respiratory depression, and headache, and the patients often require careful monitoring after administration.

Adapted from Park HM, Duncan K: Nonradioactive pharmaceuticals in nuclear medicine. J Nucl Med Technol 22:240–249, 1994.

SUGGESTED READINGS

Saremi F, Jadvar H, Siegel ME: Pharmacologic
    Interventions in Nuclear Radiology:
    Indications, Imaging Protocols, and Clinical
    Results. RadioGraphics 22:447, 2002.

Pregnancy and Breastfeeding

Appendix

G

PREGNANCY

Many clinicians are concerned about ordering radionuclide scans for a pregnant patient. The question most frequently arises in connection with lung and hepatobiliary scans. In general, if the scan is medically indicated and would be performed on a nonpregnant female, it is indicated during pregnancy. There are some facts to be kept in mind when considering this issue:

1. Radiation-induced fetal abnormalities have not been reported at fetal absorbed dose levels below 10 rads (0.1 Gy). The risk of spontaneous congenital abnormalities is between 3% and 6%.
2. The risk of radiation carcinogenesis may be higher in for the embryo/fetus and children than adults, but the risk is not likely to exceed 1 in a 1000 per rad (10 mGy). The spontaneous cancer risk in the United States is about one in three (33%).

3. Iodine will cross the placenta. The fetal thyroid does not concentrate iodine before about 12 weeks of gestation. After this, the fetal thyroid will avidly accumulate iodine, which can be blocked by administering stable iodine (potassium iodide, 130 mg) to the mother.
4. It is unlikely that the fetal absorbed dose from xenon-133 (^{133}Xe) or a technetium-99m (^{99m}Tc) radiopharmaceutical would exceed 0.5 rad (5 mGy). See Table G–1.
5. A large portion of the fetal absorbed dose from most radiopharmaceuticals comes from the maternal bladder, so hydration and frequent voiding should be encouraged.
6. In many instances, the administered activity can be reduced by half and imaging time increased without significant degradation of the information obtained.

TABLE G–1.	Estimated Absorbed Dose to Embryo for Selected Radiopharmaceuticals
RADIOPHARMACEUTICAL	**ABSORBED DOSE IN rad/mCi (mGy/MBq)**
^{18}F-FDG	0.600 (0.162)
^{67}Ga-citrate	0.250 (0.067)
^{99m}Tc-human serum albumin	0.020 (0.005)
^{99m}Tc-macroaggregated albumin	0.035 (0.009)
^{99m}Tc-diphosphonate	0.040 (0.011)
^{99m}Tc-sodium pertechnetate	0.040 (0.011)
^{99m}Tc-glucoheptonate	0.040 (0.011)
^{99m}Tc-DTPA (intravenous or aerosol)	0.035 (0.009)
^{99m}Tc-sulfur colloid	0.035 (0.009)
^{99m}Tc-DISIDA	0.030 (0.008)
^{99m}Tc red blood cells*	0.060 (0.016)
^{111}In leukocytes*	0.400 (0.110)
^{123}Na iodide (15% uptake)	0.035 (0.009)

Continued

553

TABLE G–1.	Estimated Absorbed Dose to Embryo for Selected Radiopharmaceuticals—cont'd
RADIOPHARMACEUTICAL	**ABSORBED DOSE IN rad/mCi (mGy/MBq)**
^{131}Na iodide (15% uptake)	0.100 (0.027)
^{201}Tl chloride*	0.300 (0.080)
^{133}Xe⁺	0.001 (0.0003)

*In instances in which no data on embryonic or fetal absorbed dose were available, either the maternal whole-body dose or the gonadal dose was used. To be conservative, the largest of these two quantities was chosen.
⁺Value of 0.10 before 10 weeks' gestational age.
^{18}F-FDG, fluorine-18 fluorodeoxyglucose; ^{67}Ga, gallium-67; ^{99m}Tc, technetium-99m; DTPA, diethylene triamine pentaacetic acid; DISIDA, diisopropyl iminodiacetic acid; ^{111}In, indium-111l; ^{123}Na, sodium-123; ^{131}Na, sodium-131; ^{201}Tl, thallium-201; ^{133}Xe, xenon-133.
Data adapted from Protection in Nuclear Medicine and Ultrasound Diagnostic Procedures in Children, report no. 73. Washington, DC, National Council on Radiation Protection and Measurements, 1983; and from Smith EM, Warner GG: Estimates of radiation dose to the embryo from nuclear medicine procedures. J Nucl Med 17:836, 1976.

BREASTFEEDING

Federal regulations (10 CFR 35.75) require that if the dose to a breastfeeding infant or child could exceed 100 mrem (1 mSv), assuming there was no interruption of breastfeeding, the licensee must give (1) guidance on the interruption or cessation of breastfeeding and (2) information on the consequences of failure to follow guidance. In general, diagnostic procedures involving radionuclides other than radioiodine would have no measurable consequences, and instructions would be directed at keeping doses as low as reasonable achievable. Specific requirements are shown in Table G–2.

TABLE G–2.	Activities of Radiopharmaceuticals that Require Instructions and Records When Administered to Patients Who are Breast-Feeding an Infant or Child

RADIOPHARMACEUTICAL	COLUMN 1 ACTIVITY ABOVE WHICH INSTRUCTIONS ARE REQUIRED, MBq (mCi)	COLUMN 2 ACTIVITY ABOVE WHICH A RECORD IS REQUIRED, MBq (mCi)	COLUMN 3 EXAMPLES OF RECOMMENDED DURATION OF INTERRUPTION OF BREAST FEEDING
^{131}I NaI	0.01 (0.0004)	0.07 (0.002)	Complete cessation (for this infant or child)
^{123}I NaI	20 (0.5)	100 (3)	Cessation*
^{123}I-MIBG	70 (2)	400 (10)	24 hr for 370 MBq (10 mCi) 12 hr for 150 MBq (4 mCi) Cessation*
^{125}I-OIH	3 (0.08)	10 (0.4)	12 hr*
^{131}I-OIH	10 (0.30)	60 (1.5)	12 hr*
^{99m}Tc-DTPA	1,000 (30)	6,000 (150)	Not necessary
^{99m}Tc-MAA	50 (1.3)	200 (6.5)	12 hr for 150 MBq (4 mCi)
^{99m}Tc pertechnetate	100 (3)	600 (15)	24 hr for 1100 MBq (30 mCi) 12 hr for 440 MBq (12 mCi)
^{99m}Tc-DISIDA	1,000 (30)	6,000 (150)	Not necessary
^{99m}Tc-glucoheptonate	1,000 (30)	6,000 (170)	Not necessary
^{99m}Tc-MIBI	1,000 (30)	6,000 (150)	Not necessary
^{99m}Tc-MDP	1,000 (30)	6,000 (150)	Not necessary
^{99m}Tc-RBC in vivo labeling	400 (10)	2,000 (50)	6 hr for 740 MBq (20 mCi) 12 hr*
^{99m}Tc-RBC in vitro labeling	1,000 (30)	6,000 (150)	Not necessary
^{99m}Tc-sulfur colloid	300 (7)	1,000 (35)	6 hr for 440 MBq (12 mCi)
^{99m}Tc-DTPA aerosol	1,000 (30)	6,000 (150)	Not necessary
^{99m}Tc-MAG3	1,000 (30)	6,000 (150)	Not necessary

Continued

TABLE G–2.	Activities of Radiopharmaceuticals that Require Instructions and Records When Administered to Patients Who are Breast-Feeding an Infant or Child—cont'd		

RADIOPHARMACEUTICAL	COLUMN 1 ACTIVITY ABOVE WHICH INSTRUCTIONS ARE REQUIRED, MBq (mCi)	COLUMN 2 ACTIVITY ABOVE WHICH A RECORD IS REQUIRED, MBq (mCi)	COLUMN 3 EXAMPLES OF RECOMMENDED DURATION OF INTERRUPTION OF BREAST FEEDING
^{67}Ga-citrate	1 (0.04)	7 (0.2)	1 mo for 150 MBq (4 mCi)
^{99m}Tc-white blood cells	100 (4)	600 (15)	4 hr for 1100 MBq (5 mCi)
			12 hr for 440 MBq (2 mCi)
			2 wk for 50 MBq (1.3 mCi)
			1 wk for 7 MBq (0.2 mCi)
			Cessation*
^{51}Cr-EDTA	60 (1.6)	300 (8)	
^{111}In-white blood cells	10 (0.2)	40 (1)	1 wk for 20 MBq (0.5 mCi)
			Not necessary*
^{111}In-Octreotide			Not necessary*
^{201}Tl-chloride	40 (1)	200 (5)	2 wk for 110 MBq (3 mCi), 48 hr*
^{18}F-FDG			Not necessary*

The duration of interruption of breast feeding is selected to reduce the maximum dose to a newborn infant to less than 1 mSv (0.1 rem), although the regulatory limit is 5 mSv (0.5 rem). The actual doses that would be received by most infants would be far below 1 mSv (0.1 rem). Of course, the physician may use discretion in the recommendation, increasing or decreasing the duration of interruption.

NOTES: Activities are rounded to one significant figure, except when it was considered appropriate to use two significant figures. Details of the calculations are shown in NUREG-1492, "Regulatory Analysis on Criteria for the Release of Patients Administered Radioactive Material."

If there is no recommendation in the third column of this table, the maximum activity normally administered is below the activities that require instructions on interruption or discontinuation of breastfeeding.

Although non–by-product materials are not regulated by the Nuclear Regulatory Commission, information on non–by-product material is included in this regulatory guide for the convenience of the licensee.

Agreement state regulations may vary. Agreement state licensees should check with their state regulations before using these values.

*2004 Proposal by International Commission on Radiological Protection Task Group on Radiation Dose to Patients from Radiopharmaceuticals also based on infant dose and potential for contaminants.

^{131}I, iodine 131; NaI, sodium-iodide; ^{123}I, iodine-131; MIBG, metaiodobenzylguanidine; ^{175}I, iodine-125; OIH, ortho-iodohippurate; ^{131}I, iodine-131; ^{99m}Tc, technetium-99m; DTPA, diethylene triamine pentaacetic acid; MAA, macroaggregated albumin; DISIDA, diisopropyl iminodiacetic acid; MIBI, metaiodo benzylguanidine; MDP, methylene diphosphonate; RBC, red blood cell; MAG3, mertiatide; ^{67}Ga, gallium-67; ^{51}Cr, chromium-51; EDTA, ethylenediaminetetra-acetic acid; ^{111}In, indium 111; ^{201}Tl, thallium 201; ^{18}F-FDG, fluorine-18 fluorodeoxyglucose.

General Considerations for Patients Receiving Radionuclide Therapy

1. It is important for the patient to understand the nature of the radionuclide treatment. Patient cooperation is important in minimizing unnecessary incidents and exposure.

2. Before administration of the radionuclide, the procedures and special precautions should be reviewed with the nursing staff. The nursing staff must have specific written instructions for each procedure and should review them before the patient arrives in the room.

3. Immediately after the return of the treated patient to the hospital room from the nuclear medicine department, a radiation safety officer (RSO) should survey the patient and surrounding areas to determine distance and time restrictions for hospital personnel and visitors in the patient's room. These distances and times are recorded on a form in the patient's chart and listed on the caution sign on the patient's door. These signs and labels should remain posted until removal is ordered by the RSO.

4. Hospital personnel and allowed visitors should position themselves as far from the patient as is reasonable except for necessary bedside care. A distance of 2 m is normally acceptable. In some cases, the RSO may determine that mobile lead shields are needed to reduce exposure to others in adjacent areas. Specific restrictions are noted by the RSO on the room door and in the hospital chart.

5. It is not advisable for pregnant women or children younger than 18 years to enter the hospital room.

6. Dosimeters are required for all hospital personnel who are likely to receive in excess of 25% of the dose-equivalent limit for radiation workers. The RSO identifies hospital personnel within this category and issues the appropriate dosimeters to them.

7. Pregnant personnel should not routinely be assigned to the care of patients under treatment with radioactive materials.

8. Patients receiving radionuclide therapy should be assigned a private room and restricted to the room unless an exception is authorized by the RSO.

9. Limits for release of radionuclide therapy patients from hospitals are given in the U.S. Nuclear Regulatory Commission regulatory guide 0.39 published in April 1997. Patient release criteria have been outlined in Chapter 14. Patients may be released on the basis of administered activity or dose rate. The specifics for common radionuclides are shown in Table H–1A. There are patients who may be released but who have a level of activity that requires the patient to be supplied with written instructions on how to maintain doses to other individuals as low as reasonably achievable. These activities and dose rates are shown in Table H–1B. Patients may also be released if the calculated maximum likely effective dose to another individual is no greater than 0.5 rem (5 mSv). This method requires use of a formula. The recordkeeping requirements are shown in Table H–1C.

TABLE H–1A.	Activities and Dose Rates for Authorizing Patient Release*	
RADIONUCLIDE	COLUMN 1 ACTIVITY AT OR BELOW WHICH PATIENTS MAY BE RELEASED, GBq (mCi)	COLUMN 2 DOSE RATE AT 1 M AT OR BELOW WHICH PATIENTS MAY BE RELEASED, mSv/hr (mrem/hr)[†]
^{198}Au	3.5 (93)	0.21 (21)
^{51}Cr	4.8 (130)	0.02 (2)
^{67}Ga	8.7 (240)	0.18 (18)
^{123}I	6.0 (160)	0.26 (26)
^{125}I	0.25 (7)	0.01 (1)
^{131}I	1.2 (33)	0.07 (7)
^{111}In	2.4 (64)	0.2 (20)
^{32}P	—[‡]	—[‡]
^{186}Re	28 (770)	0.15 (15)
^{188}Re	29 (790)	0.20 (20)
^{47}Sc	11 (310)	0.17 (17)
^{153}Sm	26 (700)	0.3 (30)
^{117m}Sn	1.1 (29)	0.04 (4)
^{89}Sr	—[‡]	—[‡]
^{99m}Tc	28 (760)	0.58 (58)
^{201}Tl	16 (430)	0.19 (19)
^{90}Y	—[‡]	—[‡]
^{169}Yb	0.37 (10)	0.02 (2)

*The activity values were computed based on 5 mSv (0.5 rem) total effective dose equivalent.
[†]If the release is based on the dose rate at 1 m in Column 2, the licensee must maintain a record as required by 10 CFR 35.75(c) because the measurement includes shielding by tissue. See Regulatory Position 3.1, "Records of Release," for information on records.
[‡]Activity and dose rate limits are not applicable in this case because of the minimal exposures to members of the public resulting from activities normally administered for diagnostic or therapeutic purposes.
The gigabecquerel values were calculated based on the millicurie values and the conversion factor from millicuries to gigabecquerels. The dose rate values are calculated based on the millicurie values and the exposure rate constants.
In general, the values are rounded to two significant figures. However, values less than 0.35 GBq (10 mCi) or 0.1 mSv (10 mrem) per hour are rounded to one significant figure. Details of the calculations are provided in NUREG-1492.
Although non–by-product materials are not regulated by the Nuclear Regulatory Commission, information on non–by-product material is included in this regulatory guide for the convenience of the licensee.
Agreement state regulations may vary. Agreement state licensees should check with their state regulations prior to using these values.
^{198}Au, gold-198; ^{51}Cr, chromium-51; ^{67}Ga, gallium-67; ^{123}I, iodine-123; ^{125}I, iodine-125; ^{131}I, iodine-131; ^{111}In, indium-111; ^{32}P, phosphorus-32; ^{186}Re, rhenium-186; ^{188}Re, rhenium-188; ^{47}Sc, scandium-47; ^{153}Sm, samarium-153; ^{117m}Sn, tin-177m; ^{89}Sr, strontium-89; ^{99m}Tc, technetium-99m; ^{201}Tl, thallium-201; ^{90}Y, yttrium-90; ^{169}Yb, ytterbium-169.

| TABLE H–1B. | **Activities and Dose Rates Above which Instructions should be given when Authorizing Patient Release*** | |

RADIONUCLIDE	COLUMN 1 ACTIVITY ABOVE WHICH INSTRUCTIONS ARE REQUIRED, GBq (mCi)	COLUMN 2 DOSE RATE AT 1 M ABOVE WHICH INSTRUCTIONS ARE REQUIRED, mSv/hr (mrem/hr)
^{198}Au	0.69 (19)	0.04 (4)
^{51}Cr	0.96 (26)	0.004 (0.4)
^{67}Ga	1.7 (47)	0.04 (4)
^{123}I	1.2 (33)	0.05 (5)
^{125}I	0.05 (1)	0.002 (0.2)
^{131}I	0.24 (7)	0.02 (2)
^{111}In	0.47 (13)	0.04 (4)
^{32}P	—†	—†
^{186}Re	5.7 (150)	0.03 (3)
^{188}Re	5.8 (160)	0.04 (4)
^{47}Sc	2.3 (62)	0.03 (3)
^{153}Sm	5.2 (140)	0.06 (6)
^{117m}Sn	0.21 (6)	0.009 (0.9)
^{89}Sr	—†	—†
^{99m}Tc	5.6 (150)	0.12 (12)
^{201}Tl	3.1 (85)	0.04 (4)
^{90}Y	—†	—†
^{169}Yb	0.073 (2)	0.004 0.4

*The activity values were computed based on 1 mSv (0.1 rem) total effective dose equivalent.

†Activity and dose rate limits are not applicable in this case because of the minimal exposures to members of the public resulting from activities normally administered for diagnostic or therapeutic purposes.

The gigabecquerel values were calculated based on the millicurie values and the conversion factor from millicuries to gigabecquerels. The dose rate values were calculated based on the millicurie values and the exposure rate constants.

In general, the values are rounded to two significant figures. However, values less than 0.37 GBq (10 mCi) or 0.1 mSv (10 mrem) per hour are rounded to one significant figure. Details of the calculations are provided in NUREG-1492.

Although non–by-product materials are not regulated by the Nuclear Regulatory Commission, information on non–by-product material is included in this regulatory guide for the convenience of the licensee.

Agreement state regulations may vary. Agreement state licensees should check with their state regulations prior to using these values.

Abbreviations are the same as in Table H–1A.

TABLE H–1C.   Summary of Release Criteria, Required Instructions to Patients, and Records to be Maintained

PATIENT GROUP	BASIS FOR RELEASE	CRITERIA FOR RELEASE	INSTRUCTIONS NEEDED	RELEASE RECORD REQUIRED
All patients, including patients who are breastfeeding an infant or child	Administered activity	Administered activity ≤ Column 1 of Table H1–A	Yes—if administered activity > Column 1 of Table H1–B	No
	Retained activity	Retained activity ≤ Column 1 of Table H1–A	Yes—if retained activity > Column 1 of Table H1–B	Yes
	Measured dose rate	Measured dose rate ≤ Column 2 of Table H1–A	Yes—if dose > Column 2 of Table H1–B	Yes
	Patient-specific calculations	Calculated effective dose to other individuals ≤5 mSv (0.5 rem)	Yes—if calculated effective dose to other individuals >1 mSv (0.1 rem)	Yes
Patients who are breastfeeding an infant or child	All the above bases for release		Additional instructions required if administered activity > Column 1 of Table G–2, or licensee calculated dose from breastfeeding >1 mSv (0.1 rem) to the infant or child	Records that instructions were provided are required if administered activity > Column 2 of Table G–2, or licensee calculated dose from breastfeeding >5 mSv (0.5 rem) to the infant or child

Special Considerations and Requirements for Iodine-131 Therapy

The following are useful for hospitalized patients and these can be adapted for home use if patients with over 33 mCi (1.2 GBq) of iodine-131 (^{131}I) are released.

1. All patients in the above category shall be in a private room with a toilet.
2. The door must be posted with a radioactive materials sign, and note must be made on the door or in the patient's chart where and how long visitors may stay in the patient's room.
3. Visits by people younger than 18 years should be authorized only on a patient-by-patient basis with approval of the authorized user and after consultation with the radiation safety officer (RSO).
4. A survey of the patient's room and surrounding areas should be conducted as soon as practicable after administration of treatment dose. The results of daily surveys can be used to recalculate permitted staying times of different visitors. Film or thermoluminescent dosimeter badges should be worn by the nurses attending the patient.
5. Patients containing ^{131}I shall be confined to their rooms except for special medical or nursing purposes approved by the nuclear medicine or radiation therapy departments and the RSO. The patient should remain in bed during visits.
6. If possible, there should be no pregnant visitors or nurses attending the patient.
7. Staff should wear disposable gloves, discard them in a designated waste container located just inside the room, and wash their hands after leaving the room.
8. Disposable plates and cups and other disposables should be used, and after use these should discarded in a specifically designated container.
9. All items such as clothing, bed linens, and surgical dressings may be either surveyed before removal from the room or placed in a designated container and held for decay.
10. Urine, feces, and vomitus from ^{131}I therapy patients may be disposed of by way of the sewer or stored for decay in the radioactive waste storage area. The method of disposal should be determined by the RSO.
11. If the urine from ^{131}I patients is to be collected (not a Nuclear Regulatory Commission requirement), special containers should be provided by the RSO. The patient should be encouraged to collect his or her urine in the container. If the patient is bedridden, the urinal or bedpan should be flushed several times with hot soapy water after each use.
12. The same toilet should be used by the patient at all times and should be flushed several times after each use.
13. Precautions should be taken to ensure that no urine or vomitus is spilled on the floor or bed. If any part of the patient's room is

suspected of being contaminated, the RSO should be notified.

14. If a therapy patient needs emergency surgery or dies, the RSO and the nuclear medicine or radiation therapy departments should be notified immediately.

15. After the patient is released from the room, the room should be surveyed and may not be reassigned until removable contamination is less than 2000 disintegrations/minute/100 cm^2. Final survey of the room should include areas likely to have been contaminated, such as the toilet area, and items likely to have been touched by the patient, such as the telephone and doorknobs.

16. The thyroid burden of each person who helped prepare or administer a liquid dosage of ^{131}I should be measured within 3 days after administration of the doses. The records should include each thyroid burden measurement, the date of measurement, the name of the person measured, and the initials of the person who made the measurements. These records must be maintained indefinitely.

NURSING INSTRUCTIONS

1. Only that amount of time required for ordinary nursing care should be spent near the patient.

2. Visitors should be limited to those 18 years of age or older unless specified.

3. The patient should remain in bed. All visitors should remain at least 2 m from the patient.

4. The patient should be confined to the room, except by special approval of the RSO.

5. No pregnant nurse, visitor, or attendant should be permitted in the room, if possible. Attending personnel should wear disposable gloves.

6. If a spill of urine or radioactive material is encountered, the RSO should be notified.

Emergency Procedures for Spills of Radioactive Materials

Accidental spillage of radioactive material is rare; however, spills may occur in the laboratory, in public areas such as the hall, in the freight elevator, or in any hospital room or ward through contamination by a patient's body fluids. Spill procedures should be posted in the restricted areas where radioactive materials are used or stored and should specifically state the names and telephone numbers of persons to be notified (e.g. RSO). They should also include instructions about area evacuation, spill containment, decontamination and reentry.

Major radiation accidents or serious spills of radioactive contamination have rarely involved medical or allied health personnel. Usually, spills in hospitals involve only small amounts of radioactivity, in which the main concern is the spread of the contamination (e.g., from shoes or contaminated clothing into public areas). The following is a general outline of the procedure to be followed in the event of a radioactive spill.

MINOR SPILLS*

1. Notify persons in the area that a spill has occurred.
2. Prevent the spread of contamination by covering the spill with absorbent paper.
3. Wearing gloves and protective clothing such as a lab coat and booties, clean up the spill using absorbent paper. Carefully fold the absorbent paper with clean side out and place in a "caution radioactive material" labeled plastic bag for transfer to a radioactive waste container. Also put contaminated gloves and any other contaminated disposable material in the bag.
4. Survey the area with a low-range radiation detection survey instrument sufficiently sensitive to detect the radionuclide. Check for removable contamination to ensure contamination levels are below trigger levels. Check the area around the spill as well as hands, clothing and shoes for contamination.
5. Report the incident to the RSO.

MAJOR SPILLS

1. Clear the area. Notify all persons not involved in the spill to vacate the room.
2. Prevent the spread of contamination by covering the spill with "caution radioactive material" labeled absorbent paper, but do not attempt to clean it up. To prevent the spread of contamination, clearly indicate the boundaries of the spill and limit the movement of all personnel who may be contaminated.
3. Shield the source if possible. Do this only if it can be done without further contamination or a significant increase in radiation exposure.
4. Close the room and lock or otherwise secure the area to prevent entry.
5. Notify the RSO immediately.
6. Decontaminate the personnel by removing contaminated clothing and flushing contaminated skin with lukewarm water, then washing it with mild soap. If contamination remains, the RSO may consider inducing perspiration. Then wash the affected area again to remove any contamination that was released.

---

* The differentiation of major and minor and which procedure to implement is incident specific and dependent on a number of variables (e.g. number of individuals involved or other hazards present).

TABLE I–1. General Guidance on the Amount of Radioactivity that Differentiates Minor from Major Spills

RADIONUCLIDE	MILLICURIES	RADIONUCLIDE	MILLICURIES
Phosphorus-32	1	Technetium-99m	100
Chromium-51	100	Indium-111	10
Cobalt-57	10	Iodine-123	10
Cobalt-58	10	Iodine-125	1
Iron-59	1	Iodine-131	1
Cobalt-60	1	Samarium-153	10
Gallium-67	10	Ytterbium-169	10
Selenium-75	1	Mercury-197	10
Strontium-85	10	Gold-198	10
Strontium-89	1	Thallium-201	100

For short-lived radionuclides, decay may be used rather than decontamination. A report to the NRC may be required.

SURFACE CONTAMINATION LIMITS

Recommended limits for surface contamination in restricted areas are 2000 dpm/100cm^2 for iodine and indium and 20,000 dpm/100 cm^2 for gallium-67, technetium-99m and thallium-201. Limits for unrestricted areas are an average of 1000 dpm (16.7 Bq)/100 cm^2 for iodine and 5,000 dpm (83.3 Bq)/100 cm^2 for gallium-67, technetium-99m and thallium-201. With regard to removable contamination in unrestricted areas the limits are 100 dpm (1.67 Bq) and 200 dpm (3.3 Bq)/100 cm^2 respectively.

EMERGENCY SURGERY OF PATIENTS WHO HAVE RECEIVED THERAPEUTIC AMOUNTS OF RADIONUCLIDES

The following procedure may be used.
1. If surgery is performed within the first 24 hours following the administration of iodine-131, fluids (e.g. blood, urine) will be carefully removed and contained in a closed system.
2. Protective eyewear will be worn.

3. The radiation safety staff will direct personnel in methods to keep doses as low as reasonably achievable in a practical fashion.
4. If an injury (such as a cut) or a tear in a glove occurs, the individual will be monitored to see if contamination occurred and if any action is necessary.

EMERGENCY AUTOPSY OF PATIENTS WHO HAVE RECEIVED THERAPEUTIC AMOUNTS OF RADIONUCLIDES

The following procedure may be used.
1. Immediately notify the authorized user in charge of the patient and the RSO upon death of a therapy patient.
2. An autopsy will be performed only after consultation and permission from the RSO.
3. Protective eyewear will be worn. Consider the need for protection against exposure from high energy beta rays in cases involving therapy with phosphorus-32 and yttrium-90.
4. Remove tissues containing large activities early to help reduce exposure. Shield and dispose of tissues in accord with license conditions.
5. If an injury (such as a cut) or a tear in a glove occurs, the individual will be monitored to see if contamination occurred and if any action is necessary.

Index

Note: Page numbers followed by t refer to tables. Page numbers that are italic refer to figures.

E

ECG. *See* Electrocardiogram
ECT. *See* Emission computed tomography
Ectopic thyroid tissue, abnormal images of, 80–81, *81*
EDV. *See* End-diastolic volume
Effective half-life, 5
Ejection fraction, in cardiac function imaging, 140
Electrocardiogram (ECG) studies, of coronary artery disease, 130
Electron capture, 3
Emission computed tomography (ECT)
    of osteomyelitis, *401*
    with PET imaging, 376–378, *377*
    of pulmonary embolism, 185–186, *187–190*
    of spleen, 214
End-diastolic counts, of computers, in cardiac function imaging, 140
End-diastolic volume, *509*
Endochondroma, 254–255, *258*
Epididymitis, 320, *320*
Epilepsy
    PET imaging in, 388–391, 389t, *390, 391*
    SPECT imaging in, 62–64
Equilibrium radionuclide angiography. *See also* Gated blood pool ventriculography
    of cardiac function, 138
Esophageal cancer, whole-body PET imaging of, 410–411, *411*
Esophageal transit
    in gastric emptying studies, 233
    sample techniques of, 534
Ewing's sarcoma, bone imaging in, 254, *256*

F

Fat embolism, ventilation-perfusion imaging of, 200, *201*
Fatigue, fractures, *274–275*
Fatty liver, ventilation imaging of, 166, *167*
FDG. *See* Flourine-18 fluorodeoxyglucose
Fever
    indium-111 oxine leukocytes, imaging in, 349
    of unknown origin, 343–344, *445*
^{18}F-FDG. *See* Flourine-18 fluorodeoxyglucose
Fibrous dysplasia, 255, *260, 492*
Field uniformity
    assessment, 37–39, *38, 39*
    of gamma cameras, 23, 37–38, *38*, 41t
    for quality control, 37–38, *38*, 41t
    for SPECT, 39, 39–42, *40, 41*
Filtered back projection, in tomographic image production, 29–30
Filters, for SPECT imaging, 24–25, *25*, 29–30, *31*
Fissure signs, in pulmonary perfusion imaging, *165*, 183, *450*
Flare phenomenon
    in bone imaging, 252, *253*
    in breast imaging, 410
Flood field image, of gamma camera, 37–38, *38, 39*
Flourine-18 fluorodeoxyglucose (^{18}F-FDG)
    absorbed doses of, 374t
    imaging
        of bone marrow, 387
        of brain, 381
        of breast, 385
        of genitourinary tract, 387, *387*
        of GI tract, 385, *386*
        of heart, 383, 385, *385*
        interpretation of, 387–388, 389t
        of lungs, 385

of lymph nodes, 387
of muscle and fat, 382, *382–384*
normal distribution of, 379, 380t, *381*
in oncology, 402t–403t
patient preparation for, 379
of spleen, 388
of submandibular glands, 381, *382*
of thymus, 382
for PET, 388–392, 389t, *390–393*, 393t, 545–546
    in cardiac imaging, 393–395, *396*, 545
as radiopharmaceutical, 371–372, *372*, 373t, 544–546
radiopharmaceutical affinity for, 336t
Fluorine, as radionuclide, properties of, 511t
Focal lesions
    in bone imaging, 244t, *251*, 252, *252, 254*, 254t
    in liver, 205–206, 206t, 210–211, *471*
    pulmonary perfusion imaging of, 161, *162*, 199
    space-occupying, 313–314
    spleen scans of, 212–214, *213, 214*, 215t
    valvular, 137
Focal nodular hyperplasia
    colloidal imaging of, 210, *211*
    imaging of, 210, *211*
Foot infections, diabetic, imaging of, with indium-111 oxine leukocyte, 354
Fractures
    occult, 269–270, *271*, 272
    phases of, 269, 270t
    rib, 269–270, *271*
    stress, 269–270, 270t, *464*
        fatigue, *274–275*
        insufficiency, *276*
Frame mode, for measuring cardiac functioning, 139–140
Functional images, in cardiac function imaging, 140–141
Functional renal imaging, 295

G

Gall bladder, imaging of. *See* Hepatobiliary imaging
Gallium-67
    activity in kidneys, 327t
    biologic behavior of, 326, 511t
    citrate
        in bone imaging, 279
        lung uptake of, 327t, 344t
        radiopharmaceutical affinity for, 336t
    for imaging, with thallium-201 chloride, 346
    for imaging bronchogenic carcinoma, 330
    for imaging hepatoma, 329–330, *331, 452*
    for imaging infection and inflammation
        abdominal, 327t, 343
        in fever, 343–344
        in immunocompromised patient, 344–346, *345*
        mechanism of, 341, 342t, 343
        technique of, 343
        thoracic, 343, 344t
    for imaging lymphoma, *328*, 328–329, *329, 330, 445, 482*
    imaging technique for, 326
    localization in neoplasm, 326
    normal image use, 326–327, *327*, 327t
    physical characteristics of, 326
    as radionuclide
        in liver-spleen imaging, 210
        properties of, 9
Gallium-avid adenopathy, 347, *459*